FIRST AID FOR THE®

USMLE STEP 2 CK

Sixth Edition

TAO T. LE, MD, MHS

Assistant Clinical Professor
Chief, Section of Allergy and Clinical Immunology
Department of Medicine
University of Louisville

VIKAS BHUSHAN, MD

Diagnostic Radiologist

JULIA SKAPIK

Johns Hopkins University School of Medicine
Class of 2007

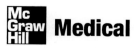 **Medical**

New York / Chicago / San Francisco / Lisbon / London / Madrid / Mexico City
Milan / New Delhi / San Juan / Seoul / Singapore / Sydney / Toronto

The McGraw·Hill Companies

First Aid for the® USMLE Step 2 CK, Sixth Edition

2 3 4 5 6 7 8 9 0   QPD/QPD   0 9 8

ISBN-13: 978-0-07-148795-5
ISBN-10: 0-07-148795-6
ISSN 1532-320X

NOTICE

Medicine is an ever-changing science. As new research and clinical experience broaden our knowledge, changes in treatment and drug therapy are required. The authors and the publisher of this work have checked with sources believed to be reliable in their efforts to provide information that is complete and generally in accord with the standards accepted at the time of publication. However, in view of the possibility of human error or changes in medical sciences, neither the authors nor the publisher nor any other party who has been involved in the preparation or publication of this work warrants that the information contained herein is in every respect accurate or complete, and they disclaim all responsibility for any errors or omissions or for the results obtained from use of the information contained in this work. Readers are encouraged to confirm the information contained herein with other sources. For example and in particular, readers are advised to check the product information sheet included in the package of each drug they plan to administer to be certain that the information contained in this work is accurate and that changes have not been made in the recommended dose or in the contraindications for administration. This recommendation is of particular importance in connection with new or infrequently used drugs.

This book was set in Electra LH by Rainbow Graphics.
The editor was Catherine A. Johnson.
The production supervisor was Phil Galea.
Project management was provided by Rainbow Graphics.
Quebecor Dubuque was printer and binder.

This book is printed on acid-free paper.

DEDICATION

To our families, friends, and loved ones, who supported and assisted in the task of assembling this guide.

and

To the contributors to this and future editions, who took time to share their knowledge, insight, and humor for the benefit of students.

CONTENTS

SECTION 3   TOP-RATED REVIEW RESOURCES   493

CONTRIBUTING AUTHORS

Hannah Alphs

Johns Hopkins University School of Medicine
Class of 2007
Gynecology, Obstetrics

J. Peter Campbell

Johns Hopkins University School of Medicine
Class of 2007
Book reviews, Infectious Disease

Barbara Chubak

Johns Hopkins University School of Medicine
Class of 2008
Hematology/Oncology, Epidemiology, Dermatology

Carrie Klotz

Johns Hopkins University School of Medicine
Class of 2007
Emergency Medicine, Musculoskeletal

Marisa North

Johns Hopkins University School of Medicine
Class of 2007
Cardiovascular, Pediatrics

Soroush Rais-Bahrami

Johns Hopkins University School of Medicine
Class of 2007
Book reviews, Renal/Genitourinary, Ethics

Sarah K. Tighe

Johns Hopkins University School of Medicine
Class of 2007
Psychiatry, Neurology

Tinsay A. Woreta

Johns Hopkins University School of Medicine
Class of 2007
Gastrointestinal, Pulmonary

FACULTY REVIEWERS

Mohamad E. Allaf, MD

Assistant Professor
Department of Urology
Johns Hopkins University School of Medicine

Emmanuel S. Antonarakis, MD

Senior Resident
Department of Medicine
Johns Hopkins University

Brad Astor, PhD, MPH

Assistant Professor
Departments of Epidemiology and Medicine
Johns Hopkins University

Patrice M. Becker, MD

Associate Professor of Medicine
Division of Pulmonary and Critical Care Medicine
Johns Hopkins University School of Medicine

Roger S. Blumenthal, MD, FACC

Associate Professor of Medicine
Johns Hopkins University School of Medicine
Director, The Johns Hopkins Ciccarone Center for the Prevention of
Heart Disease

Teresa Diaz-Montes, MD, MPH

Assistant Professor
Kelly Gynecologic Oncology Service
Department of Gynecology and Obstetrics
Johns Hopkins Hospital

John A. Flynn, MD, MBA

D. William Schlott MD Associate Professor of Medicine
Clinical Director, Division of General Internal Medicine
Johns Hopkins Hospital

Lillian Graf, MD

Department of Dermatology
New York University

Mary L. Harris, MD

Associate Professor of Medicine
Division of Gastroenterology
Johns Hopkins University School of Medicine

Matthias Holdhoff, MD, PhD

Senior Resident
Department of Medicine
Johns Hopkins University

Nancy Hueppchen, MD

Assistant Professor
Department of Gynecology and Obstetrics
Johns Hopkins Hospital

J. Lee Jenkins, MD, MSc

Assistant Chief of Service
Department of Emergency Medicine
Johns Hopkins Hospital

Matthew I. Kim, MD

Assistant Professor
Division of Endocrinology and Metabolism
Johns Hopkins University School of Medicine

Scott Yung Kim, MD

Department of Infectious Diseases
Johns Hopkins Hospital

Brian J. Krabak, MD, MBA

Assistant Professor
Department of Physical Medicine and Rehabilitation
Johns Hopkins Hospital

Cindy Le, MD

Chief Resident
Department of Psychiatry and Behavioral Sciences
Johns Hopkins Hospital

Peter McPhedran, MD

Emeritus Professor
Departments of Medicine and Laboratory Medicine
Yale University School of Medicine

Kristen Nelson, MD

Johns Hopkins Clinical Fellow
Pediatric Critical Care Medicine
Johns Hopkins University School of Medicine

Katherine Peters, MD, PhD

Chief Resident
Department of Neurology
Johns Hopkins Hospital

Véronique Taché, MD

Chief Resident
Department of Obstetrics and Gynecology
University of California, Davis Medical Center

Peter Terry, MD, MA

Professor of Medicine
Division of Pulmonary and Critical Care Medicine
Johns Hopkins University School of Medicine

PREFACE

With the sixth edition of *First Aid for the USMLE Step 2 CK*, we continue our commitment to providing students with the most useful and up-to-date preparation guide for the USMLE Step 2 CK. The sixth edition represents a thorough revision in many ways and includes:

- A revised and updated exam preparation guide for the USMLE Step 2 CK. Includes updated study and test-taking strategies for the FRED computer-based testing (CBT) format.
- Revisions and new material based on student experience with the 2006 and 2007 administrations of the USMLE Step 2 CK.
- Concise summaries of over 300 heavily tested clinical topics written for fast, high-yield studying.
- Topics integrate clinically relevant high-yield basic science facts from *First Aid for the USMLE Step 1*.
- A "rapid review" that tests your knowledge of each topic.
- A high-yield collection of over 120 glossy photos similar to those appearing on the USMLE Step 2 CK exam.
- A completely revised, in-depth guide to clinical science review and sample examination books.

The sixth edition would not have been possible without the help of the many students and faculty members who contributed their feedback and suggestions. We invite students and faculty to continue sharing their thoughts and ideas to help us improve *First Aid for the USMLE Step 2 CK*. (See How to Contribute, p. xv.)

Louisville	Tao Le
Los Angeles	Vikas Bhushan
Baltimore	Julia Skapik

ACKNOWLEDGMENTS

This has been a collaborative project from the start. We gratefully acknowledge the thoughtful comments, corrections, and advice of the many medical students, international medical graduates, and faculty who have supported the authors in the continuing development of *First Aid for the USMLE Step 2 CK*.

For support and encouragement throughout the process, we are grateful to Thao Pham, Selina Franklin, and Louise Petersen. Thanks also to those who supported the authors through the revision process.

Thanks to our publisher, McGraw-Hill, for the valuable assistance of their staff. For enthusiasm, support, and commitment for this challenging project, thanks to our editor, Catherine Johnson. For outstanding editorial work, we thank Andrea Fellows. A special thanks to David Hommel (Rainbow Graphics) for remarkable production work, and Silas Wang for creating the web survey. Thanks to Elizabeth Sanders and Ashley Pound for the interior design.

For contributions, corrections, and surveys we thank Laura Allen, Brett Anderson, Marcus Bachhuber, Celeste Bernacki, May Chan, A. Fishbein, Neal Goldenberg, GwenAudrey Kesselring, Anh Le, Joseph Lee, Kit Lu, Sasha Massachi, Jennifer Nguyen, Jackie Ogutha, Ben Paxton, Teresa Phan, Debbie Rohner, Inna Rozov, Elizabeth Salisbury, and Natasha Wehrli.

Louisville	Tao Le
Los Angeles	Vikas Bhushan
Baltimore	Julia Skapik

HOW TO CONTRIBUTE

To continue to produce a high-yield review source for the Step 2 CK exam, you are invited to submit any suggestions or corrections. We also offer **paid internships** in medical education and publishing ranging from three months to one year (see below for details). Please send us your suggestions for

- Study and test-taking strategies for the Step 2 CK exam.
- New facts, mnemonics, diagrams, and illustrations.
- Low-yield topics to remove.

For each entry incorporated into the next edition, you will receive a $10 gift certificate, as well as personal acknowledgment in the next edition. Diagrams, tables, partial entries, updates, corrections, and study hints are also appreciated, and significant contributions will be compensated at the discretion of the authors. Also let us know about material in this edition that you feel is low yield and should be deleted.

The **preferred way** to submit entries, suggestions, or corrections is via e-mail. Please include name, address, school affiliation, phone number, and e-mail address (if different from the address of origin). If there are multiple entries, please consolidate into a single e-mail or file attachment. Please send submissions to:

firstaidteam@yahoo.com

Otherwise, please send entries, neatly written or typed or on disk (Microsoft Word), to:

First Aid for the USMLE Step 2 CK
914 North Dixie Avenue, Suite 100
Elizabethtown, KY 42701
Attention: Contributions

NOTE TO CONTRIBUTORS

All entries become property of the authors and are subject to editing and reviewing. Please verify all data and spellings carefully. In the event that similar or duplicate entries are received, only the first entry received will be used. Include a reference to a standard textbook to facilitate verification of the fact. Please follow the style, punctuation, and format of this edition if possible.

INTERNSHIP OPPORTUNITIES

The author team is pleased to offer part-time and full-time paid internships in medical education and publishing to motivated physicians. Internships may range from three months (e.g., a summer) up to a full year. Participants will have an opportunity to author, edit, and earn academic credit on a wide variety of projects, including the popular First Aid series. Writing/editing experience, familiarity with Microsoft Word, and Internet access are desired. For more information, e-mail a résumé or a short description of your experience along with a cover letter to the authors at their e-mail address above.

Guide to Efficient Exam Preparation

The United States Medical Licensing Examination (USMLE) Step 2 allows you to pull together your clinical experience on the wards with the numerous "factoids" and classical disease presentations that you have memorized over the years. Whereas Step 1 stresses basic disease mechanisms and principles, Step 2 places more emphasis on clinical diagnosis and management, disease pathogenesis, and preventive medicine.

The Step 2 exam is now composed of two parts:

- The Step 2 Clinical Knowledge examination (Step 2 CK)
- The Step 2 Clinical Skills examination (Step 2 CS)

The USMLE Step 2 CK is the second of three examinations that you must pass in order to become a licensed physician in the United States. The computerized Step 2 CK is a one-day (nine-hour) multiple-choice exam.

Students are also required to take the Step 2 CS, which is a one-day live exam in which students examine 12 standardized patients. The goal of the Step 2 CS is to ensure that students from more than 1600 medical schools worldwide, with varying curricula and educational standards, can collect and interpret a history, perform a physical exam, and communicate with patients at a comparable level. For more information on this examination, please refer to *First Aid for the USMLE Step 2 CS*. Information about the Step 2 CS format and about eligibility, registration, and scoring can be found at www.nbme.org.

The information found in this section as well as in the remainder of the book will address only the Step 2 CK.

How Will the CBT Be Structured?

The goal of the Step 2 CK is to apply your knowledge of medical facts to clinical scenarios you may encounter as a resident.

The Step 2 CK is a computer-based test (CBT) administered by Prometric, Inc. It is a one-day exam with 368 questions divided into eight 60-minute blocks of 46 questions each. A new form of testing software called **FRED** is now being used by the USMLE. FRED is different from the Step 1 exam you took in that you can now **highlight** and **strike out** test choices as well as make **brief notes** to yourself. During the time allotted for each block, the examinee can answer test questions in any order as well as review responses and change answers just as in the Step 1 exam—but examinees cannot go back and change answers from previous blocks. Once an examinee finishes a block, he or she must click on a screen icon to continue to the next block. Time not used during a testing block will be added to your overall break time, but it cannot be used to complete other testing blocks. Expect to spend up to nine hours at the test center.

Testing Conditions: What Will the CBT Be Like?

Even if you're familiar with CBT and the Prometric test centers, FRED is a new testing format that you should access from the USMLE CD-ROM or Web site (www.usmle.org) and try out prior to the exam.

If you familiarize yourself with the FRED testing interface ahead of time, you can skip the 15-minute tutorial offered on exam day and add those minutes to your allotted break time of 45 minutes.

For security reasons, examinees are not allowed to bring personal electronic equipment into the testing area—which means that digital watches, watches with computer communication and/or memory capability, cellular telephones, and electronic paging devices are all prohibited. Food and beverages are prohibited as well. Examinees are given laminated writing surfaces for note taking, but these must be returned after the examination. The testing centers are monitored by audio and video surveillance equipment.

You should become familiar with a typical question screen (see Figure 1-1). A window to the left displays all the questions in the block and shows you the unanswered questions (marked with an "i"). Some questions will contain figures or color illustrations adjacent to the question. Although the contrast and brightness of the screen can be adjusted, there are no other ways to manipulate the picture (e.g., zooming, panning). Larger images are accessed with an "**exhibit**" button. The examinee can also call up a window displaying normal **lab values**. You may **mark** questions to review at a later time by clicking the check mark at the top of the screen. The **annotation** feature functions like the provided erasable dry boards and allows you to jot down notes during

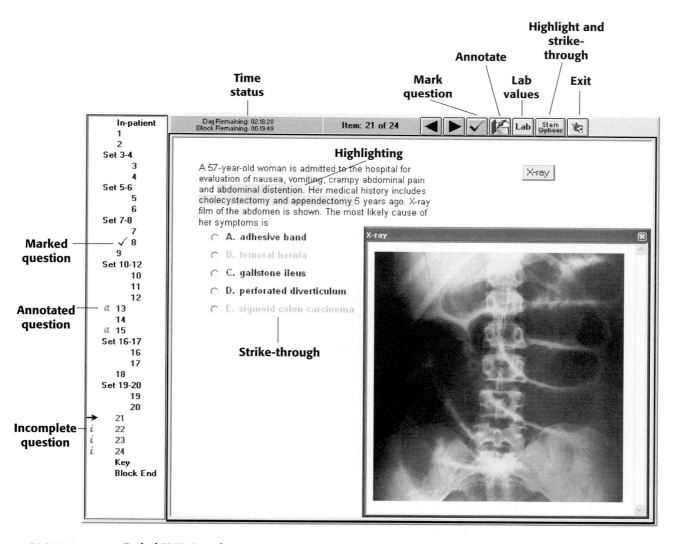

FIGURE 1-1. Typical FRED Question Screen

Keyboard shortcuts:
A–E–Letter choices.
Enter or Spacebar–Move to
next question.
Esc–Exit pop-up Lab and
Exhibit windows.
Alt-T–Countdown timers
for current session and
overall test.

the exam. Play with the **highlighting/strike-out** and annotation feature with the vignettes and multiple answers.

You should also do a few practice blocks to get a feel for which tools actually help you process questions more efficiently and accurately. If you find that you are not using the marking, annotation, or highlighting tools, then **keyboard shortcuts** can save you time over using a mouse.

What Does the CBT Format Mean for Me?

The CBT format is the same format as that of the USMLE Step 1. If you are uncomfortable with this testing format, spend some time playing with a Windows-based system and pointing and clicking icons or buttons with a mouse.

The USMLE also offers an opportunity to take a simulated test, or practice session, at a Prometric center. The session is divided into three one-hour blocks of 50 test items each. The USMLE Step 2 CK sample test items (150 questions) that are available on the CD-ROM or on the USMLE Web site (www.usmle.org) are the same as those used at CBT practice sessions. **No new items will be presented.** The cost is about $42 for U.S. and Canadian students but is higher for international students. The student receives a printed percent-correct score after completing the session. No explanations of questions are provided. You may register for a practice session online at www.usmle.org.

How Do I Register to Take the Exam?

Information on Step 2 CK format, content, and registration requirements can be found on the USMLE Web site. To register for the exam in the United States and Canada, apply online at the National Board of Medical Examiners (NBME) Web site (www.nbme.org). A printable version of the application is also available on this site.

The preliminary registration process for the USMLE Step 2 CK is as follows:

- Complete a registration form and send examination fees to the NBME (online).
- Select a three-month block in which you wish to be tested (e.g., June/July/August).
- Attach a passport-type photo to your completed application form.
- Complete a Certification of Identification and Authorization Form. This must be signed by an official at your medical school (e.g., the registrar's office) to verify your identity. This is a new form and is valid for five years, allowing you to use only your USMLE identification number for future transactions.
- Send your certified application form to the NMBE for processing. (Applications may be submitted more than six months before the test date, but examinees will not receive their scheduling permits until six months prior to the eligibility period.)
- The NBME will process your application within four to six weeks and will send you a fluorescent orange slip of paper that will serve as your scheduling permit.
- Once you have received your orange scheduling permit, decide when and where you would like to take the exam. For a list of Prometric locations nearest you, visit www.prometric.com.

- Call Prometric's toll-free number or visit www.prometric.com to arrange a time to take the exam.
- The Step 2 CK is offered on a year-round basis except for the first two weeks in January. For the most up-to-date information on available testing days at your preferred testing location, refer to www.usmle.org.

Your orange scheduling permit will contain the following important information:

- Your USMLE identification number
- The eligibility period in which you may take the exam
- Your "scheduling number," which you will need to make your exam appointment with Prometric
- Your candidate identification number, or CIN, which you must enter at your Prometric workstation in order to access the exam

Prometric has no access to the codes and will not be able to supply these numbers. **Do not lose your permit!** You will not be allowed to take the Step 2 CK unless you present your permit along with an unexpired, government-issued photo identification that contains your signature (e.g., driver's license, passport). Make sure the name on your photo ID exactly matches the name that appears on your scheduling permit.

Because the exam is scheduled on a "first-come, first-served" basis, you should be sure to call Prometric as soon as you receive your scheduling permit!

What If I Need to Reschedule the Exam?

You can change your date and/or center within your three-month period without charge by contacting Prometric. If space is available, you may reschedule up to five days before your test date. If you need to reschedule outside your initial three-month period, you can apply for a single three-month extension (e.g., April/May/June can be extended through July/August/September) after your eligibility period has begun (visit www.nbme.org for more information). This extension currently costs $50. For other rescheduling needs, you must submit a new application along with another application fee.

What About Time?

Time is of special interest on the CBT exam. Here is a breakdown of the exam schedule:

Tutorial	15 minutes
60-minute question blocks (46 questions per block)	8 hours
Break time (includes time for lunch)	45 minutes
Total test time	9 hours

The computer will keep track of how much time has elapsed during the exam. However, the computer will show you only how much time you have remaining in a given block. Therefore, it is up to you to determine if you are pacing yourself properly.

The computer will not warn you if you are spending more than the 45 minutes allotted for break time. However, you can elect not to use all of your break time, or you can gain extra break time either by skipping the tutorial or by finishing a block ahead of the allotted time.

If I Leave During the Exam, What Happens to My Score?

You are considered to have started the exam once you have entered your CIN onto the computer screen. In order to receive an official score, you must finish the entire exam. This means that you must start and either finish or run out of time for each block of the exam. If you do not complete all the blocks, your exam will be documented on your USMLE score transcript as an incomplete attempt, but no actual score will be reported.

The exam ends when all blocks have been completed or time has expired. As you leave the testing center, you will receive a written test-completion notice to document your completion of the exam.

What Types of Questions Are Asked?

- Almost all questions on the Step 2 CK are case based. A substantial amount of extraneous information may be given, or a clinical scenario may be followed by a question that could be answered without actually requiring that you read the case. It is your job to determine which information is superfluous and which is pertinent to the case at hand.
- Subject areas vary randomly from question to question.
- Most questions have a **single best answer**, but some **matching sets** call for multiple responses (the number to select will be specified). The part of the vignette that actually asks the question—the stem—is usually found at the end of the scenario. From student experience, there are a few stems that are consistently addressed throughout the exam:
  - What is the most likely diagnosis? (40%)
  - Which of the following is the most appropriate initial step in management? (20%)
  - Which of the following is the most appropriate next step in management? (20%)
  - Which of the following is the most likely cause of . . . ? (5%)
  - Which of the following is the most likely pathogen . . . ? (3%)
  - Which of the following would most likely prevent . . . ? (2%)
  - Other (10%)
- Note the age and race of the patient in each clinical scenario. When ethnicity is given, it is often relevant. Know these well (see high-yield facts), especially for more common diagnoses.
- Be able to recognize key facts that distinguish major diagnoses.
- Questions often describe clinical findings instead of naming eponyms (e.g., they cite "audible hip click" instead of "positive Ortolani's sign").
- Questions about acute patient management (e.g., trauma) in an emergency setting are common.

The cruel reality of the Step 2 CK is that no matter how much you study, there will still be questions you will not be able to answer with confidence. If you recognize that a question is not solvable in a reasonable period of time, make an educated guess and move on; you will not be penalized for guessing. Also keep in mind that 10–20% of the USMLE exam questions are "experimental" and will not count toward your score.

How Long Will I Have to Wait Before I Get My Scores?

The USMLE reports scores three to four weeks after the examinee's test date. During peak times, however, reports may take up to six weeks to be scored.

Official information concerning the time required for score reporting is posted on the USMLE Web site, www.usmle.org.

How Are the Scores Reported?

Like the Step 1 score report, your Step 2 CK report includes your pass/fail status, two numeric scores, and a performance profile organized by discipline and disease process (see Figures 1-2A and 1-2B). The first score is a three-digit scaled score based on a predefined proficiency standard. In 2006, the required passing score was 182, which required answering 60–70% of questions correctly. The second score scale, the two-digit score, defines 75 as the minimum passing score (equivalent to a score of 182 on the first scale). This score is not a percentile. Any adjustments in the required passing score will be available on the USMLE Web site.

US·MLE
United States
Medical
Licensing
Examination

UNITED STATES MEDICAL LICENSING EXAMINATION™

USMLE Step 2 is administered to students and graduates of U.S. and Canadian medical schools by the
NATIONAL BOARD OF MEDICAL EXAMINERS® (NBME®)
3750 Market Street, Philadelphia, Pennsylvania 19104-3190.
Telephone: (215) 590-9700

STEP 2 SCORE REPORT

Schmoe, Joe T
Anytown, CA 12345

USMLE ID: 1-234-567-8
Test Date: August 2006

The USMLE is a single examination program for all applicants for medical licensure in the United States; it has replaced the Federation Licensing Examination (FLEX) and the certifying examinations of the National Board of Medical Examiners (NBME Parts I, II and III). The program consists of three Steps designed to assess an examinee's understanding of and ability to apply concepts and principles that are important in health and disease and that constitute the basis of safe and effective patient care. **Step 2** is designed to assess whether an examinee possesses the medical knowledge and understanding of clinical science considered essential for the provision of patient care under supervision, including emphasis on health promotion and disease prevention. The inclusion of Step 2 in the USMLE sequence ensures that attention is devoted to principles of clinical science that undergird the safe and competent practice of medicine. Results of the examination are reported to medical licensing authorities in the United States and its territories for use in granting an initial license to practice medicine. The two numeric scores shown below are equivalent; each state or territory may use either score in making licensing decisions. These scores represent your results for the administration of Step 2 on the test date shown above.

PASS	This result is based on the minimum passing score set by USMLE for Step 2. Individual licensing authorities may accept the USMLE-recommended pass/fail result or may establish a different passing score for their own jurisdictions.

200	This score is determined by your overall performance on Step 2. For recent administrations, the mean and standard deviation for first-time examinees from U.S. and Canadian medical schools are approximately 208 and 23, respectively, with most scores falling between 140 and 260. A score of 170 is set by USMLE to pass Step 2. The standard error of measurement (SEM)‡ for this scale is approximately six points.

82	This score is also determined by your overall performance on the examination. A score of 82 on this scale is equivalent to a score of 200 on the scale described above. A score of 75 on this scale, which is equivalent to a score of 170 on the scale described above, is set by USMLE to pass Step 2. The SEM‡ for this scale is one point.

‡Your score is influenced both by your general understanding of clinical science and the specific set of items selected for this Step 2 examination. The standard error of measurement (SEM) provides an estimate of the range within which your scores might be expected to vary by chance if you were tested repeatedly using similar tests.

267PU007

NOTE: Original score report has copy-resistant watermark.

FIGURE 1-2A.   Sample Score Report—Front Page

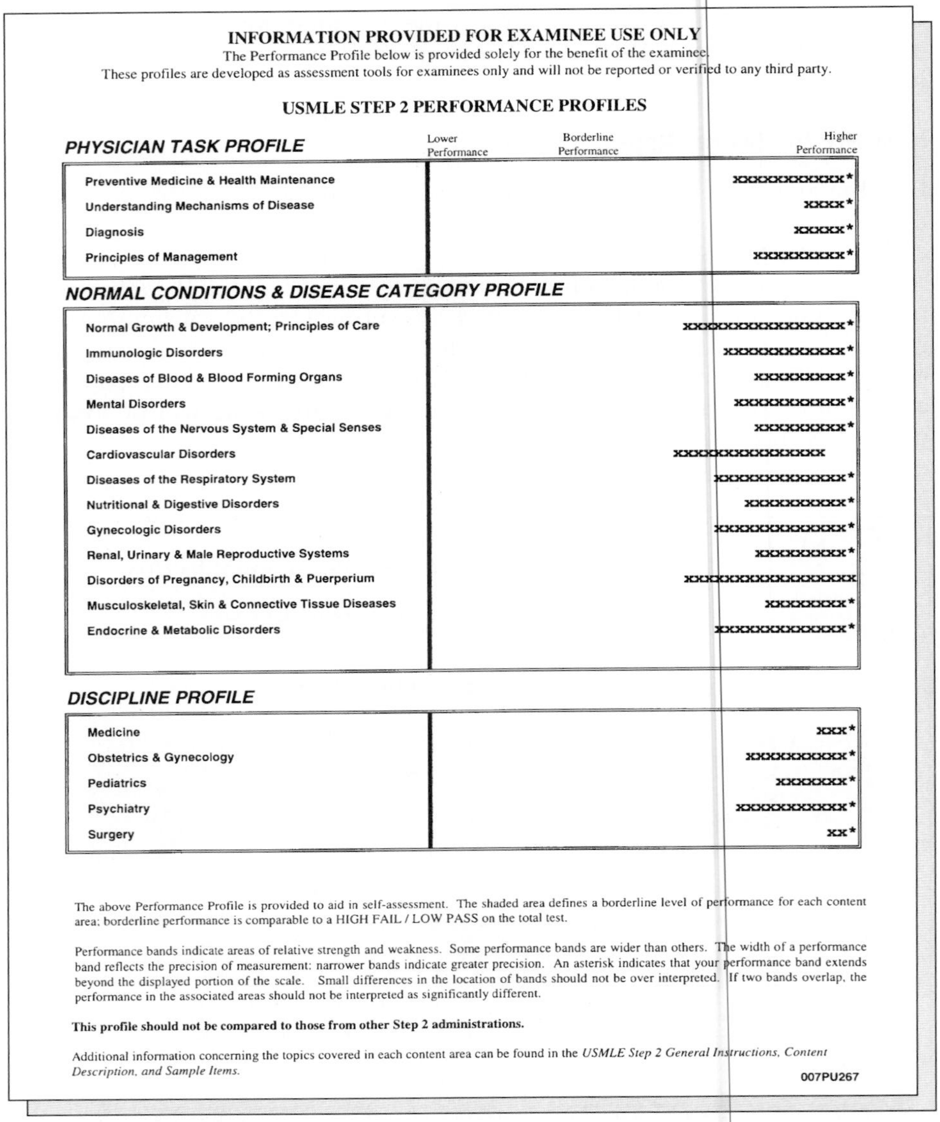

INFORMATION PROVIDED FOR EXAMINEE USE ONLY

The Performance Profile below is provided solely for the benefit of the examinee.
These profiles are developed as assessment tools for examinees only and will not be reported or verified to any third party.

USMLE STEP 2 PERFORMANCE PROFILES

PHYSICIAN TASK PROFILE	Lower Performance	Borderline Performance	Higher Performance
Preventive Medicine & Health Maintenance			xxxxxxxxxxx*
Understanding Mechanisms of Disease			xxxx*
Diagnosis			xxxxx*
Principles of Management			xxxxxxxxxx*

NORMAL CONDITIONS & DISEASE CATEGORY PROFILE

	Lower Performance	Borderline Performance	Higher Performance
Normal Growth & Development; Principles of Care			xxxxxxxxxxxxxxxx*
Immunologic Disorders			xxxxxxxxxxxx*
Diseases of Blood & Blood Forming Organs			xxxxxxxxxx*
Mental Disorders			xxxxxxxxxxx*
Diseases of the Nervous System & Special Senses			xxxxxxxxxx*
Cardiovascular Disorders		xxxxxxxxxxxxxxxx	
Diseases of the Respiratory System			xxxxxxxxxxxxx*
Nutritional & Digestive Disorders			xxxxxxxxxx*
Gynecologic Disorders			xxxxxxxxxxxx*
Renal, Urinary & Male Reproductive Systems			xxxxxxxxxx*
Disorders of Pregnancy, Childbirth & Puerperium			xxxxxxxxxxxxxxxxxxxx
Musculoskeletal, Skin & Connective Tissue Diseases			xxxxxxxxx*
Endocrine & Metabolic Disorders			xxxxxxxxxxxxxx*

DISCIPLINE PROFILE

	Lower Performance	Borderline Performance	Higher Performance
Medicine			xxx*
Obstetrics & Gynecology			xxxxxxxxxxx*
Pediatrics			xxxxxxxx*
Psychiatry			xxxxxxxxxxx*
Surgery			xx*

The above Performance Profile is provided to aid in self-assessment. The shaded area defines a borderline level of performance for each content area; borderline performance is comparable to a HIGH FAIL / LOW PASS on the total test.

Performance bands indicate areas of relative strength and weakness. Some performance bands are wider than others. The width of a performance band reflects the precision of measurement: narrower bands indicate greater precision. An asterisk indicates that your performance band extends beyond the displayed portion of the scale. Small differences in the location of bands should not be over interpreted. If two bands overlap, the performance in the associated areas should not be interpreted as significantly different.

This profile should not be compared to those from other Step 2 administrations.

Additional information concerning the topics covered in each content area can be found in the *USMLE Step 2 General Instructions, Content Description, and Sample Items.*

007PU267

FIGURE 1-2B. Sample Score Report—Back Page

DEFINING YOUR GOAL

The first and most important thing to do in your Step 2 CK preparation is define how well you want to do on the exam, as this will ultimately determine the extent of preparation that will be necessary. The amount of time spent in preparation for this exam varies widely among medical students. Possible goals include the following:

- **"Simply passing."** This goal may be sufficient for the majority of U.S. medical students, especially if you are entering a less competitive specialty.
- **Beating the mean.** This signifies an ability to integrate your clinical and factual knowledge to an extent that is superior to that of your peers (between 200 and 220 for recent exam administrations). Others redefine this goal as achieving a score one SD above the mean (usually in the range of 220 to 240). Highly competitive residency programs may use your Step 1

and Step 2 (if available) scores as a screening tool or as selection criteria (see Figure 1-3). International medical graduates (IMGs) should aim to beat the mean, as USMLE scores are likely to be a selection factor even for less competitive U.S. residency programs.

- **Acing the exam.** Perhaps you are one of those individuals for whom nothing less than the best will do—and for whom excelling on standardized exams is a source of pride and satisfaction. A high score on the Step 2 CK might also represent a way to strengthen your application and "make up" for a less-than-satisfactory score on Step 1, especially if you are taking the exam in the fall before applying for residency.

- **Evaluating your clinical knowledge.** In many ways, this goal should serve as the ultimate rationale for taking the exam, since it is technically the reason the exam was initially designed. The case-based nature of the Step 2 CK differs significantly from the more fact-based Step 1 exam in that it more thoroughly examines your ability to recognize classic clinical presentations, deal with acute emergent situations, and follow the step-by-step thought processes involved in the treatment of particular diseases.

- **Preparing for internship.** Studying for the USMLE Step 2 CK is an excellent way to review and consolidate all of the information you have learned in preparation for internship, especially if the exam is taken in the spring.

When to Take the Exam

With the CBT, you now have a wide variety of options regarding when to take the Step 2 CK. Here are a few factors to consider:

- **The nature of your objectives,** as defined above.

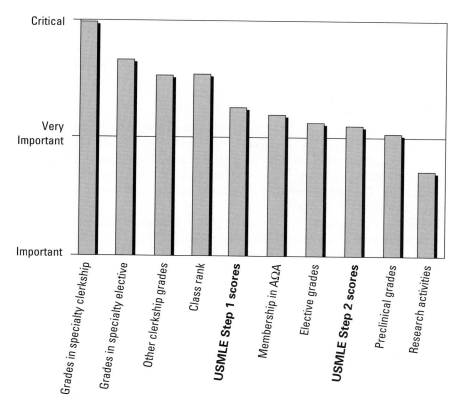

FIGURE 1-3. **Academic Factors Important to Residency Directors**

The Step 2 CK is an opportunity to consolidate your clinical knowledge and prepare for internship.

- **The specialty to which you are applying.** Some competitive residency programs may request your Step 2 CK scores, so you should consider taking the exam in the fall. If you already have a strong application and do not need Step 2 CK scores for residency applications, taking the exam in the fall could potentially hurt your application if you do poorly.
- **Prerequisite to graduation.** If passing the USMLE Step 2 CK is a prerequisite to graduation at your medical school, you will need to take the exam in the fall or winter.
- **Proximity to clerkships.** Many students feel that the core clerkship material is fresher in their minds early in the fourth year, making a good argument for taking the Step 2 CK earlier in the fall.
- **The nature of your schedule.**

STUDY RESOURCES

Quality Considerations

Although an ever-increasing number of USMLE Step 2 review books and software packages are available on the market, the quality of this material is highly variable (see Section 3). Some common problems include the following:

- Some review books are too detailed to be reviewed in a reasonable amount of time or cover subtopics that are not emphasized on the exam (e.g., a 400-page anesthesiology book).
- Many sample question books have not been updated to reflect current trends on the Step 2 CK.
- Many sample question books use poorly written questions, contain factual errors in their explanations, give overly detailed explanations, or offer no explanations at all.
- Software for boards review is of highly variable quality, may be difficult to install, and may be fraught with bugs.

Clinical Review Books

Many review books are available, so you must decide which ones to buy by evaluating their relative merits. Toward this goal, you should weigh different opinions from other medical students against each other; read the reviews and ratings in Section 3 of this guide; and examine the various books closely in the bookstore. Do not worry about finding the "perfect" book, as many subjects simply do not have one.

There are two types of review books: those that are stand-alone titles and those that are part of a series. Books in a series generally have the same style, and you must decide if that style is helpful for you and optimal for a given subject.

The best review book for you reflects the way you like to learn. If a given review book is not working for you, stop using it no matter how highly rated it may be.

Texts and Notes

Most textbooks are too detailed for high-yield boards review and should be avoided. When using texts or notes, engage in active learning by making tables, diagrams, new mnemonics, and conceptual associations whenever possible. If you already have your own mnemonics, do not bother trying to memorize someone else's. Textbooks are useful, however, to supplement incomplete or unclear material.

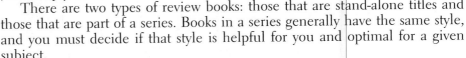

Commercial Courses

Commercial preparation courses can be helpful for some students, as they offer an effective way to organize study material. However, multiweek courses are costly and require significant time commitment, leaving limited time for independent study. Also note that some commercial courses are designed for first-time test takers, students who are repeating the examination, or IMGs.

Practice Tests

Taking practice tests can serve multiple functions for examinees, including the following:

- Provide information about strengths and weaknesses in your fund of knowledge
- Add variety to your study schedule
- Serve as the main form of study
- Improve test-taking skills
- Familiarize examinees with the style of the USMLE Step 2 CK exam

Students report that many practice tests have questions that are, on average, shorter and less clinically oriented than those on the current Step 2 CK. Step 2 CK questions demand fast reading skills and application of clinical facts in a problem-solving format. Approach sample examinations critically, and do not waste time with low-quality questions until you have exhausted better sources.

After you have taken a practice test, try to identify concepts and areas of weakness, not just the facts that you missed. Use this experience to motivate your study and to prioritize the areas in which you need the most work. Analyze the pattern of your responses to questions to determine if you have made systematic errors in answering questions. Common mistakes include reading too much into the question, second-guessing your initial impression, and misinterpreting the question.

Use practice tests to identify concepts and areas of weakness, not just facts that you missed.

NBME/USMLE Publications

We strongly encourage students to use the free materials provided by the testing agencies and to study the following NBME publications:

- **USMLE *Bulletin of Information.*** This publication provides you with nuts-and-bolts details about the exam (included on the Web site www.usmle.org; free to all examinees).
- **USMLE *Step 2 Computer-Based Content and Sample Test Questions.*** This is a hard copy of test questions and test content also found on the CD-ROM.
- **NBME Test Delivery Software (FRED) and Tutorial.** This includes 168 valuable practice questions. The questions are available on the USMLE CD-ROM and on the USMLE Web site. Make sure you are using the new FRED version and not the older Prometric version.
- **USMLE Web site (www.usmle.org).** In addition to allowing you to become familiar with the CBT format, the sample items on the USMLE Web site provide the only questions that are available directly from the test makers. Student feedback varies as to the similarity of these questions to those on the actual exam, but they are nonetheless worthwhile to know.

Things to Bring with You to the Exam

- Be sure to bring your orange scheduling permit and a photo ID with signature. (You will not be admitted to the exam if you fail to bring your permit, and Prometric will charge a rescheduling fee.)
- A watch can help you pace yourself (but do not bring a digital watch).
- Remember to bring lunch, snacks (for a little "sugar rush" on breaks), and fluids.
- Bring clothes to layer to accommodate temperature variations at the testing center.
- Earplugs will be provided at the Prometric center.

TESTING AGENCIES

National Board of Medical Examiners (NBME)
Department of Licensing Examination Services
3750 Market Street
Philadelphia, PA 19104-3102
(215) 590-9500
www.nbme.org

USMLE Secretariat
3750 Market Street
Philadelphia, PA 19104-3190
(215) 590-9700
www.usmle.org

Educational Commission for Foreign Medical Graduates (ECFMG)
3624 Market Street
Philadelphia, PA 19104-2685
(215) 386-5900
Fax: (215) 386-9196
www.ecfmg.org
email: info@ecfmg.org

Federation of State Medical Boards (FSMB)
P.O. Box 619850
Dallas, TX 75261-9850
(817) 868-4041
Fax: (817) 868-4099
www.fsmb.org
email: usmle@fsmb.org

Special Situations

"International medical graduate" (IMG) is the term now used to describe any student or graduate of a non-U.S., non-Canadian, non–Puerto Rican medical school, regardless of whether he or she is a U.S. citizen. The old term "foreign medical graduate" (FMG) was replaced because it was misleading when applied to U.S. citizens attending medical schools outside the United States.

The IMG's Steps to Licensure in the United States

If you are an IMG, you must go through the following steps (not necessarily in this order) to become licensed to practice in the United States. You must complete these steps even if you are already a practicing physician and have completed a residency program in your own country.

- Complete the basic sciences program of your medical school (equivalent to the first two years of U.S. medical school).
- Take the USMLE Step 1. You can do this while still in school or after graduating, but in either case your medical school must certify that you completed the basic sciences part of your school's curriculum before taking the USMLE Step 1.
- Complete the clinical clerkship program of your medical school (equivalent to the third and fourth years of U.S. medical school).
- Take the USMLE Step 2 Clinical Knowledge (CK) exam. If you are still in medical school, you must have completed two years of school.
- Take the Step 2 Clinical Skills (CS) exam.
- Graduate with your medical degree.
- Then, send the ECFMG a copy of your degree and transcript, which they will verify with your medical school.
- Obtain an ECFMG certificate. To do this, candidates must accomplish the following:
  - Graduate from a medical school that is listed in the International Medical Education Directory (IMED). The list can be accessed at www.ecfmg.org.
  - Pass Step 1, the Step 2 CK, and the Step 2 CS within a seven-year period.
  - Have their medical credentials verified by the ECFMG.
- The standard certificate is usually sent two weeks after all the above requirements have been fulfilled. You must have a valid certificate before entering an accredited residency program, although you may begin the application process before you receive your certification.
- Apply for residency positions in your field of interest, either directly or through the Electronic Residency Application Service (ERAS) and the National Residency Matching Program, or NRMP ("the Match"). To be entered into the Match, you need to have passed all the examinations necessary for ECFMG certification (i.e., Step 1, the Step 2 CK, and the Step 2 CS) by the rank order list deadline (typically mid-February each year). If you do not pass these exams by the deadline, you will be withdrawn from the Match.

More detailed information can be found in the 2007 edition of the ECFMG Information Booklet, available at www.ecfmg.org/ pubshome.html.

Applicants may apply online for the USMLE Step 2 CK or Step 2 CS or request an extension of the USMLE eligibility period at www.ecfmg.org/usmle/ index.html or www.ecfmg.org/usmle/ step2cs/index.html.

- Obtain a visa that will allow you to enter and work in the United States if you are not already a U.S. citizen or a green-card holder (permanent resident).
- If required for IMGs by the state in which your residency is located, obtain an educational/training/limited medical license. Your residency program may assist you with this application. Note that medical licensing is the prerogative of each individual state, not of the federal government, and that states vary with respect to their laws about licensing (although all 50 states recognize the USMLE).
- In order to begin your residency program, make sure your scores are valid.
- Once you have the ECFMG certification, take the USMLE Step 3 during your residency, and then obtain a full medical license. Once you have a license in any state, you are permitted to practice in federal institutions such as VA hospitals and Indian Health Service facilities in any state. This can open the door to "moonlighting" opportunities and possibilities for an H1B visa application. For details on individual state rules, write to the licensing board in the state in question or contact the FSMB.
- Complete your residency and then take the appropriate specialty board exams in order to become board certified (e.g., in internal medicine or surgery). If you already have a specialty certification in your home country (e.g., in surgery or cardiology), some specialty boards may grant you six months' or one year's credit toward your total residency time.
- Currently, many residency programs are accepting applications through ERAS. For more information, see *First Aid for the Match* or contact:

ECFMG/ERAS Program
P.O. Box 11746
Philadelphia, PA 19101-0746
(215) 386-5900
Fax: (215) 222-5641
e-mail: eras-support@ecfmg.org
www.ecfmg.org/eras

The USMLE and the IMG

The USMLE is a series of standardized exams that give IMGs a level playing field. It is the same exam series taken by U.S. graduates even though it is administered by the ECFMG rather than by the NBME. This means that passing marks for IMGs for Step 1, the Step 2 CK, and the Step 2 CS are determined by a statistical process that is based on the scores of U.S. medical students. For example, to pass Step 1, you will probably have to score higher than the bottom 8–10% of U.S. and Canadian graduates.

Timing of the USMLE

For an IMG, the timing of a complete application is critical. It is extremely important that you send in your application early if you are to garner the maximum number of interview calls. A rough guide would be to complete all exam requirements by August of the year in which you wish to apply. This would translate into sending both your score sheets and your ECFMG certificate with your application.

In terms of USMLE exam order, arguments can be made for taking the Step 1 or the Step 2 CK exam first. For example, you may consider taking the Step 2 CK exam first if you have just graduated from medical school and the clinical topics are still fresh in your mind. However, keep in mind that there is a large overlap between Step 1 and Step 2 CK topics in areas such as pharmacology, pathophysiology, and biostatistics. You might therefore consider taking the Step 1 and Step 2 CK exams close together to take advantage of this overlap in your test preparation.

USMLE Step 1 and the IMG

What Is the USMLE Step 1? It is a computerized test of the basic medical sciences that consists of 350 multiple-choice questions divided into seven blocks.

Content. Step 1 includes test items in the following content areas:

- Anatomy
- Behavioral sciences
- Biochemistry
- Microbiology and immunology
- Pathology
- Pharmacology
- Physiology
- Interdisciplinary topics such as nutrition, genetics, and aging

Significance of the Test. Step 1 is required for the ECFMG certificate as well as for registration for the Step 2 CS. Since most U.S. graduates apply to residency with their Step 1 scores only, it may be the only objective tool available with which to compare IMGs with U.S. graduates.

Official Web Sites. www.usmle.org and www.ecfmg.org/usmle.

Eligibility. Both students and graduates from medical schools that are listed in IMED are eligible to take the test. Students must have completed at least two years of medical school by the beginning of the eligibility period selected.

Eligibility Period. A three-month period of your choice.

Fee. The fee for Step 1 is $695 plus an international test delivery surcharge (if you choose a testing region other than the United States or Canada).

Retaking the Exam. In the event that you failed the test, you can reapply and select an eligibility period that begins at least 60 days after the last attempt. You cannot take the same Step more than three times in any 12-month period. You cannot retake the exam if you passed. The minimum score to pass the exam is 75 on a two-digit scale. To pass, you must answer roughly 60–70% of the questions correctly.

Statistics. In 2005, only 68% of ECFMG candidates passed Step 1 on their first attempt, compared with 93% of U.S. and Canadian medical students and graduates. Of note, 1994–1995 data showed that USFMGs (U.S. citizens attending non-U.S. medical schools) performed 0.4 SD lower than IMGs (non-U.S. citizens attending non-U.S. medical schools). Although their overall scores were lower, USFMGs performed better than IMGs on behavioral sciences. In general, students from non-U.S. medical schools perform worst in behavioral science and biochemistry (1.9 and 1.5 SDs below U.S. students) and comparatively better in gross anatomy and pathology (0.7 and 0.9 SD below U.S. students). Although derived from data collected in 1994–1995, these data may help you focus your studying efforts.

Tips. Although few if any students feel totally prepared to take Step 1, IMGs in particular require serious study and preparation to reach their full potential on this exam. It is also imperative that IMGs do their best on Step 1, as a poor score on Step 1 is a distinct disadvantage in applying for most residencies. Remember that if you pass Step 1, you cannot retake it in an attempt to improve your score. Your goal should thus be to beat the mean, because you can then confidently assert that you have done better than average for U.S. students. Good Step 1 scores will also lend credibility to your residency application and help you get into highly competitive specialties such as radiology, orthopedics, and dermatology.

Commercial Review Courses. Do commercial review courses help improve your scores? Reports vary, and such courses can be expensive. Many IMGs decide to try the USMLE on their own and then consider a review course only if they fail. Just keep in mind that many states require that you pass the USMLE within three attempts. (For more information on review courses, see Section 3.)

USMLE Step 2 CK and the IMG

What Is the Step 2 CK? It is a computerized test of the clinical sciences consisting of 368 multiple-choice questions divided into eight blocks. It can be taken at Prometric centers in the United States and several other countries.

Content. The Step 2 CK includes test items in the following content areas:

- Internal medicine
- Obstetrics and gynecology
- Pediatrics
- Preventive medicine
- Psychiatry
- Surgery
- Other areas relevant to the provision of care under supervision

Significance of the Test. The Step 2 CK is required for the ECFMG certificate. It reflects the level of clinical knowledge of the applicant. It tests clinical subjects, primarily internal medicine. Other areas that are tested are surgery, obstetrics and gynecology, pediatrics, orthopedics, psychiatry, ENT, ophthalmology, and medical ethics.

Official Web Sites. www.usmle.org and www.ecfmg.org/usmle.

Eligibility. Students and graduates from medical schools that are listed in IMED are eligible to take the Step 2 CK. Students must have completed at least two years of medical school. This means that students must have completed the basic medical science component of the medical school curriculum by the beginning of the eligibility period selected.

Eligibility Period. A three-month period of your choice.

Fee. The fee for the Step 2 CK is $695 plus an international test delivery surcharge (if you choose a testing region other than the United States or Canada).

Retaking the Exam. In the event that you fail the Step 2 CK, you can reapply and select an eligibility period that begins at least 60 days after the last attempt. You cannot take the same Step more than three times in any 12-month period. You cannot retake the exam if you passed.

Statistics. In 2004–2005, 77% of ECFMG candidates passed the Step 2 CK on their first attempt, compared with 94% of U.S. and Canadian candidates.

Tips. It's better to take the Step 2 CK after you have completed your internal medicine rotation because most of the questions give clinical scenarios and ask you to make medical diagnoses and clinical decisions. In addition, because this is a clinical sciences exam, cultural and geographic considerations play a greater role than is the case with Step 1. For example, if your medical education gave you ample exposure to malaria, brucellosis, and malnutrition but little to alcohol withdrawal, child abuse, and cholesterol screening, you must work to familiarize yourself with topics that are more heavily emphasized in U.S. medicine. You must also have a basic understanding of the legal and social aspects of U.S. medicine, because you will be asked questions about communicating with and advising patients.

USMLE Step 2 CS and the IMG

What Is the Step 2 CS? The Step 2 CS is a test of clinical and communication skills administered as a one-day, eight-hour exam. It includes 10 to 12 encounters with standardized patients (15 minutes each, with 10 minutes to write a note after each encounter). Test results are valid indefinitely.

Content. The Step 2 CS tests the ability to communicate in English as well as interpersonal skills, data-gathering skills, the ability to perform a physical exam, and the ability to formulate a brief note, a differential diagnosis, and a list of diagnostic tests. The areas that are covered in the exam are as follows:

- Internal medicine
- Surgery
- Obstetrics and gynecology
- Pediatrics
- Psychiatry
- Family medicine

Unlike the USMLE Step 1, Step 2 CK, or Step 3, there are no numerical grades for the Step 2 CS—it's simply either a pass or a fail. To pass, a candidate must demonstrate a passing performance in **each** of the following three components:

- **Integrated Clinical Encounter (ICE)**: Includes Data Gathering, the Physical Exam, and the Patient Note.
- **Spoken English Proficiency (SEP)**.
- **Communication and Interpersonal Skills (CIS)**.

According to the NBME, the most common component that IMGs fail on the Step 2 CS is the CIS component.

Significance of the Test. The Step 2 CS is required for the ECFMG certificate. It has eliminated the Test of English as a Foreign Language (TOEFL) as a requirement for ECFMG certification.

Official Web Site. www.ecfmg.org/usmle/step2cs.

Eligibility. Students must have completed at least two years of medical school in order to take the test. That means students must have completed the basic medical science component of the medical school curriculum at the time they apply for the exam.

Fee. The fee for the Step 2 CS is $1200.

Scheduling. You must schedule the Step 2 CS within **four months** of the date indicated on your notification of registration. You must take the exam within 12 months of the date indicated on your notification of registration. It is generally advisable to take the Step 2 CS as soon as possible in the year before your Match, as the results often arrive too late to allow you to retake the test and pass it before the Match.

Retaking the Exam. There is no limit to the number of attempts you can make to pass the Step 2 CS. However, you cannot retake the exam within 60 days of a failed attempt, and you cannot take it more than three times in a 12-month period.

Test Site Locations. The Step 2 CS is currently administered at the following five locations:

- Philadelphia, PA
- Atlanta, GA
- Los Angeles, CA
- Chicago, IL
- Houston, TX

For more information about the Step 2 CS exam, please refer to *First Aid for the Step 2 CS.*

USMLE Step 3 and the IMG

What Is the USMLE Step 3? It is a two-day computerized test in clinical medicine consisting of 480 multiple-choice questions and nine computer-based case simulations (CCS). The exam aims at testing your knowledge and its application to patient care and clinical decision making (i.e., this exam tests if you can safely practice medicine independently and without supervision).

Significance of the Test. Taking Step 3 before residency is critical if an IMG is seeking an H1B visa and is a bonus that can be added to the residency application. Step 3 is also required to obtain a full medical license in the United States and can be taken during residency for this purpose.

Official Web Site. www.usmle.org.

Fee. The fee for Step 3 is $590 (the total application fee can vary among states).

Eligibility. Most states require that applicants have completed one, two, or three years of postgraduate training (residency) before they apply for Step 3 and permanent state licensure. The exceptions are the 13 states mentioned below, which allow IMGs to take Step 3 at the beginning of or even before residency. So if you don't fulfill the prerequisites to taking Step 3 in your state of choice, simply use the name of one of the 13 states in your Step 3 application. You can take the exam in any state you choose regardless of the state that you mentioned on your application. Once you pass Step 3, it will be recognized by all states. Basic eligibility requirements for the USMLE Step 3 are as follows:

- Obtaining an MD or DO degree (or its equivalent) by the application deadline.
- Obtaining an ECFMG certificate if you are a graduate of a foreign medical school or are successfully completing a "fifth pathway" program (at a date no later than the application deadline).
- Meeting the requirements imposed by the individual state licensing authority to which you are applying to take Step 3. Please refer to www.fsmb.org for more information.

The following states do not have postgraduate training as an eligibility requirement to apply for Step 3:

- Arkansas
- California
- Connecticut
- Florida
- Louisiana
- Maryland
- Nebraska*
- New York
- South Dakota
- Texas
- Utah*
- Washington
- West Virginia

* Requires that IMGs obtain a "valid indefinite" ECFMG certificate.

The Step 3 exam is not available outside the United States. Applications can be found online at www.fsmb.org and must be submitted to the FSMB.

Residencies and the IMG

It is becoming increasingly difficult for IMGs to obtain residencies in the United States given the rising concern about an oversupply of physicians in the United States. Official bodies such as the Council on Graduate Medical Education (COGME) have recommended that the total number of residency slots be reduced. Furthermore, changes in immigration law have made it harder for noncitizens or legal residents of the United States to remain in the country after completing a residency.

In the residency Match, the number of U.S.-citizen IMG applications has been stable for the past few years, while the percentage accepted has slowly increased. For non-U.S.-citizen IMGs, applications fell from 7977 in 1999 to 5556 in 2005, while the percentage accepted significantly increased (see Table 1-1). This decrease in the total number of IMGs applying for the Match may be attributed to several factors:

- Introduction of the Step 2 CS as a requirement.
- Increased difficulty obtaining U.S. visas.
- Increased expenses associated with the USMLE exams, ERAS, and travel to the United States.
- An increase in the number of IMGs who are withdrawing from the Match to sign a separate "pre-Match" contract with programs.

More information about residency programs can be obtained at www.ama-assn.org.

TABLE 1-1. IMGs in the Match.

APPLICANTS	2003	2004	2005
U.S.-citizen IMGs	1987	2015	2091
% U.S.-citizen IMGs accepted	55	55	55
Non-U.S.-citizen IMGs	5029	5671	5554
% non-U.S.-citizen IMGs accepted	56	52	56
U.S. graduates (non-IMGs)	14,332	14,609	14,719
% U.S. graduates accepted	93	93	94

The Match and the IMG

Given the increasing number of IMG candidates with strong applications, IMGs should bear in mind that good USMLE scores are not the only way to gain a competitive edge. However, USMLE Step 1 and Step 2 CK scores continue to be used as the initial screen for considering candidates for interviews.

Based on accumulated IMG Match experiences over recent years, here are a few pointers to help IMGs maximize their chances for a residency interview.

The IMG Checklist

- **Apply early.** Programs offer a limited number of interviews and often select candidates on a first-come, first-served basis. In view of this, IMGs should aim to complete the entire process of applying for the ERAS token, registering with the Association of American Medical Colleges (AAMC), mailing necessary documents to ERAS, and completing the ERAS application, including the Common Application Form (CAF), before September (see Figure 1-5). Community programs usually send out interview offers earlier than university and university-affiliated programs.
- **U.S. clinical experience helps.** Externships and observerships in a U.S. hospital setting have emerged as an important credential on an IMG application. Externships are like short-term medical school internships and offer hands-on clinical experience. Observerships, also called "shadowing," involve following a physician and observing how he or she manages patients. Externships are considered superior to observerships, but having either of them is always better than having none. Some programs require students to have participated in an externship or observership before applying. It is best to get such an experience before or at the time you apply to the various programs so that you can include it on your ERAS application. If such an experience or opportunity comes up after you apply, be sure to inform the programs.

FIGURE 1-5. IMG Timeline for Application

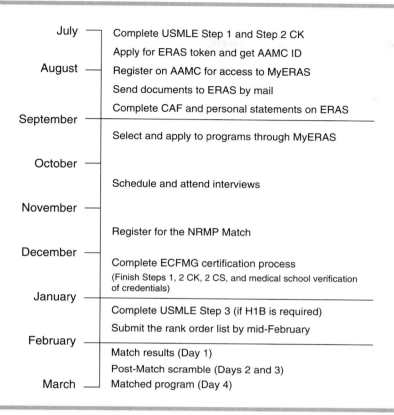

July	Complete USMLE Step 1 and Step 2 CK
	Apply for ERAS token and get AAMC ID
August	Register on AAMC for access to MyERAS
	Send documents to ERAS by mail
	Complete CAF and personal statements on ERAS
September	
	Select and apply to programs through MyERAS
October	
	Schedule and attend interviews
November	
	Register for the NRMP Match
December	
	Complete ECFMG certification process
	(Finish Steps 1, 2 CK, 2 CS, and medical school verification of credentials)
January	
	Complete USMLE Step 3 (if H1B is required)
	Submit the rank order list by mid-February
February	
	Match results (Day 1)
	Post-Match scramble (Days 2 and 3)
March	Matched program (Day 4)

- **Clinical research helps.** University programs are attracted to candidates who show a strong interest in clinical research and academics. They may even relax their application criteria for individuals with unique backgrounds and strong research experience. Publications in well-known journals are an added bonus.

- **Time the Step 2 CS well.** The ECFMG has published the new Step 2 CS score-reporting schedule for the years 2006–2007 at http://ecfmg.org/announce.htm#reportsched. Most program directors would like to see passing scores on the Step 1, Step 2 CK, and Step 2 CS exams before they rank an IMG on their rank order list in mid-February. Too many candidates have missed out on a position on the rank order list—and have thus lost a Match—because their Step 2 CS scores were delayed or because they neglected to retake the test on time after having failed. It is also difficult for candidates to predict their results on the Step 2 CS, since the grading process is not very transparent. Therefore, it is advisable that candidates take the Step 2 CS as early as possible in the application year.

- **U.S. letters of recommendation (LORs) help.** LORs from clinicians practicing in the United States carry more weight than recommendations from home countries.

- **Step up the Step 3.** If H1B visa sponsorship is desired, aim to have Step 3 results by January of the Match year. Besides the visa advantage, an early and good Step 3 score may benefit those IMGs who have been away from clinical medicine for a while as well as those who have low scores on the Step 1 and Step 2 CK exams.

- **Verify medical credentials in a timely manner.** Do not overlook the medical school credential verification process. The ECFMG certificate arrives only after credentials have been verified, so it's good to keep track of the process and keep checking with the ECFMG from time to time about your status.
- **Schedule interviews with prematches in mind.** Schedule interviews with your favorite programs first. This will leave you better prepared to make a decision in the event that you are offered a pre-Match position.

Visa Options for the IMG

If you are living outside the United States, you will need to apply for a visa that will allow you lawful entry into the United States in order to take the Step 2 CS and/or do your interviews for residency. A B1 or B2 visitor visa may be issued by the U.S. consulate in your country. Citizens of some countries may have to undergo an additional security check that could take up to six months. Upon your entry into the United States, either the B1 or, more commonly, the B2 will be issued on your I-94. Both visas allow you a limited period within which to stay in the United States (two to six months) in order to take the exam. If the given period is not sufficient, you may apply for an extension before the expiration of your I-94.

Documents that are recommended to facilitate this process include the following:

- The Step 2 CS admission permit and a letter from the ECFMG (which explains why the applicant must enter the United States)
- Your medical diploma
- Transcripts from your medical school
- Your USMLE score sheets
- A sponsor letter or affidavit of support stating that you (if you are sponsoring yourself) or your sponsor will bear the expense of your trip and that you have sufficient funds to meet that expense
- An alien status affidavit

Individuals from certain countries may be allowed to enter the United States for up to 90 days without a visa under the Visa Waiver Program. See www.uscis.gov.

As an IMG, you need a visa to work or train in the United States unless you are a U.S. citizen or a permanent resident (i.e., hold a green card). Two types of visas enable you to accept a residency appointment in the United States: J1 and H1B. Most sponsoring residency programs (SRPs) prefer a J1 visa. Above all, this is because SRPs are authorized by the Department of Homeland Security (DHS) to issue a Form DS-2019 directly to an IMG. By contrast, SRPs must complete considerable paperwork, including an application to the Immigration and Labor Department, to apply to the DHS for an H1B visa on behalf of an IMG.

The J1 Visa

Also known as the Exchange Visitor Program, the J1 visa was introduced to give IMGs in diverse specialties the chance to use their training experience in the United States to improve conditions in their home countries. As mentioned above, the DHS authorizes most SRPs to issue Form DS-2019 in the same manner that I-20s are issued to regular international students in the United States.

To enable an SRP to issue a DS-2019, you must obtain a certificate from the ECFMG indicating that you are eligible to participate in a residency program in the United States. First, however, you must ask the Ministry of Health in your country to issue a statement indicating that your country needs physicians with the skills you propose to acquire from a U.S. residency program. This statement, which must bear the seal of your country's government and must be signed by a duly designated government official, is intended to satisfy the U.S. Secretary of Health and Human Services (HHS) that there is such a need. The Health Ministry in your country should send this statement to the ECFMG (or they may allow you to mail it to the ECFMG).

How can you find out if the government of your country will issue such a statement? In many countries, the Ministry of Health maintains a list of medical specialties in which there is a need for further training abroad. You can also consult seniors in your medical school. A word of caution: If you are applying for a residency in internal medicine and internists are not in short supply in your country, it may help to indicate an intention to pursue a subspecialty after completing your residency training.

The text of your statement of need should read as follows:

> Name of applicant for visa: _____. There currently exists in _____ (your country) a need for qualified medical practitioners in the specialty of _____. (Name of applicant for visa) has filed a written assurance with the government of this country that he/she will return to _____ (your country) upon completion of training in the United States and intends to enter the practice of medicine in the specialty for which training is being sought.
>
> Stamp (or seal and signature) of issuing official of named country. Dated _____

To facilitate the issuing of such a statement by the Ministry of Health in your country, you should submit a certified copy of the agreement or a contract from your SRP in the United States. The agreement or contract must be signed by you and the residency program official responsible for the training.

Armed with Form DS-2019, you should then go to the U.S. consulate closest to the residential address indicated in your passport. As for other nonimmigrant visas, you must show that you have a genuine nonimmigrant intent to return to your home country. You must also show that all your expenses will be paid.

When you enter the United States, bring your Form DS-2019 along with your visa. You are usually admitted to the United States for the length of the Jl program, designated as "D/S," or duration of status. The duration of your program is indicated on the DS-2019.

In the wake of the terrorist attacks of September 11, 2001, a number of new regulations have been introduced to improve the monitoring of exchange visitors during their time in the United States. All SRPs and students are currently required to register with the Student and Exchange Visitor Program (SEVP) via the Student and Exchange Visitor Information System (SEVIS). SEVIS allows the DHS to maintain up-to-date information (e.g., enrollment status, current address) on exchange visitors. SEVIS Form DS-2019 is used for visa applications, admission, and change of status. Procedural details for this new legislation are still being hammered out, so contact your SRP or check www.uscis.gov for the most current information.

Duration of Participation. The duration of a resident's participation in a program of graduate medical education or training is limited to the time normally required to complete such a program. If you would like to get an idea of the typical training time for the various medical subspecialties, you may consult the *Directory of Medical Specialties*, published by Marquis Who's Who for the American Board of Medical Specialties. The authority charged with determining the duration of time required by an individual IMG is the State Department. The maximum amount of time for participation in a training program is ordinarily limited to seven years unless the IMG has demonstrated to the satisfaction of the ECFMG and the State Department that his or her home country has an exceptional need for the specialty in which he or she will receive further training. An extension of stay may be granted in the event that an IMG needs to repeat a year of clinical medical training or needs time for training or education to take an exam required for board certification.

Requirements after Entry into the United States. Each year, all IMGs participating in a residency program on a Jl visa must furnish the Attorney General of the United States with an affidavit (Form I-644) attesting that they are in good standing in the program of graduate medical education or training in which they are participating and that they will return to their home countries upon completion of the education or training for which they came to the United States.

Restrictions under the Jl Visa. No later than two years after the date of entry into the United States, an IMG participating in a residency program on a Jl visa is allowed one opportunity to change his or her designated program of graduate medical education or training if his or her director approves that change.

The J1 visa includes a condition called the "two-year foreign residence requirement." The relevant section of the Immigration and Nationality Act states:

> Any exchange visitor physician coming to the United States on or after January 10, 1977, for the purpose of receiving graduate medical education or training is automatically subject to the two-year home-country physical presence requirement of section 212(e) of the Immigration and Nationality Act, as amended. Such physicians are not eligible to be considered for section 212(e) waivers on the basis of "No Objection" statements issued by their governments.

The law thus requires that a J1 visa holder, upon completion of the training program, leave the United States and reside in his or her home country for a period of at least two years. Currently, the American Medical Association (AMA) is advocating that this period be extended to five years.

An IMG on a J1 visa is ordinarily not allowed to change from a J1 to most other types of visas or (in most cases) to change from J1 to permanent residence while in the United States until he or she has fulfilled the "foreign residence requirement." The purpose of the foreign residence requirement is to ensure that an IMG uses the training he or she obtained in the United States for the benefit of his or her home country. The U.S. government may, however, waive the two-year foreign residence requirement under the following circumstances:

- If you as an IMG can prove that returning to your country would result in "exceptional hardship" to you or to members of your immediate family who are U.S. citizens or permanent residents;
- If you as an IMG can demonstrate a "well-founded fear of persecution" due to race, religion, or political opinions if forced to return to your country;
- If you obtain a "no objection" statement from your government; or
- If you are sponsored by an "interested governmental agency" or a designated state Department of Health in the United States.

Applying for a J1 Visa Waiver. IMGs who have sought a waiver on the basis of the last alternative have found it beneficial to approach the following potentially "interested government agencies":

- **The Department of Health and Human Services.** Recently, HHS has expanded its role in reviewing J1 waiver applications. HHS's considerations for a waiver have classically been as follows: (1) the program or activity in which the IMG is engaged is "of high priority and of national or international significance in an area of interest" to HHS; (2) the IMG must be an "integral" part of the program or activity "so that the loss of his/her services would necessitate discontinuance of the program or a major phase of it"; and (3) the IMG "must possess outstanding qualifications, training, and experience well beyond the usually expected accomplishments at the graduate, postgraduate, and residency levels and must clearly demonstrate the capability to make original and significant contributions to the program." Under these criteria, HHS waivers are granted to physicians working in high-level biomedical research.

New rules will also allow HHS to review J1 waiver applications from community health centers, rural hospitals, and other health care providers. In the past, the U.S. Department of Agriculture (USDA) served as the interested federal government agency that reviewed waiver applications to allow foreign doctors to serve in rural underserved communities outside Appalachia, while the Appalachian Regional Commission (ARC) played that role for Appalachian communities. The USDA is no longer handling applications for J1 waivers. HHS will now review waiver applications for primary care practitioners and psychiatrists who have completed residency training within one year of application to practice in designated Health Professional Shortage Areas (HPSAs), Medically Underserved Areas and Populations (MUA/Ps), and Mental Health Professional Shortage Areas (MHPSAs). HHS waiver applications should be mailed to Joyce E. Jones, Executive Secretary, Exchange Visitor Waiver Review Board, Room 639-H, Hubert H. Humphrey Building, Department of Health and Human Services, 200 Independence Avenue, S.W., Washington, D.C. 20201; phone (202) 690-6174; fax (202) 690-7127.

■ **The Department of Veterans Affairs.** With more than 170 health care facilities located in various parts of the United States, the VA is a major employer of physicians in this country. In addition, many VA hospitals are affiliated with university medical centers. The VA sponsors IMGs working in research, patient care (regardless of specialty), and teaching. The waiver applicant may engage in teaching and research in conjunction with clinical duties. The VA's latest guidelines (issued on June 22, 1994) provide that it will act as an interested government agency only when the loss of an IMG's services would necessitate the discontinuance of a program or a major phase of it and when recruitment efforts have failed to locate a U.S. physician to fill the position.

The procedure for obtaining a VA sponsorship for a J1 waiver is as follows: (1) the IMG should deal directly with the Human Resources Department at the local VA facility; and (2) the facility must request that the VA's chief medical director sponsor the IMG for a waiver. The waiver request should include the following documentation: (1) a letter from the director of the local facility describing the program, the IMG's immigration status, the health care needs of the facility, and the facility's recruitment efforts; (2) recruitment efforts, including copies of all job advertisements run within the preceding year; and (3) copies of the IMG's licenses, test results, board certifications, IAP-66 or SEVIS DS-2019 forms, and the like. The VA contact person in Washington, D.C., should be contacted by the local medical facility rather than by IMGs or their attorneys.

- **The Appalachian Regional Commission.** ARC sponsors physicians in certain places in the eastern and southern United States—namely, in Alabama, Georgia, Kentucky, Maryland, Mississippi, New York, North Carolina, Ohio, Pennsylvania, South Carolina, Tennessee, Virginia, and West Virginia. Since 1992, ARC has sponsored approximately 200 primary care IMGs annually in counties within its jurisdiction that have been designated as HPSAs by HHS.

  In accordance with its February 1994 revision of its J1 waiver policies, ARC requires that waiver requests initially be submitted to the ARC contact person in the state of intended employment. Contact information for each state can be found on the ARC Web site (www.arc.gov). If the state concurs, a letter from the state's governor recommending the waiver must be addressed to Anne B. Pope, the new federal cochair of ARC. The waiver request should include the following: (1) a letter from the facility to Ms. Pope stating the proposed dates of employment, the IMG's medical specialty, the address of the practice location, an assertion that the IMG will practice primary care for at least 40 hours per week in the HPSA, and details as to why the facility needs the services of the IMG; (2) a J1 Visa Data Sheet; (3) the ARC federal cochair's J1 Visa Waiver Policy and the J1 Visa Waiver Policy Affidavit and Agreement with the notarized signature of the IMG; (4) a contract of at least three years' duration; (5) evidence of the IMG's qualifications, including a résumé, medical diplomas and licenses, and IAP-66 or SEVIS DS-2019 forms; and (6) evidence of unsuccessful attempts to recruit qualified U.S. physicians within the preceding six months. Copies of advertisements, copies of résumés received, and reasons for rejection must also be included. ARC will not sponsor IMGs who have been out of status for six months or longer.

  Requests for ARC waivers are then processed in Washington, D.C. (ARC, 1666 Connecticut Avenue, N.W., Washington, D.C. 20009). ARC is usually able to forward a letter confirming that a waiver has been recommended to the requesting facility or attorney within 30 days of the request.

- **The Department of Agriculture.** At the time of publication, the USDA is no longer sponsoring J1 waivers. The scope of the HHS J1 waiver program has been expanded to fill the gap.

- **State Departments of Public Health.** There is no application form for a state-sponsored J1 waiver. However, regulations specify that an application must include the following documents: (1) a letter from the state Department of Public Health identifying the physician and specifying that it would be in the public interest to grant him or her a J1 waiver; (2) an employment contract that is valid for a minimum of three years and that states the name and address of the facility that will employ the physician and the geographic areas in which he or she will practice medicine; (3) evidence that these geographic areas are located within HPSAs; (4) a statement by the physician agreeing to the contractual requirements; (5) copies of all IAP-66 or SEVIS DS-2019 forms; and (6) a completed U.S. Information Agency (USIA) Data Sheet. Applications are numbered in the order in which they are received, since only 30 physicians per year may be granted waivers in a particular state under the Conrad State 30 program. Individual states may elect to participate or not to participate in this program. At the time of publication, nonparticipating states included Idaho, Oklahoma, and Wyoming, while Texas had suspended its J1 waiver program pending new legislation.

The H1B Visa

Since 1991, the law has allowed medical residency programs to sponsor foreign-born medical residents for H1B visas. There are no restrictions on changing the H1B visa to any other kind of visa, including permanent resident status (green card), through employer sponsorship or through close relatives who are U.S. citizens or permanent residents. It is advisable for SRPs to apply for H1B visas as soon as possible in the official year (beginning October 1) when the new quota officially opens up.

According to the Web site www.immihelp.com, as of October 17, 2000, the following beneficiaries of approved H1B petitions are exempt from the H1B annual cap:

- Beneficiaries who are in J1 nonimmigrant status in order to receive graduate medical education or training, and who have obtained a waiver of the two-year home residency requirement;
- Beneficiaries who are employed at, or who have received an offer of employment at, an institution of higher education or a related or affiliated nonprofit entity;
- Beneficiaries who are employed by, or who have received an offer of employment from, a nonprofit research organization;
- Beneficiaries who are employed by, or who have received an offer of employment from, a governmental research organization;
- Beneficiaries who are currently maintaining, or who have held within the last six years, H1B status, and are ineligible for another full six-year stay as an H1B; and
- Beneficiaries who have been counted once toward the numerical limit and are the beneficiary of multiple petitions.

H1B visas are intended for "professionals" in a "specialty occupation." This means that an IMG intending to pursue a residency program in the United States with an H1B visa needs to clear all three USMLE Steps before becoming eligible for the H1B. The ECFMG administers Steps 1 and 2, whereas Step 3 is conducted by the individual states. You will need to contact the FSMB or the medical board of the state where you intend to take Step 3 for details.

H1B Application. An application for an H1B visa is filed not by the IMG but rather by his or her employment sponsor—in your case, by the SRP in the United States. If an SRP is willing to do so, you will be told about it at the time of your interview for the residency program.

Before filing an H1B application with the DHS, an SRP must file an application with the U.S. Department of Labor affirming that the SRP will pay at least the normal salary for your job that a U.S. professional would earn. After receiving approval from the Labor Department, your SRP should be ready to file the H1B application with the DHS. The SRP's supporting letter is the most important part of the H1B application package; it must describe the job duties to make it clear that the physician is needed in a "specialty occupation" (resident) under the prevalent legal definition of that term.

Most SRPs prefer to issue a SEVIS Form DS-2019 for a J1 visa rather than file papers for an H1B visa because of the burden of paperwork and the attorney costs involved in securing approval of an H1B visa application. Even so, a sizable number of SRPs are willing to go through the trouble, particularly if an IMG is an excellent candidate or if the SRP concerned finds it difficult to fill all the available residency slots (although this is becoming rarer with continuing cuts in residency slots). If an SRP is unwilling to file for an H1B visa because of attorney costs, you could suggest that you would be willing to bear the burden of such costs. The entire process of getting an H1B visa can take anywhere from 10 to 20 weeks.

H1B Premium Processing Service. According to the Web site www.myvisa.com, the DHS offers the opportunity to obtain processing of an H1B visa application within 15 calendar days. Within 15 days of receiving Form I-907, the DHS will mail you a notice of approval, request for evidence, intent to deny, or notice of investigation for fraud or misrepresentation. If the notice requires the submission of additional evidence or indicates an intent to deny, a new 15-day period will begin upon delivery to the DHS of a complete response to the request for evidence or notice of intent to deny. The fee for this service is $1000. With this service, the total time needed to obtain an H1B visa has become significantly shorter than that required for the J1.

Although an H1B visa can be stamped by any U.S. consulate abroad, it is advisable that you have it stamped at the U.S. consulate where you first applied for a visitor visa to travel to the United States for interviews.

A Final Word

IMGs should also be aware of a new program called the National Security Entry-Exit Registration System, which aims to tighten up homeland security by keeping closer tabs on nonimmigrants residing in or entering the United States on temporary visas.

Male citizens or nationals of specific countries who are already residing in the United States may be required to report to a designated DHS office for registration, which includes being fingerprinted, photographed, and interviewed under oath. The official list of countries includes Bangladesh, Egypt, Indonesia, Jordan, Kuwait, Pakistan, Saudi Arabia, Afghanistan, Algeria, Bahrain, Eritrea, Lebanon, Morocco, North Korea, Oman, Qatar, Somalia, Tunisia, the United Arab Emirates, Yemen, Iran, Iraq, Libya, Sudan, and Syria. Different registration deadlines and criteria have been assigned to citizens of the above-mentioned countries, so please refer to www.uscis.gov for details.

If you are entering the United States, you may be registered at the port of entry if you are (1) a citizen or national of Iran, Iraq, Libya, Sudan, or Syria; (2) a nonimmigrant who has been designated by the State Department; or (3) any other nonimmigrant identified by immigration officers at airports, seaports, and land ports of entry in accordance with new regulation 8 CFR 264.1(f)(2). If you will be staying in the United States for more than 30 days, you will then be required to register in person at a DHS district office within 30 days for an interview and will be required to reregister annually.

Once you are registered, certain special procedures will apply. If you leave the United States for any reason, you must appear in person before a DHS inspecting officer at a preapproved airport, seaport, or land port and leave the United States from that port on the same day. If you change your address, employment, or school, you must report to the DHS in writing within 10 days using Form AR-11 SR. If any of these regulations are not followed, you may be considered out of status and subject to arrest, detention, fines, and/or removal from the United States, and any further application for immigration may be affected.

For the most up-to-date information regarding policies and procedures, please consult www.uscis.gov.

Summary

Despite some significant obstacles, a number of viable methods are available to IMGs who seek visas to pursue a residency program or eventually practice medicine in the United States. There is no doubt that the best alternative for an IMG is to obtain an H1B visa to pursue a medical residency. However, in cases where an IMG joins a residency program with a J1 visa, there are some possibilities for obtaining waivers of the two-year foreign residency requirement, particularly for those who are willing to make a commitment to perform primary care medicine in medically underserved areas.

Resources for the IMG

- **ECFMG**
  3624 Market Street, Fourth Floor
  Philadelphia, PA 19104-2685
  (215) 386-5900
  Fax: (215) 386-9196
  www.ecfmg.org

  The ECFMG telephone number is answered only between 9:00 A.M. and 12:30 P.M. and between 1:30 P.M. and 5:00 P.M. Monday through Friday EST. The ECFMG often takes a long time to answer the phone, which is frequently busy at peak times of the year, and then gives you a long voice-mail message—so it is better to write or fax early than to rely on a last-minute phone call. Do not contact the NBME, as all IMG exam matters are conducted by the ECFMG. The ECFMG also publishes an information booklet on ECFMG certification and the USMLE program, which gives details on the dates and locations of forthcoming USMLE and English tests for IMGs together with application forms. It is free of charge and is also available from the public affairs offices of U.S. embassies and consulates worldwide as well as from Overseas Educational Advisory Centers. You may order single copies of the handbook by calling (215) 386-5900, preferably on weekends or between 6 P.M. and 6 A.M. Philadelphia time, or by faxing to (215) 387-9963. Requests for multiple copies must be made by fax or mail on organizational letterhead. The full text of the booklet is also available on the ECFMG's Web site at www.ecfmg.org.

- **FSMB**
  P.O. Box 619850
  Dallas, TX 75261-9850
  (817) 868-4000
  Fax: (817) 868-4099
  www.fsmb.org

  The FSMB has a number of publications available, including *The Exchange, Section I*, which gives detailed information on examination and licensing requirements in all U.S. jurisdictions. The cost is $30. (Texas residents must add 8.25% state sales tax.) To obtain these publications, submit the online order form. Payment options include Visa or MasterCard. Alternatively, write to Federation Publications at the above address. All orders must be prepaid with a personal check drawn on a U.S. bank, a cashier's check, or a money order payable to the federation. Foreign orders must be accompanied by an international money order or the equivalent, payable in U.S. dollars through a U.S. bank or a U.S. affiliate of a foreign bank. For Step 3 inquiries, the telephone number is (817) 868-4041. You may e-mail the FSMB at usmle@fsmb.org or write to Examination Services at the address above.

- Immigration information for IMGs is available from the sites of Siskind Susser, a firm of attorneys specializing in immigration law: www.visalaw.com/IMG/resources.html.
- Another source of immigration information can be found on the Web site of the law offices of Carl Shusterman, a Los Angeles attorney specializing in medical immigration law: www.shusterman.com.
- The AMA has dedicated a portion of its Web site to information on IMG demographics, residencies, immigration, and the like: www.ama-assn.org/ama/pub/category/17.html.
- International Medical Placement Ltd., a U.S. company specializing in recruiting foreign physicians to work in the United States, has a site at www.intlmedicalplacement.com.
- Two more useful Web sites are www.myvisa.com and www.immihelp.com.
- *First Aid for the International Medical Graduate,* 2nd ed., by Keshav Chander (2002; 313 pages; ISBN 0071385320), is an excellent resource written by a successful IMG. The book includes interviews with successful IMGs and students gearing up for the USMLE, complete "getting settled" information for new residents, and tips for dealing with possible social and cultural transition difficulties. The book provides useful advice on the U.S. curriculum, the health care delivery system, and ethical issues—and the differences IMGs should expect. Dr. Chander points out the weaknesses often found in IMG hopefuls and suggests ways to improve their performance on standardized tests as well as on academic and clinical evaluations. As a bonus, the guide contains information on how to get good fellowships after residency. The bottom line is that this is a reassuring guide that can help IMGs boost their confidence and proficiency. A great "first of its kind" that will empower IMGs with information that they need to succeed.

Other books that may be useful and of interest to IMGs are as follows:

- *International Medical Graduates in U.S. Hospitals: A Guide for Directors and Applicants,* by Faroque A. Khan and Lawrence G. Smith (1995; ISBN 094312641x).
- *Insider's Guide for the International Medical Graduate to Obtain a Medical Residency in the U.S.A.,* by Ahmad Hakemi (1999; ISBN 1929803001).

The USMLE provides accommodations for students with documented disabilities. The basis for such accommodations is the Americans with Disabilities Act (ADA) of 1990. The ADA defines a disability as "a significant limitation in one or more major life activities." This includes both "observable/physical" disabilities (e.g., blindness, hearing loss, narcolepsy) and "hidden/mental disabilities" (e.g., attention-deficit hyperactivity disorder, chronic fatigue syndrome, learning disabilities).

To provide appropriate support, the administrators of the USMLE must be informed of both the nature and the severity of an examinee's disability. Such documentation is required for an examinee to receive testing accommodations. Accommodations include extra time on tests, low-stimulation environments, extra or extended breaks, and zoom text.

Who Can Apply for Accommodations?

Students or graduates of a school in the United States or Canada that is accredited by the Liaison Committee on Medical Education (LCME) or the American Osteopathic Association (AOA) may apply for test accommodations directly from the NBME. Requests are granted only if they meet the ADA definition of a disability. If you are a disabled student or a disabled graduate of a foreign medical school, you must contact the ECFMG (see below).

Who Is Not Eligible for Accommodations?

Individuals who do not meet the ADA definition of disabled are not eligible for test accommodations. Difficulties not eligible for test accommodations include test anxiety, slow reading without an identified underlying cognitive deficit, English as a second language, and learning difficulties that have not been diagnosed as a medically recognized disability.

Understanding the Need for Documentation

Although most learning-disabled medical students are all too familiar with the often exhausting process of providing documentation of their disability, you should realize that **applying for USMLE accommodation is different from these previous experiences.** This is because the NBME determines whether an individual is disabled solely on the basis of the guidelines set by the ADA. Previous accommodation does not in itself justify provision of an accommodation, so be sure to review the NBME guidelines carefully.

Getting the Information

The first step in applying for USMLE special accommodations is to contact the NBME and obtain a guidelines and questionnaire booklet. This can be obtained by calling or writing to:

Testing Coordinator
Office of Test Accommodations
National Board of Medical Examiners
3750 Market Street
Philadelphia, PA 19104-3102
(215) 590-9700

Internet access to this information is also available at www.nbme.org. This information is also relevant for IMGs, since the information is the same as that sent by the ECFMG.

Foreign graduates should contact the ECFMG to obtain information on special accommodations by calling or writing to:

ECFMG
3624 Market Street, Fourth Floor
Philadelphia, PA 19104-2685
(215) 386-5900

When you get this information, take some time to read it carefully. The guidelines are clear and explicit about what you need to do to obtain accommodations.

Database
of High-Yield Facts

The sixth edition of *First Aid for the USMLE Step 2 CK* contains a revised and expanded database of clinical material that student authors and faculty have identified as high yield for boards review. The facts are organized according to subject matter, whether medical specialty (e.g., Cardiovascular, Renal) or high-yield topic (e.g., Ethics) in medicine. Each subject is then divided into smaller subsections of related facts. Individual facts are generally presented in a logical approach, from basic definitions and epidemiology to **History/Physical Exam, Diagnosis,** and **Treatment.** Lists, mnemonics, and tables are used when helpful in forming key associations.

The content is mostly useful for reviewing material already learned. This section is not ideal for learning complex or highly conceptual material for the first time. Black-and-white images appear throughout the text. In some cases, reference is made to the "clinical image" section at the end of Section 2, which contains full-color glossy plates of histology and patient pathology by topic. At the end of Section 2, we also feature a Rapid Review chapter of key facts and classic associations to cram a day or two before the exam.

The Database of High-Yield Facts is not comprehensive. Use it to complement your core study material and not as your primary study source. The facts and notes have been condensed and edited to emphasize the essential material. Work with the material, add your own notes and mnemonics, and recognize that not all memory techniques work for all students.

We update Section 2 biannually to keep current with new trends in boards content as well as to expand our database of high-yield information. However, we must note that inevitably many other very high-yield entries and topics are not yet included in our database.

We actively encourage medical students and faculty to submit entries and mnemonics so that we may enhance the database for future students. We also solicit recommendations of additional tools for study that may be useful in preparing for the examination, such as diagrams, charts, and computer-based tutorials (see How to Contribute, page xiii).

Disclaimer

The entries in this section reflect student opinions of what is high yield. Owing to the diverse sources of material, no attempt has been made to trace or reference the origins of entries individually. We have regarded mnemonics as essentially in the public domain. All errors and omissions will be gladly corrected if brought to the attention of the authors, either through the publisher or directly by e-mail.

HIGH-YIELD FACTS IN

Cardiovascular

To evaluate patients for cardiac abnormalities, methodically assess the electrocardiogram (ECG) for rate, rhythm, axis, intervals, waveforms, and chamber enlargement (see Figure 2.1-1).

Rate

The normal heart rate is 60–100 bpm. A rate < 60 bpm constitutes bradycardia; > 100 bpm is tachycardia.

Rhythm

Look for sinus rhythm (P before every QRS and QRS after every P), irregular rhythms, and junctional or ventricular rhythms (no P before a QRS).

Axis

- **Normal:** An upright QRS in leads I and aVF.
- **Left-axis deviation:** An upright QRS in lead I and a downward QRS in lead aVF.
- **Right-axis deviation:** A downward QRS in lead I and an upright QRS in lead aVF.

An upright QRS in leads I and aVF—the "double thumbs-up" sign—signifies a normal axis.

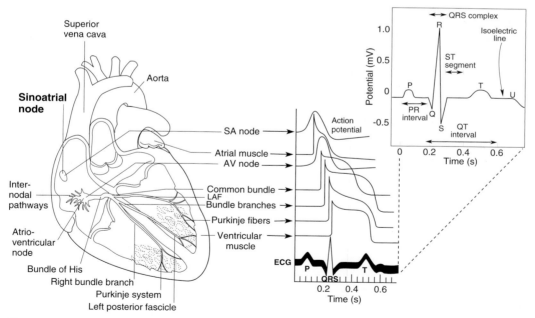

SA node "pacemaker" inherent dominance with slow phase of upstroke
AV node - 100-msec delay - atrioventricular delay

FIGURE 2.1-1. **Electrocardiogram measurements.**

(Adapted, with permission, from Ganong WF et al. *Review of Medical Physiology*, 20th ed. New York: McGraw-Hill, 2001.)

Intervals

- **Atrioventricular (AV) block:** PR interval > 200 msec, or P with no QRS afterward.
- **Left bundle branch block (LBBB):** QRS duration > 120 msec; no R wave in V_1; wide, tall R waves in I, V_5, and V_6.
- **Right bundle branch block (RBBB):** QRS duration > 120 msec; RSR′ complex with a wide R wave in V_1; QRS pattern with a wide S wave in I, V_5, and V_6.
- **Long QT syndrome:** QTc > 440 msec. An underdiagnosed congenital disorder that predisposes to ventricular tachyarrhythmias.

Waveforms

Look for significant Q waves (> 40 msec or more than one-third of the QRS amplitude) indicating past MIs, inverted T waves indicating possible ischemia, and changes in the ST segment (elevation or depression).

Chamber Enlargement

- **Atrial hypertrophy:** Right atrial abnormality (RAA) if P-wave amplitude in lead II > 2.5 mm; left atrial abnormality (LAA) if P-wave width in lead II > 120 msec.
- **Ventricular hypertrophy:** LVH can be diagnosed by the Cornell criteria if the amplitude of the R wave in aVL plus the amplitude of the S wave in $V_3 \geq 24$ mm in males or > 20 mm in females. RVH can be diagnosed with right-axis deviation and an R wave in V_1 > 7 mm.

ARRHYTHMIAS

Bradyarrhythmias and Conduction Abnormalities

Table 2.1-1 outlines the etiologies, clinical presentation, and treatment of common bradyarrhythmias and conduction abnormalities.

Tachyarrhythmias

Tables 2.1-2 and 2.1-3 outline the etiologies, clinical presentation, and treatment of common supraventricular and ventricular tachyarrhythmias.

CARDIOMYOPATHY

Myocardial disease; categorized as dilated, hypertrophic, or restrictive (see Table 2.1-4).

Dilated Cardiomyopathy

The most common cardiomyopathy. Left ventricular dilation and systolic dysfunction (low EF) must be present for diagnosis. Most cases are idiopathic, but known causes include alcohol, wet beriberi, coxsackievirus, Chagas' disease, parasites, cocaine, myocarditis, doxorubicin, HIV, and AZT use. The two most common causes of 2° dilated cardiomyopathy are ischemia and long-standing hypertension.

TABLE 2.1-1.   Bradyarrhythmias and Conduction Abnormalities

TYPE	ETIOLOGY	SIGNS/SYMPTOMS	ECG FINDINGS	TREATMENT
Sinus bradycardia	Normal response to cardiovascular conditioning; can also result from sinus node dysfunction or from β-blocker or calcium channel blocker (CCB) excess.	May be asymptomatic, but can also present with lightheadedness, syncope, chest pain, and hypotension.	Ventricular rate < 60 bpm; normal P wave before every QRS complex.	None necessary if asymptomatic; atropine may be used to ↑ heart rate; pacemaker placement is the definitive treatment in severe cases.
First-degree AV block	Can occur in normal individuals; associated with ↑ vagal tone and with β-blocker or CCB use.	Asymptomatic.	PR interval > 200 msec.	None necessary.
Second-degree AV block (Mobitz I/ Wenckebach)	Drug effects (digoxin, β-blockers, CCBs) or ↑ vagal tone.	Usually asymptomatic.	PR interval ↑ until a dropped beat occurs; PR interval then resets.	Stop the offending drug.
Second-degree AV block (Mobitz II)	Results from fibrotic disease of the conduction system or from a previous septal myocardial infarction (MI).	Occasionally syncope or progression to third-degree AV block.	Unexpected dropped beat without a change in PR interval.	Pacemaker placement.
Third-degree AV block (complete)	No electrical communication between the atria and ventricles.	Syncope, dizziness, acute heart failure, hypotension, cannon A waves.	No relationship between P waves and QRS complexes.	Pacemaker placement.

HISTORY/PE

- Presents with gradual development of congestive heart failure (CHF) symptoms.
- Exam may reveal cardiomegaly and an S3 gallop as well as tricuspid and mitral regurgitation.

DIAGNOSIS

- Echocardiography is diagnostic.
- ECG may show nonspecific ST-T changes, low-voltage QRS, sinus tachycardia, and ectopy. LBBB is common.
- CXR shows an enlarged, balloon-like heart and pulmonary congestion.

An S3 gallop signifies the end of rapid ventricular filling in the setting of fluid overload and is associated with dilated cardiomyopathy.

HIGH-YIELD FACTS

CARDIOVASCULAR

TABLE 2.1-2. Supraventricular Tachyarrhythmias

TYPE	ETIOLOGY	SIGNS/SYMPTOMS	ECG FINDINGS	TREATMENT
Atrial				
Sinus tachycardia	Normal physiologic response to fear, pain, and exercise. Can also be due to hyperthyroidism, dehydration, infection, or pulmonary embolism.	Palpitations, shortness of breath.	Ventricular rate > 100 bpm; normal P waves before every QRS complex.	Treat the underlying cause.
Atrial fibrillation (AF)	**PIRATES:** **P**ulmonary disease **I**schemia **R**heumatic heart disease **A**nemia/**A**trial myxoma **T**hyrotoxicosis **E**thanol **S**epsis	Often asymptomatic, but may present with shortness of breath, chest pain, or palpitations. Physical exam reveals irregularly irregular pulse.	Wavy baseline without discernible P waves, with variable and irregular QRS response (see Figure 2.1-2).	Anticoagulation if > 48 hours (to prevent CVA); rate control (CCBs, β-blockers, digoxin). Cardioversion only if new onset (< 48 hours) and transesophageal echocardiogram (TEE) shows no left atrial clot, or after six weeks of warfarin treatment with satisfactory INR.
Atrial flutter	Circular movement of electrical activity around the atrium at a rate of 300 times per minute.	Usually asymptomatic, but can present with palpitations, syncope, and lightheadedness.	Regular rhythm; "sawtooth" appearance of P waves (see Figure 2.1-2).	Anticoagulation and rate control. Cardiovert according to atrial fibrillation criteria.
Multifocal atrial tachycardia	Multiple atrial pacemakers or reentrant pathways; COPD, hypoxemia.	May be asymptomatic.	Three or more unique P-wave morphologies; rate > 100 bpm.	Treat the underlying disorder; verapamil or β-blockers for rate control and suppression of atrial pacemakers.
AV junction				
Atrioventricular nodal reentry tachycardia (AVNRT)	A reentry circuit in the AV node depolarizes the atrium and ventricle simultaneously.	Palpitations, shortness of breath, angina, syncope, lightheadedness.	Rate 150–250 bpm; P wave is often **buried in** QRS or shortly after.	Carotid massage, Valsalva, or adenosine can stop the arrhythmia. Cardiovert if hemodynamically unstable.

TABLE 2.1-2 (continued).   Supraventricular Tachyarrhythmias

TYPE	ETIOLOGY	SIGNS/SYMPTOMS	ECG FINDINGS	TREATMENT
AV junction (continued)				
Atrioventricular reciprocating tachycardia (AVRT)	Circular movement of an impulse between the AV node and the atrium through a bypass tract. Seen in Wolff-Parkinson-White syndrome.	Palpitations, shortness of breath, angina, syncope, lightheadedness.	Retrograde P wave is often seen **after** a normal QRS.	Same as that for AVNRT.
Paroxysmal atrial tachycardia	Rapid ectopic pacemaker in the atrium (not sinus node).	Palpitations, shortness of breath, angina, syncope, lightheadedness.	Rate > 100 bpm; P wave with an unusual axis **before** each normal QRS.	Adenosine can be used to unmask underlying atrial activity.

HIGH-YIELD FACTS

CARDIOVASCULAR

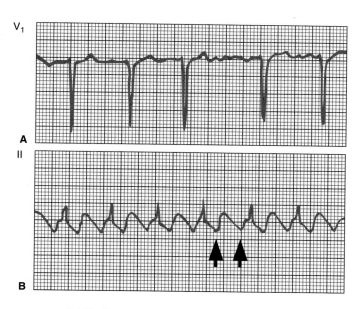

FIGURE 2.1-2.   Atrial fibrillation and atrial flutter.

(A) Lead V₁ demonstrates an irregular ventricular rhythm associated with poorly defined irregular atrial activity consistent with AF. (B) Lead II demonstrates atrial flutter, identified by the regular "sawtooth-like" activity (arrows) at an atrial rate of 300 bpm with 2:1 ventricular response. (Reproduced, with permission, from Kasper DL et al [eds]. *Harrison's Principles of Internal Medicine*, 16th ed. New York: McGraw-Hill, 2005, p. 1345.)

TABLE 2.1-3. **Ventricular Tachyarrhythmias**

TYPE	ETIOLOGY	SIGNS/SYMPTOMS	ECG FINDINGS	TREATMENT
Premature ventricular contraction (PVC)	Ectopic beats arise from ventricular foci. Associated with hypoxia, electrolyte abnormalities, and hyperthyroidism.	Usually asymptomatic, but may → palpitations.	Early, wide QRS not preceded by a P wave. PVCs are followed by a compensatory pause.	Treat the underlying cause. If symptomatic, give β-blockers or occasionally other antiarrhythmics.
Ventricular tachycardia	Associated with coronary artery disease (CAD), MI, and structural heart disease.	Nonsustained ventricular tachycardia is often asymptomatic; sustained ventricular tachycardia can → palpitations, hypotension, angina, and syncope. Can progress to VF.	Three or more consecutive PVCs; wide QRS complexes in a regular rapid rhythm; AV dissociation (see Figure 2.1-3).	Cardioversion and antiarrhythmics (e.g., amiodarone, lidocaine, procainamide).
Ventricular fibrillation (VF)	Associated with CAD and MI.	Syncope, hypotension, pulselessness.	Totally erratic tracing (see Figure 2.1-3).	Immediate electrical cardioversion and ACLS protocol.
Torsades de pointes	Associated with long QT syndrome, hypokalemia, and congenital deafness.	Can present with sudden cardiac death; typically associated with palpitations, dizziness and syncope.	Polymorphous QRS; ventricular tachycardia with rates between 150 and 250 bpm.	Correct hypokalemia; withdraw offending drugs. Give magnesium initially and cardiovert if unstable.

TABLE 2.1-4. **Differential Diagnosis of Cardiomyopathies**

	DILATED	HYPERTROPHIC	RESTRICTIVE
Major abnormality	Impaired contractility	Impaired relaxation	Impaired elasticity
Left ventricular cavity size (end diastole)	↑↑	↓	↑
Left ventricular cavity size (end systole)	↑↑	↓↓	↑
Ejection fraction (EF)	↓↓	↑ or ↔	↓ or ↔
Wall thickness	↓	↑↑	↑

A. Ventricular tachycardia

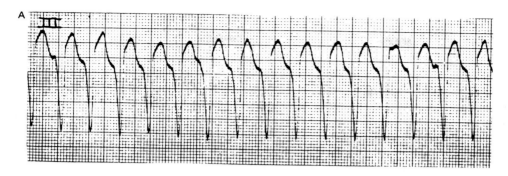

B. Ventricular fibrillation

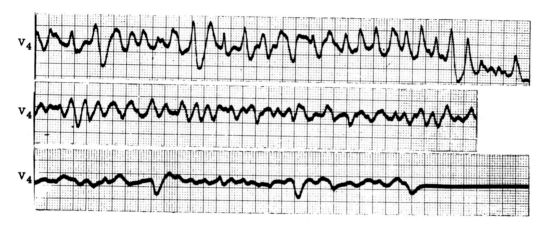

FIGURE 2.1-3.   **Ventricular tachycardia and ventricular fibrillation.**

(A) Ventricular tachycardia. Note the regular, wide-complex rhythm with no discernible P waves. **(B)** Ventricular fibrillation. Note the erratic nature of the tracing. (Reproduced, with permission, from Saunders CE. *Current Emergency Diagnosis & Treatment*, 4th ed. Stamford, CT: Appleton & Lange, 1992, pp. 515, 517.)

TREATMENT

- Stop all alcohol use.
- Treat symptoms of CHF and prevent disease progression (diuretics, ACEIs, β-blockers). Consider anticoagulation to ↓ thrombus risk.
- Consider an implantable cardiac defibrillator (ICD) if EF < 35%.

Hypertrophic Cardiomyopathy

LVH results in impaired left ventricular relaxation and filling (diastolic dysfunction). Hypertrophy frequently involves the interventricular septum → left ventricular outflow tract obstruction and impaired ejection of blood. The congenital form, formerly known as idiopathic hypertrophic subaortic stenosis (IHSS), is inherited as an autosomal-dominant trait in 50% of patients and is the most common cause of sudden death in young, healthy athletes in the United States. Other causes of marked hypertrophy include hypertension and aortic stenosis.

An S4 gallop signifies a stiff ventricle and ↑ "atrial kick" and may be associated with hypertrophic cardiomyopathy.

Hypertrophic cardiomyopathy is the most common cause of sudden death in young, healthy athletes in the United States.

HISTORY/PE

- Patients may be asymptomatic but may also present with syncope, dyspnea, palpitations, angina, or sudden cardiac death.
- Exam may reveal mitral regurgitation, a sustained apical impulse, an S4 gallop, and a systolic ejection crescendo-decrescendo murmur that gets louder with ↓ preload (Valsalva, squatting).
- Obstruction is worsened by ↑ myocardial contractility or by ↓ left ventricular filling (e.g., exercise, Valsalva maneuvers, vasodilators, dehydration).

DIAGNOSIS

- Echocardiography is diagnostic and shows thickened left ventricular walls and dynamic obstruction of blood flow.
- ECG may show signs of left ventricular hypertrophy.
- CXR may reveal left atrial enlargement due to mitral regurgitation.

TREATMENT

- β-blockers are initial therapy for symptomatic relief; CCBs are second-line agents.
- Surgical options for IHSS include dual-chamber pacing, partial excision of the myocardial septum, and ICD placement.
- Patients should avoid intense athletic competition and training.

Restrictive Cardiomyopathy

Defined as ↓ elasticity of myocardium → impaired diastolic filling without significant systolic dysfunction (normal or slightly ↓ EF). Caused by infiltrative disease (sarcoidosis, hemochromatosis, amyloidosis) or by scarring and fibrosis (due to radiation or doxorubicin).

HISTORY/PE

Signs and symptoms of left-sided and right-sided heart failure occur, but symptoms of right-sided heart failure (JVD, peripheral edema) often predominate.

DIAGNOSIS

- CXR and echocardiography are often nondiagnostic.
- Cardiac biopsy may reveal fibrosis or evidence of infiltration.
- ECG frequently shows LBBB.

TREATMENT

Generally symptomatic. Medical treatment includes cautious use of diuretics for fluid overload, vasodilators to ↓ filling pressure, and anticoagulation if not contraindicated.

CONGESTIVE HEART FAILURE (CHF)

Defined as a clinical syndrome caused by the inability of the heart to pump enough blood to meet the O_2 requirements of the heart and peripheral tissues. Risk factors include CAD, hypertension, cardiomyopathy, valvular heart disease, and diabetes. The American Heart Association/American College of Cardiology (AHA/ACC) guidelines classify heart failure according to clinical syndromes, but alternative classification systems include functional severity, left-sided vs. right-sided failure, and systolic vs. diastolic failure (see Tables 2.1-5 through 2.1-8).

Systolic Dysfunction

Heart failure caused by systolic dysfunction is defined by a ↓ EF (< 50%) and ↑ left ventricular end-diastolic volumes. It is caused by inadequate left ventricular contractility or ↑ afterload. The heart compensates for low EF and ↑ preload through hypertrophy and ventricular dilation (Frank-Starling law) but ultimately fails, leading to ↑ myocardial work and worsening systolic function.

HISTORY/PE

- Dyspnea is the earliest and most common presenting symptom.
- Chronic cough, fatigue, lower extremity edema, orthopnea, paroxysmal nocturnal dyspnea (PND), Cheyne-Stokes respirations, and/or abdominal fullness may be seen.
- Look for signs to distinguish between left- and right-sided heart failure (see Table 2.1-7).

DIAGNOSIS

- CHF is a **clinical syndrome** whose diagnosis is based on signs and symptoms.

Causes of CHF—

HEART FAILED

Hypertension
Endocrine
Anemia
Rheumatic heart disease
Toxins
Failure to take meds
Arrhythmia
Infection
Lung (embolism)
Electrolytes
Diet (excess Na⁺)

The most common cause of right-sided heart failure is left-sided heart failure.

TABLE 2.1-5. **AHA/ACC Classification and Treatment of CHF**

STAGE	DESCRIPTION	TREATMENT
A	Patients who are at high risk of developing CHF because of the presence of risk factors, but who have no identified structural or functional abnormalities and no signs or symptoms of CHF.	Manage treatable risk factors (hypertension, smoking, hyperlipidemia, obesity, exercise, alcohol abuse). ACEIs can be used in patients with atherosclerotic vascular disease, DM, or hypertension.
B	Patients with structural heart disease (e.g., a history of MI, left ventricular systolic dysfunction, valvular disease) who have never had symptoms of CHF.	ACEIs, β-blockers.
C	Patients with structural heart disease who have prior or current symptoms of CHF (shortness of breath, fatigue, ↓ exercise tolerance).	Treatment includes diuretics, ACEIs, β-blockers, digitalis, and dietary salt restriction.
D	Patients with marked symptoms of CHF at rest despite maximal medical therapy.	Treatment options include mechanical assist devices, heart transplantation, continuous IV inotropic drugs, and hospice care for end-stage patients.

TABLE 2.1-6. NYHA Functional Classification of CHF

CLASS	DESCRIPTION
I	No limitation of activity; no symptoms with normal activity.
II	Slight limitation of activity; comfortable at rest or with mild exertion.
III	Marked limitation of activity; comfortable only at rest.
IV	Confined to complete rest in bed or chair, as any physical activity brings on discomfort; symptoms present at rest.

- **CXR:** Look for cardiomegaly, cephalization of pulmonary vessels, pleural effusions, vascular plumpness, and prominent hila.
- **Echocardiogram:** Look for ↓ EF and ventricular dilation.
- **Lab abnormalities:** BNP, ↑ creatinine, ↓ sodium.
- **ECG:** Usually nondiagnostic, but MI or AF may precede acute exacerbations.

TREATMENT

- **Acute:**
  - Correct underlying causes (e.g., arrhythmias, alcohol-induced failure, thyroid and valvular disease).
  - Diurese aggressively with loop and thiazide diuretics (see Table 2.1-9).
  - Use ACEIs in all patients who can tolerate them. If a patient cannot tolerate an ACEI, an angiotensin receptor blocker (ARB) should be considered. β-blockers should not be used during decompensated CHF, as they may cause hypotension. Once the patient is euvolemic, carvedilol, bisoprolol, or extended-release metoprolol should be started and the dose should be gradually ↑.
  - Treat acute pulmonary congestion with **LMNOP** (see mnemonic).
- **Chronic:**
  - Control comorbid conditions (e.g., diabetes, hypertension, obesity) and limit dietary sodium and fluid intake.
  - Long-term β-blockers and ACEIs/ARBs together help prevent neurohormonal remodeling of the heart. All of these agents ↓ mortality for New York Heart Association (NYHA) class II–IV patients.
  - Daily aspirin and a statin are recommended for ischemic heart disease to prevent further ischemic events.

> *Acute CHF management–*
>
> **LMNOP**
>
> **L**asix
> **M**orphine
> **N**itrates
> **O**xygen
> **P**ulmonary ventilation

TABLE 2.1-7. Left-Sided vs. Right-Sided Heart Failure

LEFT-SIDED CHF SYMPTOMS	RIGHT-SIDED CHF SYMPTOMS
Bilateral basilar rales	JVD
S3 gallop	Hepatomegaly
Pleural effusions	Hepatojugular reflex
Pulmonary edema	Bipedal edema

TABLE 2.1-8. Comparison of Systolic and Diastolic Dysfunction

	SYSTOLIC DYSFUNCTION	DIASTOLIC DYSFUNCTION
Patient age	Often < 65 years of age.	Often > 65 years of age.
Comorbidities	Dilated cardiomyopathy, valvular heart disease.	Restrictive or hypertrophic cardiomyopathy; renal disease or hypertension.
Physical findings	Displaced PMI, S3 gallop.	Sustained PMI, S4 gallop.
CXR	Pulmonary congestion, cardiomegaly.	Pulmonary congestion, normal heart size.
ECG/echocardiography	Q waves, ↓ EF (< 40%).	LVH, normal EF (> 55%).

- Chronic diuretic therapy (loop diuretic ± thiazide) can prevent volume overload.
- Low-dose spironolactone has been shown to ↓ mortality risk when given with ACEIs and loop diuretics in patients with left ventricular systolic dysfunction and NYHA class III–IV heart failure. Monitor for hyperkalemia.
- Anticoagulate patients with AF, those with an EF < 30%, and those with a history of previous embolic events. Consider an ICD in patients with both an EF < 30% and CAD.
- CHF that is unresponsive to maximal medical therapy may require a mechanical left ventricular assist device or cardiac transplantation.

Loops lose calcium, whereas thiazides save it.

TABLE 2.1-9. Types of Diuretics

CLASS	EXAMPLES	SITE OF ACTION	MECHANISM OF ACTION	SIDE EFFECTS
Osmotic agents	Mannitol	Proximal tubule	Creates ↑ tubular fluid osmolarity → ↑ urine flow.	Pulmonary edema, dehydration. Contraindicated in anuria and CHF.
Carbonic anhydrase inhibitors	Acetazolamide	Proximal convoluted tubule	$NaHCO_3$ diuresis ↓ total body $NaHCO_3$.	Hyperchloremic metabolic acidosis, neuropathy, NH_3 toxicity, sulfa allergy.
Loop diuretics	Furosemide, ethacrynic acid, bumetanide, torsemide.	Loop of Henle	↓ $Na^+/K^+/2Cl^-$ cotransporter; ↓ urine concentration; ↑ Ca^{2+} excretion.	Ototoxicity, hypokalemia, hypocalcemia, dehydration, gout.
Thiazide diuretics	HCTZ, chlorothiazide, chlorthalidone	Early distal tubule	↓ NaCl reabsorption → ↓ diluting capacity of nephron; ↓ Ca^{2+} excretion.	Hypokalemic metabolic alkalosis, hyponatremia, hyperglycemia, hyperlipidemia, hyperuricemia, hypercalcemia.
K^+-sparing agents	Spironolactone, triamterene, amiloride	Cortical collecting tubule	Spironolactone is an aldosterone receptor antagonist; triamterene and amiloride block Na^+ channels.	Hyperkalemia, gynecomastia, hirsutism, sexual dysfunction.

Diastolic Dysfunction

Defined by ↓ ventricular compliance with normal systolic function. The ventricle has either impaired active relaxation (due to ischemia, aging, and/or hypertrophy) or impaired passive filling (scarring from prior MI; restrictive cardiomyopathy). Left ventricular end-diastolic pressure ↑, cardiac output remains essentially normal, and EF is normal or ↑.

History/PE

Associated with stable and unstable angina, shortness of breath, dyspnea on exertion, arrhythmias, MI, heart failure, and sudden death.

Treatment

- Diuretics are first-line therapy (see Table 2.1-9).
- Maintain rate and BP control via β-blockers, ACEIs, ARBs, or CCBs.
- Digoxin is not useful in these patients.

CORONARY ARTERY DISEASE (CAD)

Clinical manifestations of CAD include stable and unstable angina, shortness of breath, dyspnea on exertion, arrhythmias, MI, heart failure, and sudden death. Risk factors include DM, a family history of premature CAD, smoking, obesity, and hypertension.

Major risk factors for CAD include age, male gender, hyperlipidemia, DM, hypertension, obesity, a ⊕ family history, and smoking.

The classic triad of angina consists of retrosternal chest pain that is provoked by exertion and relieved by rest or nitrates.

Angina Pectoris

Substernal chest pain due to myocardial ischemia (↑ O_2 demand and/or ↓ O_2 supply). Prinzmetal's (variant) angina mimics angina pectoris but is caused by vasospasm of coronary vessels. It classically affects young women at rest in the early morning and is associated with ST-segment elevation but not with cardiac enzyme elevation.

History/PE

- The classic triad consists of substernal chest pain or pressure that is precipitated by exertion and relieved by rest or nitrates.
- Pain can radiate to the arms, jaw, and neck and may be associated with shortness of breath, nausea/vomiting, diaphoresis, or lightheadedness.
- Examination of patients experiencing stable angina is generally unremarkable. Look for bruits and hypertension.

Diagnosis

Rule out pulmonary, GI, or other cardiac causes of chest pain. Significant ST-segment changes on exercise stress test with ECG monitoring is diagnostic of CAD.

Treatment

- Treat acute symptoms with O_2 and/or IV nitroglycerin, IV morphine, and IV β-blockers. Use of nondihydropyridine CCBs (diltiazem, verapamil) and ACEIs has also been validated.
- Patients with a suspected MI must be admitted and monitored until acute MI is ruled out by serial cardiac enzymes.

- Treat chronic symptoms with nitrates, β-blockers, and CCBs. ASA ↓ the risk of MI.
- Risk factor reduction (e.g., smoking, cholesterol, hypertension).

ACUTE CORONARY SYNDROMES

A spectrum of clinical syndromes caused by plaque disruption or vasospasm → acute myocardial ischemia.

Unstable Angina/Non-ST-Elevation Myocardial Infarction (NSTEMI)

Unstable angina describes chest pain that is new onset, is accelerating (i.e., occurs with less exertion, lasts longer, or is less responsive to medications), or occurs at rest; it is distinguished from stable angina by patient history. It signals an area of myocardial ischemia that has **not yet produced necrosis** but could acutely progress to complete occlusion and MI. In contrast, **NSTEMI** indicates myocardial necrosis marked by **elevations in troponin I, troponin T, or CK-MB.**

Think unstable angina if chest pain is new onset, accelerating, or occurring at rest.

DIAGNOSIS

- Patients should be risk stratified according to the TIMI (Thrombolysis in Myocardial Infarction study) criteria to determine the likelihood of adverse cardiac events (see Table 2.1-10).
- Unstable angina is not associated with elevated cardiac markers, but ST changes may be seen on ECG and are indicative of high-risk occlusions.
- NSTEMI is diagnosed by serial cardiac enzymes.

TREATMENT

- Acute treatment of symptoms is as described for stable angina; ASA, clopidogrel, unfractionated heparin or enoxaparin, and glycoprotein IIb/IIIa inhibitors (e.g., eptifibatide, tirofiban, abciximab) should also be considered.
- Patients with chest pain refractory to medical therapy, a TIMI score of ≥ 3, a troponin elevation, or ST changes > 1 mm should be given heparin and scheduled for angiography and possible revascularization (PCI or CABG).

ST-Elevation Myocardial Infarction (STEMI)

Defined as ST elevations and cardiac enzyme release 2° to prolonged cardiac ischemia.

HISTORY/PE

- Presents with acute-onset substernal chest pain, commonly described as a pressure or tightness that can radiate to the arms (more often the left arm), neck, or jaw.
- Associated symptoms may include diaphoresis, shortness of breath, lightheadedness, anxiety, nausea/vomiting, and syncope.
- Physical exam may reveal arrhythmias, new mitral regurgitation (ruptured papillary muscle), hypotension (cardiogenic shock), and evidence of new CHF (rales, peripheral edema, S3 gallop).
- The best predictor of survival is left ventricular EF.

Women, diabetics, elderly, and postorthotopic heart transplant patients may have atypical, clinically silent MIs.

TABLE 2.1-10. TIMI Risk Score for Unstable Angina/NSTEMI

CHARACTERISTICS	POINT	RISK OF CARDIAC EVENTS (%) WITHIN 14 DAYS		
		RISK SCORE	DEATH OR MI	DEATH, MI, OR URGENT REVASCULARIZATION
History				
Age ≥ 65 years	1	0/1	3	5
≥ 3 CAD risk factors (family history, DM, tobacco, hypertension, ↑ cholesterol)	1	2	3	8
Known CAD (stenosis > 50%)	1	3	5	13
ASA use in past seven days	1	4	7	20
Presentation		5	12	26
Severe angina (≥ 2 episodes within 24 hours)	1	6/7	19	41
ST deviation ≥ 0.5 mm	1	Higher-risk patients (risk score ≥ 3) benefit more from enoxaparin (vs. unfractionated heparin), glycoprotein IIb/IIIa inhibitors, and early angiography.		
+ cardiac marker	1			
RISK SCORE—TOTAL POINTS	(0–7)			

DIAGNOSIS

- **ECG:** Look for ST-segment elevations or new LBBB.
- **Sequence of ECG changes:** Peaked T waves → ST-segment elevation → Q waves → T-wave inversion → ST-segment normalization → T-wave normalization.
- **Cardiac enzymes:** Troponin I is most sensitive; CK-MB is more specific. Both can take up to six hours to rise after the onset of chest pain.
- **ST-segment abnormalities:**
  - ST-segment elevation in leads **II, III,** and **aVF** is consistent with an **inferior MI** (see Figure 2.1-4).
  - ST-segment elevation in leads V_1–V_4 usually indicates an **anterior MI** (see Figure 2.1-5).
  - ST-segment elevation in leads **I, aVL,** and V_5–V_6 points to a **lateral MI.**

Time is myocardium.

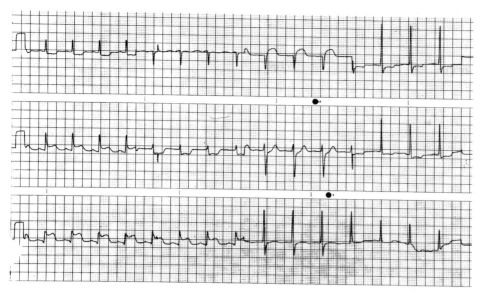

FIGURE 2.1-4. **Inferior wall MI.**

In this patient with acute chest pain, the ECG demonstrated acute ST-segment elevation in leads II, III, and aVF with reciprocal ST-segment depression and T-wave flattening in leads I, aVL, and V_4–V_6. (Reproduced, with permission, from Stobo J et al. *The Principles and Practice of Medicine*, 23rd ed. Stamford, CT: Appleton & Lange, 1996, p. 20.)

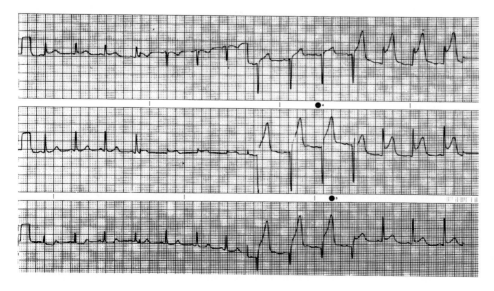

FIGURE 2.1-5. **Anterior wall MI.**

This patient presented with acute chest pain. The ECG showed acute ST-segment elevation in leads aVL and V_1–V_6, and hyperacute T waves. (Reproduced, with permission, from Stobo J et al. *The Principles and Practice of Medicine*, 23rd ed. Stamford, CT: Appleton & Lange, 1996, p. 19.)

TREATMENT

- Six key medications should be considered: aspirin, β-blockers, clopidogrel, morphine, nitrates, and oxygen.
- If the patient is in heart failure or in cardiogenic shock, do not give β-blockers; give ACEIs instead, provided that the patient is not hypotensive.
- If the patient presents within three hours, PCI cannot be performed within 90 minutes, and there are no contraindications to thrombolysis (e.g., a history of hemorrhagic stroke or recent ischemic stroke, severe heart failure, cardiogenic shock), thrombolysis with tPA, reteplase, or streptokinase should be performed instead of PCI.
- Otherwise, **emergent angiography and PCI** should be performed; if possible the patient should undergo PCI on the lesion thought to be responsible for STEMI.
- If there is three-vessel disease, left main coronary artery disease, discrete lesions not amenable to PCI, or diffuse disease with good target vessels, **PCI should be attempted immediately** on the lesion thought to be responsible for STEMI; the patient is a candidate for CABG afterwards.
- Long-term treatment includes ASA, ACEIs, β-blockers, high-dose statins, and clopidogrel (if PCI was performed). Modify risk factors with dietary changes, exercise, and tobacco cessation.

> **Indications for CABG—**
>
> **DUST**
>
> **D**epressed ventricular function
> **U**nable to perform PCI (diffuse disease)
> **S**tenosis of left main coronary artery
> **T**riple-vessel disease

COMPLICATIONS

- Arrhythmia is the most common complication following acute MI; lethal arrhythmia is the most common cause of death following acute MI.
- Less common complications include reinfarction, left ventricular wall rupture, VSD, pericarditis, papillary muscle rupture (with mitral regurgitation), left ventricular aneurysm or pseudoaneurysm, and mural thrombi.
- Dressler's syndrome, an autoimmune process occurring 2–10 weeks post-MI, presents with fever, pericarditis, pleural effusion, leukocytosis, and ↑ ESR.

HYPERCHOLESTEROLEMIA

↑ blood cholesterol (defined as a total cholesterol level > 200 mg/dL), ↑ LDL, ↑ triglycerides, and ↓ HDL are risk factors for CAD. Etiologic factors include obesity, DM, alcoholism, hypothyroidism, nephrotic syndrome, hepatic disease, Cushing's disease, OCP use, high-dose diuretic use, and familial hypercholesterolemia.

HISTORY/PE

- Most patients have **no specific signs or symptoms.**
- Patients with extremely high triglycerides or LDL levels may have xanthomas (eruptive nodules in the skin over the tendons), xanthelasmas (yellow fatty deposits in the skin around the eyes), and lipemia retinalis (creamy appearance of retinal vessels).

Hypercholesterolemia is usually asymptomatic.

Dyslipidemia =
- *LDL > 130 mg/dL or*
- *HDL < 40 mg/dL*

DIAGNOSIS

- Conduct a fasting lipid profile for patients > 20 years of age and repeat **every five years.**
- Total serum cholesterol > 200 mg/dL on two different occasions is diagnostic of hypercholesteremia.
- LDL > 130 mg/dL or HDL < 40 mg/dL, even if total serum cholesterol is < 200 mg/dL, is diagnostic of dyslipidemia.

TABLE 2.1-11. Risk Stratification and Target LDL

RISK CATEGORY	TARGET LDL (mg/dL)
0–1 risk factor	< 160
≥ 2 risk factors	< 130
CAD or risk equivalent	< 70

TREATMENT

- Based on risk stratification (see Table 2.1-11). Risk factors include diabetes (considered a CAD risk equivalent), smoking, hypertension, HDL < 40 mg/dL, age > 45 (males), age > 55 (females), and early CAD in first-degree relatives (males < 55 and females < 65).
- The **first intervention** should be a **12-week trial of diet and exercise** in a patient with no known atherosclerotic vascular disease. Commonly used lipid-lowering agents are listed in Table 2.1-12.

TABLE 2.1-12. Lipid-Lowering Agents

CLASS	EXAMPLES	MECHANISM OF ACTION	EFFECT ON LIPID PROFILE	SIDE EFFECTS
HMG-CoA reductase inhibitors (statins)	Atorvastatin, simvastatin, lovastatin, pravastatin	Inhibit the rate-limiting step in cholesterol synthesis.	↓ LDL, ↓ triglycerides	↑ LFTs, myositis, warfarin potentiation.
Lipoprotein lipase stimulators (fibrates)	Gemfibrozil	↑ lipoprotein lipase → ↑ VLDL and triglyceride catabolism.	↓ triglycerides, ↑ HDL	GI upset, cholelithiasis, myositis, LFT abnormalities.
Cholesterol absorption inhibitors	Ezetimibe (Zetia)	↓ absorption of cholesterol at the small intestine brush border.	↓ LDL	Diarrhea, abdominal pain. Can cause angioedema.
Niacin	Extended-release niacin (Niaspan)	↓ fatty acid release from adipose tissue; ↓ hepatic synthesis of LDL.	↑ HDL, ↓ LDL	Skin flushing (can be prevented with aspirin), paresthesias, pruritus, GI upset, ↑ LFTs.
Bile acid resins	Cholestyramine, colestipol, colesevelam	Bind intestinal bile acids → ↓ bile acid stores and ↑ catabolism of LDL from plasma.	↓ LDL	Constipation, GI upset, LFT abnormalities, myalgias. Can ↓ absorption of other drugs from the small intestine.

The BP goal in uncomplicated hypertension is < 140/< 90. For diabetics or patients with renal disease, the goal is < 130/< 80.

Treatment of hypertension—

ABCD

ACEIs/**A**RBs
β-blockers
Calcium channel blockers
Diuretics

Defined as a systolic BP > 140 and/or a diastolic BP > 90 based on three measurements separated in time (see Table 2.1-13). Classified as 1° or 2°.

1° (Essential) Hypertension

Represents **95% of cases** of hypertension. Risk factors include a family history of hypertension or heart disease, a high-sodium diet, smoking, obesity, race (blacks > whites), and advanced age.

HISTORY/PE

- **Hypertension is asymptomatic until complications develop.**
- Patients should be evaluated for end-organ damage to the brain (stroke, dementia), eye (cotton wool exudates), heart (LVH), and kidney (proteinuria, chronic kidney disease). Renal bruits may signify renal artery stenosis as the cause of hypertension.

DIAGNOSIS

- Conduct cardiovascular, neurologic, ophthalmologic, and abdominal exams.
- Obtain a head and/or abdominal CT, UA, BUN/creatinine, CBC, and electrolytes to assess the extent of end-organ damage.

TREATMENT

- Rule out 2° causes of hypertension.
- Begin with lifestyle modifications (e.g., weight loss, smoking cessation, salt reduction). The BP goal in otherwise healthy patients is < 140/< 90. The goal in diabetics or patients with renal disease with proteinuria is < 130/< 80.
- **Diuretics** (inexpensive and particularly effective in African-Americans), **ACEIs**, and **β-blockers** (beneficial for patients with CAD) have been shown to ↓ mortality in uncomplicated hypertension. They are **first-line agents** unless a comorbid condition requires another medication.

TABLE 2.1-13. JNC-7 Classification and Management of Hypertension

BP CLASSIFICATION	SYSTOLIC BP	DIASTOLIC BP	MANAGEMENT
Normal	< 120	< 80	None.
Prehypertension	120–139	80–89	Lifestyle modifications.
Stage I hypertension	140–159	90–99	Thiazide diuretic; may consider ACEIs, β-blockers, CCBs, or a combination.
Stage II hypertension	≥ 160	≥ 100	Two-drug combination (usually a thiazide diuretic and an ACEI, an ARB, a β-blocker, or a CCB).

- Conduct periodic tests for end-organ complications, including renal (BUN, creatinine, urine protein-to-creatinine ratio) and cardiac (ECG evidence of hypertrophy) complications.

2° Hypertension

Hypertension due to an identifiable organic cause. See Table 2.1-14 for the diagnosis and treatment of common causes.

Hypertensive Crises

A spectrum of clinical presentations in which elevated BPs → end-organ damage.

TABLE 2.1-14. **Common Causes of 2° Hypertension**

	DESCRIPTION	MANAGEMENT
1° renal disease	Often unilateral renal parenchymal disease.	Treat with ACEIs, which slow the progression of renal disease.
Renal artery stenosis	Especially common in patients < 25 and > 50 years of age with recent-onset hypertension. Etiologies include fibromuscular dysplasia (usually in younger patients) and atherosclerosis (usually in older patients).	Diagnose with MRA or renal artery Doppler ultrasound. Treat with angioplasty and stenting if possible. Consider ACEIs as adjunctive or temporary therapy in unilateral disease. (In bilateral disease, ACEIs can accelerate kidney failure by preferential vasodilation of the efferent arteriole.) Open surgery is a second option if angioplasty is not effective or feasible.
OCP use	Common in women > 35 years of age, obese women, and those with long-standing use.	Discontinue OCPs (effect may be delayed).
Pheochromocytoma	An adrenal gland tumor that secretes epinephrine and norepinephrine → episodic headache, sweating, and tachycardia.	Diagnose with urinary metanephrines and catecholamine levels or plasma metanephrine. Surgical removal of tumor after treatment with both α-blockers and β-blockers.
Conn's syndrome (hyperaldosteronism)	Most often due to an aldosterone-producing adrenal adenoma. Causes the triad of hypertension, unexplained hypokalemia, and metabolic alkalosis.	Surgical removal of tumor.
Cushing's syndrome	Due to an ACTH-producing pituitary tumor, an ectopic ACTH-secreting tumor, or cortisol secretion by an adrenal adenoma or carcinoma.	Surgical removal of tumor.
Coarctation of the aorta	See the Pediatrics section.	Surgical repair.

Hypertensive crises are diagnosed on the basis of the extent of end-organ damage, not BP measurement.

HISTORY/PE

End-organ damage may be revealed by chest pain (ischemia or MI), back pain (aortic dissection), or changes in mental status (hypertensive encephalopathy).

DIAGNOSIS

- Hypertensive urgency is diagnosed on the basis of an elevated BP with only mild to moderate symptoms (headache, chest pain, syncope) and without end-organ damage.
- Hypertensive emergency is diagnosed by a significantly elevated BP with signs or symptoms of impending end-organ damage such as ARF, intracra-

TABLE 2.1-15. **Major Classes of Antihypertensive Agents**

CLASS	AGENTS	MECHANISM OF ACTION	SIDE EFFECTS
Diuretics	Thiazide, loop, K^+ sparing	↓ extracellular fluid volume and thereby ↓ vascular resistance.	Hypokalemia, hyperglycemia, hyperlipidemia, hyperuricemia, azotemia.
β-adrenergic blockers (β-blockers)	Propranolol, metoprolol, nadolol, atenolol, timolol, carvedilol, labetalol	↓ cardiac contractility and renin release.	Bronchospasm (in severe asthma), bradycardia, CHF exacerbation, impotence, fatigue, depression.
Centrally acting adrenergic agonists	Methyldopa, clonidine	Inhibit the sympathetic nervous system via central α_2-adrenergic receptors.	Somnolence, orthostatic hypotension, impotence, rebound hypertension.
α_1-adrenergic blockers	Prazosin, terazosin, phenoxybenzamine	Cause vasodilation by blocking actions of norepinephrine on vascular smooth muscle.	Orthostatic hypotension.
Ca^{2+} channel blockers	Dihydropyridines (nifedipine, felodipine, amlodipine), nondihydropyridines (diltiazem, verapamil)	↓ smooth muscle tone and cause vasodilation; may also ↓ cardiac output.	**Dihydropyridines:** Headache, flushing, peripheral edema. **Nondihydropyridines:** ↓ contractility.
Vasodilators	Hydralazine, minoxidil	↓ peripheral resistance by dilating arteries/arterioles.	**Hydralazine:** Headache, lupus-like syndrome. **Minoxidil:** Orthostasis, facial hirsutism.
ACEIs	Captopril, enalapril, fosinopril, benazepril, lisinopril	Block aldosterone formation, reducing peripheral resistance and salt/water retention.	Cough, rashes, leukopenia, hyperkalemia.
ARBs	Losartan, valsartan, irbesartan	Block aldosterone effects, reducing peripheral resistance and salt/water retention.	Rashes, leukopenia, and hyperkalemia but no cough.

TABLE 2.1-16. Antihypertensive Medications Indicated in Specific Patient Populations

POPULATIONS	TREATMENT
Diabetes with proteinuria	ACEIs or ARBs.
CHF	β-blockers, ACEIs or ARBs, diuretics (including spironolactone).
Isolated systolic hypertension	Diuretics preferred; long-acting dihydropyridine CCBs.
MI	β-blockers without intrinsic sympathomimetic activity; ACEIs.
Osteoporosis	Thiazide diuretics.
BPH	α_1-adrenergic blockers.

- nial hemorrhage, papilledema, and ECG changes suggestive of ischemia or pulmonary edema.
- Malignant hypertension is diagnosed on the basis of progressive renal failure and/or encephalopathy with papilledema.

TREATMENT

- Hypertensive urgencies can be treated with oral antihypertensives (e.g., β-blockers, clonidine, ACEIs) with the goal of gradually lowering BP over 24–48 hours (see Tables 2.1-15 and 2.1-16).
- Hypertensive emergencies should be treated with IV medications (labetalol, nitroprusside, nicardipine) with the goal of lowering mean arterial pressure by no more than 25% over the first two hours to avoid cerebral hypoperfusion or coronary insufficiency.

PERICARDIAL DISEASE

Results from acute or chronic pericardial insults; can → pericardial effusion.

Pericarditis

Inflammation of the pericardial sac, often with an effusion. Can compromise cardiac output via tamponade or constrictive pericarditis. Most commonly idiopathic, although known etiologies include viral infection, TB, SLE, uremia, drugs, radiation, and neoplasms. May also occur after MI (either within days after MI or as a delayed phenomenon, i.e., Dressler's syndrome) or open heart surgery.

HISTORY/PE

- May present with pleuritic chest pain, dyspnea, cough, and fever.
- Chest pain tends to worsen in the supine position and with inspiration.
- Examination may reveal a pericardial friction rub, elevated JVP, and pulsus paradoxus (a ↓ in systolic BP > 10 mmHg on inspiration).

> *Look for signs of* **PERICarditis—**
>
> **P**ulsus paradoxus
> **E**CG changes
> **R**ub
> **I**ncreased JVP
> **C**hest pain

Beck's triad can diagnose acute cardiac tamponade:

- *Look for **JVD***
- *Measure **hypotension***
- *Listen for **distant heart sounds***

DIAGNOSIS

- CXR, ECG, and echocardiogram to rule out MI and pneumonia.
- ECG changes include PR-segment depressions and diffuse ST-segment elevation followed by T-wave inversions.
- Pericardial thickening or effusion may be evident on echocardiography.

TREATMENT

- Treat the underlying cause (e.g., steroids/immunosuppressants for SLE, dialysis for uremia) or symptoms (e.g., aspirin for post-MI pericarditis, aspirin/NSAIDs for viral pericarditis). Avoid steroids within a few days after MI, as they can predispose to ventricular wall rupture.
- Pericardial effusions without symptoms can be followed, but evidence of tamponade requires pericardiocentesis, with continuous drainage if necessary.

Cardiac Tamponade

Excess fluid in the pericardial sac → compromised ventricular filling and ↓ cardiac output. The condition is more closely related to the rate of fluid formation than to the size of the effusion. Risk factors include pericarditis, malignancy, SLE, TB, and trauma (commonly stab wounds medial to the left nipple).

HISTORY/PE

- Presents with fatigue, dyspnea, anxiety, tachycardia, and tachypnea that can rapidly progress to shock and death.
- Examination of a patient with acute tamponade may reveal Beck's triad (hypotension, distant heart sounds, and distended neck vein), a narrow pulse pressure, pulsus paradoxus, and Kussmaul's sign (JVD on inspiration).

DIAGNOSIS

- Echocardiogram shows right atrial and right ventricular diastolic collapse. CXR shows an enlarged, globular heart.
- If present on ECG, electrical alternans is diagnostic.

TREATMENT

- Aggressive volume expansion with IV fluids.
- Urgent pericardiocentesis (aspirate will be nonclotting blood).
- Decompensation may warrant balloon pericardotomy and pericardial window.

VALVULAR HEART DISEASE

Until recently, rheumatic fever (which affects the mitral valve more often than the aortic valve) was the most common cause of valvular heart disease in U.S. adults; the leading cause is now mechanical degeneration.

Aortic Stenosis

Most often seen in elderly individuals, although unicuspid and bicuspid valves can → symptoms in childhood and adolescence.

HISTORY/PE

- May be asymptomatic for many years even with a significant degree of stenosis.
- Once patients develop symptoms, they usually progress from angina to syncope to CHF to death within five years.
- Physical exam may reveal pulsus parvus et tardus (weak, delayed carotid upstroke) and a paradoxically split S2 sound.

DIAGNOSIS

Echocardiography.

TREATMENT

Primarily interventional; balloon valvuloplasty can bridge patients to aortic valve replacement.

Aortic Regurgitation

Acute cases are typically linked to infective endocarditis, aortic dissection, and chest trauma. Chronic cases are more frequently associated with valve malformations, rheumatic fever, and connective tissue disorders.

HISTORY/PE

- Chronic regurgitation is a slowly progressive disorder characterized by dyspnea on exertion, orthopnea, and PND.
- Three murmurs can be evident on exam: a blowing diastolic murmur at the left sternal border, a mid-diastolic rumble (Austin Flint murmur), and a midsystolic apical murmur.
- Acute regurgitation rapidly → pulmonary congestion, cardiogenic shock, and severe dyspnea.

DIAGNOSIS

The widened pulse pressure of aortic regurgitation is also associated with numerous signs evident on physical exam, including de Musset's sign (head bob with heartbeat), Corrigan's sign (water-hammer pulse), and Duroziez's sign (femoral bruit heard with compression of the femoral artery).

TREATMENT

Vasodilator therapy (CCBs or ACEIs) can be used to maintain patients with isolated aortic regurgitation until symptoms become severe enough to warrant valve replacement therapy.

Mitral Valve Stenosis

- The most common etiology continues to be rheumatic fever.
- **Hx/PE:** Symptoms range from dyspnea, orthopnea, and PND to infective endocarditis and arrhythmias. Physical exam may reveal an opening snap and pulmonary edema.
- **Tx:** Antiarrhythmic agents (digoxin, β-blockers) may be used for symptomatic relief; mitral balloon valvotomy and valve replacement are effective for severe cases.

Aortic stenosis complications—

ARC

Angina
Syncope
Congestive heart failure

Causes of aortic regurgitation—

CREAM

Congenital
Rheumatic damage
Endocarditis
Aortic dissection/**A**ortic root dilatation
Marfan's syndrome

HIGH-YIELD FACTS

CARDIOVASCULAR

Mitral Valve Regurgitation

- Primarily caused by rheumatic fever or chordae tendineae rupture after MI.
- **Hx/PE:** Patients present with dyspnea, orthopnea, and fatigue. Exam reveals a holosystolic murmur that often radiates to the axillae.
- **Dx:** CXR may show an enlarged left atrium (puts patients at risk for AF). Echocardiography will demonstrate regurgitant flow; angiography can assess the severity of disease.
- **TX:** Antiarrhythmics if necessary; nitrates and diuretics to ↓ preload.

Infective Endocarditis

Transient bacteremia → seeding of heart valves. Cases can be divided into native valve endocarditis, prosthetic valve endocarditis, and endocarditis associated with IV drug use.

HISTORY/PE

- **Constitutional symptoms are most common** (fever, fatigue, weight loss).
- Specific embolic signs include focal neurologic deficits from embolic stroke, Roth's spots (retinal hemorrhages), splinter hemorrhages in the nail beds, and Osler's nodes (tender nodules on the distal surfaces of the fingers and toes).

DIAGNOSIS

Three sets of blood cultures are highly sensitive for bacteremia; TEE is sensitive and specific for cardiac valve vegetations.

TREATMENT

- Antibiotic therapy is administered before definitive speciation on the basis of the most likely infectious organism: native valve (streptococci), prosthetic valve (staphylococci), or IV drug associated (staphylococci).
- High-risk patients should undergo antibiotic prophylaxis before any invasive procedure, including dental interventions.

> **Classic presentation of endocarditis—**
>
> **FAME**
>
> **F**ever
> **A**nemia (splenomegaly)
> **M**urmur (new onset)
> **E**mboli (systemic)

VASCULAR DISEASE

Aortic Aneurysm

Aortic aneurysms are most commonly **associated with atherosclerosis.** Most are abdominal, and > 90% originate below the renal arteries.

HISTORY/PE

- **Usually asymptomatic** and discovered incidentally on exam or radiologic study.
- Risk factors include hypertension, high cholesterol, other vascular disease, a ⊕ family history, smoking, gender (males > females), and age.
- Exam demonstrates a **pulsatile abdominal mass or abdominal bruits.**
- Ruptured aneurysm → hypotension and severe, tearing abdominal pain radiating to the back.

DIAGNOSIS

Abdominal ultrasound for diagnosis or to follow an aneurysm over time. CT may be a useful adjunct to determine the precise anatomy.

Aortic aneurysm is most often associated with atherosclerosis, while aortic dissection is commonly linked to hypertension.

TREATMENT

- In asymptomatic patients, monitoring is appropriate for lesions < 5 cm.
- Surgical repair is indicated if the lesion is > 5.5 cm (abdominal) or > 6 cm (thoracic) or smaller but rapidly enlarging.
- Emergent surgery for symptomatic or ruptured aneurysms.

Aortic Dissection

A transverse tear in the intima of a vessel → blood entering the media, creating a false lumen and → a hematoma that propagates longitudinally. **Most commonly due to hypertension.** The most common sites of origin are above the aortic valve and distal to the left subclavian artery. Most often occurs in those 40–60 years of age, with a greater frequency in men than in women.

HISTORY/PE

- Sudden tearing/ripping pain in the anterior chest in ascending dissection; interscapular back pain in descending dissection.
- The patient is typically hypertensive. If a patient is hypotensive, consider pericardial tamponade, hypovolemia from blood loss, or acute MI from involvement of the coronary arteries.
- **Asymmetric pulses and BP measurements** are indicative of aortic dissection.
- Signs of pericarditis or pericardial tamponade may be seen; a murmur of aortic regurgitation may be heard if the aortic valve is involved. **Neurologic deficits** may be seen if the **aortic arch or spinal arteries** are involved.

DIAGNOSIS

- ECG, CXR (widening of the mediastinum, cardiomegaly or new left pleural effusion); CT angiography is the gold standard of imaging.
- TEE can provide details of the thoracic aorta, the proximal coronary arteries, the origins of arch vessels, the presence of a pericardial effusion, and aortic valve integrity.
- There are two systems of classification for aortic dissection:
    - **DeBakey system:** Classifies dissections as involving both the ascending and descending aorta (type I), confined to the ascending aorta (type II), or confined to the descending aorta (type III).
    - **Stanford system:** Classifies dissection of the ascending aorta as type A and all others as type B.

TREATMENT

- Monitor and medically manage BP and heart rate as necessary.
- Do not use thrombolytics.
- If the dissection involves the ascending aorta, it is a surgical emergency; descending dissections can often be managed with BP and heart rate control.

Deep Venous Thrombosis (DVT)

Clot formation in the large veins of the extremities or pelvis. The classic **Virchow's triad** of risk factors includes venous stasis (e.g., plane flights, bed rest, incompetent venous valves in the lower extremities), endothelial trauma (injury to the lower extremities), and hypercoagulable states (e.g., malignancy, pregnancy, OCP use).

Ascending aortic dissections are surgical emergencies, but descending dissections can often be treated medically.

A negative D-dimer test can be used to rule out the possibility of pulmonary embolism in low-risk patients.

HISTORY/PE

- Generally presents with unilateral lower extremity pain, erythema, and swelling.
- **Homans' sign** is calf tenderness with passive foot dorsiflexion (poor sensitivity and specificity for DVT).

DIAGNOSIS

Doppler ultrasound; spiral CT or V/Q scan may be used to evaluate for pulmonary embolism.

TREATMENT

- Initial anticoagulation with IV unfractionated heparin or SQ low-molecular-weight heparin followed by PO warfarin for a total of 3–6 months.
- Consider an IVC filter in patients with contraindications to anticoagulation.
- Hospitalized patients should receive DVT prophylaxis consisting of exercise as tolerated, antithromboembolic stockings, and SQ unfractionated heparin or low-molecular-weight heparin.

Peripheral Vascular Disease

Occlusion of the blood supply to the extremities by atherosclerotic plaques. The lower extremities are most commonly affected. Clinical manifestations depend on the vessels involved, the extent and rapidity of obstruction, and the presence of collateral blood flow.

HISTORY/PE

- Initially presents with **intermittent claudication** (reproducible leg pain that occurs with walking and is always relieved with rest). As the disease worsens, there is progression to pain at rest and ischemia that affects the distal aspects of the extremities. Dorsal foot ulcerations may develop. A painful, cold, numb foot is characteristic of severe ischemia.
- Disease-specific presentations are as follows:
    - **Aortoiliac disease:** Associated with **Leriche's syndrome** (buttock claudication, ↓ femoral pulses, male impotence).
    - **Femoropopliteal disease:** Calf claudication is present; pulses below the femoral artery are absent.
    - **Acute ischemia:** Most often caused by embolization from the heart; acute occlusions commonly occur at bifurcations distal to the last palpable pulse.
    - **Severe chronic ischemia:** Lack of blood perfusion → muscle atrophy, pallor, cyanosis, hair loss, and gangrene/necrosis.

DIAGNOSIS

- Careful palpation of pulses and auscultation for bruits.
- Measurement of ankle and brachial systolic BP (ankle-brachial index, or ABI) can provide objective evidence of atherosclerosis (rest pain usually occurs with an ABI < 0.4).
- Doppler ultrasound helps identify stenosis and occlusion. Doppler ankle systolic pressure readings that are > 90% of brachial readings are normal.
- Arteriography and digital subtraction angiography are necessary for surgical evaluation.

The 6 P's of acute ischemia:

Pain
Pallor
Pulselessness
Paralysis
Paresthesia
Poikilothermia

TREATMENT

- Control underlying conditions (e.g., DM); eliminate tobacco and institute careful hygiene and foot care. Exercise helps to develop collateral circulation.
- Aspirin, cilostazol, and thromboxane inhibitors may improve symptoms; anticoagulants may prevent clot formation.
- Angioplasty and stenting have a variable success rate that is dependent on the area of occlusion.
- Surgery (arterial bypass) or amputation can be employed when conservation treatment fails.

SYNCOPE

Defined as a sudden, temporary loss of consciousness and postural tone due to cerebral hypoperfusion. Etiologies fall into cardiac and noncardiac categories:

- **Cardiac:** Valvular lesions, arrhythmias, pulmonary embolism, cardiac tamponade, aortic dissection.
- **Noncardiac:** Orthostatic hypotension, TIA, metabolic abnormalities, vasovagal syndromes (e.g., micturition syncope).

History/PE

- Patient history can rule out many potential etiologies; triggering factors, the presence or absence of prodromal symptoms, and associated symptoms should be investigated.
- Cardiac causes of syncope are typically associated with very brief or absent prodromal symptoms, a ⊕ history of exertion, and lack of association with changes in position.

Diagnosis

Depending on the suspected etiology, Holter monitors or event recorders (arrhythmias), echocardiograms (structural abnormalities), and stress tests (ischemia) can be useful diagnostic tools.

Cardiac syncope is associated with one-year sudden cardiac death rates of up to 40%.

Dermatology

LAYERS OF THE SKIN

The skin consists of three layers: the epidermis, dermis, and subcutaneous tissue (see Figure 2.2-1). Table 2.2-1 describes pertinent components of the epidermis, the dermis, and the various skin appendages.

COMMON TERMINOLOGY

Table 2.2-2 outlines terms frequently used to describe common manifestations of dermatologic disease.

ALLERGIC AND IMMUNE-MEDIATED DISEASES

Hypersensitivity Reactions

Table 2.2-3 outlines the types and mechanisms of hypersensitivity reactions. Descriptions of common allergic and immune-mediated disorders follow.

Atopic Dermatitis (Eczema)

A **relapsing** inflammatory skin disorder that is common in infancy and presents differently in different age groups. It is characterized by **pruritus** that → **lichenification** (see Figure 2.2-2). Although genetic factors are important, the exact etiology of the condition is unclear. Triggers are nongenetic and include climate, food, contact with allergens or physical or chemical irritants, and emotional factors.

HISTORY/PE

- Atopic dermatitis is commonly associated with asthma and allergic rhinitis, but unlike these conditions, it is not clearly affected by seasonal changes or extrinsic allergens. Patients are at risk of 2° bacterial and viral infection.
- Clinical manifestations by age group are as follows:
  - **Infants:** Erythematous, weeping, pruritic patches on the face, scalp, and diaper area.
  - **Children:** Dry, scaly, pruritic, excoriated patches in the flexural areas and neck.
  - **Adults:** Lichenification and dry, fissured skin, often limited to the hands.

Eczema is the "itch that rashes."

TABLE 2.2-1. Components of Skin Layers

EPIDERMIS	DERMIS	SKIN APPENDAGES
Keratinocytes	Fibroblasts (synthesize collagen,	Nails (nail matrix, nail fold, nail
Melanocytes	elastin, and ground substance)	plate, nail bed)
Langerhans cells	Mast cells	Hair complex (hair follicles,
Merkel cells	Monocytes/macrophages	sebaceous glands, apocrine
	Vessels/lymphatics	glands)
	Nerves	Eccrine gland
	Smooth muscle	

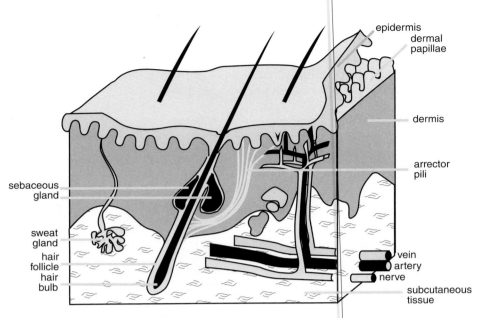

FIGURE 2.2-1. Layers of the skin.

(Adapted, with permission, from Hardman JG et al. *Goodman and Gilman's The Pharmacological Basis of Therapeutics*, 10th ed. New York: McGraw-Hill, 2001, p. 1805.)

DIAGNOSIS

Diagnosis is made clinically. Patients may have mild eosinophilia and an elevated IgE. Rule out seborrheic dermatitis, contact dermatitis, pityriasis rosea, drug eruption, and cutaneous T-cell lymphoma.

TREATMENT

- Prophylactic measures include use of nondrying soaps, use of **moisturizers,** and avoidance of known triggers.
- Treat with topical corticosteroids (avoid systemic steroids in light of their side effect profile), PUVA, and topical immunomodulators (e.g., tacrolimus, pimecrolimus).

Contact Dermatitis

A **type IV hypersensitivity reaction** that results from contact with an allergen to which the patient has **previously been exposed and sensitized.** Its pathogenesis involves allergenic molecules that are passed through the epidermis and taken up by **Langerhans cells,** which carry them to the lymph nodes and expose them to T lymphocytes. Dermatitis develops when the patient is reexposed to the allergen or to a cross-reactive compound. More common in adults than in children.

HISTORY/PE

- Commonly implicated allergens include poison ivy, poison oak, nickel, soaps, detergents, cosmetics, and rubber gloves.

TABLE 2.2-2.   **Common Terms Used to Describe Skin Lesions**

TERM	DEFINITION
Macule	A flat lesion that differs in color from surrounding skin.
Papule	An elevated, solid lesion that is generally small (< 5 mm in diameter).
Patch	A small circumscribed area differing in color or structure from the surrounding surface (> 1 cm in diameter).
Plaque	A large-diameter, broad-based papule.
Cyst	An epithelial-lined sac containing fluid or semisolid material.
Vesicle	A fluid-filled, very small (< 0.5-mm), elevated lesion.
Bulla	A large vesicle (> 5 mm).
Wheal (or hive)	An area of localized edema that follows vascular leakage and usually disappears within hours.
Erosion	A circumscribed, superficial depression resulting from the loss of some or all of the epidermis.
Ulcer	A deeper depression resulting from destruction of the epidermis and upper dermis.
Scale	Abnormal shedding or accumulation of stratum corneum in flakes.
Crust	A hardened deposit of dried serum, blood, or purulent exudates.
Lichenification	Thickening of the epidermis.
Scar	A healing defect of the dermis (the epidermis alone heals without a scar).

- The dermatitis begins in the area of contact with the antigen, with its appearance varying with the acuity of the lesion.
  - **Acute:** Approximately 24–48 hours after an allergic contact, the skin becomes erythematous, presenting with tiny blisters followed by scale and crusts. Lesions are intensely pruritic.
  - **Subacute:** Results from episodic exposure or a weak allergen. Lesions are less "angry appearing" than those of an acute inflammatory rash, and some lichenification is seen.
  - **Chronic:** Results from extended exposure to an allergen. Characterized by erythema and lichenification with fissuring, often with superimposed acute dermatitis.
- The overall shape of the rash often mimics that of the exposing object (see Figure 2.2-3), but it can also spread over the body via transfer of allergen by the hands or via circulating T lymphocytes. Patients are at ↑ risk of 2° infection.

DIAGNOSIS

Diagnosed by clinical impression. A **patch test** can be used to establish the causative allergen after the acute-phase rash has been treated. The differential includes atopic dermatitis, seborrheic dermatitis, impetigo, HSV, herpes zoster, and fungal infection.

TABLE 2.2-3.   Types and Mechanisms of Hypersensitivity Reactions

TYPE	MECHANISM	COMMENTS
Type I	**Anaphylactic and atopic:** Antigen cross-links IgE on presensitized mast cells and basophils, triggering the release of vasoactive amines (i.e., histamine). Reaction develops rapidly after antigen exposure as a result of preformed antibody. Examples include anaphylaxis, asthma, and local wheal and flare.	First and Fast (anaphylaxis). Types I, II, and III are all antibody mediated.
Type II	**Cytotoxic:** IgM and IgG bind to antigen on an "enemy" cell → lysis (by complement) or phagocytosis. Examples include autoimmune hemolytic anemia, Rh disease (erythroblastosis fetalis), Goodpasture's syndrome, and rheumatic fever.	Cy-2-toxic. Antibody and complement → membrane attack complex (MAC).
Type III	**Immune complex:** Antigen-antibody complexes activate complement, which attracts neutrophils; neutrophils release lysosomal enzymes. Examples include polyarteritis nodosa, immune complex glomerulonephritis, SLE, and rheumatoid arthritis. **Serum sickness:** An immune complex disease (type III) in which antibodies to the foreign proteins are produced (takes five days). Immune complexes form and are deposited in membranes, where they fix complement (→ tissue damage). More common than Arthus reaction. **Arthus reaction:** A local subacute antibody-mediated hypersensitivity (type III) reaction. Intradermal injection of antigen induces antibodies, which form antigen-antibody complexes in the skin. Characterized by edema, necrosis, and activation of complement. Examples include hypersensitivity pneumonitis and thermophilic actinomycetes.	Imagine an immune complex as three things stuck together: antigen-antibody complement. Most serum sickness is now caused by drugs (not serum). Fever, urticaria, arthralgias, proteinuria, and lymphadenopathy occur 5–10 days after antigen exposure. Antigen-antibody complexes cause the Arthus reaction.
Type IV	**Delayed (cell-mediated) type:** Sensitized T lymphocytes encounter antigen and then release lymphokines (→ macrophage activation). Examples include TB skin tests, transplant rejection, and contact dermatitis (e.g., poison ivy, poison oak).	**4th** and last—delayed. Cell mediated; therefore, it is not transferable by serum.

TREATMENT

- Prophylaxis consists of avoidance of the offending allergen.
- Treat with topical or systemic corticosteroids as needed and with cool, wet compresses to relieve and debride the skin.

Seborrheic Dermatitis

A common disease that is especially prevalent and particularly severe in AIDS patients. It has a predilection for **areas with oily skin** such as the scalp, eyebrows, nasolabial folds, and midchest. It may be caused by *Pityrosporum ovale*, a normally harmless yeast found in sebum and hair follicles.

HISTORY/PE

- The appearance of rash varies with age:
  - **Infants:** Presents as a severe, red diaper rash with yellow scale, erosions, and blisters. A thick crust ("cradle cap") may be seen on the scalp.

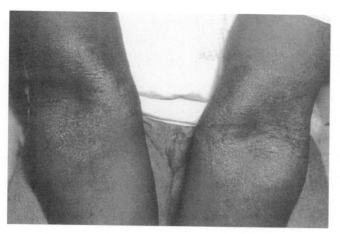

FIGURE 2.2-2. **Atopic dermatitis.**

Hyperpigmentation, lichenification, and scaling are seen in the antecubital fossae. (Courtesy of Robert Swerlick, MD.)

- **Children/adults:** Red, scaly patches are seen around the ears, eyebrows, nasolabial fold, midchest, and scalp. The rash is more localized and less dramatic than that seen in infants.
- Patients with **HIV/AIDS can develop an overlapping syndrome** of severe seborrheic dermatitis, psoriasis, psoriatic arthritis, and even Reiter's syndrome.

Suspect HIV in a young person with severe seborrheic dermatitis.

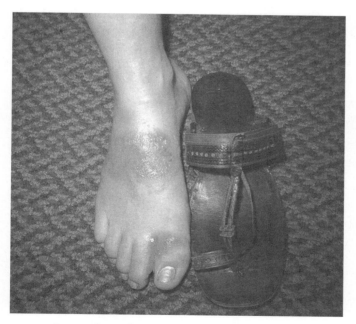

FIGURE 2.2-3. **Contact dermatitis.**

Shown above are erythematous papules and vesicles with serous weeping localized to areas of contact with the offending agent. (Reproduced, with permission, from Hurwitz RM. *Pathology of the Skin: Atlas of Clinical-Pathological Correlation*, 2nd ed. Stamford, CT: Appleton & Lange, 1998, p. 3.)

DIAGNOSIS

Diagnosed by clinical impression. Rule out contact dermatitis and psoriasis.

TREATMENT

Treatment consists of tar shampoo, topical ketoconazole or other imidazoles, and topical corticosteroids.

Psoriasis

A dermatosis characterized by **erythematous patches** and **silvery scales** due to dermal inflammation and epidermal hyperplasia. Five percent of patients also have a **seronegative arthritis.** There are a number of types, including vulgaris (chronic or guttate) and pustular. The disease has a polygenic inheritance pattern and may appear in childhood but usually starts in puberty or young adulthood. Its incidence is 2–4%.

HISTORY/PE

- Psoriatic lesions can be provoked by local irritation or by trauma (**Koebner's phenomenon**). A streptococcal infection can → cutaneous immune complex deposition, which triggers guttate psoriasis. Some medications, such as β-blockers, lithium, and ACEIs, can also induce psoriasis.
- The typical lesion is a round, sharply bordered erythematous patch with silvery scales (see Figure 2.2-4A). Lesions are classically found on **extensor surfaces,** including the elbows, knees, scalp, and lumbosacral regions.
- Lesions may initially appear very small (guttate) but may slowly enlarge and become confluent. Psoriatic nails feature pitting, "oil spots," and **onycholysis,** or lifting of the nail plate (see Figure 2.2-4B).
- **Psoriatic arthritis** usually begins in the hands with **"sausage fingers,"** but the lumbosacral region is also commonly affected. Arthritic patients are usually HLA-B27 ⊕.

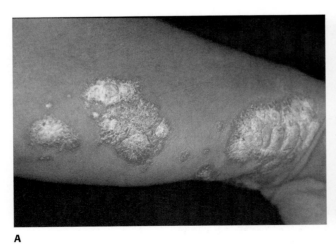

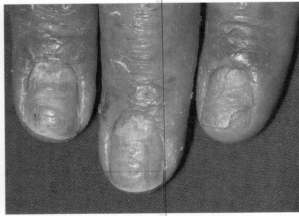

A   B

FIGURE 2.2-4.   Psoriasis.

(A) Skin changes. The classic sharply demarcated plaques with silvery scales are commonly located on the extensor surfaces (e.g., elbows, knees). (B) Nail changes. Note the pitting, onycholysis, and "oil spots." (Reproduced, with permission, from Hurwitz RM. *Pathology of the Skin: Atlas of Clinical-Pathological Correlation,* 2nd ed. Stamford, CT: Appleton & Lange, 1998, pp. 15, 18.)

- Patients with the less common pustular type have sterile intraepidermal collections of neutrophils on their palms and soles or in wider areas. When pustular psoriasis is generalized, it can be life-threatening, presenting with fever, electrolyte abnormalities, and loss of serum proteins.

DIAGNOSIS

- Clinical impression is usually sufficient for diagnosis, as no other disease presents with silvery erythematous patches on the knees and elbows.
- Classically presents with the **Auspitz sign** (bleeding capillaries when scale is scraped), but biopsy can be useful when the diagnosis is unclear.
- Histologic findings include a thickened epidermis, an absent granular cell layer, and preservation of nuclei and a sterile neutrophilic infiltrate (**Munro's microabscess**) in the stratum corneum.

TREATMENT

- Treat with topical steroids combined with keratolytic agents, tar, or anthralin along with UV therapy, including PUVA. Methotrexate may be used for severe cases. Retinoids (vitamin A derivatives) are especially effective in pustular psoriasis
- Arthritis should be treated first with NSAIDs and then with methotrexate if necessary. Systemic corticosteroids should be avoided, as tapering can induce psoriatic flares.
- Recently, biologic agents such as TNF-α inhibitors have proven effective in severe psoriatic arthritis and psoriasis.

Urticaria (Hives)

Both **a clinical description and a disease,** urticaria is characterized by superficial, intense edema in a localized area. It is usually acute but can also be chronic (lasting > 6 weeks). The condition results from the release of vasoactive substances (histamine, prostaglandins) from mast cells in a **type I hypersensitivity response.** Acute urticaria is a response to a trigger that may be a food, drug, virus, insect bite, or physical stimulus. Chronic urticaria is usually idiopathic.

HISTORY/PE

- Hives can range in severity from a few itchy bumps to life-threatening anaphylaxis.
- The typical lesion is an elevated papule or plaque that is reddish or white and variable in size. Lesions are widespread and last a few hours.
- In severe allergic reactions, **extracutaneous manifestations** can include tongue swelling, angioedema (deeper, more diffuse swelling), asthma, GI symptoms, joint swelling, and fever.
- Some forms of urticaria are associated with neutrophilic vasculitis. Such forms are typically seen in patients with arthritis, renal disease, or hypocomplementemia and often last > 24 hours.

DIAGNOSIS

Diagnosed by clinical impression and patient report. Biopsy demonstrates perivascular edema. It can often be difficult to determine the cause.

TREATMENT

Treat with systemic antihistamines. Topical medications are of no benefit.

Drug Eruption

Twenty percent of patients hospitalized for five or more days develop a cutaneous drug reaction. Such reactions can take many forms, including urticarial, lupus-like, vasculitic, purpuric, lichenoid, and blistered. Drugs can cause **all four types of hypersensitivity reactions,** and sometimes the same drug may cause different types of reactions in different patients.

History/PE

- Eruptions occur **7–14 days after exposure,** so if a patient reacts within a day or two of starting a new drug, it is probably not the causative agent.
- Eruptions are generally **widespread, relatively symmetrical,** and **pruritic.** Most are relatively short-lived, disappearing within 1–2 weeks following removal of the offending agent.
- The exception is **fixed drug eruption,** which consists of reddish macules or papules that develop in the same area (usually the genitalia, face, or extremities) each time the patient is exposed to the triggering agent. After these lesions resolve, there is often a persistent brown pigmentation. Extreme complications of drug eruptions include erythroderma and toxic epidermal necrolysis (TEN).

Diagnosis

Diagnosed by clinical impression. Patients may have eosinophilia and a cutaneous infiltrate.

Treatment

Discontinue the offending agent; treat symptoms with antihistamines.

Toxic Epidermal Necrolysis (TEN)

May be confused with staphylococcal scalded-skin syndrome (SSSS), another disease in which patients **lose widespread sheets of skin.** Whereas SSSS is usually seen in children and is infectious in etiology, however, TEN is usually seen in **adults** and is caused by a **drug reaction.** The main drugs that cause TEN are sulfonamides, allopurinol, phenytoin (Dilantin), and carbamazepine.

History/PE

- TEN may be preceded by a maculopapular drug reaction or by erythema multiforme. In other cases, patients rapidly develop widespread erythema and begin to shed large sheets of skin.
- Damage involves the **entire epidermis,** and **the mucous membranes** of the eyes, mouth, and genitals can become eroded and hemorrhagic.

Diagnosis

Biopsy can distinguish TEN from SSSS; TEN shows full-thickness epidermal damage, whereas SSSS has only superficial damage. The differential also includes graft-vs.-host reaction (usually after bone marrow transplant), radiation therapy, and burns.

Treatment

Patients have the **same complications as burn victims,** including thermoregulatory difficulties, electrolyte disturbances, and 2° infections. Therapy includes skin coverage and maintenance of fluid and electrolyte balance. Controversial treatments include systemic steroids in the early stages of TEN or IVIG. There is a high risk of mortality.

Erythema Multiforme

An **annular, pruritic** cutaneous reaction pattern that has many triggers and is often recurrent. Although some cases are idiopathic, most are triggered by recurrent HSV infection of the lip. Other triggers are mycoplasmal infections and drugs.

Think HSV infection with recurrent erythema multiforme.

HISTORY/PE

- The characteristic lesion has a **target appearance** (see Figure 2.2-5), but other types of lesions may be seen as well.
- The disease can occur on mucous membranes, where erosions are seen. Typically, lesions start as erythematous macules that become centrally clear and then develop a blister. The **palms and soles** are often affected.
- In its minor form, the disease is uncomplicated and localized to the skin. However, severe erythema multiforme can → **TEN or Stevens-Johnson syndrome,** in which patients are very ill with involvement of at least two mucosal surfaces.

DIAGNOSIS

Diagnosed by clinical impression. A **history of recurrent labial herpes** should be sought in all recurrent rashes.

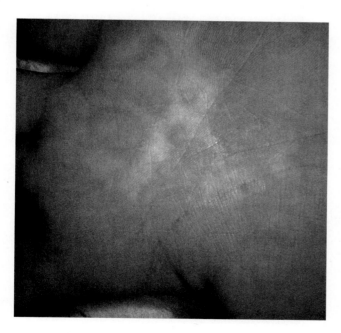

FIGURE 2.2-5. Erythema multiforme.

Evolving erythematous plaques and papules are seen with a target appearance consisting of a dull red center, a pale zone, and a darker outer ring. (Reproduced, with permission, from Hurwitz RM. *Pathology of the Skin: Atlas of Clinical-Pathological Correlation,* 2nd ed. Stamford, CT: Appleton & Lange, 1998, p. 24.)

TREATMENT

Symptomatic treatment is all that is necessary; systemic corticosteroids are of no benefit. Minor cases can be treated with antipruritics; major cases should be treated as burns. In patients with HSV, suppressive acyclovir may ↓ the frequency of rashes.

Erythema Nodosum

A **panniculitis** whose triggers include **infection** (e.g., *Streptococcus*, *Coccidioides*, *Yersinia*, TB), **drug reactions** (e.g., sulfonamides, various antibiotics, OCPs), and **chronic inflammatory diseases** (e.g., sarcoidosis, Crohn's disease, ulcerative colitis, Behçet's disease).

HISTORY/PE

Painful, erythematous nodules appear on the patient's lower legs (see Figure 2.2-6) and slowly spread, turning brown or gray. Patients may present with **fever and joint pain.**

DIAGNOSIS

Diagnosed by clinical impression. Histology shows nonspecific septal panniculitis.

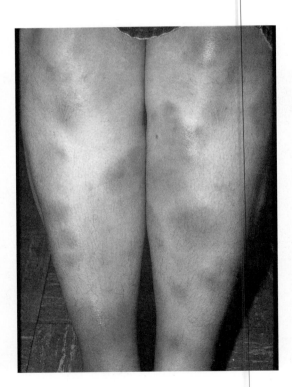

FIGURE 2.2-6. **Erythema nodosum.**

Erythematous plaques and nodules are commonly located on pretibial areas. Lesions are painful and indurated but heal spontaneously without ulceration. (Reproduced, with permission, from Hurwitz RM. *Pathology of the Skin: Atlas of Clinical-Pathological Correlation*, 2nd ed. Stamford, CT: Appleton & Lange, 1998, p. 132.)

Remove the triggering factor and treat the underlying disease where possible. NSAIDs can be used but may → erythema nodosum.

Pemphigus

The most common version is pemphigus vulgaris. Characterized by an **intraepidermal blister that → widespread painful erosions** of the skin and mucous membranes. Antibodies are directed against desmoglein molecules responsible for keratinocyte adherence, leading to loss of cellular attachment. These antibodies also stimulate cellular proteinases and complement, resulting in inflammation that hastens cellular separation. Patients are generally **middle-aged (40–60)**.

HISTORY/PE

Rarely, an intact blister may be seen, but generally presents only with erosions, often accompanied by crusting, weeping, and 2° infections. Mucous membranes are involved.

DIAGNOSIS

- Along with the clinical picture, a ⊕ **Nikolsky's sign** (the ability to produce a blister by rubbing skin adjacent to a natural blister) and skin biopsy are highly suggestive.
- Biopsy shows **acantholysis** (intraepidermal split with free-floating keratinocytes in the blister). Immunofluorescence and ELISA are confirmatory for antidesmoglein antibodies.

TREATMENT

Local wound treatment with burn care and high doses of systemic corticosteroids. Corticosteroid side effects are unavoidable at such high doses. Steroid-sparing agents include azathioprine and other antimetabolites.

Bullous Pemphigoid

The pemphigoid diseases are **acquired blistering diseases** that → **separation at the epidermal basement membrane.** Bullous pemphigoid is a chronic condition that is most commonly seen in patients **60–80 years of age.** Its pathogenesis involves **antibodies** that are developed against the bullous pemphigoid antigen, which lies superficially in the basement membrane zone (BMZ). Antigen-antibody complexes activate complement and eosinophil degranulation that provoke an inflammatory reaction and → separation at the BMZ. The **blisters are stable** because their roof consists of nearly normal epidermis.

HISTORY/PE

Presents with firm, stable blisters that arise on erythematous skin, often preceded by urticarial lesions. **Nikolsky's sign is** ⊖. The blisters form crusts and erosions (see Figure 2.2-7). Mucous membranes are less commonly involved than is the case in pemphigus.

DIAGNOSIS

Diagnosed according to the clinical picture. Skin biopsy shows a subepidermal blister, often with an eosinophil-rich infiltrate. Immunofluorescence

Less common forms of pemphigus are the foliaceous and paraneoplastic types.

HIGH-YIELD FACTS

DERMATOLOGY

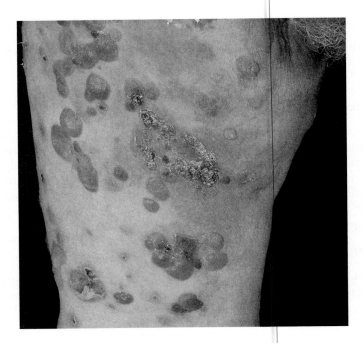

FIGURE 2.2-7. **Bullous pemphigoid.**

Multiple tense serous and partially hemorrhagic bullae can be seen. (Reproduced, with permission, from Fitzpatrick TB. *Color Atlas & Synopsis of Clinical Dermatology,* 4th ed. New York: McGraw-Hill, 2001, p. 100.)

demonstrates a band of immunoglobulin and complement at the epidermal-dermal junction. Patients occasionally have eosinophilia.

TREATMENT

Systemic corticosteroids. Topical corticosteroids can help prevent blister formation when applied to early lesions.

INFECTIOUS DISEASE MANIFESTATIONS

Viral Diseases

HERPES SIMPLEX

A painful, recurrent vesicular eruption of the mucocutaneous surfaces due to infection with HSV. **HSV-1 usually produces oral-labial lesions, while HSV-2 usually causes genital lesions.** The initial infection is passed by direct contact, after which the herpesvirus remains in local nerves. The virus spreads through epidermal cells, causing them to fuse into **giant cells.** The local host inflammatory response → erythema and swelling. The mechanism for disease recurrence is unclear.

HISTORY/PE

- **1° episodes** are generally longer and more severe than recurrences. Clinical presentation varies according to type.
  - **HSV-1:** Typically presents in infancy with widespread, severe herpetic gingivostomatitis with oral erosions.

- **HSV-2:** Typically affects adults, presenting with bilateral, erosive vesicular lesions accompanied by edema and lymphadenopathy. Patients may be unaware of their first infection.
- **Recurrences** vary according to site.
  - **Recurrent oral herpes:** Typically consists of the common **"cold sore,"** which presents as a cluster of crusted vesicles on an erythematous base (see Figure 2.2-8A). It is often triggered by sun and fever.
  - **Recurrent genital herpes:** Unilateral and characterized by a cluster of blisters on an erythematous base, but with less pain and systemic involvement than the 1° infection.

DIAGNOSIS

Diagnosed primarily by the clinical picture. **Multinucleated giant cells** on **Tzanck smear** (see Figure 2.2-8B) yield a presumptive diagnosis, but VZV has the same appearance on Tzanck, so culture or direct fluorescence antibody staining is needed for definitive diagnosis.

TREATMENT

- The mainstay of treatment is oral or IV acyclovir (IV for severe cases or for immunocompromised patients), which ↓ both the frequency and the severity of recurrences. Daily acyclovir suppressive therapy may be used in patients with > 6 outbreaks per year or for those with erythema multiforme.
- Acyclovir ointment is somewhat effective in reducing the duration of viral shedding but does not prevent recurrence.
- In AIDS patients, HSV can persist, with ulcers remaining resistant to antiviral therapy. Any persistent genital or perianal ulcer in an AIDS patient should thus be regarded as genital herpes. Symptomatic HSV infection lasting > 1 month can be considered an AIDS-defining illness.

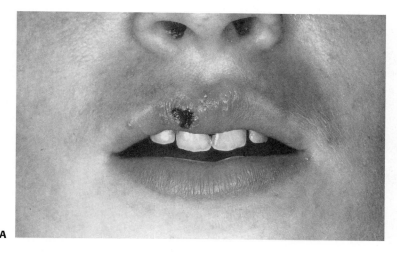
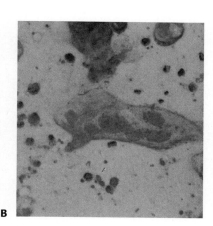

A   B

FIGURE 2.2-8.   Herpes simplex.

(A) 1° infection. Grouped vesicles on an erythematous base on the patient's lips and oral mucosa may progress to pustules before resolving. (B) Tzanck smear. The multinucleated giant cells from vesicular fluid provide a presumptive diagnosis of HSV infection. The Tzanck smear cannot distinguish between HSV and VZV infection. (Reproduced, with permission, from Hurwitz RM. *Pathology of the Skin: Atlas of Clinical-Pathological Correlation*, 2nd ed. Stamford, CT: Appleton & Lange, 1998, p. 145.)

VARICELLA-ZOSTER VIRUS (VZV)

VZV causes two very different diseases—**varicella and herpes zoster**—with transmission occurring via respiratory droplet or by direct contact. VZV has an incubation period of 10–20 days, with contagion beginning 24 hours before the eruption appears and lasting until lesions have crusted. It is unclear how patients who have recovered from the 1° infection of varicella (**chickenpox**) develop the recurrent infection of herpes zoster (**shingles**).

HISTORY/PE

- Varicella:
    - In varicella, a prodrome consisting of malaise, fever, headache, and myalgia occurs 24 hours before the onset of the rash. Pruritic lesions appear in crops over a period of 2–3 days, evolving from red macules to grouped central vesicles (**"dewdrop on a rose petal"**) and then crusting over.
    - At any given time, patients have all stages of lesions over their entire body. The trunk, face, scalp, and mucous membranes are involved, but the **palms and soles are spared.**
    - In adults, chickenpox is often more severe, with **systemic complications** such as pneumonia and encephalitis.
- Zoster:
    - Herpes zoster represents the recurrence of VZV in a specific nerve, with lesions cropping up along the nerve's **dermatomal** distribution. Outbreaks are usually preceded by intense local pain and then arise as grouped blisters on an erythematous base (see Figure 2.2-9).
    - In immunocompromised patients, zoster can → severe local disease, disseminated cutaneous disease, and systemic diseases that mimic varicella. Older patients with severe zoster may develop **postherpetic neuralgia.**

DIAGNOSIS

Diagnosed by the clinical picture.

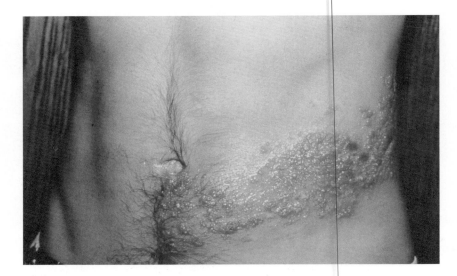

FIGURE 2.2-9. Varicella zoster.

The unilateral dermatomal distribution of the grouped vesicles on an erythematous base is characteristic.

TREATMENT

Varicella is self-limited in healthy children, but adults should be treated with systemic acyclovir. A **vaccine** is available for infants, children, and adults and is routinely used for disease prevention. Although acyclovir may speed the cutaneous course of zoster, **pain control** is most important for patients with this disease.

MOLLUSCUM CONTAGIOSUM

A poxvirus infection that is most common in **young children** and in **AIDS patients.** It is spread by physical contact.

HISTORY/PE

- The rash is composed of **tiny waxy papules,** frequently with **central umbilication.** In children, lesions are found on the trunk, extremities, or face (see Figure 2.2-10). In adults, they are commonly found on the genitalia and in the perineal region.
- In AIDS patients, lesions often appear on the face and can become quite large.
- **Lesions are asymptomatic** unless they become inflamed or irritated.

DIAGNOSIS

Diagnosed by the clinical picture, and confirmed by expressing and staining the contents of the papules. **Giemsa or Wright's stain** allows for the identification of **large inclusion or molluscum bodies.**

TREATMENT

Any local destructive method is effective, including curetting, freezing, or applying trichloroacetic acid to the lesions. Lesions resolve spontaneously over months to years and are often left untreated in children.

If you see giant molluscum contagiosum, think HIV.

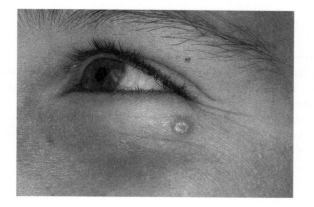

FIGURE 2.2-10. **Molluscum contagiosum.**

The dome-shaped, fleshy, umbilicated papule on the child's eyelid is characteristic. (Reproduced, with permission, from Hurwitz RM. *Pathology of the Skin: Atlas of Clinical-Pathological Correlation,* 2nd ed. Stamford, CT: Appleton & Lange, 1998, p. 149.)

VERRUCAE (WARTS)

Warts are caused by **many different types of HPV** and can occur on skin, mucous membranes, and other epithelia. Although usually benign, **some subtypes of HPV (especially 16 and 18)** → squamous **malignancies.** Spread is by direct contact. HPV → hyperproliferation of infected cells.

HISTORY/PE

- Common warts are the most prevalent HPV infection. Although most often seen on the hands, they can occur anywhere. On plantar and palmar surfaces, warts tend to grow downward into the skin rather than outward, giving them a flatter appearance.
- The classic genital wart is a cauliflower-like papule or nodule appearing on the glans penis, the vulva, or the perianal region. Warts on mucous membranes are generally velvety and white, appearing on oral, genital, and even laryngeal mucosa. Laryngeal warts are transmitted to infants by mothers with genital HPV.

DIAGNOSIS

Diagnosed by the clinical picture. **Acetowhitening** can be helpful in visualizing mucosal lesions. There is a long latency period, with children sometimes acquiring HPV at birth and not manifesting any lesions until years later.

TREATMENT

Treatment centers on destruction of the tissue by curettage, cryotherapy, or acid keratolytics. Genital warts are treated locally with podophyllin, trichloroacetic acid, imiquimod, or 5-FU. HPV lesions on the cervix must be monitored cytologically and histologically for evidence of malignancy.

Bacterial Infections

IMPETIGO

A superficial, weeping local infection that primarily occurs in **children** and is caused by both **group A streptococcal and staphylococcal** organisms. It is transmitted by direct contact.

HISTORY/PE

- There are two kinds of impetigo. The **common type,** which features pustules and honey-colored crusts on an erythematous base, commonly appears on the face (see Figure 2.2-11). The **bullous type,** which is usually acral, is characterized by stable blisters that are often large.
- Bullous impetigo is almost always caused by S. *aureus* and can evolve into SSSS. Streptococcal impetigo can be complicated by streptococcal acute glomerulonephritis.

DIAGNOSIS

Diagnosed by the clinical picture.

TREATMENT

Treat with antibiotics with antistaphylococcal activity. Topical antibiotics are often sufficient, but systemic agents can hasten recovery and prevent spread to other patients.

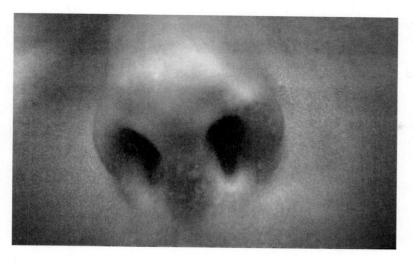

FIGURE 2.2-11. Impetigo.

Dried pustules with a superficial golden-brown crust are most commonly found around the nose and mouth. (Reproduced, with permission, from Hurwitz RM. *Pathology of the Skin: Atlas of Clinical-Pathological Correlation,* 2nd ed. Stamford, CT: Appleton & Lange, 1998, p. 165.)

CELLULITIS

A **deep, local infection** involving the connective tissue, subcutaneous tissue, or muscle in addition to the skin. It is commonly caused by **staphylococci** or by **group A streptococci** originating from an area of damaged skin or from a systemic source of infection. **Community-acquired MRSA** is an increasingly common cause of virulent cellulitis. Risk factors include diabetes, IV drug use, venous stasis, and immune compromise.

HISTORY/PE

Presents with **red, hot, swollen, tender skin.** Fever and chills are also common.

DIAGNOSIS

Diagnosed by the clinical picture. Wound culture may aid in diagnosis and help determine antibiotic sensitivities for treatment. Blood cultures should be obtained when bacteremia is suspected. Culture and sensitivities are important in case of MRSA. Rule out abscess, urticaria, contact dermatitis, osteomyelitis, and necrotizing fasciitis.

TREATMENT

Treat with 7–10 days of oral antibiotics for mild cases or with IV antibiotics if there is evidence of systemic toxicity, comorbid conditions, DM, extremes of age, hand or orbital involvement, or other concerns.

FOLLICULITIS

Inflammation of the hair follicle. Although typically caused by infection with *Staphylococcus, Streptococcus,* and **gram-⊖ bacteria,** folliculitis is occasionally caused by **yeast** such as *Candida albicans* or *P. ovale.* It may also be **mechanical,** arising from ingrown hairs (most common in patients with curly hair).

HISTORY/PE

- Each lesion is a **tiny pustule** that appears at the opening of a hair follicle and usually has a hair penetrating it. When the infection is deeper, a **furuncle,** or hair follicle abscess, develops.
- Furuncles are larger and more painful than folliculitic lesions and may disseminate to adjacent follicles to form a **carbuncle.** Patients with diabetes or immunosuppression are at ↑ risk.
- Folliculitis can be a major problem in AIDS patients, in whom the disease is intensely pruritic and resistant to therapy.

DIAGNOSIS

Diagnosed by the clinical picture.

TREATMENT

Topical antibiotics can be used to treat mild disease, but severe cases require systemic antibiotics. Large lesions must be incised, drained, and cultured to rule out MRSA. Patients who are prone to ingrown hairs should be advised not to shave.

ACNE VULGARIS

An endogenous skin disease that is common among adolescents. The pathogenesis is complex, involving hormonal activation of sebaceous glands, the development of the comedo or plugged sebaceous follicle, and involvement of *Propionibacterium acnes* in the follicle. Follicular bacteria cause much of the inflammation associated with the disease, and their metabolic activity produces substances that irritate the skin. Comedones may be caused by medications (e.g., lithium, corticosteroids) or by topical occlusion (e.g., cosmetics).

HISTORY/PE

- There are three stages of acne lesions:
  - **Comedo:** May be open ("**blackheads**") or closed ("**whiteheads**"); present in large quantities but with little inflammation.
  - **Inflammatory:** The comedo ruptures, creating a pustule that can be large and nodular.
  - **Scar:** As the inflammation heals, scars may develop. Picking at papules exacerbates scarring.
- Two types of cysts can occur in acne: inflammatory cysts, which are large, fluctuant pustules, and epidermoid cysts, which develop along the eyebrows and behind the ears.
- Acne first develops at puberty and typically persists for several years. Males are more likely to have severe, cystic acne than are females. Women in their 20s tend to have a variant that flares cyclically with menstruation, featuring fewer comedones and more painful lesions on the chin. Androgenic stimulation may contribute to these lesions.

DIAGNOSIS

Diagnosed by the clinical picture.

TREATMENT

- Treat comedones with topical **tretinoin** (Retin-A) and benzoyl peroxide.
- Inflammatory lesions should be treated with topical antibiotics (e.g., erythromycin, clindamycin) or systemic agents (e.g., tetracycline, erythromycin).

- Isotretinoin (**Accutane**) → marked improvement in > 90% of acne patients and has greatly improved the treatment of severe acne. It is, however, a teratogen that → transient elevations in cholesterol, triglycerides, and LFTs, and it may also be associated with depression. Patients on isotretinoin should thus be carefully monitored.

PILONIDAL CYSTS

Abscesses in the sacrococcygeal region that usually occur near the top of the natal cleft. Their name may not be appropriate, as not all such cysts contain hair, and not all are true cysts. Although the etiology is unclear, repetitive trauma to the region plays a role. Cysts are thought to start as a folliculitis that becomes an abscess complicated by perineal microbes, especially *Bacteroides*. The disorder most commonly occurs between the ages of 20 and 40, affecting men more often than women. Risk factors include deep and hairy natal clefts, obesity, and a sedentary lifestyle.

HISTORY/PE

Patients present with an abscess at the natal cleft that can be tender, fluctuant, warm, and indurated and is sometimes associated with purulent drainage or cellulitis. Systemic symptoms are uncommon, but cysts may develop into perianal fistulas.

DIAGNOSIS

Diagnosed by the clinical picture. Rule out perirectal and anal abscess.

TREATMENT

- Treatment consists of incision and drainage of the abscess under local anesthesia followed by sterile packing of the wound. Abscesses should be allowed to heal by 2° intention.
- Antibiotics are not needed unless cellulitis is present; if they are prescribed, both aerobic and anaerobic coverage is required.
- Good local hygiene and shaving of the sacrococcygeal skin can help prevent recurrence. Patients should follow up with a surgeon.

Fungal Infections

TINEA VERSICOLOR

Caused by *Pityrosporum orbiculare*, a yeast that is part of the normal skin flora. It is unclear what leads the organism to overgrow on the skin surface and become a pathogen. The pathogenic form has been called *Malassezia furfur*. Cushing's syndrome, immunosuppression, and hot, humid conditions are all risk factors.

HISTORY/PE

- Patients present with small, scaly patches of varying color, usually on the chest or back.
- Lesions may be hypopigmented as a result of interference with melanin production, or they may be hyperpigmented by virtue of thickened scale.

DIAGNOSIS

Diagnosed by clinical impression, and confirmed by **KOH preparation** of scale that reveals a **"spaghetti and meatballs"** pattern of hyphae and spores.

TREATMENT

Treat lesions with topical selenium sulfide daily for one week, followed by application once weekly for prophylaxis.

DERMATOPHYTE INFECTIONS

Dermatophytes **live only in tissues with keratin** (i.e., the skin, nails, and hair) and are a common cause of infection. Causative organisms include *Microsporum, Trichophyton,* and *Epidermophyton.* The immune response to the dermatophyte, rather than the organism itself, is responsible for many of the symptoms. **Pets** are a reservoir for *Microsporum.* Other risk factors include diabetes, ↓ peripheral circulation, immune compromise, and chronic maceration of skin (e.g., from athletic activities).

HISTORY/PE

Presentation varies according to subtype:

- **Tinea corporis:** Presents as a scaly, pruritic eruption with a sharp, irregular border, often with central clearing. May be seen in immunocompromised patients or in children following contact with infected pets.
- **Tinea pedis/manuum:** Presents as chronic interdigital scaling with erosions between the toes (**"athlete's foot"**) or as a thickened, scaly skin on the soles. Asymmetric involvement of the hands is typical.
- **Tinea cruris ("jock itch"):** A chronic infection of the groin (typically sparing the scrotum) that is usually associated with tinea pedis.
- **Tinea capitis ("ringworm"):** A diffuse, scaly scalp eruption similar to seborrheic dermatitis.

DIAGNOSIS

Diagnosed by the clinical picture; confirmed by scales prepared in **KOH showing mold hyphae.**

TREATMENT

Patients can be treated with topical or systemic antifungals. Tinea capitis must be treated with systemic drugs.

Parasitic Infections

LICE

Lice live off blood and on specific parts of the body, depending on their species. The **head louse** lives on the scalp and lays its eggs as nits attached to hair; the **body louse** lives in clothing and bites only the body. The **pubic louse** lives on pubic hair. Lice are spread through body contact or by the sharing of bedclothes and other garments. They secrete local toxins that → pruritus.

HISTORY/PE

- Patients with lice often experience severe pruritus, and 2° bacterial infection of the excoriations is a risk. **Classroom epidemics** of head lice are common.
- Body lice are seen in people with inadequate hygiene or in those with crowded living conditions. Pubic lice (called "crabs" because of their

squat, crablike body shape) contain anticoagulant in their saliva, so their bites often turn **blue.**

DIAGNOSIS

Lice can be seen on hairs or in clothes.

TREATMENT

- **Head lice:** Treat with OTC pyrethrin (RID) and mechanical removal of nits.
- **Body lice:** Wash body, clothes, and bedding thoroughly.
- **Pubic lice:** Treat with RID.

SCABIES

Caused by *Sarcoptes scabiei,* a tiny arthropod that mates on the skin surface, after which the female digs a passage into the stratum corneum and lays her eggs. The **burrowing** → **pruritus** that ↑ in intensity once an allergy to the mite or its products develops. Scabies mites are spread through close contact.

HISTORY/PE

Patients present with intense pruritus, especially at **night.** The most commonly affected sites are the hands, axillae, and genitals. On exam, the mite's **track** can sometimes be seen along with **erythematous, excoriated papules.** 2° bacterial infection is common.

DIAGNOSIS

A history of pruritus in several family members is suggestive. The mite may be identifiable by scraping an intact tunnel and looking under the microscope, but this is often difficult.

TREATMENT

Patients should be treated with 1–2 applications of **permethrin,** and their contacts should be treated as well. Oral **ivermectin** is also effective. Pruritus may persist for two weeks after treatment, so symptomatic treatment should be provided.

ISCHEMIC DISEASES

Decubitus Ulcers

Results from ischemic necrosis following continuous pressure on an area of skin that restricts microcirculation to the area. Ulcers are most commonly seen in **bedridden patients** who lie in one spot for too long. An underlying bony prominence or lack of fat ↑ the likelihood of ulcer formation. Patients who lack mobility or cutaneous sensation are also at ↑ risk. Incontinence of urine or stool may macerate the skin, facilitating ulceration.

HISTORY/PE

Ulcers are graded by degree of damage:

- **Grade I:** Characterized by persistent redness.
- **Grade II:** Marked by ulceration.

- **Grade III:** Involves destruction of structures beneath the skin such as muscle or fat.

DIAGNOSIS

Diagnosed by the history and clinical appearance.

TREATMENT

Prevention is key and involves routinely moving bedridden patients and using special beds that distribute pressure. Once an ulcer has developed, low-grade lesions can be treated with routine **wound care,** including hydrocolloid dressings. High-grade lesions require **surgical debridement.**

Gangrene

Defined as necrosis of body tissue. There are three subtypes: **dry, wet, and gas.** The presence of one subtype does not exclude the others. Etiologies are as follows:

- **Dry gangrene:** Due to insufficient blood flow to tissue, typically from atherosclerosis.
- **Wet gangrene:** Involves bacterial infection, usually with skin flora.
- **Gas gangrene:** Due to *Clostridium perfringens* infection.

HISTORY/PE

- **Dry gangrene:** Early signs are a dull ache, cold, and pallor of the flesh. As necrosis sets in, the tissue (usually a toe) becomes bluish-black, dry, and shriveled. Diabetes, vasculopathy, and smoking are risk factors.
- **Wet gangrene:** The tissue appears bruised, swollen, or blistered with pus.
- **Gas gangrene:** Typically occurs at a site of recent injury or surgery, presenting with swelling around the injury and with skin that turns pale and then dark red. Bacteria are rapidly destructive of tissue, producing gas that separates healthy tissue and exposes it to infection. **A medical emergency.**

DIAGNOSIS

Diagnosed by clinical impression.

TREATMENT

- Surgical **debridement,** with amputation if necessary, is the mainstay of treatment. **Antibiotics alone do not suffice** by virtue of inadequate blood flow, but they should be given as an adjuvant to surgery.
- **Gas gangrene can be treated with hyperbaric oxygen,** which is toxic to the anaerobic *C. perfringens.* Susceptible patients should maintain careful **foot care** and should avoid trauma.

MISCELLANEOUS SKIN DISEASES

Acanthosis Nigricans

- A condition in which the skin in the **intertriginous zones** (genital and axillary regions and especially the nape of the neck) is hyperkeratotic and hyperpigmented with a **velvety** appearance (see Figure 2.2-12).

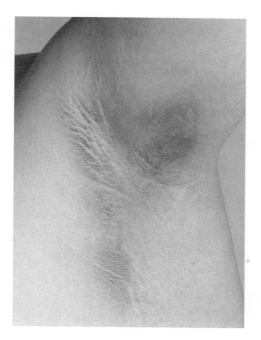

FIGURE 2.2-12.   Acanthosis nigricans.

Velvety, dark brown epidermal thickening of the armpit with prominent skin fold and feathered edges. (Reproduced, with permission, from Wolff K, Johnson RA, Suurmond D. *Fitzpatrick's Color Atlas & Synopsis of Clinical Dermatology*, 5th ed. New York: McGraw-Hill, 2005, p. 87.)

- The condition may be inherited with insulin resistance, may be 2° to obesity, or, when it occurs in previously normal adults, may represent a paraneoplastic sign of underlying adenocarcinoma (most often in the GI tract).
- **Dx:** Clinical appearance
- **Tx:** May be treated with topical steroids or retinoid. Patients should be encouraged to lose weight.

Lichen Planus

- A chronic, intensely pruritic disease of unknown etiology.
- **Hx/PE:**
  - Presents with **violaceous, flat-topped, polygonal papules.** Lesions may have **Wickham's striae** (white stripes), especially on the mucous membranes (see Figure 2.2-13), as well as prominent **Koebner's phenomena** (lesions that appear at the site of trauma). The initial lesions often appear on the genitalia, where they are ulcerated.
  - Although most cases resolve spontaneously over 6–18 months, those with oral involvement have a more chronic course.
- **Dx:** Histology reveals a "lichenoid pattern"—i.e., a band of **T lymphocytes at the epidermal-dermal junction with damage to the basal layer.**
- **Tx:** Mild cases are treated with topical corticosteroids. For severe disease, systemic steroids may be used. Tretinoin gel may be helpful on oral mucosa.

Lichen planus is the "P" disease: Planar, Purple, Pruritic, Persistent, Polygonal, Penile, Perioral, Puzzling, and Koebner's Phenomenon.

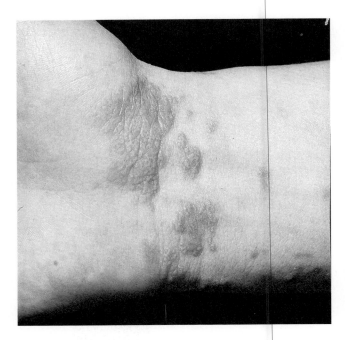

FIGURE 2.2-13. **Lichen planus.**

Flat-topped, polygonal, sharply defined papules of violaceous color are grouped and confluent. The surface is shiny and reveals fine white lines (Wickham's striae). (Reproduced, with permission, from Wolff K, Johnson RA, Suurmond D. *Fitzpatrick's Color Atlas & Synopsis of Clinical Dermatology*, 5th ed. New York: McGraw-Hill, 2005, p. 125.)

Rosacea

A disease of unclear etiology that is inflammatory but not infectious.

HISTORY/PE

- Patients are generally **middle-aged** and often have an **abnormal flushing** response to various substances.
- Early in the disease, **central facial erythema** is seen with telangiectasias. Later, papules and pustules may develop.
- Associated findings include **ocular keratitis** and **rhinophyma** (sebaceous gland hyperplasia of the nose).

DIAGNOSIS

Diagnosed by the clinical picture. Rosacea can be confused with acne but is not follicular in origin and involves an older age group.

TREATMENT

Treat with low-potency topical corticosteroids or topical metronidazole. In more severe disease, systemic antibiotics may be used. Extremely severe cases can be treated with short-term oral metronidazole.

Pityriasis Rosea

An acute dermatitis that is pink and scaly. Its etiology is unknown but is thought to represent a reaction to a viral **infection with human herpesvirus**

7 (HHV-7) because it tends to occur in **mini-epidemics among young adults.**

HISTORY/PE

- The initial lesion is a **herald patch** that is several centimeters in diameter and erythematous with a peripheral scale.
- Days to weeks later, a 2° exanthem appears, presenting with multiple tiny, symmetric papules with a fine **"cigarette paper"** scale (see Figure 2.2-14). Papules are arranged along skin lines, giving a classic **"Christmas tree pattern"** on the patient's back.
- Patients are generally asymptomatic, although the disease may be more extensive, pruritic, and chronic in African-Americans.

DIAGNOSIS

Diagnosed by clinical impression and confirmed by KOH exam to rule out fungus (the herald patch may be mistaken for tinea corporis). The differential also includes 2° syphilis (RPR should be ordered), guttate psoriasis, and drug eruptions.

TREATMENT

Patients usually heal without treatment in 2–3 weeks, but skin lubrication, topical antipruritics, and systemic antihistamines may occasionally be necessary. Severe cases can be treated with a short course of systemic corticosteroids.

Vitiligo

A disease of **depigmentation** whose pathogenesis is unknown. The mechanism may be autoimmune, neurologic, or both.

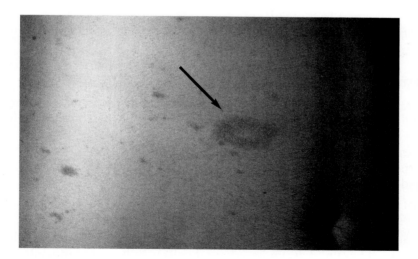

FIGURE 2.2-14.   Pityriasis rosea.

The round to oval erythematous plaques are often covered with a fine white scale ("cigarette paper") and are often found on the trunk and proximal extremities. Plaques are often preceded by a larger herald patch (arrow). (Reproduced, with permission, from Hurwitz RM. *Pathology of the Skin: Atlas of Clinical-Pathological Correlation*, 2nd ed. Stamford, CT: Appleton & Lange, 1998, p. 13.)

HISTORY/PE

- Patients develop **small, sharply demarcated white spots** on otherwise normal skin, often on the hands, face, or genitalia. These spots then spread, sometimes in dermatomal patterns, to include large segments of skin. The disease is usually **chronic and progressive,** with some patients becoming completely depigmented.
- Many patients have **serologic markers of autoimmune disease** (e.g., antithyroid antibodies, DM, pernicious anemia) but seldom present with these diseases. Patients with malignant melanoma may develop an **antimelanocyte immune response** that → vitiligo.

DIAGNOSIS

History and clinical picture; **pathology demonstrates total absence of melanocytes.** Conditions to rule out include postinflammatory hypopigmentation, scleroderma, piebaldism, and toxic exposure (phenolated cleansers are toxic to melanocytes).

TREATMENT

Topical or systemic psoralens and exposure to sunlight or PUVA may be helpful. Patients must wear **sunscreens** because depigmented skin lacks inherent sun protection. Dyes and makeup may be used to color skin, or the skin may be chemically bleached to produce a uniformly white color.

DYSPLASIAS

Seborrheic Keratosis

The most common skin tumor, appearing in almost all patients after age 40. The etiology is unknown. When many seborrheic keratoses erupt suddenly, they may be part of a **paraneoplastic syndrome** due to tumor production of epidermal growth factors. Lesions have no malignant potential but may be a cosmetic problem.

HISTORY/PE

- Present as **exophytic, waxy brown papules and plaques** with prominent follicle openings (see Figure 2.2-15). They often appear in great numbers and **look as if they could be scraped off.**
- Lesions may become irritated either spontaneously or by external trauma, especially in the groin, breast, or axillae. Irritated lesions are smoother and redder.

DIAGNOSIS

Diagnosed by the clinical picture; can be confirmed by histology showing **hyperplasia of benign, basaloid epidermal cells** with **horn pseudocysts** (prominent follicular openings). Rule out actinic keratosis, lentigo (focal ↑ in melanocytes), squamous cell carcinoma (SCC), and basal cell carcinoma (BCC).

TREATMENT

Cryotherapy or curettage is curative.

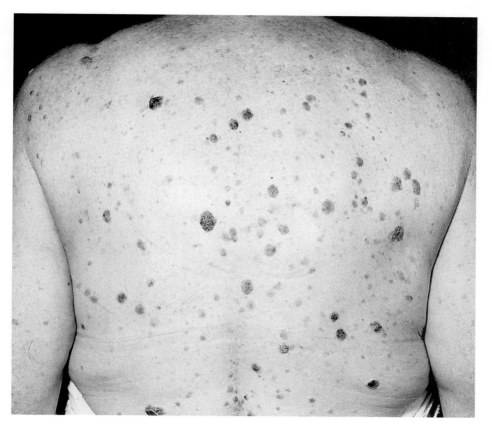

FIGURE 2.2-15. Seborrheic keratoses.

Multiple brown, warty papules and nodules are seen on the back, characterized by a "stuck-on" appearance. (Reproduced, with permission, from Fitzpatrick TB. *Color Atlas & Synopsis of Clinical Dermatology*, 4th ed. New York: McGraw-Hill, 2001, p. 195.)

Actinic Keratosis

Actinic keratosis is **a precursor of SCC in situ** and can slowly evolve into an invasive tumor. Lesions are caused by **sunlight.**

HISTORY/PE

Lesions appear on sun-exposed areas (especially the face and arms) and primarily affect **older patients,** who rarely have a solitary lesion. They are erythematous and sharply demarcated, with a light scale that can become thick and crusted (see Figure 2.2-16). Early lesions may be difficult to visualize and may be easier to find by palpation.

DIAGNOSIS

Diagnosed by clinical impression. Biopsy is seldom necessary but shows intraepidermal atypia over a sun-damaged dermis. The differential includes **Bowen's disease,** another form of SCC in situ that may be idiopathic or due to carcinogen exposure (especially arsenic).

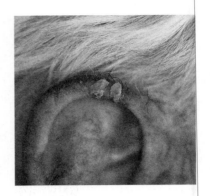

FIGURE 2.2-16. **Actinic keratosis.**

The discrete patch above has an erythematous base and a rough white scale. (Reproduced, with permission, from Hurwitz RM. *Pathology of the Skin: Atlas of Clinical-Pathological Correlation,* 2nd ed. Stamford, CT: Appleton & Lange, 1998, p. 359.)

TREATMENT

Cryosurgery or topical 5-FU is used to destroy the lesion. If carcinoma is suspected, biopsy followed by excision or curettage is appropriate. Patients should be advised to use sun protection.

Squamous Cell Carcinoma (SCC)

The second most common skin tumor, with locally destructive effects as well as the potential for **metastasis and death. UV light** is the most common causative factor, but exposure to **chemical carcinogens,** prior **radiation** therapy, and the presence of **chronically draining infectious sinuses** (as in osteomyelitis) also predispose patients to developing SCC. Most SCCs occur in older adults with sun-damaged skin, arising from actinic keratoses.

HISTORY/PE

- SCCs have a variety of forms, and a single patient will often have multiple variants (see Table 2.2-4).
- SCCs that arise from actinic keratoses rarely metastasize, but those that arise on the lips and on ulcers are more likely to do so.

TABLE 2.2-4. **Types of Squamous Cell Carcinoma**

TYPE	PRESENTATION
SCC with cutaneous horn	A nodular tumor with a hyperkeratotic growth on top.
Nodular SCC	A thick papule or nodule, often with central ulceration.
Exophytic SCC	A red, friable nodule that bleeds easily and usually arises from Bowen's disease (see Figure 2.2-17).
Verrucous carcinoma	A low-grade SCC that resembles a wart and is usually found on mucous membranes and plantar surfaces.

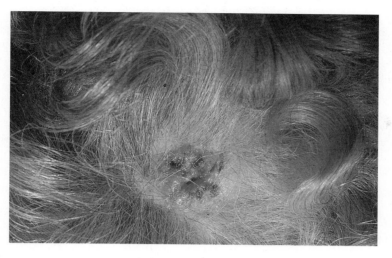

FIGURE 2.2-17.   Squamous cell carcinoma.

Note the crusting and ulceration of this erythematous plaque. Most lesions are exophytic nodules with erosion or ulceration. (Reproduced, with permission, from Hurwitz RM. *Pathology of the Skin: Atlas of Clinical-Pathological Correlation*, 2nd ed. Stamford, CT: Appleton & Lange, 1998, p. 360.)

DIAGNOSIS

- Diagnosed by clinical suspicion and confirmed by **biopsy,** which is necessary for accurate diagnosis and appropriate therapeutic planning.
- Histology shows intraepidermal atypical keratinocytes, with penetration of the basement membrane by malignant epidermal cells growing into the dermis. SCCs are **graded histologically.**

TREATMENT

Surgical excision. Lesions with high metastatic potential may require additional radiation or chemotherapy.

Basal Cell Carcinoma (BCC)

The most common malignant skin tumor, BCC is slow growing and locally destructive but has **virtually no metastatic potential. Chronic UV light** exposure is the main risk factor. Multiple lesions on non-sun-exposed areas are suggestive of **arsenic exposure** or **inherited BCC nevus syndrome.** Most lesions appear on the face and on other sun-exposed areas.

HISTORY/PE

There are many types of BCC with varying degrees of pigmentation, ulceration, and depth of growth (see Table 2.2-5).

DIAGNOSIS

Diagnosed by clinical impression; confirmed by biopsy showing islands of proliferating epithelium resembling the basal layer of the epidermis. The differential includes benign tumors, hypopigmented melanocytic nevi, melanoma, dermatitis, psoriasis, and Paget's disease.

TABLE 2.2-5. **Types of Basal Cell Carcinoma**

TYPE	PRESENTATION
Nodular BCC	The classic, most common type. Presents as a nodular, pearly tumor with telangiectasias, often with central ulceration (see Figure 2.2-18).
Ulcerated BCC	Patients present with a lesion that frequently crusts and bleeds and then heals over. Dramatic tissue destruction may be seen.
Sclerosing BCC	Presents with a scarred area that looks as though it has been previously treated but has actually occurred spontaneously.
Superficial BCC	Appears as a flat patch that occasionally bleeds or peels. Lesions usually occur on the trunk. Can be 2° to arsenic exposure.
Pigmented BCC	2° proliferation of melanocytes gives the lesion a pigmented appearance. Most common among African-Americans.
BCC nevus syndrome	An autosomal-dominant disorder in which patients have multiple BCCs from childhood. Patients also have frontal bossing, jaw cysts, and CNS tumors.

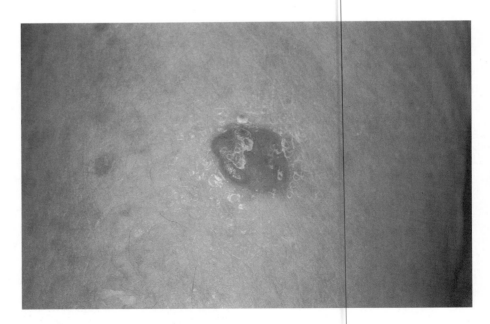

FIGURE 2.2-18. **Basal cell carcinoma.**

Seen above is an erythematous, fleshy, telangiectatic nodule with a translucent surface. (Reproduced, with permission, from Hurwitz RM. *Pathology of the Skin: Atlas of Clinical-Pathological Correlation*, 2nd ed. Stamford, CT: Appleton & Lange, 1998, p. 362.)

TREATMENT

Options include excision, curettage and electrodesiccation/cautery, deep cryotherapy, superficial radiation therapy, and Mohs' surgery. **Cure rates are > 95%.**

Melanoma

The **most common life-threatening problem in dermatology,** with an increasing incidence throughout the world. Although its pathogenesis is unclear, certain risk factors have been established, including **short, intense bursts of sun exposure** (especially in childhood) and the presence of **congenital melanocytic or dysplastic nevi.** Affected patients are thought to have melanocytes that are more likely to evolve into malignant melanoma. Immunosuppression also ↑ risk. Some patients inherit a predisposition to melanoma, with the **familial atypical mole and melanoma (FAM-M) syndrome.** There are several subtypes (see Table 2.2-6).

HISTORY/PE

- All malignant melanomas begin in the epidermal basal layer, where melanocytes are normally found.
- The first growth phase is horizontal-intraepidermal, presenting with a lesion that is flat but increasing in diameter (typical of lentigo maligna or melanoma in situ). Later, there is a vertical growth phase with dermal invasion.
- Lesion characteristics that are suggestive of melanoma include **irregular pigment, irregular contour and border, nodule and ulcer formation,** and **changes in size/shape/color/contour/surface** noted by the patient (see Figure 2.2-19).
- Malignant melanoma may metastasize, and 10% of patients with metastatic melanoma have no known 1° lesion. Metastasis may be local (to

TABLE 2.2-6. **Types of Melanoma**

TYPE	PRESENTATION
Lentigo maligna	Arises in a lentigo maligna that develops a nodule and ulcerates. Usually found on sun-damaged skin of the face.
Superficial spreading	Typically affects younger adults, presenting on the trunk in men and on the legs in women. A relatively prolonged horizontal growth phase helps identify the disease early, when it is still confined to the epidermis.
Nodular	Lesions have a rapid vertical growth phase and appear as a rapidly growing reddish-brown nodule with ulceration or hemorrhage.
Acral lentiginous	Begins on the hands and feet as a slowly spreading, pigmented patch. More common in Asians and African-Americans.
Amelanotic	Presents as a lesion without clinical pigmentation. Extremely difficult to identify.

nearby skin), regional (between the original lesion and its regional lymph nodes), or distant (via lymphatic or hematogenous spread to almost every organ in the body).

DIAGNOSIS

- Early recognition and treatment are essential. All adults should be examined for lesions that are suspicious for melanoma according to the **ABCD criteria,** which were developed by the American Cancer Society to identify dysplastic nevi and superficial spreading melanoma (see mnemonic).
- The onset of **pruritus** is also an early sign of malignant change. An **excisional biopsy** should be performed on any suspicious lesion. **Malignancy is determined histologically.**
- Malignant melanomas are characterized by **Clark's levels** and by tumor-node-metastasis (**TNM**) **staging** (see Tables 2.2-7 and 2.2-8).

TREATMENT

- Lesions confined to the skin are treated by **excision with margins.** Lymph node dissection is useful for staging but does not ↑ survival. Chemotherapy and radiation therapy may be used but are not likely to be successful.
- Malignant melanoma has the potential to **relapse after several years;** patients with early melanoma are at low risk for relapse but are at high risk for the development of **subsequent melanomas. Patient surveillance** is thus essential.

Kaposi's Sarcoma (KS)

A vascular proliferative disease. It is attributed to a herpesvirus, HHV-8, also called Kaposi's sarcoma–associated herpesvirus (KSHV).

> *The **ABCD**s of melanoma:*
>
> **A**symmetric
> Irregular **B**order
> Irregular **C**olor
> **D**iameter > 6 mm

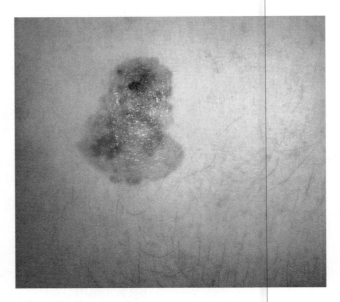

FIGURE 2.2-19. Melanoma.

Note the asymmetry, border irregularity, color variation, and large diameter of this plaque. (Reproduced, with permission, from Hurwitz RM. *Pathology of the Skin: Atlas of Clinical-Pathological Correlation,* 2nd ed. Stamford, CT: Appleton & Lange, 1998, p. 432.)

TABLE 2.2-7. Characterization of Melanoma by Clark's Levels

LEVEL	DEPTH OF LESION	FIVE-YEAR SURVIVAL (%)
I	Within the epidermis	99
II	Into the papillary dermis	95
III	Filling the papillary dermis	90
IV	Into the reticular dermis	65
V	To subcutaneous fat	25

HISTORY/PE

There are several types of KS:

- The **classic variant** is characterized by multicentric vascular macules and coalescent papules and plaques on the lower extremities. It usually occurs in the elderly, with a preponderance of cases in patients of Ashkenazi Jewish or Mediterranean descent.
- More disseminated cases occur in **African KS (endemic KS)** and in **immunocompromised** patients.
- **Epidemic HIV-associated KS** is an aggressive form of the disease, and although less common since the advent of HAART, it remains the **most common HIV-associated malignancy.**

DIAGNOSIS

History and clinical impression, which are confirmed by biopsy showing spindle cells (elongated tumor cells) and the presence of the viral protein LANA in the cells.

TREATMENT

Treatment is palliative. Local lesions may be treated with radiation or cryotherapy; surgery is not recommended. Widespread or internal disease is treated with systemic chemotherapy (anthracyclines, paclitaxil, or IF-α).

Mycosis Fungoides (Cutaneous T-Cell Lymphoma)

Not a fungus but rather a slow, progressive proliferation of T cells. Its pathogenesis is unclear but is thought to be related to chronic immunostimulation

TABLE 2.2-8. TNM Staging of Melanoma

STAGE	EXTENT OF DISEASE	FIVE-YEAR SURVIVAL (%)
I	1° skin melanoma	70
II	Local or regional metastasis	30
III	Distant metastasis	0

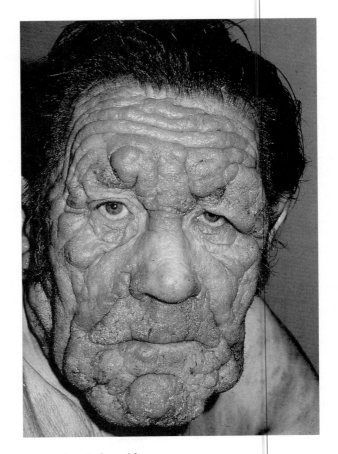

FIGURE 2.2-20. **Mycosis fungoides.**

Massive nodular infiltration of the face → a leonine facies. (Reproduced, with permission, from Fitzpatrick TB. *Color Atlas & Synopsis of Clinical Dermatology*, 4th ed. New York: McGraw-Hill, 2001, p. 541.)

that leads **helper T cells to gather in the epidermis.** Industrial exposure to irritating chemicals appears to ↑ risk. The disease is **chronic** and is more common in men than in women.

HISTORY/PE

- The early lesion is a nonspecific, psoriatic-appearing plaque that is palpable and often pruritic.
- **Stage I** is a patchy, plaque-like skin disease, whereas **stage II** is characterized by skin tumors with multicentric, often confluent reddish-brown nodules (see Figure 2.2-20). Rarely, patients skip the plaque stage and present directly with tumors.
- Patients may have dermatopathic lymphadenopathy without actual tumor involvement of the node. However, the **internal organs can be involved,** including the nodes, liver, and spleen.

DIAGNOSIS

- Diagnosed by clinical features and histology, with immunologic characterization and electron microscopy showing the typical **Sézary or Lutzner cells** (cerebriform lymphocytes).

- The early lesion is clinically indistinguishable from dermatitis, so **histologic diagnosis is indicated for any dermatitis that is chronic and resistant to treatment.**
- Once clinical tumors have evolved, histology is useful for showing the type of cells present.

TREATMENT

Stage I disease is treated topically with steroids, retinoids, chemotherapy, or PUVA. **Stage II is treated systemically** with retinoids, interferon, monoclonal antibodies, or chemotherapy.

Endocrinology

Type 1 Diabetes Mellitus (Type 1 DM)

Due to autoimmune pancreatic β-cell destruction → insulin deficiency and abnormal fuel metabolism.

HISTORY/PE

- Classically presents with **polyuria** (especially nocturia), **polydipsia, polyphagia,** and rapid, unexplained weight loss. Patients may also present with **ketoacidosis.**
- Usually affects nonobese children or young adults.
- Associated with HLA-DR3 and -DR4.

DIAGNOSIS

At least one of the following is required to make the diagnosis:

- A fasting (> 8-hour) plasma glucose of ≥ 126 mg/dL on two separate occasions.
- A random plasma glucose of ≥ 200 mg/dL plus symptoms.
- A two-hour postprandial glucose of ≥ 200 mg/dL after a glucose tolerance test on two separate occasions if the results of initial testing are equivocal.

TREATMENT

- Insulin (see Table 2.3-1) and self-monitoring of blood glucose in the normal range (80–120 mg/dL). Higher blood glucose levels (≥ 200 mg/dL) can be tolerated, particularly in the very young, in light of the ↑ risk of hypoglycemia.
- Routine HbA_{1c} testing (with a goal HbA_{1c} < 8 in children), frequent BP checks, foot checks, annual dilated-eye exams, annual microalbuminuria screening, and a lipid profile every 2–5 years.

COMPLICATIONS

Table 2.3-2 outlines the acute, chronic, and treatment-related complications of DM.

TABLE 2.3-1. Types of Insulin[a]

INSULIN	ONSET	PEAK EFFECT	DURATION
Regular	30–60 minutes	2–4 hours	5–8 hours
Humalog (lispro)	5–10 minutes	0.5–1.5 hours	6–8 hours
NovoLog (aspart)	10–20 minutes	1–3 hours	3–5 hours
Apidra (glulisine)	5–15 minutes	1.0–1.5 hours	1.0–2.5 hours
Exubera (inhaled)	10–12 minutes	0.5–1.5 hours	6 hours
NPH	2–4 hours	6–10 hours	18–28 hours
Levemir (detemir)	2 hours	No discernible peak	20 hours
Lantus (glargine)	1–4 hours	No discernible peak	20–24 hours

[a]Combination preparations mix longer-acting and shorter-acting types of insulin together to provide immediate and extended coverage in the same injection, e.g., 70 NPH/30 regular = 70% NPH + 30% regular.

TABLE 2.3-2.   Complications of DM

COMPLICATION	DESCRIPTION
Complications of treatment	
Dawn phenomenon	Early-morning hyperglycemia caused by ↓ effectiveness of insulin and ↑ secretion of growth hormone (GH) and other hormones overnight. **Move P.M. insulin closer to bedtime to treat.**
Acute complications	
Diabetic ketoacidosis (DKA)	Hyperglycemia-induced crisis that occurs most commonly in **type 1 DM.** Often precipitated by stress (including infections, MI, trauma, or alcohol) or by noncompliance with insulin therapy. May present with **abdominal pain, vomiting, Kussmaul respirations,** and a **fruity, acetone breath odor.** Patients are severely dehydrated with many electrolyte abnormalities and may also develop mental status changes. Treatment includes fluids, potassium, **insulin,** and treatment of the initiating event or underlying disease process.
Hyperosmolar hyperglycemic state (HHS)	Presents as **profound dehydration,** mental status changes, hyperosmolarity, and extremely high plasma glucose (> 600 mg/dL) without acidosis. Occurs in **type 2 DM;** precipitated by acute stress (dehydration, infections) and often can be fatal. Treatment includes **aggressive fluid and electrolyte replacement** and insulin. Treat the initiating event.
Chronic complications	
Retinopathy (nonproliferative, proliferative)	Appears when diabetes has been present for at least **3–5 years.** Preventive measures include control of hyperglycemia and hypertension, annual eye exams, and **laser photocoagulation therapy for retinal neovascularization.**
Diabetic nephropathy	Characterized by glomerular hyperfiltration followed by **microalbuminuria.** Preventive measures include **ACEIs** and BP and glucose control.
Neuropathy	Peripheral, symmetric, sensorimotor neuropathy → burning pain, foot trauma, infections, and diabetic ulcers. Treat with preventive **foot care** and **analgesics.** Late complications due to autonomic dysfunction include delayed gastric emptying, esophageal dysmotility, impotence, and orthostatic hypotension.
Macrovascular complications	Cardiovascular, cerebrovascular, and peripheral vascular disease. Cardiovascular disease is the most common cause of death in diabetic patients. Goal BP is < 130/< 75; ↓ LDL to < 100 mg/dL; ↓ triglycerides to < 150 mg/dL. Patients should also be started on low-dose ASA.

HIGH-YIELD FACTS

ENDOCRINOLOGY

Type 2 Diabetes Mellitus (Type 2 DM)

A dysfunction in glucose metabolism that is best characterized as varying degrees of insulin resistance that may → β-cell burnout and insulin dependence.

HISTORY/PE

- Patients typically present with symptoms of hyperglycemia.
- Onset is more **insidious** than that of type 1 DM, and patients often present with complications.
- **Nonketotic hyperglycemia** may be seen in the setting of poor glycemic control.
- Usually occurs in older adults with obesity (often truncal); has a strong genetic predisposition.

DIAGNOSIS

- Diagnostic criteria are the **same as those for type 1 DM.**

- Follow-up testing:
  - **Patients with no risk factors:** Test at 45 years of age; retest every three years.
  - **Patients with impaired fasting glucose** (> 110 mg/dL but < 126 mg/dL): Follow up with frequent retesting.

TREATMENT

The goal of treatment is tight glucose control—i.e., blood sugars ranging from 80 to 120 mg/dL and HbA_{1c} levels < 6.5. Treatment measures include the following:

- Diet, weight loss, and exercise.
- **Oral agents** (monotherapy or combination if uncontrolled) include the following:
  - **Sulfonylureas (glipizide, glyburide, and glimepiride):** Insulin secretagogues. Hypoglycemia and weight gain are side effects.
  - **Meglitinides (repaglinide and nateglinide):** Short-acting agents whose mechanism of action is similar to that of sulfonylureas.
  - **Metformin:** Inhibits hepatic gluconeogenesis; ↑ peripheral sensitivity to insulin. Side effects include weight loss, GI upset, and, rarely, lactic acidosis. Contraindicated in the elderly (those > 80 years of age) and in patients with renal disease.
  - **Thiazolidinediones (the "glitazones"):** ↑ insulin sensitivity. Side effects include weight gain, edema, and potential hepatotoxicity.
  - **α-glucosidase inhibitors:** ↓ intestinal absorption of carbohydrates. Rarely used owing to the side effect of flatulence.
- Insulin (alone or in conjunction with oral agents).
- Statins for hypercholesterolemia (goal LDL < 100); glucose control and fibric acid derivatives for hypertriglyceridemia.
- **Strict BP control to < 130/80;** ACEIs/ARBs are usually first-line agents.
- **Antiplatelet agents** (ASA) for patients at risk of cardiovascular disease or for those > 40 years of age.
- Regular screening for cardiovascular disease, nephropathy, retinopathy, neuropathy, and smoking cessation.

COMPLICATIONS

See Table 2.3-2 for an outline of the complications of DM. Note that the presence of **diabetes is equivalent to the highest risk for cardiovascular disease** regardless of all other risk factors.

Metabolic Syndrome

- Also known as insulin resistance syndrome or syndrome X. Associated with an ↑ risk of CAD and mortality from a cardiovascular event.
- **Hx/PE:** Presents with **abdominal obesity, high BP, impaired glycemic control,** and **dyslipidemia.**
- **Dx:** Three out of five of the following criteria must be met:
  - Abdominal obesity (↑ waist girth).
  - Triglycerides ≥ 150 mg/dL.
  - HDL cholesterol < 40 mg/dL in men and < 50 mg/dL in women.
  - BP ≥ 130/85 mmHg or administration of antihypertensive drugs.
  - Fasting glucose ≥ 110 mg/dL.
- **Tx:** Intensive weight loss, aggressive cholesterol lowering, and BP control. Metformin has been shown to slow the onset of diabetes in this high-risk population.

Testing of Thyroid Function

TFTs include the following (see also Table 2.3-3):

- **Radioactive iodine uptake (RAIU) and scan:** Determines the level of iodine uptake by the thyroid. Useful in differentiating thyrotoxic states.
- **Total T_4 measurement:** Not an adequate screening test. Ninety-nine percent of circulating T_4 is bound to thyroxine-binding globulin (TBG). Total T_4 levels can be altered by changes in levels of the binding proteins.
- **T_3 resin uptake (T3RU):** Used with total T_4 or T_3 to correct for changes in TBG levels (e.g., the free thyroxine index = total $T_4 \times$ T3RU).
- **Free T_4 measurement:** The preferred screening test for thyroid hormone levels; more useful for unstable thyroid states.
- **TSH measurement: The single best test for assessing thyroid function.** High TSH levels → 1° hypothyroidism; low TSH levels → 1° hyperthyroidism.

Hyperthyroidism

Causes of thyrotoxicosis (↑ levels of T_3/T_4 due to any cause) in which the thyroid overproduces thyroid hormone, including **Graves' disease,** toxic multinodular goiter (TMNG), and toxic adenomas.

- **Hx/PE:**
    - Presents with **weight loss, heat intolerance, nervousness, palpitations, ↑ bowel frequency,** insomnia, and menstrual abnormalities.
    - Exam reveals warm, moist skin, goiter, sinus **tachycardia** or **atrial fibrillation,** fine **tremor, lid lag,** and hyperactive reflexes. **Exophthalmos,** pretibial myxedema, and thyroid bruits are seen only in Graves' disease (see Figure 2.3-1).
- **Dx:** See Table 2.2-3.
- **Tx:**
    - 1° therapy is **radioactive ^{131}I thyroid ablation;** thyroidectomy and antithyroid drugs (methimazole or propylthiouracil) may also be used if radioactive iodine is not indicated.
    - Give **propranolol** for adrenergic symptoms while awaiting the resolution of hyperthyroidism.

TSH receptor antibodies are seen in patients with Graves' disease.

HIGH-YIELD FACTS

ENDOCRINOLOGY

TABLE 2.3-3. Common Thyroid Function Abnormalities

DIAGNOSIS	TSH	T_4	T_3	CAUSES
1° hyperthyroidism	↓	↑	↑	Graves' disease, TMNG, toxic adenoma, amiodarone, molar pregnancy, postpartum thyrotoxicosis, postviral thyroiditis.
1° hypothyroidism	↑	↓	↓	Hashimoto's thyroiditis, hypothyroid phase of thyroiditis, iatrogenic factors (radioactive thyroid ablation or excision with inadequate supplementation, external radiation), lithium, amiodarone, iodide, infiltrative disease.

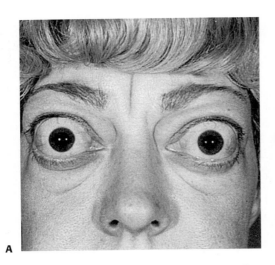
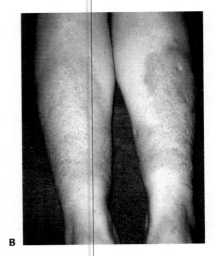

FIGURE 2.3-1. **Physical signs of Graves' disease.**

(A) Graves' ophthalmopathy. (B) Pretibial myxedema. (Reproduced, with permission, from Greenspan FS, Strewler GJ [eds]. *Basic and Clinical Endocrinology,* 5th ed. Stamford, CT: Appleton & Lange, 1997.)

- Administer levothyroxine to prevent hypothyroidism in patients who have undergone ablation or surgery.

Hypothyroidism

- **Hashimoto's thyroiditis** is the most common cause of hypothyroidism (see Table 2.3-3). Anti-TPO antibodies are ⊕.
- **Myxedema coma** refers to severe hypothyroidism with ↓ mental status, hypothermia, and other parasympathetic symptoms. Mortality is 30–60%.
- **Hx/PE:** Presents with weakness, fatigue, **cold intolerance, constipation,** weight gain, **depression,** menstrual irregularities, and **hoarseness.** Exam may reveal **dry, cold, puffy skin** accompanied by edema, **bradycardia,** and delayed relaxation of DTRs.
- **Dx:** See Table 2.2-3.
- **Tx:**
  - **Uncomplicated hypothyroidism (e.g., Hashimoto's disease):** Administer levothyroxine.
  - **Myxedema coma:** IV levothyroxine and IV hydrocortisone (if adrenal insufficiency has not been excluded).

Thyroiditis

- Inflammation of the thyroid gland. Common subtypes include subacute granulomatous, radiation-induced, autoimmune (lymphocytic), postpartum, and drug-induced (e.g., amiodarone) thyroiditis.
- **Hx/PE: Subacute and radiation-induced** forms present with a **tender thyroid** accompanied by malaise and URI symptoms. Other forms are associated with painless goiter.
- **Dx:** Thyroid dysfunction (typically thyrotoxicosis followed by hypothyroidism), with ↓ uptake on RAIU during the thyrotoxic phase.
- **Tx:**
  - **β-blockers for hyperthyroidism; levothyroxine for hypothyroidism.**
  - **Subacute thyroiditis:** Usually self-limited; treat with **NSAIDs** or with oral **steroids** for severe cases.

Thyroid Neoplasms

Thyroid nodules are very common and show an ↑ incidence with age. Most are benign.

HISTORY/PE

- Usually **asymptomatic** on initial presentation.
- **Hyperfunctioning nodules** present with hyperthyroidism and local symptoms (dysphagia, dyspnea, cough, choking sensation) and are associated with a family history (especially **medullary thyroid cancer**).
- An ↑ risk of malignancy is associated with a **history of neck irradiation, "cold" nodules** (on radionuclide scan), male sex, age < 20 or > 70, firm and fixed solitary nodules, a ⊕ family history (especially medullary thyroid cancer), and **rapidly growing nodules** with **hoarseness**.
- Check for anterior cervical lymphadenopathy. Carcinoma (see Table 2.3-4) may be **firm and fixed**.
- Medullary thyroid carcinoma is associated with multiple endocrine neoplasia (MEN) type 2 and familial medullary thyroid cancer.

DIAGNOSIS

- **TFTs** (TSH to exclude hyperfunction).
- **Ultrasound** determines if the nodule is solid or cystic; a radioactive scan determines whether it is hot or cold (cancers are usually cold and solid). Hot nodules are never cancerous and should not be biopsied.
- The best method of assessing a nodule for malignancy is **fine-needle aspiration** (FNA), which has high sensitivity and moderate specificity.

TREATMENT

- **Benign FNA:** Follow with physical exam/ultrasound or a trial of levothyroxine suppression treatment.
- **Malignant FNA:** Surgical resection is first-line treatment; adjunctive radioiodine ablation following excision is appropriate for follicular lesions.

> **Thyroid neoplasms—**
>
> **The most Popular is Papillary:**
>
> **P**apillae (branching)
> **P**alpable lymph nodes
> "**P**upil" nuclei ("Orphan Annie" nuclei)
> **P**sammoma bodies within lesion (often)
> Also has a **P**ositive **P**rognosis

TABLE 2.3-4. Types of Thyroid Carcinoma

TYPE[a]	CHARACTERISTICS	PROGNOSIS
Papillary	Represents 75–80% of thyroid cancers. The female-to-male ratio is 3:1. Slow growing; found in thyroid hormone–producing cells.	Ninety percent of patients survive 10 years or more after diagnosis; the prognosis is worse in elderly patients or those with large tumors.
Follicular	Accounts for 17% of thyroid cancers; found in thyroid hormone–producing cells.	Ninety percent of patients survive 10 years or longer after diagnosis; the prognosis is worse in elderly patients or those with large tumors.
Medullary	Responsible for 6–8% of thyroid cancers; found in calcitonin-producing C cells; the prognosis is related to degree of vascular invasion.	Eighty percent of patients survive at least 10 years after surgery.
Anaplastic	Accounts for fewer than 2% of thyroid cancers; rapidly enlarges and metastasizes.	Ten percent of patients will survive for > 3 years.

[a]Tumors may contain mixed papillary and follicular pathologies.

- **Indeterminate FNA:** Remove the nodule by surgical excision and wait for final pathology.
- Medullary thyroid cancer has a poorer prognosis than papillary and follicular types. Anaplastic thyroid cancer has an extremely poor prognosis.

Multiple Endocrine Neoplasia (MEN)

Associated with autosomal-dominant inheritance. Subtypes are as follows:

- **MEN type 1 (Wermer's syndrome):** Pancreatic islet cell tumors (e.g., Zollinger-Ellison syndrome, insulinomas, VIPomas), parathyroid hyperplasia, and pituitary adenomas.
- **MEN type 2A (Sipple's syndrome):** Medullary carcinoma of the thyroid, pheochromocytoma or adrenal hyperplasia, parathyroid gland hyperplasia.
- **MEN type 2B:** Medullary carcinoma of the thyroid, pheochromocytoma, oral and intestinal ganglioneuromatosis (mucosal neuromas), marfanoid habitus.

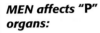

> **MEN affects "P" organs:**
>
> **P**ancreas
> **P**ituitary
> **P**arathyroid

BONE AND MINERAL DISORDERS

Osteoporosis

A common metabolic bone disease characterized by low bone mass and microarchitectural disruption, with bone mineral density > 2.5 SDs below normal peak bone mass. Most often affects thin, postmenopausal women (17%), especially Caucasians and Asians, with risk doubling (30%) after age 65.

Osteoporosis is the most common cause of pathologic fractures in elderly, thin women.

HISTORY/PE

- Commonly asymptomatic even in the presence of a vertebral fracture.
- Exam may reveal **hip fractures, vertebral compression fractures** (loss of height and progressive thoracic kyphosis), and/or distal radius fractures following minimal trauma (see Figure 2.3-2).
- Bone pain unrelated to fracture is most likely osteomalacia rather than osteoporosis.
- **Smoking,** excessive caffeine or alcohol intake, a history of amenorrhea, thyroid dysfunction, and **steroid use** are associated with an ↑ risk.

DIAGNOSIS

- **Labs:** Markers of bone turnover (↑ urinary N-telopeptides and deoxypyridinoline) can facilitate diagnosis in equivocal cases but are not routinely used; rule out 2° causes with TFTs, CMP, serum 25-hydroxyvitamin D, CBC, and testosterone (in men).
- **X-rays:** Global demineralization is apparent only after > 30% of bone density is lost.
- **DEXA:** Reveals significant osteopenia (bone mineral density < 2.5 SDs from normal peak level), most commonly in the vertebral bodies, proximal femur, and distal radius.

TREATMENT

- Prevention with **calcium supplementation** and vitamin D.
- Smoking cessation and weight-bearing exercises help maintain bone density.
- Bisphosphonates (e.g., alendronate, risedronate, ibandronate, zoledronic acid), selective estrogen receptor modulators (e.g., raloxifene), and in-

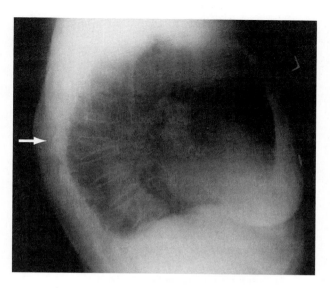

FIGURE 2.3-2. **Radiographic findings in osteoporosis.**

Lateral spine x-ray shows severe osteopenia and a severe wedge-type deformity (severe anterior compression). (Reproduced, with permission, from Kasper DL et al [eds]. *Harrison's Principles of Internal Medicine*, 16th ed. New York: McGraw-Hill, 2005, p. 2269.)

tranasal calcitonin may be used to prevent resorption and stabilize bone mineral density.
- Estrogen replacement therapy may be indicated for short-term treatment in the symptomatic perimenopausal period.
- Recombinant PTH may be used in patients with the highest level of risk.

Paget's Disease

- Characterized by an ↑ rate of bone turnover. Causes both excessive resorption and excessive formation of bone → a "mosaic" lamellar bone pattern. Suspected to be due to latent viral infection in genetically susceptible individuals. Found in roughly 4% of men and women > 40 years of age and associated with 1° hyperparathyroidism in up to one-fifth of patients.
- **Hx/PE:** Usually asymptomatic, but may present with **aching bone or joint pain,** headaches, skull deformities, fractures, or nerve entrapment → loss of hearing in 37% of cases.
- **Dx:**
  - Based on clinical history, characteristic radiographic changes (see Figure 2.3-3), and lab findings.
  - Radionuclide bone scan is the most sensitive test.
  - Lab abnormalities include ↑ serum alkaline phosphatase with normal calcium and phosphate levels; urinary pyridolines may be helpful. Must be differentiated from metastatic bone disease.
- **Tx: The majority of patients are asymptomatic and require no treatment.** There is no cure for Paget's disease. Bisphosphonates and calcitonin are used to slow osteoclastic bone resorption; NSAIDs and acetaminophen are given for arthritis pain.
- **Cx:** Pathologic fractures, cardiac complications, osteosarcoma (up to 1%).

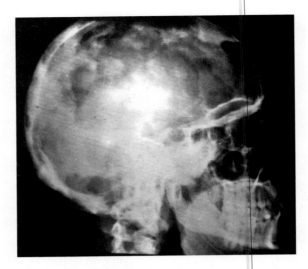

FIGURE 2.3-3. **Radiographic findings in Paget's disease.**

Skull of a 58-year-old woman with Paget's disease of bone. (Reproduced, with permission, from Kasper DL et al [eds]. *Harrison's Principles of Internal Medicine*, 16th ed. New York: McGraw-Hill, 2005, p. 2280.)

Hyperparathyroidism

- Eighty percent of 1° cases are due to a single **adenoma** and 15% to parathyroid hyperplasia. The most common 2° cause is phosphate retention in chronic renal failure, which → renal osteodystrophy. 3° hyperparathyroidism occurs when chronic 2° hyperparathyroidism progresses to an unregulated state, resulting in hypercalcemia.
- **Hx/PE:** Most cases are **asymptomatic,** but signs and symptoms may be mild and include **stones** (nephrolithiasis), **bones** (bone pain, myalgias, arthralgias, fractures), abdominal **groans** (abdominal pain, nausea, vomiting, PUD, pancreatitis), and **psychiatric overtones** (fatigue, depression, anxiety, sleep disturbances). Chronic renal insufficiency and gout are also associated with 1° hyperparathyroidism.
- **Dx:**
    - Labs reveal **hypercalcemia, hypophosphatemia,** and hypercalciuria. Intact PTH is inappropriately ↑ relative to ionized calcium (see Table 2.3-5). Vitamin D deficiency may obscure mild cases.
    - A radionuclide parathyroid scan may help with localization of an adenoma, although localization is not always necessary. Cancer is the most likely alternative diagnosis and must be ruled out, but with carcinoma PTH is usually < 25 pg/mL unless hyperparathyroidism is also present. Lithium and thiazides may exacerbate hyperparathyroidism.
- **Tx:**
    - **Parathyroidectomy** if symptomatic or if certain criteria are met. For acute hypercalcemia, give **IV fluids (with a loop diuretic in the setting of renal or heart failure), IV bisphosphonate, and calcitonin.**
    - Oral phosphate binders (aluminum hydroxide, calcium salts, sevelamer hydrochloride, and lanthanum carbonate) and dietary phosphate restriction are used in patients with 2° hyperparathyroidism regardless of dialysis status.
    - Cinacalcet ↓ PTH as well as calcium and phosphate and may be a helpful adjunct in ESRD.

TABLE 2.3-5.   Functions and Mechanisms of PTH

SOURCE	FUNCTIONS	MECHANISMS	REGULATION
Chief cells of parathyroid.	↑ bone resorption of calcium and phosphate. ↑ kidney resorption of calcium in the distal convoluted tubule. ↓ kidney resorption of phosphate. ↑ 1,25-$(OH)_2$ vitamin D (cholecalciferol) production by stimulating kidney 1α-hydroxylase.	PTH ↑ serum Ca^{2+}, ↓ serum $(PO_4)^{3-}$, and ↑ urine $(PO_4)^{3-}$. PTH stimulates both osteoclasts and osteoblasts.	↓ in free serum Ca^{2+} ↑ PTH secretion.

- **Cx:** Hypercalcemia is the most severe complication, presenting acutely with coma or altered mental status, bone disease, nephrolithiasis, and abdominal pain with nausea and vomiting.

PITUITARY AND HYPOTHALAMIC DISORDERS

Cushing's Syndrome

The most common endogenous cause is hypersecretion of ACTH from a pituitary adenoma (known as Cushing's disease, or **central** hypercortisolism). Other endogenous causes include ectopic ACTH secretion from neoplasia (e.g., carcinoid tumor, small cell lung cancer) or excess adrenal secretion of cortisol (e.g., bilateral adrenal hyperplasia, adenoma, adrenal cancer). Most commonly iatrogenic due to treatment with exogenous corticosteroids.

HISTORY/PE

- Presents with **hypertension, central obesity,** muscle wasting, thin skin with purple **striae,** psychological disturbances, **hirsutism, moon facies,** and "**buffalo hump.**"
- Exam reveals **depression,** oligomenorrhea, growth retardation, proximal weakness, acne, **excessive hair growth,** symptoms of **diabetes** (2° to glucose intolerance), and ↑ susceptibility to infection. **Headache** or cranial nerve deficits are also seen with increasing size of the pituitary mass.

DIAGNOSIS

Diagnosis is as follows (see also Table 2.3-6):

- **Screen:** A 24-hour free urine cortisol or overnight low-dose dexamethasone suppression test is considered **abnormal if A.M. cortisol is persistently elevated following overnight suppression.**
- **Differentiate between ACTH-dependent and -independent causes:** Cushing's disease or ectopic ACTH is likely if late-afternoon ACTH levels are elevated.
- Hyperglycemia, glycosuria, and **hypokalemia** may also be present.

TABLE 2.3-6. Laboratory Findings in Cushing's Syndrome

	CUSHING'S DISEASE (PITUITARY HYPERSECRETION)	EXOGENOUS STEROID USE	ECTOPIC ACTH SECRETION	ADRENAL CORTISOL HYPERSECRETION
ACTH	↑	↓	↑	↓
Urinary free cortisol	↑	↑	↑	↑

TREATMENT

- **Surgical resection** of the hypersecretory source (pituitary, adrenal).
- Pituitary radiotherapy may also be considered.
- Blockers of adrenal steroidogenesis (**ketoconazole, aminoglutethimide**).

Acromegaly

An adult condition due to a benign pituitary GH adenoma. Children with excess GH production present with **gigantism.**

HISTORY/PE

- Presents with **enlargement of the jaw, hands, and feet and coarsening of facial features.** May → carpal tunnel syndrome, diastolic dysfunction, hypertension, and arthritis.
- **Bitemporal hemianopia** may result from compression of the optic chiasm by a pituitary adenoma.
- Excess GH may also → **glucose intolerance** or **diabetes.**

DIAGNOSIS

- MRI of the pituitary shows a sellar lesion.
- Screen by measuring insulin-like growth factor 1 (IGF-1) levels (↑ with acromegaly); confirm the diagnosis with an oral glucose suppression test (GH levels will remain elevated despite glucose stimulation; baseline GH is not a reliable test).

TREATMENT

- Transsphenoidal surgical resection or external beam radiation of the tumor.
- Octreotide can be used to suppress GH secretion.
- Pegvisomant can be used to block GH receptors in refractory cases.

Prolactinoma

- The **most common functioning pituitary tumor.**
- **Hx/PE:** Hypogonadism is manifested by infertility, oligomenorrhea, or amenorrhea. Galactorrhea, gynecomastia, or bitemporal hemianopia may be prominent.
- **Dx:** The serum prolactin level is typically > 200 mg/mL.
- **Tx:**
  - **Dopamine agonists (first-line therapy):** Cabergoline, bromocriptine, or pergolide.

- **Surgery:** Should be considered when medical treatment has failed, when the patient desires future pregnancies, or in the presence of visual field defects.

Adrenal Insufficiency (AI)

May be 1° or 2°. Etiologies are as follows:

- **1°:**
  - Most commonly caused by autoimmune adrenal cortical destruction (**Addison's disease**) → deficiencies of mineralocorticoids and glucocorticoids. **Autoimmune destruction** may occur as part of a polyglandular autoimmune syndrome (hypothyroidism, type 1 DM, vitiligo, premature ovarian failure, testicular failure, pernicious anemia).
  - Other causes of 1° AI include congenital enzyme deficiencies, adrenal hemorrhage, TB, and other infections.
- **2°:** Caused by ↓ ACTH production by the pituitary; most often due to **cessation of long-term glucocorticoid treatment.**

HISTORY/PE

- Most symptoms are nonspecific.
- **Weakness, fatigue,** and **anorexia with weight loss** are common. GI manifestations, hypotension, and salt craving are also seen.
- **Hyperpigmentation** (due to ↑ ACTH secretion) is seen in Addison's disease, especially in areas of sun exposure or friction.

DIAGNOSIS

- Labs show **hyponatremia** and **eosinophilia** (1° or 2°).
- **Hyperkalemia** is specific to 1° AI.
- Hypercalcemia is seen in up to one-third of cases.
- Diagnosis is confirmed with plasma **cortisol levels:**
  - Low plasma cortisol levels (< 20 < μg/dL) during a period of high physiologic stress is confirmatory.
  - A random plasma cortisol level > 20 μg/dL excludes the diagnosis.
  - **Confirmatory test with synthetic ACTH stimulation test:** A plasma cortisol level > 20 μg/dL excludes the diagnosis.

TREATMENT

- **Glucocorticoid replacement, with mineralocorticoid** replacement if 1°.
- In adrenal crisis, correct electrolyte abnormalities as needed; provide 50% dextrose to correct hypoglycemia; and initiate volume resuscitation.
- ↑ steroids during periods of stress (e.g., major surgery, trauma, infection). Avoid 2° AI by tapering steroids slowly.

> **The 4 S's of adrenal crisis management:**
>
> **S**alt: 0.9% saline
> **S**teroids: IV hydrocortisone 100 mg q 8 hours
> **S**upport
> **S**earch for the underlying illness

Pheochromocytoma

- Tumors of chromaffin tissue of either the adrenal medulla or extra-adrenal sites that secrete catecholamines. May be associated with von Hippel–Lindau syndrome, neurofibromatosis, or MEN 2 syndromes.
- **Hx/PE:** Presents with intermittent tachycardia, palpitations, chest pain, diaphoresis, hypertension, headache, tremor, and anxiety. Crisis may be precipitated by anesthesia.

> **Pheochromocytoma rule of 10's:**
>
> 10% extra-adrenal
> 10% bilateral
> 10% malignant
> 10% occur in children
> 10% familial

- **Dx:** CT or MRI often demonstrates a suprarenal mass. Screen with plasma free metanephrines (metanephrine and normetanephrine) or 24-hour urine metanephrines. MIBG scan is sometimes helpful.
- **Tx: Surgical resection.** Preoperatively, **use α-adrenergic blockade first** to control hypertension, followed by β-blockade to control tachycardia. Never give β-blockade first; otherwise, unopposed α-adrenergic stimulation → refractory hypertension.

Hyperaldosteronism

- Results from excessive secretion of aldosterone from the zona glomerulosa of the adrenal cortex. Usually due to unilateral adrenal adenoma (**Conn's syndrome**), but can also be due to adrenocortical hyperplasia.
- **Hx/PE:**
  - Presents with **hypertension, headache, polyuria,** and **muscle weakness.**
  - Tetany, paresthesias, and peripheral edema are seen in severe cases.
- **Dx:** Labs show **hypokalemia, mild hypernatremia,** metabolic alkalosis, hypomagnesemia, and ↑ **aldosterone/plasma renin activity ratio.** CT or MRI may reveal an adrenal mass.
- **Tx:** Laparoscopic or open **adrenalectomy** for adrenal tumors (after correcting BP and potassium). Treat with **spironolactone** (an aldosterone receptor antagonist) for bilateral hyperplasia.

Congenital Adrenal Hyperplasia

- A family of inherited disorders → **cortisol deficiency.** Most cases are due to **21-hydroxylase deficiency (autosomal recessive)** → ↓ cortisol production with elevated cortisol precursors (e.g., 17-OH progesterone). In severe cases, mineralocorticoid deficiency with salt wasting may develop.
- Other causes include 11- and 17-hydroxylase deficiencies. Cortisol deficiency stimulates ACTH synthesis and → overproduction of adrenal androgens.
- **Hx/PE:**
  - **Ambiguous genitalia** in female infants; **virilization** (if manifested later in life).
  - **Macrogenitosomia** in male infants; precocious puberty (if manifested later in life); hypertension (with 11- and 17-hydroxylase deficiencies).
- **Dx:** High levels of cortisol precursors and androgens in blood and urine.
- **Tx:**
  - **Medical: Immediate fluid resuscitation and salt repletion.** Cortisol administration to ↓ ACTH and adrenal androgens. Fludrocortisone for severe 21-hydroxylase deficiency.
  - **Surgical:** May be required in the case of ambiguous genitalia in female infants.

Epidemiology

■ The **prevalence** of a disease is the number of existing cases in the population at a moment in time.
■ The **incidence** of a disease is the number of new cases in the disease-free population that develop over a period of time.
■ Prevalent cases are incident cases that have persisted in a population for various reasons:

$$\text{Prevalence} = \text{Incidence} \times \text{Average duration of disease}$$

Prevalence Studies

A **prevalence study** is one in which people in a population are examined for the presence of a disease of interest at a given point in time.

■ The **advantages** of prevalence studies are as follows:
  ■ They provide an efficient means of examining a population, allowing cases and noncases to be assessed all at once.
  ■ They can be used as a basis for diagnostic testing.
  ■ They can be used to plan which health services to offer and where.
■ Their **disadvantages** include the following:
  ■ One cannot determine causal relationships, because information is obtained only at a single point in time (a chi-square test can be used to estimate causal relationships).
  ■ The risk or incidence of disease cannot be directly measured (an odds ratio can be used to estimate relative risk or exposure).

Sensitivity and Specificity

Physicians often use tests to try to ascertain a diagnosis, but because no test is perfect, a given result may be falsely ⊕ or ⊖ (see Figure 2.4-1). When deciding whether to administer a test, one should thus consider both its sensitivity and its specificity.

■ **Sensitivity** is the probability that a patient with a disease will have a ⊕ test result. **A sensitive test will rarely miss people with the disease and is therefore good at ruling people out.**

$$\text{False-}\ominus\text{ ratio} = 1 - \text{sensitivity}$$

■ **Specificity** is the probability that a patient without a disease will have a ⊖ test result. **A specific test will rarely determine that someone has the disease when in fact they do not and is therefore good at ruling people in.**

$$\text{False-}\oplus\text{ ratio} = 1 - \text{specificity}$$

Incidence is measured with a cohort study; prevalence is measured with a prevalence study.

Another name for a prevalence study is a cross-sectional study.

SnOUT: Sensitive tests rule **OUT** disease.
SpIN: Specific tests rule **IN** disease.

	Disease Present	No Disease	
Positive test	a	b	$PPV = a / (a + b)$
Negative test	c	d	$NPV = d / (c + d)$
	Sensitivity = a / (a + c)	Specificity = d / (b + d)	

FIGURE 2.4-1. **Sensitivity, specificity, PPV, and NPV.**

- The ideal test is both sensitive and specific, but a trade-off must often be made between sensitivity and specificity.
  - **High sensitivity** is particularly desirable when there is a significant penalty for missing a disease. It is also desirable early in a diagnostic workup, when it is necessary to reduce a broad differential.
  - **High specificity** is useful for confirming a likely diagnosis or for situations in which false-$\oplus$ results may prove harmful.

Positive and Negative Predictive Values

Once a test has been administered and a patient's result has been made available, that result must be interpreted through use of predictive values (or posttest probabilities):

- The **positive predictive value (PPV)** is the probability that a patient with a $\oplus$ test result truly has the disease. The more specific a test, the higher its PPV. The higher the disease prevalence, the higher the PPV of the test for that disease.
- The **negative predictive value (NPV)** is the probability that a patient with a $\ominus$ test result truly does not have the disease. The more sensitive a test, the higher its NPV. The lower the disease prevalence, the higher the NPV of the test for that disease.

Likelihood Ratio

Another way to describe the performance of a diagnostic test involves the use of **likelihood ratios (LRs),** which express how much more or less likely a given test result is in diseased as opposed to nondiseased people:

$$\oplus\,LR = \frac{\text{Diseased people with a } \oplus \text{ test result}}{\text{Nondiseased people with a } \oplus \text{ test result}} = \frac{\text{Sensitivity}}{1 - \text{specificity}}$$

$$\ominus\,LR = \frac{\text{Diseased people with a } \ominus \text{ test result}}{\text{Nondiseased people with a } \ominus \text{ test result}} = \frac{1 - \text{sensitivity}}{\text{Specificity}}$$

ASSESSMENT OF RISK

Knowledge of risk factors may be used to predict future disease in a given patient. Risk factors may be causal (immediate or distant causes of disease) or disease markers (in which removing the risk factor does not necessarily ↓ the likelihood of disease). Risk factors can be difficult to discover for a variety of reasons, including the following:

- A disease may have a long latency period, with risky exposures remote and forgotten.
- A risky exposure may be so common that its impact is hard to discern.
- Disease incidence may be low, and it is hard to draw conclusions from infrequent events.
- Risk associated with any individual exposure is small and hard to parse out.
- There is seldom a close, constant relationship between a risk factor and a disease.

Because the predictive value of a test is affected by disease prevalence, it is advantageous to apply diagnostic tests to patients with an ↑ likelihood of having the disease being sought (i.e., an at-risk population).

If a test has an LR of 1, it does not change the pretest probability of disease. If the LR is 10, it makes disease 45% more likely. If the LR is 0.1, disease is 45% less likely.

Pretest probability = disease prevalence.

The best way to determine whether an exposure actually ↑ disease risk is with a study. The ideal study for risk factor assessment would be an experiment in which the researcher controls risk exposure and then relates it to disease incidence. Doing so, however, may be unethical as well as prohibitively intrusive, time-consuming, and expensive. Instead, observational studies such as cohort or case-control studies are used to determine risk.

Cohort Studies

In a **cohort study**, a group of people is assembled, **none of whom have the outcome of interest** (i.e., the disease), but **all of whom could potentially experience that outcome.** For each possible risk factor, the members of the cohort are classified as either exposed or unexposed. All the cohort members are then followed over time, and **rates of outcome events are compared in the two exposure groups.**

- **Advantages** of cohort studies are as follows:
    - They follow the same logic as the clinical question (if people are exposed, will they get the disease?).
    - They are the only way to directly establish incidence (i.e., absolute risk).
    - They can be used to assess the relationship of a given exposure to many diseases.
    - In prospective studies, exposure is elicited without bias from a known outcome.
- The **disadvantages** of such studies include the following:
    - They can be time-consuming and expensive, especially in the case of prospective studies.
    - Studies assess only the relationship of the disease to the few exposure factors recorded at the start of the study.
    - They require many subjects and are thus inefficient and cannot be used to study rare diseases.

Case-Control Studies

Case-control studies are essentially cohort studies in reverse. In such studies, a researcher selects **two groups—one with the disease in question (cases) and one without (controls)—and then looks back in time to measure the comparative frequency of exposure to a possible risk factor** in the two groups.

- The validity of a case-control study depends on **appropriate selection of cases and controls, the manner in which exposure is measured, and the manner in which extraneous variables (confounders) are dealt with.**
    - Cases and controls should be comparable—i.e., they are members of the same base population with an equal opportunity of risk factor exposure.
    - Cases should be newly diagnosed using explicit criteria for diagnosis.
    - Exposures should be assessed in as unbiased a fashion as possible.
    - Confounding may be ↓ by matching subjects or through the stratification/standardization of subjects. Multivariable analysis may be helpful in this context.

Cohort studies are also known as longitudinal studies, prospective studies, and incidence studies.

Cohort studies may be prospective—in which a cohort is assembled in the present and followed into the future—or they may be retrospective, in which a cohort is identified from past records and followed to the present.

- **Advantages** of such studies are as follows:
  - Studies use small groups, thereby reducing expense.
  - They can be used to study rare diseases and can easily examine multiple risk factors.
- **Disadvantages** include the following:
  - Studies cannot calculate disease prevalence, incidence, or relative risk, because the numbers of subjects with and without a disease are determined artificially by the investigator rather than by nature (an odds ratio can be used to estimate relative risk).
  - Retrospective data may be inaccurate owing to recall or survivorship biases.

Another name for a case-control study is a retrospective study.

MEASURES OF EFFECT

There are several ways to express and compare risk. These include the following:

- **Absolute risk:** Defined as the incidence of disease.
- **Attributable risk (or risk difference):** The additional incidence of disease that is due to a risky exposure, on top of the background incidence from other causes.

Attributable risk = Incidence of disease in exposed − Incidence in unexposed

- **Relative risk (or risk ratio):** Expresses how much more likely an exposed person is to get disease in comparison to an unexposed person. This indicates the **strength of the association between exposure and disease**, making it useful when one is considering disease etiology.

$$\text{Relative risk} = \frac{\text{Incidence in exposed}}{\text{Incidence in unexposed}}$$

- **Odds ratio:** An estimate of relative risk that is used in case-control studies. The odds ratio tells how much more likely it is that a person with a disease has been exposed to a risk factor than someone without the disease. The lower the disease incidence, the more closely it approximates relative risk (see Figure 2.4-2).

$$\text{Odds ratio} = \frac{\text{Odds that a diseased person is exposed}}{\text{Odds that a nondiseased person is exposed}}$$

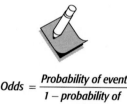

$$Odds = \frac{Probability\ of\ event}{1 - probability\ of\ event}$$

$$Probability = \frac{Odds}{1 + odds}$$

	Disease Develops	No Disease	
Exposure	a	b	$RR = \dfrac{a/(a+b)}{c/(c+d)}$
No exposure	c	d	$OR = ad/bc$

FIGURE 2.4-2. Relative risk (RR) vs. odds ratio (OR).

Once a diagnosis has been established, it is important to be able to describe the associated prognosis. **Survival analysis is used to summarize the average time from one event (e.g., presentation, diagnosis, or start of treatment) to any outcome that can occur only once during follow-up (e.g., death or recurrence of cancer).** The usual method is with a Kaplan-Meier curve (see Figure 2.4-3) describing the survival (or time-to-event if the measured outcome is not death) in a cohort of patients, with the probability of survival decreasing over time as patients die or drop out (are censored) from the study.

TREATMENT

Studies may be used to judge the best treatment for a disease. Although the gold standard for such evaluation is a randomized controlled trial, other types of studies may be used as well (e.g., an observational study, in which the exposure in question is a therapeutic intervention).

Randomized Controlled Trials

A randomized controlled trial is **an experimental, prospective study in which subjects are randomly assigned to a treatment or control group.** Random assignment helps ensure that the two groups are truly comparable. The control group may be treated with a placebo or with the accepted standard of care. The study **may be blinded** in one of two ways: single-blind, in which patients do not know which treatment group they are in, or double-blind, in which neither the patients nor their physicians know who is in which group. Double-blind studies are the gold standard for studying treatment effects.

- **Advantages** of randomized controlled trials are as follows:
    - They involve minimal bias.
    - They have the potential to demonstrate causal relationships.

Randomization minimizes bias and confounding; double-blinded studies prevent observation bias.

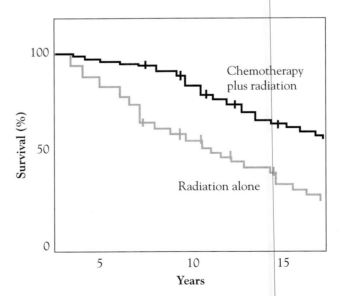

FIGURE 2.4-3. **Example of a Kaplan-Meier curve.**

- **Disadvantages** include the following:
  - They are costly and time-intensive.
  - Informed consent may be difficult to obtain.
  - Some interventions (e.g., surgery) are not amendable to blinding.

Bias

Defined as **any process that → results systematically differing from the truth.** Good studies and data analyses seek to minimize potential bias. Observational studies are particularly susceptible to bias, whereas studies that are blinded and randomized are better protected from the effects of bias. There are a number of types of biases, including the following:

- **Selection bias:** Occurs when comparisons are made between groups of patients that differ in determinants of outcome other than the one being studied.
- **Measurement bias:** A type of bias in which the measurement or data-gathering methods used differ in different groups of patients, thereby distorting the data.
- **Confounding bias:** Occurs when variables are associated with each other such that the effect of one is confused with that of the other.
- **Recall bias:** Bias that may occur in retrospective studies as a result of errors of memory.
- **Lead-time bias:** Bias in which disease is identified earlier, giving an appearance of prolonged survival when in fact the natural course is not altered.
- **Length bias:** Occurs when screening tests detect a disproportionate number of slowly progressive diseases but miss rapidly progressive ones → overestimation of the benefit of the screen.

Chance

Even with bias reduction, unsystematic random error is unavoidable owing to chance variation in studied data. Types of errors are as follows:

- **Type I (α) error:**
  - Defined as the probability of saying that there is a difference in treatment effects between groups when in fact there is not (i.e., a false-$\oplus$ conclusion).
  - The **p-value** is an estimate of the probability that differences in treatment effects in a study could have happened by chance alone. Classically, differences associated with a $p < 0.05$ are statistically significant.
- **Type II (β) error:**
  - Defined as the probability of saying that there is no difference in treatment effects (i.e., a false-$\ominus$ conclusion).
  - **Power** is the probability that a study will find a statistically significant difference when one is truly there. It relates directly to the number of subjects. Power (β) = 1 – type II error.
- The **confidence interval (CI)** is a way of expressing statistical significance (p-value) that shows the size of the effect and the statistical power. CIs are interpreted as follows:
  - There is a 95% chance that the interval contains the true effect size, which is likely to be closest to the point estimate near the center of the interval.
  - If the CI includes the value corresponding to a relative risk of 1.0 (i.e., zero treatment difference), the results are not statistically significant.
  - If the CI is wide, power is low.

- There are three levels of prevention:
  - **1° prevention** includes measures to ↓ the incidence of disease.
  - **2° prevention** includes measures that detect disease early, when it is asymptomatic or mild, and can thus halt or slow disease progression.
  - **3° prevention** includes measures that ↓ morbidity or mortality resulting from the presence of disease.
- Prevention may be accomplished by a **combination of immunization, chemoprevention, behavioral counseling, and screening.** A good screening test has the following characteristics:
  - It has high sensitivity and specificity.
  - It has a high PPV.
  - It is inexpensive, easy to administer, and safe.
  - Treatment after screening is more effective than subsequent treatment without screening.

Vaccination

- Vaccines work by mimicking infections and triggering an immune response in which memory cells are formed to recognize and fight any future infection. There are several different vaccine formulations, as indicated in Table 2.4-1.
- Recommended vaccination schedules for children and adults are outlined in Figures 2.4-4 and 2.4-5.
- **Live vaccines should not be administered to immunosuppressed patients.** Such vaccines are also **contraindicated in pregnant women** owing to a theoretical risk of transmission of the virus to the fetus.

Chemoprevention

Defined as the use of drugs to prevent disease. Examples include supplementation of water and food with healthful vitamins and minerals; aspirin prophylaxis for heart disease; statin treatment for hypercholesterolemia; and perioperative β-blockade.

TABLE 2.4-1. Types of Vaccinations

VACCINE TYPE	TARGETED DISEASES
Live, attenuated	Measles, mumps, rubella, polio (Sabin), yellow fever.
Inactivated (killed)	Cholera, influenza, HAV, polio (Salk), rabies.
Toxoid	Diphtheria, tetanus.
Subunit	HBV, pertussis, *Streptococcus pneumoniae*, HPV, meningococcus.
Conjugate	Hib, *S. pneumoniae.*

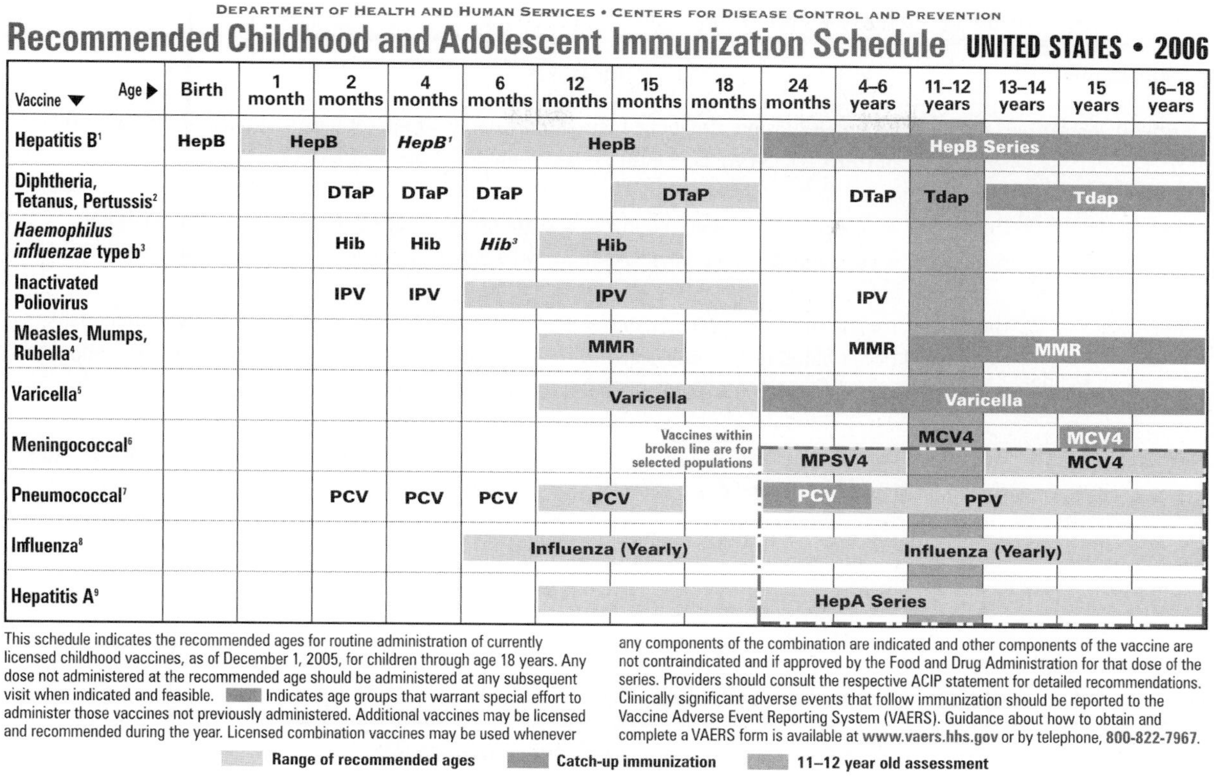

Recommended Childhood and Adolescent Immunization Schedule UNITED STATES • 2006

Vaccine ▼ Age ▶	Birth	1 month	2 months	4 months	6 months	12 months	15 months	18 months	24 months	4–6 years	11–12 years	13–14 years	15 years	16–18 years
Hepatitis B[1]	HepB	HepB		HepB[1]		HepB					HepB Series			
Diphtheria, Tetanus, Pertussis[2]			DTaP	DTaP	DTaP		DTaP			DTaP	Tdap	Tdap		
Haemophilus influenzae type b[3]			Hib	Hib	Hib[3]	Hib								
Inactivated Poliovirus			IPV	IPV		IPV				IPV				
Measles, Mumps, Rubella[4]						MMR				MMR	MMR			
Varicella[5]						Varicella				Varicella				
Meningococcal[6]							Vaccines within broken line are for selected populations		MPSV4		MCV4	MCV4	MCV4	
Pneumococcal[7]			PCV	PCV	PCV	PCV			PCV	PPV				
Influenza[8]						Influenza (Yearly)				Influenza (Yearly)				
Hepatitis A[9]						HepA Series								

This schedule indicates the recommended ages for routine administration of currently licensed childhood vaccines, as of December 1, 2005, for children through age 18 years. Any dose not administered at the recommended age should be administered at any subsequent visit when indicated and feasible. ▓▓▓▓ Indicates age groups that warrant special effort to administer those vaccines not previously administered. Additional vaccines may be licensed and recommended during the year. Licensed combination vaccines may be used whenever

any components of the combination are indicated and other components of the vaccine are not contraindicated and if approved by the Food and Drug Administration for that dose of the series. Providers should consult the respective ACIP statement for detailed recommendations. Clinically significant adverse events that follow immunization should be reported to the Vaccine Adverse Event Reporting System (VAERS). Guidance about how to obtain and complete a VAERS form is available at www.vaers.hhs.gov or by telephone, 800-822-7967.

▓ Range of recommended ages   ▓ Catch-up immunization   ▓ 11–12 year old assessment

FIGURE 2.4-4. Recommended vaccinations for children and adolescents.

(Reproduced from the Centers for Disease Control and Prevention, Atlanta, GA, www.cdc.gov/nip/recs/child-schedule-color-print.pdf.)

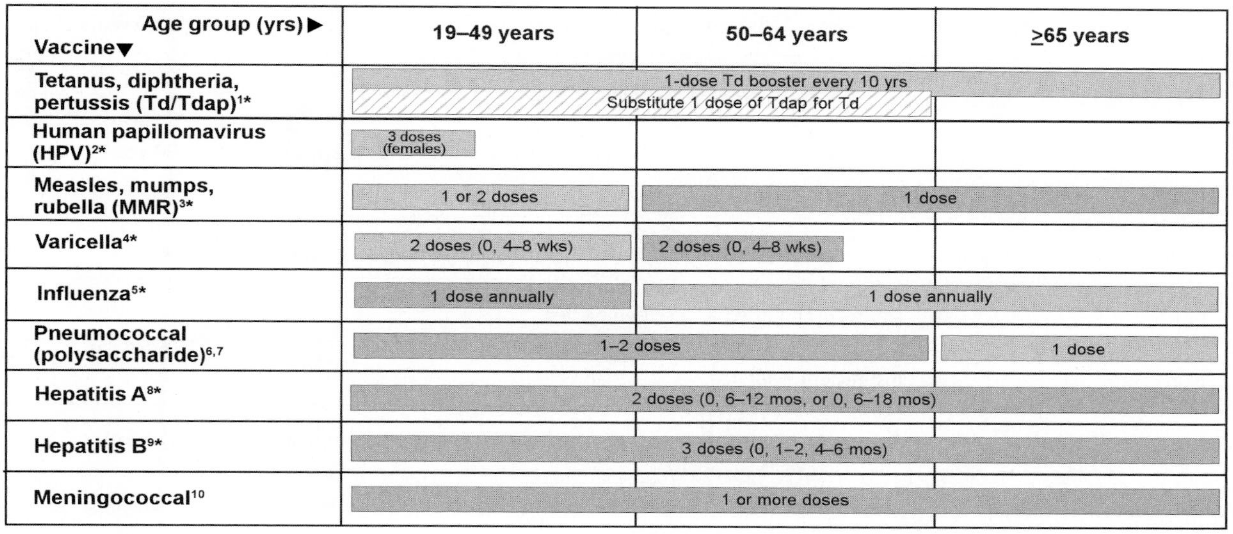

Age group (yrs) ▶ Vaccine ▼	19–49 years	50–64 years	≥65 years
Tetanus, diphtheria, pertussis (Td/Tdap)[1*]	1-dose Td booster every 10 yrs		
	Substitute 1 dose of Tdap for Td		
Human papillomavirus (HPV)[2*]	3 doses (females)		
Measles, mumps, rubella (MMR)[3*]	1 or 2 doses	1 dose	
Varicella[4*]	2 doses (0, 4–8 wks)	2 doses (0, 4–8 wks)	
Influenza[5*]	1 dose annually	1 dose annually	
Pneumococcal (polysaccharide)[6,7]	1–2 doses		1 dose
Hepatitis A[8*]	2 doses (0, 6–12 mos, or 0, 6–18 mos)		
Hepatitis B[9*]	3 doses (0, 1–2, 4–6 mos)		
Meningococcal[10]	1 or more doses		

FIGURE 2.4-5. Recommended vaccinations for adults.

(Reproduced from the Centers for Disease Control and Prevention, Atlanta, GA, http://www.cdc.gov/Nip/ home-hcp.htm.)

HIGH-YIELD FACTS

EPIDEMIOLOGY

T A B L E   2 . 4 - 2 .   Health Screening Methods by Age

AGE GROUP	MEASURES
Birth–10 years	Height and weight, BP, vision screening, hemoglobinopathy screen (at birth), phenylalanine level (at birth), TSH and/or T_4 (at birth), lead level (at least one time before six years of age).
11–24 years	Height and weight, BP, Pap smear, chlamydia and gonorrhea (GC) screen (if sexually active), rubella serology or vaccination (women only); screen for risky behaviors, including substance abuse.
25–64 years	Height and weight, BP (every two years), cholesterol (every five years), Pap smear and bimanual pelvic exam, fecal occult blood test (FOBT), sigmoidoscopy or colonoscopy, mammography, rubella serology or vaccination (women only); screen for alcohol abuse and depression.
≥ 65 years	Height and weight, BP, FOBT, sigmoidoscopy or colonoscopy, Pap smear, vision and hearing screening; screen for alcohol abuse and depression.

T A B L E   2 . 4 - 3 .   Health Screening Methods by Modality

MODALITY	RECOMMENDATION[a]
Colonoscopy	Once every 10 years in patients ≥ 50 years of age; screening ≥ 40 years for high-risk patients. Preferred modality if there is a known history of dysplasia.
Flexible sigmoidoscopy	Once every five years in patients ≥ 50 years of age; screening ≥ 40 years for high-risk patients.
FOBT	Once yearly in patients ≥ 50 years of age; screening ≥ 40 years for high-risk patients.
Bimanual pelvic exam	Once every 1–3 years in patients 20–40 years of age; once yearly in patients ≥ 40 years of age.
Pap smear	Once every 1–3 years if sexually active or ≥ 21 years of age.
Mammography	Once every 1–2 years in patients ≥ 40 years of age; once yearly in patients ≥ 50 years of age (controversial).
Endometrial tissue sampling	Not recommended as a screening test; indicated for postmenopausal bleeding.
CXR	Not recommended as a screening test.
Skin exam	Insufficient evidence.
DRE	Offer to high-risk patients at 40 years and to others at 50 years of age (controversial).
PSA	Offer to high-risk patients at 40 years and to others at 50 years of age (controversial).
Clinical breast exam	Offer to patients at 40 years of age or earlier if they are high risk (controversial).

[a] Different medical societies have various recommendations regarding cancer screening. Refer to the National Cancer Institute's Web site for a recent summary of recommendations: www.nci.nih.gov/cancer_information/testing.

Adapted from the National Guideline Clearinghouse, www.guidelines.gov.

Behavioral Counseling

- Counseling patients about their health-related behaviors to ↓ the likelihood of morbidity/mortality is an essential part of routine health care for every population. Which behaviors to address vary with the patient demographic.
  - All patients may benefit from counsel regarding maintenance of a healthy diet, exercise, and sun and injury protection.
  - Adolescent and adult patients should be offered advice about safe sex, smoking cessation, and abuse of alcohol and illicit drugs.
- In offering counsel, physicians should tailor their education and suggestions to the individual patient as well as to his or her **stage of change**—i.e., precontemplation, contemplation, preparation, action, or maintenance. Counseling is most likely to be successful when it accommodates the patient's willingness to change (or lack thereof.)

SCREENING RECOMMENDATIONS

Tables 2.4-2 and 2.4-3 outline recommended health care screening measures by age group and modality.

CAUSES OF DEATH

The leading cause of cancer mortality in the United States is lung cancer. Prostate and breast cancers are the most prevalent cancers in men and women, respectively, with lung and colorectal cancers ranking second and third most common in both sexes. Table 2.4-4 lists the principal causes of death in the United States by age group.

TABLE 2.4-4.   Leading Causes of Death by Age Group

AGE GROUP	VARIABLE
All ages	Heart disease, cancer, stroke, chronic lower respiratory disease, accidents, diabetes.
< 1 year	Congenital anomalies, disorders related to low birth weight, SIDS, maternal complications.
1–4 years	Injuries, congenital anomalies, neoplasms, homicide, heart disease.
5–14 years	Injuries, neoplasms, congenital anomalies, homicide, suicide, heart disease.
15–24 years	Injuries, homicide, suicide, neoplasms, heart disease.
25–44 years	Injuries, neoplasms, heart disease, suicide, **HIV,** homicide.
45–64 years	Neoplasms, heart disease, injuries, stroke, diabetes, chronic lower respiratory disease.
≥ 65 years	Heart disease, neoplasms, stroke, COPD, influenza and pneumonia, diabetes.

Adapted from the National Center for Health Statistics, *Health 2003.*

TABLE 2.4-5.   **Common Reportable Diseases**

DISEASE CATEGORY	EXAMPLES
STDs	HIV, AIDS, syphilis, gonorrhea, chlamydia, chancroid, HCV.
Tick-borne disease	Lyme disease, ehrlichiosis, Rocky Mountain spotted fever.
Potential bioweapons	Anthrax, smallpox, plague.
Vaccine-preventable disease	Diphtheria, tetanus, pertussis, measles, mumps, rubella, polio, varicella (death), HAV, HBV, Hib (invasive), meningococcal disease.
Water-/food-borne disease	Cholera, giardiasis, legionella, listeriosis, botulism, shigellosis, shiga toxin–producing *E. coli*, salmonellosis, trichinellosis, typhoid.
Zoonoses	Tularemia, psittacosis, brucellosis, rabies.
Miscellaneous	TB, leprosy, toxic shock syndrome, SARS, West Nile virus, MRSA, VRSA, coccidioidomycosis, cryptosporidiosis.

REPORTABLE DISEASES

By law, disease reporting is mandated at the state level, and the list of diseases that must be reported to public health authorities varies slightly by state. The CDC has a list of nationally notifiable diseases that states voluntarily report to the CDC. These diseases include but are not limited to those listed in Table 2.4-5.

Ethics and Legal Issues

GENERAL PRINCIPLES

- **Autonomy:** Clinicians are obligated to respect patients as individuals and to honor their preferences in medical care.
- **Beneficence:** Physicians have a responsibility to act in the patient's best interest ("the physician is a fiduciary"). Patient autonomy may conflict with beneficence.
- **Nonmaleficence:** "Do no harm." If the benefits of an intervention outweigh the risks, however, a patient may make an informed decision to consent and proceed.
- **Paternalism:** Physicians at times make decisions for their patients, or act to prevent a patient from carrying out a decision, on the premise that it is for the patient's benefit. Like beneficence, this may conflict with patient autonomy and thus should rarely be invoked.

INFORMED CONSENT

> **BRAIN of Informed Consent:**
>
> **B**enefits
> **R**isks
> **A**lternatives
> **I**ndications
> **N**ature

- Defined as willing acceptance (without coercion) of a medical intervention by a patient after adequate discussion with a physician about the **nature** of the intervention, **indications, risks, benefits,** and potential **alternatives** (including no treatment).
- **Patients may change their minds at any time.** Exceptions include the following:
  - When emergency treatment is required (consent is implied).
  - When patients lack decision-making capacity (consent can be obtained from a surrogate decision maker).

MINORS

- **Consent for treatment** is implied in life-threatening situations when parents cannot be contacted.
- Emancipated minors do not require parental consent for medical care. Minors are emancipated if they are married or in the armed services.
- Minors are considered emancipated for the purposes of obtaining medical care for **pregnancy, sexually transmitted infections,** or **drug or alcohol abuse.**
- If a parent requests information about an emancipated minor, confidentiality can be broken only with the patient's permission or if the minor presents a danger to him/herself or to others.
- **Refusal of treatment:** A parent has the right to refuse treatment for his/her child as long as those decisions do not pose a serious threat to the child's well-being (e.g., refusing immunizations is not considered a serious threat). If a decision is not in the best interest of the child, a physician may seek a court order to provide treatment against parental wishes. In emergent situations, if withholding treatment jeopardizes the child's safety, treatment can be initiated on the basis of legal precedent.

COMPETENCE AND DECISION-MAKING CAPACITY

- **Competence:** Refers to a person's legal capacity to make decisions and be held accountable in a court of law. Competence is assessed by the courts and may be used interchangeably with the term *decision-making capacity.*
- **Decision-making capacity:** A medical term that refers to the ability of a patient to understand relevant information, appreciate the severity of the

medical situation and its consequences, communicate a choice, and deliberate rationally about one's values in relation to the decision being made.

- Patients who have decision-making capacity have the right to refuse or discontinue treatment (e.g., Jehovah's Witnesses can refuse blood products).
- Incompetent patients, as assessed by the courts, or temporarily incapacitated patients (e.g., intoxicated patients with altered mental status) cannot decide to accept or refuse treatment.

END-OF-LIFE ISSUES

Written Advance Directives

- **Living will:** Addresses a patient's wishes to maintain, withhold, or withdraw life-sustaining treatment in the event of terminal disease or a persistent vegetative state. Examples include **DNR** (do not resuscitate) and **DNI** (do not intubate) orders.
- **Durable power of attorney (DPOA):** Legally designates a surrogate health care decision maker if a patient lacks decision-making capacity. **More flexible** than a living will. Surrogates should make decisions consistent with the person's stated wishes.
- If no living will or DPOA exists, decisions should be made by close family members (spouse, adult children, parents, and adult siblings), friends, or personal physicians, in that order.

*DNR/DNI orders do **not** mean "do not treat."*

Withdrawal of Care

- Patients and their decision makers have the right to forgo life-sustaining treatment.
- There is **no ethical distinction between withholding and withdrawing life-sustaining interventions.** These include ventilation, fluids, nutrition, and medications (e.g., antibiotics).
- It is ethical to provide palliative treatment to relieve pain and suffering even if such treatment may hasten a patient's death, provided that the intent is to relieve suffering and the medications administered are titrated for that purpose.

It is ethical to provide palliative treatment even through it may hasten a patient's death.

Euthanasia and Physician-Assisted Suicide

- **Euthanasia** is the administration of a lethal agent with the intent to end life.
  - It is opposed by the AMA Code of Medical Ethics and **is illegal.**
  - Patients who request euthanasia should be evaluated for inadequate pain control and comorbid depression.
- **Physician-assisted suicide** is prescribing a lethal agent to a patient who will self-administer it to end his/her own life. This is currently legal only in the state of Oregon.

Futility

Physicians are not ethically obligated to provide treatment and may refuse a family member's request for further intervention on the grounds of futility under the following circumstances:

- There is no pathophysiologic rationale for treatment.
- Maximal intervention is currently failing.

- A given intervention has already failed.
- Treatment will not achieve the goals of care.

Full Disclosure

- Patients have a right to know about their medical status, prognosis, and treatment options (full disclosure).
- A patient's family cannot require that a doctor withhold information from the patient.
- A doctor may withhold information only if the patient requests not to be told or in the rare case when a physician determines that disclosure would severely harm the patient or undermine their informed decision-making capacity (**therapeutic privilege**).

Medical Errors

- **Physicians are obligated to inform patients of mistakes made in their medical treatment.**
- In events where the specific error or series of errors is not known, the physician should communicate this with the family promptly and maintain contact with the patient as investigations further reveal facts of the case.

Clinical Research

- Physicians are obligated to inform patients considering involvement in a clinical research protocol about the purpose of the research study and the entire study design as it will affect the patient's treatment. This includes the possible risks, benefits, and alternatives to the research protocol.
- An informed consent form approved by the overseeing research institutional review board (IRB) should be completed for participation in any clinical research protocol, describing the possible risks and benefits of involvement in the research study.

- Information disclosed by a patient to his/her physician and information about a patient's medical condition are confidential and cannot be divulged without expressed patient consent.
- A patient may waive the right to confidentiality (e.g., with insurance companies).
- It is ethically and legally necessary to override confidentiality in the following situations:
    - **Patient intent to commit a violent crime (Tarasoff decision):** Physicians have a **duty to protect** the intended victim through reasonable means (e.g., warn the victim, notify police).
    - Suicidal patients.
    - Child and elder abuse.
    - Infectious diseases (duty to warn public officials and identifiable people at risk).
    - Gunshot and knife wounds (duty to notify the police).
    - Impaired automobile drivers (e.g., the department of motor vehicles requires that licensed drivers be seizure free for at least six months).

Tarasoff decision: Duty to warn/protect if a patient intends to commit a crime or harm others.

CONFLICT OF INTEREST

- Occurs when physicians find themselves having two interests in a given situation and their professional obligations are influenced by personal interest in another matter.
- **Example:** A physician may own stock in a pharmaceutical company (financial interest) that produces a drug he is prescribing to his patient (patient care interest).
- Physicians should disclose existing conflicts of interest to affected parties (e.g., patients, institutions, the audience of a journal article, scientific meeting).

MALPRACTICE

- The essential elements of a civil suit under negligence include the **four D's:**
  - The physician has a **D**uty to the patient.
  - **D**ereliction of duty occurs.
  - There is **D**amage to the patient.
  - Dereliction is the **D**irect cause of damage.
- Unlike a criminal suit, in which the burden of proof is "beyond a reasonable doubt," the burden of proof in a malpractice suit is "a preponderance of the evidence."

> *The 4 D's of malpractice:*
>
> **D**uty
> **D**ereliction
> **D**amage
> **D**irect cause

Gastrointestinal

Dysphagia/Odynophagia

Difficulty swallowing (dysphagia) or pain with swallowing (odynophagia) due to abnormalities of the oropharynx or esophagus. Etiologic factors include achalasia, peptic stricture, infectious esophagitis, eosinophilic esophagitis, esophageal webs, rings, or diverticula (Zenker's), carcinoma, scleroderma, spastic motility disorders, Sjögren's syndrome, medications, and radiation injury.

Squamous esophageal cancer is associated with tobacco and alcohol use.

HISTORY/PE

- Oropharyngeal dysphagia usually involves **liquids** more than solids and may be accompanied by dysarthria or dysphonia.
- Esophageal dysphagia usually involves **solids** more than liquids for most **obstructive** causes and is generally progressive; **motility** disorders (achalasia, scleroderma, esophageal spasm) present with **both** liquid and solid dysphagia.
- Examine for masses (e.g., goiter, tumor) and anatomical defects.

Esophageal webs are associated with iron deficiency anemia (Plummer-Vinson syndrome).

DIAGNOSIS

- **Oropharyngeal dysphagia:** Cine-esophagram.
- **Esophageal dysphagia:** Barium swallow followed by endoscopy, manometry, and/or pH monitoring. If an obstructive lesion is suspected, proceed directly to endoscopy with biopsy.
- **Odynophagia:** Upper endoscopy.

TREATMENT

Etiology dependent. Endoscopic dilation for benign peptic strictures.

Infectious Esophagitis

- Most often occurs in **immunosuppressed** patients. The most common pathogens are *Candida albicans*, **HSV**, and **CMV**.
- Hx/PE: Patients present with odynophagia, dysphagia, and/or substernal chest pain.
- Dx/Tx: Table 2.6-1 summarizes the diagnosis and treatment of the various causes of infectious esophagitis.

Candidal esophagitis is associated with AIDS.

TABLE 2.6-1. **Causes of Infectious Esophagitis**

ETIOLOGIC AGENT	EXAM FINDINGS	UPPER ENDOSCOPY	TREATMENT
Candida albicans	Oral thrush	Yellow-white plaques adherent to the mucosa.	Fluconazole PO
HSV	Oral ulcers	Small, deep ulcerations; multinucleated giant cells with nuclear inclusions on biopsy.	Acyclovir IV
CMV	Retinitis, colitis	Large, superficial ulcerations; intranuclear inclusions on biopsy.	Ganciclovir IV

HIGH-YIELD FACTS

GASTROINTESTINAL

Diffuse Esophageal Spasm

- Results from **nonperistaltic contractions** of the esophagus.
- Hx/PE: Presents with dysphagia, odynophagia, and/or chest pain, often precipitated by ingestion of hot or cold liquids and relieved by nitroglycerin.
- Dx: **Barium swallow** may show a **corkscrew**-shaped esophagus. **Esophageal manometry** reveals high-amplitude, simultaneous contractions.
- Tx: Nitrates and calcium channel blockers (CCBs) for symptomatic relief; surgery (esophageal myotomy) for severe, incapacitating symptoms.

Achalasia

A motor disorder of the esophagus characterized by **impaired relaxation of the lower esophageal sphincter (LES)** and loss of peristalsis in the distal two-thirds of the esophagus. Thought to result from the loss of inhibitory interneurons in Auerbach's plexus.

HISTORY/PE

- Progressive dysphagia, chest pain, regurgitation of undigested food, weight loss, and nocturnal cough are common symptoms.
- 2°causes of achalasia include **malignancy** (gastric carcinoma, lymphoma) and Chagas' disease. 2° achalasia may present with greater weight loss and a shorter duration of symptoms in older patients.

Malignancy may mimic achalasia (pseudoachalasia).

DIAGNOSIS

- **Barium swallow** reveals esophageal **dilation** with a "bird's beak" tapering of the distal esophagus (see Figure 2.6-1).
- **Manometry** shows ↑ **resting LES pressure** with **incomplete relaxation upon swallowing** and ↓ **peristalsis** in the body of the esophagus.
- Endoscopy may be helpful for excluding 2° causes of achalasia.

TREATMENT

Nitrates, CCBs, or endoscopic injection of botulinum toxin into the LES may provide short-term relief of symptoms. Pneumatic dilation or surgical myotomy may result in long-term relief.

Esophageal Cancer

- **Squamous cell carcinoma** and **adenocarcinoma** are **equally common types of esophageal cancer.** The latter is associated with Barrett's esophagus (columnar metaplasia of the distal esophagus 2° to chronic GERD).
- Risk factors include alcohol use, male gender, smoking, and age > 50 years.
- Hx/PE: Progressive dysphagia, initially to solids and later to liquids, is common. Weight loss, odynophagia, GERD, GI bleeding, and vomiting are also seen.
- Dx: Barium study shows narrowing of the esophagus with an irregular border protruding into the lumen. EGD and biopsy confirm the diagnosis. CT and endoscopic ultrasound are used for staging.
- Tx: Chemoradiation therapy is used, but the prognosis is poor. Surgical resection can be beneficial in some cases. Patients may require an endoscopically placed esophageal stent for palliation and improved quality of life.

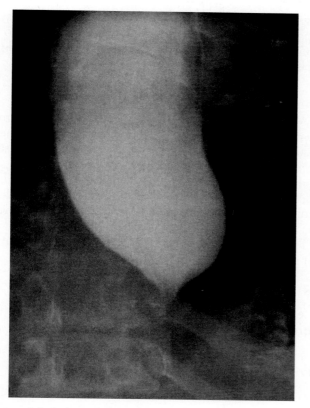

FIGURE 2.6-1. Achalasia.

Barium esophagram reveals esophageal dilation with a "bird's beak" tapering of the distal esophagus. (Reprinted from *Med Clin North Am* 65, Waters PF, DeMeester TR. Foregut motor disorders and their surgical management, page 1235, Copyright 1981, with permission from Elsevier.)

Gastroesophageal Reflux Disease (GERD)

Symptomatic reflux of gastric contents into the esophagus, most commonly as a result of **transient LES relaxation.** Can be due to an incompetent LES, gastroparesis, or hiatal hernia. Risk factors include ↑ intra-abdominal pressure (e.g., obesity, pregnancy), scleroderma, alcohol, caffeine, nicotine, chocolate, peppermint, and fatty foods.

HISTORY/PE

- Patients present with **heartburn** that commonly occurs 30–90 minutes **after a meal, worsens with reclining,** and often improves with antacids, sitting, or standing.
- Sour taste ("water brash"), laryngitis, dysphagia, and cough or wheezing are also seen.
- Exam is usually **normal** unless a systemic disease (e.g., scleroderma) is present.

DIAGNOSIS

- History and clinical impression.
- Diagnosis may include barium swallow (of limited usefulness, but can diagnose hiatal hernia), esophageal manometry, and 24-hour pH monitoring.

BARR*ett's—*

Becomes
Adenocarcinoma,
Results from **R**eflux.

Risk factors for GERD include hiatal hernia and ↑ intra-abdominal pressure.

GERD can mimic asthma.

- **EGD** with biopsies should be performed in patients with symptoms that are unresponsive to initial empiric therapy, long-standing (to rule out Barrett's esophagus and adenocarcinoma), or suggestive of complicated disease (anorexia, weight loss, dysphagia/odynophagia).

TREATMENT

- **Lifestyle:** Weight loss, head-of-bed elevation, reduction of meal size, and avoidance of nocturnal meals and substances that ↓ LES tone.
- **Health maintenance:** Monitor for Barrett's esophagus and esophageal adenocarcinoma with **serial EGD and biopsy.**
- **Pharmacologic:** Start with **antacids** in patients with mild, intermittent symptoms; use **H$_2$ receptor antagonists** (cimetidine, ranitidine) or **PPIs** (omeprazole, lansoprazole) in patients with chronic and frequent symptoms. PPIs are preferred for severe or erosive disease.
- **Surgical:** For refractory or severe disease, **Nissen fundoplication** may offer significant relief.

COMPLICATIONS

Esophagitis, esophageal stricture, aspiration of gastric contents, upper GI bleeding, **Barrett's esophagus.**

Patients with GERD should avoid caffeine, alcohol, chocolate, garlic, onions, mints, and nicotine.

Hiatal Hernia

- Herniation of a portion of the stomach upward into the chest through a diaphragmatic opening. There are two common types:
    - **Sliding hiatal hernias (95%):** The gastroesophageal junction and a portion of the stomach are displaced above the diaphragm.
    - **Paraesophageal hiatal hernias (5%):** The gastroesophageal junction remains below the diaphragm, while a neighboring portion of the fundus herniates into the mediastinum.
- **Hx/PE:** May be asymptomatic. Those with sliding hernias may present with GERD.
- **Dx:** Commonly an incidental finding on CXR, but frequently diagnosed by barium swallow or EGD.
- **Tx:**
    - **Sliding hernias:** Medical therapy and lifestyle modifications to ↓ GERD symptoms.
    - **Paraesophageal hernias:** Surgical gastropexy (attachment of the stomach to the rectus sheath and closure of the hiatus) is recommended to prevent gastric volvulus.

DISORDERS OF THE STOMACH AND DUODENUM

Gastritis

Inflammation of the stomach lining. Subtypes are as follows:

- **Acute gastritis:** Rapidly developing, superficial lesions that are often due to **NSAIDs,** alcohol, *H. pylori* infection, and stress from severe illness (e.g., burns, CNS injury).
- **Chronic gastritis:**
    - **Type A (10%):** Occurs in the fundus and is due to **autoantibodies to parietal cells.** Associated with other autoimmune disorders, including **pernicious anemia** and thyroiditis, as well as with an ↑ risk of gastric adenocarcinoma.

- **Type B (90%):** Occurs in the antrum and may be caused by NSAID use or **H. pylori infection.** Often asymptomatic, but associated with an ↑ risk of PUD and gastric cancer.

HISTORY/PE

Patients may be asymptomatic or may complain of epigastric pain, nausea, vomiting, hematemesis, or melena.

DIAGNOSIS

- Upper endoscopy can help visualize the gastric lining.
- *H. pylori* infection can be detected by urease breath test, serum IgG antibody (indicating exposure, not current infection), *H. pylori* stool antigen, or endoscopic biopsy.

TREATMENT

- ↓ intake of offending agents. Antacids, sucralfate, H_2 blockers, and/or PPIs may help.
- Use triple therapy (amoxicillin, clarithromycin, omeprazole) to treat *H. pylori* infection.
- Give a prophylactic H_2 blocker or PPI for patients at risk for stress ulcers (e.g., ICU patients).

Type A gastritis is associated with pernicious anemia due to the lack of intrinsic factor necessary for the absorption of vitamin B_{12}

Gastric Cancer

- This malignant tumor is the second most common cause of cancer-related death worldwide. Tumors are generally adenocarcinomas, which exhibit two morphologic types:
  - **Intestinal type:** Thought to arise from intestinal metaplasia of **gastric mucosal cells.** Risk factors include a diet high in nitrites and salt and low in fresh vegetables (antioxidants), *H. pylori* colonization, and chronic gastritis.
  - **Diffuse type:** Tends to be poorly differentiated and not associated with *H. pylori* infection or chronic gastritis. Risk factors are largely unknown.
- **Hx/PE:** Advanced cases generally present with abdominal pain, early satiety, and weight loss. Five-year survival is < 10%.
- **Dx:** Early gastric carcinoma is largely asymptomatic and is discovered serendipitously with endoscopic examination of high-risk individuals.
- **Tx:** Successful treatment rests entirely on early detection and surgical removal of the tumor.

Peptic Ulcer Disease (PUD)

Damage to the gastric or duodenal mucosa caused by impaired mucosal defense and/or ↑ acidic gastric contents. **H. pylori** plays a causative role in > 90% of duodenal ulcers and 70% of gastric ulcers. Other risk factors include **corticosteroid, NSAID, alcohol,** and **tobacco** use. Males are affected more often than females.

HISTORY/PE

- Classically presents with chronic or periodic **dull, burning epigastric pain** that **improves with meals** (especially duodenal ulcers), worsens 2–3 hours after eating, and can radiate to the back.

Roughly 5–7% of lower GI bleeds are from an upper GI source.

Rule out Zollinger-Ellison syndrome with serum gastrin levels in cases of GERD and PUD that are refractory to medical management.

Misoprostol can help patients with PUD who require NSAID therapy (e.g., patients with arthritis).

Complications of PUD—

HOPI

Hemorrhage
Obstruction
Perforation
Intractable pain

Zollinger-Ellison syndrome is associated with MEN 1 syndrome in roughly 25–50% of cases.

- Patients may also complain of nausea, hematemesis ("coffee-ground" emesis), or blood in the stool (melena or hematochezia).
- Exam may reveal varying degrees of **epigastric tenderness** and, if there is active bleeding, a ⊕ stool guaiac.
- An acute perforation can present with a rigid abdomen, rebound tenderness, guarding, or other signs of peritoneal irritation.

DIAGNOSIS

- **AXR to rule out perforation** (free air under the diaphragm); CBC to assess for GI bleeding (low or ↓ hematocrit).
- **Upper endoscopy** with biopsy to confirm PUD and to rule out active bleeding or gastric adenocarcinoma (10% of gastric ulcers); barium swallow is an alternative.
- *H. pylori* testing.
- In recurrent or refractory cases, serum gastrin can be used to screen for Zollinger-Ellison syndrome (patients must discontinue PPI use prior to testing).

TREATMENT

- **Acute:**
  - Rule out active bleeding with serial hematocrits, a rectal exam with stool guaiac, and NG lavage.
  - Monitor the patient's hematocrit and BP and initiate IV hydration, transfusion, IV PPIs, endoscopy, and surgery as needed for complications.
  - If perforation is likely, **emergent surgery** is indicated.
- **Pharmacologic:**
  - Involves protecting the mucosa, decreasing acid production, and eradicating *H. pylori* infection.
  - Treat mild disease with antacids or with sucralfate, bismuth, and misoprostol (a prostaglandin analog) for mucosal protection. PPIs or H₂ receptor antagonists may be used to ↓ acid secretion.
  - Patients with confirmed *H. pylori* infection should receive triple therapy (amoxicillin, clarithromycin, and omeprazole).
- Discontinue use of exacerbating agents. Patients with recurrent or severe disease may require chronic symptomatic therapy.
- **Endoscopy and surgery:**
  - Patients with symptomatic gastric ulcers for > 2 **months** that are **refractory** to medical therapy should have either endoscopy or an upper GI series with barium to rule out gastric adenocarcinoma.
  - Refractory cases may require a surgical procedure such as **parietal cell vagotomy** (the most selective and preferred surgical approach).

COMPLICATIONS

Hemorrhage (posterior ulcers that erode into the gastroduodenal artery), gastric outlet obstruction, perforation (usually anterior ulcers), intractable pain.

Zollinger-Ellison Syndrome

- A rare condition characterized by **gastrin-producing tumors** in the duodenum and/or pancreas → oversecretion of gastrin.

- ↑ gastrin → the production of high levels of **gastric acid** by the gastric mucosa → recurrent/intractable **ulcers** in the stomach and duodenum (may occur more distally).
- In 25–50% of cases, gastrinomas are associated with MEN 1.
- **Hx/PE:** Patients may present with unresponsive, recurrent **gnawing, burning abdominal pain** as well as with **diarrhea,** nausea, vomiting, fatigue, weakness, weight loss, and **GI bleeding.**
- **Dx:** ↑ fasting serum gastrin levels are characteristic. Octreotide scan and endoscopic ultrasound can be used to localize the 1° tumor.
- **Tx:**
  - Requires ↓ **acid production.** H_2 blockers are typically ineffective, but a moderate- to high-dose PPI often controls symptoms.
  - Surgical repair of peptic ulcers and/or removal of tumor can be beneficial in refractory cases.
  - Since roughly 50% of gastrinomas are malignant, close **follow-up** is mandatory.

DISORDERS OF THE SMALL BOWEL

Diarrhea

Defined as the production of **> 200 g of feces per day along with ↑ frequency or ↓ consistency of stool.** Risk factors include viral/bacterial GI infection, systemic infection, sick contacts, immunosuppression, recent antibiotic use, and recent travel.

HISTORY/PE

Common presentations of diarrhea are as follows (see also Table 2.6-2):

- **Acute diarrhea:**
  - Acute onset with < 2 weeks of symptoms; usually infectious and self-limited.
  - Causes include bacteria with preformed toxins (e.g., *S. aureus, Bacillus cereus*), noninvasive bacteria (e.g., enterotoxigenic *E. coli, Vibrio cholerae, C. difficile*), invasive bacteria (e.g., enteroinvasive *E. coli, Salmonella, Shigella, Campylobacter, Yersinia*), parasites (e.g., *Giardia, Entamoeba histolytica*), and opportunistic organisms (e.g., *Cryptosporidium, Isospora, Microsporidia,* CMV).
  - One of the most common causes of **pediatric diarrhea** is **rotavirus infection (winter).**
- **Chronic diarrhea:**
  - Insidious onset with > 4 weeks of symptoms.
  - Can be due to ↑ intestinal **secretion** (e.g., carcinoid, VIPomas), **malabsorption/osmotic** diarrhea (e.g., bacterial overgrowth, pancreatic insufficiency, mucosal abnormalities, lactose intolerance), **inflammatory bowel disease,** or altered **motility** (e.g., IBS). ↑ stool osmotic gap and resolution of diarrhea with fasting suggest osmotic diarrhea. See Figure 2.6-2 for a diagnostic algorithm.

DIAGNOSIS

- Acute diarrhea usually does not require laboratory investigation unless the patient has a high fever, bloody diarrhea, or diarrhea lasting > 4–5 days.
- Send stool for fecal leukocytes, bacterial culture, *C. difficile* toxin, and O&P.
- Consider sigmoidoscopy in patients with bloody diarrhea.

Avoid antimotility agents in patients with bloody diarrhea, high fever, or systemic toxicity.

Acute diarrhea is generally infectious and self-limited.

Organisms that cause bloody diarrhea include Salmonella, Shigella, E. coli, and Campylobacter.

TABLE 2.6-2. **Causes of Infectious Diarrhea**

INFECTIOUS AGENT	HISTORY	PE	COMMENTS	TREATMENT
Campylobacter	**The most common etiology of infectious diarrhea.** Ingestion of contaminated food or water. Affects young children and young adults. Generally lasts 7–10 days.	Fecal RBCs and WBCs.	Rule out appendicitis and IBD.	Erythromycin.
Clostridium difficile	Recent treatment with antibiotics (penicillins, cephalosporins, **clindamycin**). Affects hospitalized adult patients. **Watch for toxic megacolon.**	Fever, abdominal pain, possible systemic toxicity. Fecal RBCs and WBCs.	Most commonly in the large bowel, but can also involve the small bowel. Identify *C. difficile* toxin in the stool. Sigmoidoscopy shows pseudomembranes.	**Cessation of inciting antibiotic.** PO metronidazole or PO vancomycin; IV metronidazole if the patient cannot tolerate oral medication.
Entamoeba histolytica	Ingestion of contaminated food or water; history of travel in developing countries. Incubation period can last up to three months.	Severe abdominal pain, fever. Fecal RBCs and WBCs.	Chronic amebic colitis mimics IBD.	Steroids can → fatal perforation. Treat with metronidazole.
E. coli O157:H7	Ingestion of contaminated food (raw meat). Affects children and the elderly. Generally lasts 5–10 days.	Severe abdominal pain, low-grade fever, vomiting. Fecal RBCs and WBCs.	It is important to rule out GI bleed and ischemic colitis. HUS is a possible complication.	Avoid antibiotic therapy.
Salmonella	Ingestion of contaminated poultry or eggs. Affects young children and elderly patients. Generally lasts 2–5 days.	Prodromal headache, fever, myalgia, abdominal pain. Fecal WBCs.	Sepsis is a concern, as 5–10% of patients become bacteremic. Sickle cell patients are susceptible to invasive disease → osteomyelitis.	Treat bacteremia or at-risk patients (e.g., sickle cell patients) with oral quinolone or TMP-SMX.
Shigella	Extremely contagious; transmitted between people by fecal-oral route. Affects young children and institutionalized patients.	Fecal RBCs and WBCs.	May → severe dehydration. Can also → febrile seizures in the very young.	Treat with TMP-SMX to ↓ person-to-person spread.

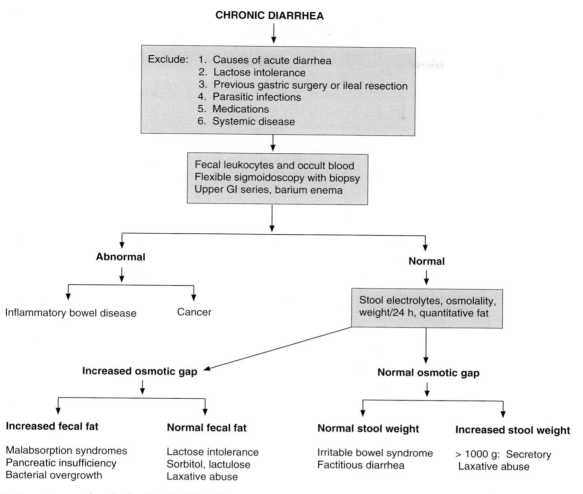

CHRONIC DIARRHEA

Exclude:
1. Causes of acute diarrhea
2. Lactose intolerance
3. Previous gastric surgery or ileal resection
4. Parasitic infections
5. Medications
6. Systemic disease

Fecal leukocytes and occult blood
Flexible sigmoidoscopy with biopsy
Upper GI series, barium enema

Abnormal

Inflammatory bowel disease   Cancer

Normal

Stool electrolytes, osmolality, weight/24 h, quantitative fat

Increased osmotic gap

Increased fecal fat

Malabsorption syndromes
Pancreatic insufficiency
Bacterial overgrowth

Normal fecal fat

Lactose intolerance
Sorbitol, lactulose
Laxative abuse

Normal osmotic gap

Normal stool weight

Irritable bowel syndrome
Factitious diarrhea

Increased stool weight

> 1000 g: Secretory
Laxative abuse

FIGURE 2.6-2. **Chronic diarrhea decision diagram.**

(Reproduced, with permission, from Tierney LM. *Current Medical Diagnosis & Treatment*, 39th ed. New York: McGraw-Hill, 2000, p. 566.)

TREATMENT

- **Acute diarrhea:**
  - When bacterial infection is not suspected, treat with antidiarrheals (e.g., loperamide, bismuth salicylate) and oral rehydration solutions.
  - If the patient has evidence of systemic infection (e.g., fever, chills, malaise), avoid antimotility agents and consider antibiotics after stool studies have been sent.
- **Chronic diarrhea:** Identify the underlying cause and treat symptoms with loperamide, opioids, octreotide, or cholestyramine.
- **Pediatric diarrhea:** For children who cannot take medication or PO fluids, hospitalize, give IV fluids, and treat the underlying cause.

Malabsorption

- Inability to absorb nutrients as a result of an underlying condition such as **bile salt deficiency** (e.g., bacterial overgrowth, ileal disease), **short bowel** syndrome, **mucosal abnormalities** (e.g., celiac disease, Whipple's disease, tropical sprue), and **pancreatic insufficiency.** The small bowel is most commonly involved.

- May result in ↓ absorption of protein, fat, carbohydrates, and the smaller vitamins and minerals.
- Hx/PE: Presents with **frequent, loose, watery stools** and/or **pale, foul-smelling, bulky stools** associated with abdominal pain, **flatus, bloating,** weight loss, **nutritional deficiencies,** and fatigue.
- Tx: Etiology dependent. Institute a gluten-free diet for patients with celiac sprue. Severely affected patients may receive TPN, immunosuppressants, and anti-inflammatory medications.

Lactose Intolerance

- Results from a **deficiency of lactase,** a brush border enzyme that hydrolyzes the disaccharide lactose into glucose and galactose.
- Lactose deficiency is common among populations of African, Asian, and Native American descent. It may also occur 2° to an acute episode of gastroenteritis or other disorders affecting the proximal small intestinal mucosa.
- Hx/PE: Presents with **abdominal bloating, flatulence, cramping,** and **watery diarrhea following milk ingestion.**
- Dx: **Hydrogen breath test** reveals ↑ breath hydrogen following ingestion of lactose load (indicates metabolism of lactose by colonic bacteria). An empiric lactose-free diet that → symptom resolution is highly suggestive of the diagnosis.
- Tx: Avoidance of dairy products; lactase enzyme replacement.

Carcinoid Syndrome

Cutaneous flushing, diarrhea, wheezing, and cardiac valvular lesions are the most common manifestations of carcinoid tumors.

- Due to liver metastasis of **carcinoid tumors** (hormone-producing enterochromaffin cells) that most commonly arise from the ileum and appendix and produce vasoactive substances such as serotonin and substance P.
- Hx/PE: **Cutaneous flushing, diarrhea, abdominal cramps, wheezing,** and right-sided **cardiac valvular lesions** are the most common manifestations. Symptoms usually follow eating, exertion, or excitement.
- Dx: High urine levels of the serotonin metabolite 5-HIAA are diagnostic. Chest and abdominal CT scans can localize the tumor.
- Tx: Treatment includes **octreotide** (for symptoms) and reduction of tumor mass.

Irritable Bowel Syndrome (IBS)

An idiopathic **functional disorder** characterized by abdominal pain and changes in bowel habits that ↑ with stress and are **relieved by bowel movements.** Most common in the second and third decades, but since the syndrome is chronic, patients may present at any age. Half of all IBS patients who seek medical care have comorbid psychiatric disorders (e.g., depression, anxiety).

- Patients present with abdominal pain, a change in bowel habits (diarrhea and/or constipation), abdominal distention, stools with mucus, and relief of pain with a bowel movement.
- IBS rarely awakens patients from sleep; vomiting, significant weight loss, and constitutional symptoms are also uncommon.
- Examination is usually unremarkable except for mild abdominal tenderness.

DIAGNOSIS

- A **diagnosis of exclusion** based on clinical history.
- Tests to rule out other GI causes include CBC, TSH, electrolytes, stool cultures, abdominal films, and barium contrast studies.
- Manometry can assess sphincter function.

TREATMENT

- **Psychological:** Patients need **reassurance** from their physicians. They should not be told that their symptoms are "all in their head."
- **Dietary:** Fiber supplements (psyllium) may help.
- **Pharmacologic:** Treat with TCAs, **antidiarrheals** (loperamide), **antispasmodics** (dicyclomine, anticholinergics), or tegaserod (for those with constipation-predominant IBS).

IBS is a diagnosis of exclusion.

Half of all patients with IBS have comorbid psychiatric disturbances.

Small Bowel Obstruction (SBO)

Defined as blocked passage of bowel contents through the small bowel. Fluid and gas can build up proximal to the obstruction → fluid and electrolyte imbalances and significant abdominal discomfort. The obstruction can be complete or partial, and ischemia or necrosis of the bowel may occur. SBO may arise from **adhesions** from a prior abdominal surgery (60% of cases) or from **hernias** (10–20%), neoplasms (10–20%), intussusception, gallstone ileus, stricture due to IBD, volvulus, or CF.

HISTORY/PE

- Patients typically experience cramping abdominal pain with a recurrent **crescendo-decrescendo pattern** at 5- to 10-minute intervals.
- **Vomiting** typically follows the pain; early emesis is bilious and nonfeculent if the obstruction is proximal but **feculent** if it is distal.
- In partial obstruction, there is continued passage of flatus but no stool, whereas in complete obstruction no flatus or stool is passed (**obstipation**).
- Abdominal exam often reveals distention, tenderness, prior surgical scars, or hernias.
- Bowel sounds are characterized by **high-pitched tinkles** and **peristaltic rushes.**
- Later in the disease, peristalsis may disappear. Fever, hypotension, rebound tenderness, and tachycardia suggest **peritonitis,** a surgical emergency.

The leading cause of SBO in adults is adhesions.

HIGH-YIELD FACTS

GASTROINTESTINAL

The leading cause of SBO in children is hernias.

Never let the sun rise or set on a complete SBO.

DIAGNOSIS

- CBC may demonstrate **leukocytosis** if there is ischemia or necrosis of bowel.
- Chemistries often reflect **dehydration** and **metabolic alkalosis** due to vomiting. Lactic acidosis is particularly worrisome, as it suggests necrotic bowel and the need for emergent surgical intervention.
- Abdominal films often demonstrate a **stepladder pattern of dilated small-bowel loops, air-fluid levels** (see Figure 2.6-3), and a paucity of gas in the colon. The presence of radiopaque material at the cecum is suggestive of gallstone ileus.

TREATMENT

- For partial obstruction, supportive care may be sufficient and should include NPO status, NG suction, IV hydration, correction of electrolyte abnormalities, and Foley catheterization to monitor fluid status.
- Surgery is required in cases of complete SBO, vascular compromise (necrotic bowel), or symptoms lasting > 3 days without resolution.
- Exploratory laparotomy may be performed with lysis of adhesions, resection of necrotic bowel, and evaluation for stricture, IBD, and hernias.
- There is a 2% mortality risk for a nonstrangulated SBO; strangulated SBO is associated with up to a 25% mortality rate depending on the time between diagnosis and treatment.
- A second-look laparotomy or laparoscopy may be performed 18–36 hours after initial surgical treatment to reevaluate bowel viability.

Ileus

Loss of peristalsis without structural obstruction. Risk factors include recent surgery/GI procedures, severe medical illness, immobility, hypokalemia or other electrolyte imbalances, hypothyroidism, DM, and medications that slow GI motility (e.g., anticholinergics, opioids).

In diagnosing ileus, look for air throughout the small and large bowel on AXR.

Anticholinergics, opioids, and hypokalemia slow GI motility.

HISTORY/PE

- Presenting symptoms include diffuse, constant, moderate abdominal discomfort; **nausea and vomiting** (especially with eating); and an **absence of flatulence or bowel movements.**
- Exam may reveal diffuse tenderness and **abdominal distention, no peritoneal signs,** and ↓ or absent bowel sounds.
- A rectal exam is required to rule out fecal impaction in elderly patients.

DIAGNOSIS

- Diffusely **distended loops of small and large bowel** are seen on **supine AXR** with air-fluid levels on upright view.
- A Gastrografin study can rule out partial obstruction; CT can rule out neoplasms.

TREATMENT

- ↓ the use of narcotics and any other drugs that reduce **bowel motility.**
- Temporarily ↓ or discontinue oral feeds.
- Initiate **NG suction/parenteral feeds** as necessary.
- Replete electrolytes as needed.

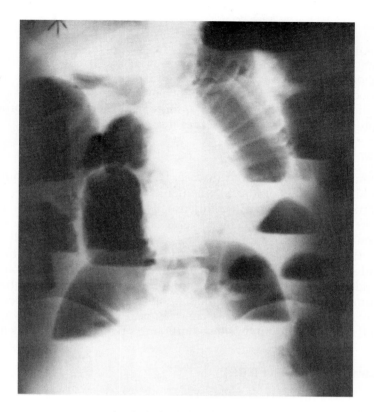

FIGURE 2.6-3. **Acute mechanical obstruction of the small intestine (upright film).**

Note the air-fluid levels, marked distention of bowel loops, and absence of colonic gas. (Reproduced, with permission, from Kasper DL et al [eds]. *Harrison's Principles of Internal Medicine*, 16th ed. New York: McGraw-Hill, 2005, p. 1804.)

DISORDERS OF THE LARGE BOWEL

Diverticular Disease

Outpouchings of mucosa and submucosa (false diverticula) that herniate through the colonic muscle layers in areas of high intraluminal pressure; most commonly found in the sigmoid colon. **Diverticulosis is the most common cause of acute lower GI bleeding in patients > 40 years of age.** Risk factors include a **low-fiber and high-fat diet,** advanced age (65% occur in those > 80 years of age), and connective tissue disorders (e.g., Ehlers-Danlos and Marfan's syndromes). **Diverticulitis** is due to inflammation and, potentially, perforation of a diverticulum 2° to fecalith impaction.

HISTORY/PE

- Diverticulosis is often **asymptomatic.**
- Bleeding is painless and sudden, generally presenting as hematochezia with symptoms of anemia (fatigue, lightheadedness, dyspnea on exertion).
- **Diverticulitis** presents with **LLQ abdominal pain, fever,** nausea, vomiting, and constipation. Perforation is a serious complication that → peritonitis and shock.

Diverticular disease is the most common cause of acute lower GI bleeding in patients > 40 years of age.

Diverticular disease must be distinguished from colon cancer with perforation.

Avoid flexible sigmoidoscopy and barium enemas in the initial stages of diverticulitis because of perforation risk.

DIAGNOSIS

- CBC may show **leukocytosis.**
- Diagnosis is based on AXR (to rule out free air, ileus, or obstruction), colonoscopy, or barium enema. Sigmoidoscopy/colonoscopy must be avoided in those with early diverticulitis owing to perforation risk.
- In patients with severe disease or in those who show lack of improvement, abdominal CT may reveal abscess or free air.

TREATMENT

- **Uncomplicated diverticular disease:** Patients can be followed and placed on a **high-fiber diet** or fiber supplements.
- **Diverticular bleeding:** Bleeding usually stops spontaneously; transfuse and hydrate as needed. If bleeding does not stop, angiography with embolization or **surgery** is indicated.
- **Diverticulitis:** Treat with **bowel rest** (NPO), NG tube placement, and **broad-spectrum antibiotics** (metronidazole and a fluoroquinolone or a second- or third-generation cephalosporin) if the patient is stable. Avoid barium enema and flexible sigmoidoscopy if diverticulitis is suspected.
- For perforation, perform immediate surgical resection of diseased bowel with temporary colostomy with a Hartmann's pouch and mucous fistula.

Large Bowel Obstruction (LBO)

Table 2.6-3 describes features that distinguish SBO from LBO. Figure 2.6-4 demonstrates the classic radiographic findings of LBO.

Colon and Rectal Cancer

The second leading cause of cancer mortality in the United States after lung cancer. There is an ↑ incidence with age, with a peak incidence at 70–80 years. Risk factors and screening protocols are summarized in Table 2.6-4.

HISTORY/PE

- In the absence of screening, colon and rectal cancer typically present with symptoms only after a prolonged period of silent growth.
- Abdominal pain is the most common presenting complaint. Other features depend on location:
  - **Right-sided lesions:** Often bulky, ulcerating masses that → **anemia from chronic occult blood loss.** Patients may complain of weight loss, anorexia, diarrhea, weakness, or vague abdominal pain. Obstruction is rare.
  - **Left-sided lesions:** Typically **"apple-core" obstructing** masses (see Figure 2.6-5). Patients complain of a **change in bowel habits** (e.g., ↓ stool caliber, constipation, obstipation), colicky abdominal pain, and/or blood-streaked stools. Obstruction is common.
  - **Rectal lesions:** Usually present with bright red blood per rectum, often with tenesmus and/or rectal pain. Can coexist with hemorrhoids, so rectal cancer must be ruled out in all patients with rectal bleeding.

DIAGNOSIS

- Order a CBC (often shows microcytic anemia) and stool occult blood.
- Perform sigmoidoscopy to evaluate rectal bleeding and all suspicious left-sided lesions.

TABLE 2.6-3. **Characteristics of Small and Large Bowel Obstruction**

	SBO	LBO
History	Moderate to severe acute abdominal pain; **copious emesis.** Cramping pain with distal SBO. Fever, signs of dehydration, and hypotension may be seen.	Constipation/obstipation, deep and cramping abdominal pain (less intense than SBO), nausea/vomiting (less than SBO but more commonly **feculent**).
PE	**Abdominal distention** (distal SBO), abdominal tenderness, visible peristaltic waves, fever, hypovolemia. Look for **surgical scars/hernias;** perform a rectal exam. **High-pitched "tinkly" bowel sounds;** later, absence of bowel sounds.	Sigificant **distention,** tympany and tenderness; examine for peritoneal irritation or mass; fever or signs of shock suggest perforation/peritonitis or ischemia/necrosis. **High-pitched "tinkly" bowel sounds;** later, absence of bowel sounds.
Causes	**Adhesions** (postsurgery), **hernias,** neoplasm, volvulus, intussusception, gallstone ileus, foreign body, Crohn's disease, CF, stricture, hematoma.	**Colon cancer,** diverticulitis, volvulus, fecal impaction, benign tumors. **Assume colon cancer until proven otherwise.**
Differential	LBO, paralytic ileus, gastroenteritis.	SBO, paralytic ileus, appendicitis, IBD.
Evaluation	CBC, lactic acid, electrolytes, AXR (see Figure 2.6-3); contrast studies (determine if it is partial or complete), CT scan.	CBC, electrolytes, lactic acid, AXR (see Figure 2.6-4), CT scan; water contrast enema (if perforation is suspected); sigmoidoscopy/colonoscopy if stable.
Treatment	Hospitalize. Partial SBO can be treated conservatively with **NG decompression** and NPO status. Patients with complete SBO should be managed aggressively with NPO status, NG decompression, IV fluids, electrolyte replacement, and **surgical correction.**	Hospitalize. Obstruction can be with a Gastrografin enema, colonoscopy, or a **rectal tube;** however, **surgery** is usually required. Ischemic colon usually requires partial colectomy with a diverting colostomy. Treat the underlying cause (e.g., neoplasm).

- Rule out synchronous right-sided lesions with colonoscopy. If colonoscopy is incomplete, rule out additional lesions with an air-contrast barium enema.
- Determine the degree of invasion in **rectal cancer** with endorectal ultrasound.
- Order a CXR, LFTs, and an abdominal/pelvic CT for metastatic workup. Metastases may arise from direct extension to local viscera, hematogenous spread (40–50% go to the liver, but spread may also occur to bone, lungs, and brain), or lymphatic spread (to pelvic lymph nodes).
- Staging is based on the depth of tumor penetration into the bowel wall and the presence of lymph node involvement and distant metastases.

TREATMENT

- Surgical resection of the 1° cancer is the treatment of choice. Regional lymph node dissection should be performed for staging purposes.

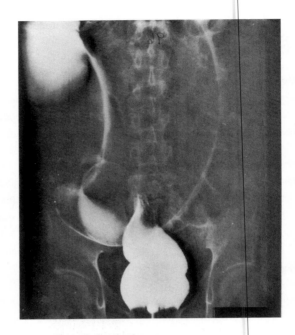

FIGURE 2.6-4. **Large bowel obstruction.**

Barium study shows the "bird-beak" sign, with juxtaposed adjacent bowel walls in the dilated loop pointing toward the site of obstruction. (Reproduced, with permission, from Way LW [ed]. *Current Surgical Diagnosis & Treatment*, 10th ed. Stamford, CT: Appleton & Lange, 1994, p. 676.)

- For **rectal lesions,** the resection technique depends on the proximity of the lesion to the anal verge (junction between the anal canal and the anal skin).
    - **Abdominoperineal resection:** For distal lesions < 10 cm from the anal verge, when the sphincter cannot be preserved, the rectum and anus are resected and a permanent colostomy is placed.

TABLE 2.6-4. **Risk Factors and Screening for Colorectal Cancer**

RISK FACTORS	SCREENING
Age.	A DRE should be performed yearly for patients ≥ 50 years of age.
Hereditary syndromes—familial adenomatous polyposis (100% risk), Gardner's disease, hereditary nonpolyposis colorectal cancer (HNPCC).	Up to 10% of all lesions are palpable with DRE. Stool guaiac should be performed every year for patients ≥ 50 years of age. Up to 50% of ⊕ guaiac tests are due to colorectal cancer.
Family history.	Colonoscopy every 10 years in those ≥ 50 years of age
IBD—ulcerative colitis carries a higher risk than does Crohn's disease.	Colonoscopy should be performed every 10 years in patients ≥ 40 years of age with a family history of colon cancer or polyps, or 10 years prior to the age at diagnosis of the youngest family member with colorectal cancer.
Adenomatous polyps—villous polyps progress more often than tubular polyps and sessile more than pedunculated polyps. Lesions > 2 cm carry an ↑ risk.	
Past history of colorectal cancer.	
High-fat, low-fiber diet.	

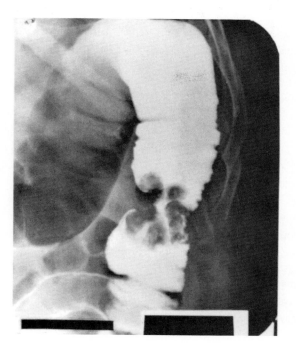

FIGURE 2.6-5. **Colon carcinoma.**

The encircling carcinoma appears as an "apple-core" filling defect in the descending colon on barium enema x-ray. (Reproduced, with permission, from Way LW [ed]. *Current Surgical Diagnosis & Treatment*, 10th ed. Stamford, CT: Appleton & Lange, 1994, p. 658.)

- **Low anterior resection:** For proximal lesions > 10 cm from the anal verge, a 1° anastomosis is created between the colon and rectum.
- **Wide local excision:** For small, low-stage, well-differentiated tumors in the lower third of the rectum.
- **Adjuvant chemotherapy:** Used in cases of colon cancer with ⊕ nodes. Radiation is ineffective for colon cancer but is a useful adjuvant in rectal cancer.
- Follow with serial CEA levels (diagnostically nonspecific, but useful for monitoring recurrence), colonoscopy, LFTs, CXR, and abdominal CT (for metastasis).

Iron deficiency anemia in an elderly male is colorectal cancer until proven otherwise.

GASTROINTESTINAL BLEEDING

Bleeding from the GI tract may present as hematemesis, hematochezia, and/or melena. Table 2.6-5 presents the features of upper and lower GI bleeding.

INFLAMMATORY BOWEL DISEASE (IBD)

Consists of **Crohn's disease and ulcerative colitis** (see Figure 2.6-6). Most common in Caucasians and **Ashkenazi Jews,** appearing most frequently during the teens to early 30s or in the 50s. Table 2.6-6 summarizes the features of IBD.

TABLE 2.6-5. **Features of Upper and Lower GI Bleeding**

Variable	Upper GI Bleeding	Lower GI Bleeding
History/PE	Hematemesis, melena > hematochezia, depleted volume status (e.g., tachycardia, lightheadedness, hypotension).	Hematochezia > melena, but can be either.
Diagnosis	NG tube and NG lavage; endoscopy if stable.	Rule out upper GI bleed with NG tube and NG lavage. Anoscopy/sigmoidoscopy for patients < 45 years of age with small-volume bleeding. Colonoscopy and/or bleeding scan if stable; arteriography or exploratory laparotomy if unstable.
Common causes	**Gastritis,** PUD, Mallory-Weiss tear, esophageal varices, vascular abnormalities, neoplasm, esophagitis.	**Diverticulosis** (most common), AVMs, neoplasm, IBD, anorectal disease, mesenteric ischemia.
Initial management	Protect the airway (may need intubation). Stabilize the patient with IV fluids and blood (hematocrit may be normal early in acute blood loss).	Similar to upper GI bleed.
Long-term management	Endoscopy followed by therapy directed at the underlying cause (e.g., high-dose PPIs for PUD; octreotide and/or banding for varices).	Depends on the underlying etiology. Endoscopic therapy (e.g., epinephrine injection), intra-arterial vasopressin infusion or embolization, or surgery for diverticular disease or angiodysplasia.

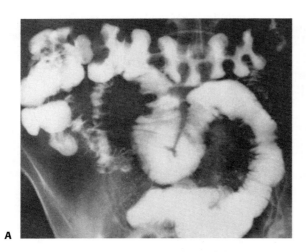

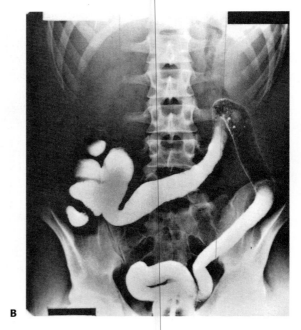

A   B

FIGURE 2.6-6. **Inflammatory bowel disease.**

(A) Crohn's disease. Barium enema x-ray reveals deep transverse fissures, ulcers, and edema of the bowel. (B) Ulcerative colitis. Barium enema x-ray demonstrates shortening of the colon, loss of haustra ("lead pipe" appearance), and fine serrations of the bowel edges from small ulcers. (Reproduced, with permission, from Stobo J et al. *The Principles and Practice of Medicine*, 23rd ed. Stamford, CT: Appleton & Lange, 1996, p. 135.)

TABLE 2.6-6. Features of Ulcerative Colitis and Crohn's Disease

VARIABLE	ULCERATIVE COLITIS	CROHN'S DISEASE
Site of involvement	The **rectum** is always involved. May extend proximally in a **continuous fashion.** Inflammation and ulceration are **limited to the mucosa and submucosa.**	May involve **any portion** of the GI tract, particularly the **ileocecal region,** in a **discontinuous pattern** ("skip lesions"). The rectum is often spared. **Transmural inflammation** is seen.
History/PE	**Bloody diarrhea,** lower abdominal cramps, tenesmus, urgency. Exam may reveal orthostatic hypotension, tachycardia, abdominal tenderness, frank blood on rectal exam, and extraintestinal manifestations.	Abdominal pain, abdominal mass, low-grade fever, weight loss, watery diarrhea. Exam may reveal fever, abdominal tenderness or mass, **perianal fissures, fistulas,** and extraintestinal manifestations.
Extraintestinal manifestations	Aphthous stomatitis, episcleritis/uveitis, arthritis, **1° sclerosing cholangitis,** erythema nodosum, and pyoderma gangrenosum.	Same as ulcerative colitis, as well as gallstones, nephrolithiasis, and fistulas to the skin, bladder, or between bowel loops.
Diagnosis	CBC, AXR, stool cultures, O&P, stool assay for *C. difficile.* Colonoscopy can show diffuse and continuous rectal involvement, friability, edema, and **pseudopolyps.** Definitive diagnosis can be made with biopsy.	Same lab workup as ulcerative colitis. Upper GI series with small bowel follow-through. Colonoscopy may show aphthoid, linear, or stellate ulcers, strictures, **"cobblestoning,"** and **"skip lesions."** "Creeping fat" may also be present. Definitive diagnosis can be made with biopsy.
Treatment	**5-ASA agents** (e.g., sulfasalazine, mesalamine), topical or oral; corticosteroids and immunomodulating agents (e.g., azathioprine) for refractory disease. **Total colectomy is curative** for long-standing or fulminant colitis or **toxic megacolon.**	**5-ASA agents;** corticosteroids and immunomodulating agents (e.g., azathioprine, infliximab) are indicated if no improvement is seen. Surgical resection may be necessary for suspected perforation, stricture, fistula, or abscess; **may recur** anywhere in the GI tract.
Incidence of cancer	**Markedly ↑ risk of colorectal cancer** in long-standing cases (monitor with frequent fecal occult blood screening and yearly colonoscopy with multiple biopsies after eight years of disease).	Incidence of 2° malignancy is lower than in ulcerative colitis.

MESENTERIC ISCHEMIA

Small Bowel Ischemia

↓ mesenteric blood supply → insufficient perfusion to intestinal tissue and ischemic injury. Causes include **acute arterial occlusion** (usually involving the SMA) from **thrombosis** (due to atherosclerosis) or **embolism** (due to atrial fibrillation or ↓ EF), nonocclusive arterial disease (low cardiac output, arteriolar vasospasm), and venous thrombosis (due to hypercoagulable states).

HISTORY/PE

- Patients present with sudden onset of **severe abdominal pain out of proportion to the exam.**
- A history of prior episodes of similar abdominal pain after eating ("intestinal angina") may be present.
- Other symptoms may include nausea, vomiting, diarrhea, and bloody stools.
- Early abdominal exam is often unremarkable; later findings may include peritoneal signs (suggests bowel infarction).

DIAGNOSIS

- Lab tests may show **leukocytosis, metabolic acidosis** with ↑ lactate, ↑ amylase, ↑ LDH, and ↑ CK.
- AXR and CT may reveal bowel-wall edema ("thumbprinting") and air within the bowel wall (pneumatosis).
- Mesenteric **angiography** is the gold standard for arterial occlusive disease.

TREATMENT

The mortality rate for acute mesenteric ischemia is > 50%.

- Volume resuscitation, broad-spectrum antibiotics, optimization of hemodynamics, and avoidance of vasoconstrictors.
- Anticoagulation for arterial or venous thrombosis or embolism.
- **Early laparotomy** for acute arterial occlusive disease or if evidence of peritonitis or clinical deterioration is present.
- Angioplasty +/− endovascular stenting for acute arterial thrombosis.
- Embolectomy for acute arterial embolism.
- Resection of infarcted bowel.

COMPLICATIONS

Sepsis/septic shock, multisystem organ failure, death.

Ischemic Colitis

Ischemic colitis is a disease of the elderly.

- Due to lack of arterial blood supply to the colon. Severity ranges from superficial mucosal involvement to full-thickness necrosis.
- The most commonly affected site is the left colon, particularly the "watershed area" at the splenic flexure. Incidence ↑ with increasing age.
- Hx/PE: Presents with crampy **lower abdominal pain** associated with **bloody diarrhea.** Fever and peritoneal signs suggest infarction.
- Dx:
  - CBC may reveal **leukocytosis.**
  - Flexible sigmoidoscopy or **colonoscopy** to assess colonic mucosa.
- Tx:
  - Supportive therapy with bowel rest, IV fluids, and broad-spectrum antibiotics.
  - Surgery with resection is indicated for infarction, fulminant colitis, or obstruction 2° to ischemic stricture.

INGUINAL HERNIAS

Abnormal **protrusions of abdominal contents** (usually the small intestine) into the inguinal region through a weakness or defect in the abdominal wall. Defined as **direct** or **indirect** on the basis of their relationship to the inguinal canal.

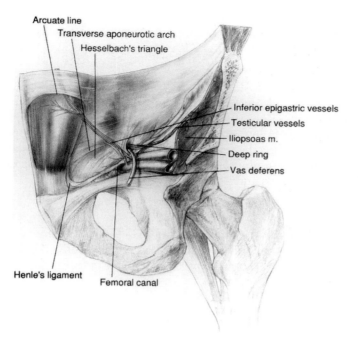

Arcuate line
Transverse aponeurotic arch
Hesselbach's triangle

Inferior epigastric vessels
Testicular vessels
Iliopsoas m.
Deep ring
Vas deferens

Henle's ligament
Femoral canal

FIGURE 2.6-7. Hesselbach's triangle.

(Reproduced, with permission, from Schwartz LS. *Principles of Surgery*, 7th ed. New York: Mc-Graw-Hill, 1999, p. 1588.)

- **Indirect:** Herniation of abdominal contents through the internal and then **external inguinal rings** and eventually into the scrotum (in males).
    - The **most common hernia in both genders.**
    - Due to a **congenital patent processus vaginalis.**
- **Direct:** Herniation of abdominal contents through the floor of **Hesselbach's triangle** (see Figure 2.6-7).
    - Hernial sac contents do not traverse the internal **inguinal ring**; they herniate directly through the abdominal wall and are contained within the **aponeurosis** of the **external oblique muscle.**
    - Most often due to an acquired defect in the **transversalis fascia** from mechanical breakdown that ↑ with age.

TREATMENT

- Because of the risk of **incarceration** and **strangulation**, surgical management (open or laparoscopic) is indicated unless specific contraindications are present.
- Repair of a direct inguinal hernia involves correcting the defect in the transversalis fascia.
- Indirect inguinal hernias are repaired by isolating and ligating the hernial sac and reducing the size of the internal inguinal ring to allow only the spermatic cord structures in males to pass through.

Hesselbach's triangle is an area bounded by the inguinal ligament, the inferior epigastric artery, and the rectus abdominis.

BILIARY DISEASE

Cholelithiasis and Biliary Colic

Colic results from transient cystic duct blockage from impacted stones. Although risk factors include the **4 F's**—Female, Fat, Fertile, and Forty—the disorder is common and can occur in any patient. Other risk factors include

OCP use, rapid weight loss, a $\oplus$ family history, chronic hemolysis (pigment stones), small bowel resection, and TPN.

Pigmented gallstones result from hemolysis.

HISTORY/PE

- Patients present with **postprandial abdominal pain** (usually in the **RUQ**) that radiates to the right subscapular area or the epigastrium.
- Pain is abrupt, is followed by gradual relief, and is often associated with **nausea and vomiting,** fatty food intolerance, dyspepsia, and flatulence.
- Gallstones may be asymptomatic in up to 80% of patients. Exam may reveal RUQ tenderness and a palpable gallbladder.

Only 10–15% of gallstones are radiopaque.

DIAGNOSIS

- Plain x-rays are rarely diagnostic; only 10–15% of stones are radiopaque.
- **RUQ ultrasound** may show gallstones (85–90% sensitive).
- Consider an upper GI series to rule out a hiatal hernia or an ulcer.

TREATMENT

- **Cholecystectomy** is curative and can be performed electively for symptomatic gallstones. Asymptomatic gallstones do not require any intervention.
- Patients may require preoperative ERCP for common bile duct stones.
- Treat nonsurgical candidates with **dietary modification** (avoid triggers such as fatty foods).

COMPLICATIONS

Recurrent biliary colic, acute cholecystitis, choledocholithiasis, acute cholangitis, gallstone ileus, gallstone pancreatitis.

Acute Cholecystitis

Prolonged blockage of the cystic duct, usually by an impacted stone, that $\rightarrow$ obstructive distention, inflammation, superinfection, and possibly gangrene of the gallbladder (acute gangrenous cholecystitis). **Acalculous cholecystitis** occurs in the absence of cholelithiasis in chronically debilitated patients, those on TPN, and trauma or burn victims.

HISTORY/PE

- Patients present with **RUQ pain, nausea, vomiting, and fever.** Symptoms are typically more severe and of longer duration than those of biliary colic.
- RUQ tenderness, inspiratory arrest during deep palpation of the RUQ **(Murphy's sign),** low-grade fever, mild icterus, and possibly guarding or rebound tenderness may be present on exam.

DIAGNOSIS

- CBC usually shows leukocytosis; serum amylase, bilirubin, alkaline phosphatase, and aminotransferase levels may be elevated.
- Ultrasound may demonstrate stones, bile sludge, pericholecystic fluid, a thickened gallbladder wall, gas in the gallbladder, and an ultrasonic Murphy's sign (see Figure 2.6-8).
- Obtain a **HIDA scan** when ultrasound is equivocal (see Figure 2.6-9); nonvisualization of the gallbladder on HIDA scan suggests acute cholecystitis.

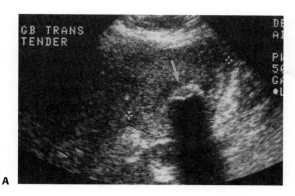
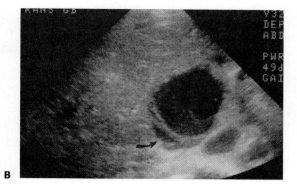

FIGURE 2.6-8. Acute cholecystitis, ultrasound.

(A) Note the sludge-filled, thick-walled gallbladder with a hyperechoic stone and acoustic shadow (arrow). (B) This patient exhibits sludge and pericholecystic fluid (arrow) but no gallstones. (Reproduced, with permission, from Grendell J. *Current Diagnosis and Treatment in Gastroenterology,* 1st ed. Stamford, CT: Appleton & Lange, 1996, p. 212.)

TREATMENT

- Hospitalize patients, administer **IV antibiotics** and **IV fluids,** and replete electrolytes.
- Perform **early cholecystectomy** (within 72 hours of symptom onset) along with either a preoperative ERCP or an **intraoperative cholangiogram** to rule out common bile duct stones.
- Since 50% of cases resolve spontaneously, hemodynamically stable patients with significant medical problems (e.g., DM) can initially be managed medically with a four- to six-week delay in surgical treatment.

COMPLICATIONS

Gangrene, empyema, perforation, emphysematous gallbladder (due to infection by gas-forming organisms), fistulization, gallstone ileus, sepsis, abscess formation.

In patients with significant medical problems (including DM), delay cholecystectomy until acute inflammation resolves.

Choledocholithiasis

- Gallstones in the common bile duct. Symptoms vary according to the degree of obstruction, the duration of the obstruction, and the extent of bacterial infection.
- **Hx/PE:** Although sometimes asymptomatic, it often presents with biliary colic, jaundice, fever, and pancreatitis.
- **Dx:** The hallmark is ↑ **alkaline phosphatase** and **total bilirubin,** which may be the only abnormal lab values.
- **Tx:** Management generally consists of ERCP with sphincterotomy followed by semielective cholecystectomy.

Acute Cholangitis

An acute bacterial infection of the biliary tree that commonly occurs 2° to **obstruction,** usually from **gallstones (choledocholithiasis)** or 1° sclerosing cholangitis (progressive inflammation of the biliary tree associated with ulcerative colitis). Other etiologies include bile duct stricture and malignancy (biliary or pancreatic). Gram-⊖ enterics (e.g., *E. coli, Enterobacter, Pseudomonas*) are commonly identified pathogens.

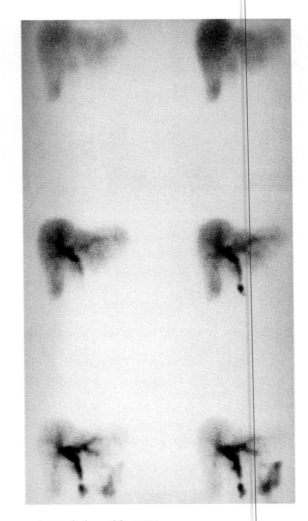

FIGURE 2.6-9. **Acute cholecystitis, HIDA scan.**

IV dye is taken up by hepatocytes and is conjugated and excreted into the common bile duct. The gallbladder is not visualized, although activity is present in the liver, common duct, and small bowel, suggesting cystic duct obstruction due to acute cholecystitis. (Reproduced, with permission, from Grendell J. *Current Diagnosis and Treatment in Gastroenterology,* 1st ed. Stamford, CT: Appleton & Lange, 1996, p. 217.)

Charcot's triad consists of RUQ pain, jaundice, and fever/chills.

Reynolds' pentad consists of RUQ pain, jaundice, fever/chills, shock, and altered mental status.

HISTORY/PE

- Charcot's triad—**RUQ pain, jaundice,** and **fever/chills**—is classic.
- Reynolds' pentad—Charcot's triad plus **shock** and **altered mental status**—may be present in acute suppurative cholangitis and suggests sepsis.

DIAGNOSIS

- Look for **leukocytosis,** ↑ **bilirubin,** and ↑ **alkaline phosphatase.**
- Obtain blood cultures to rule out sepsis. **Ultrasound** or CT may be a useful adjunct, but diagnosis is often clinical.
- **ERCP** is both diagnostic and therapeutic (biliary drainage).

- Patients often require **ICU admission** for monitoring, hydration, BP support, and broad-spectrum **IV antibiotic treatment.**
- Patients with acute suppurative cholangitis require **emergent bile duct decompression** via ERCP/sphincterotomy, percutaneous transhepatic drainage, or open decompression.

1° Sclerosing Cholangitis

- An idiopathic disorder characterized by inflammation, fibrosis, and strictures of extra- and intrahepatic bile ducts. The disease usually presents in **young men** with **IBD** (most often ulcerative colitis).
- Hx/PE: Presents with progressive **jaundice, pruritus, and fatigue.**
- Dx:
  - Laboratory findings include ↑ **alkaline phosphatase** and ↑ bilirubin.
  - MRCP/ERCP show **multiple bile duct strictures** with dilatations between strictures.
  - Liver biopsy reveals periductal sclerosis ("onion skinning").
- Tx: High-dose ursodeoxycholic acid; endoscopic dilation and short-term stenting of bile duct strictures; liver transplantation. Patients are at ↑ risk for **cholangiocarcinoma.**

LIVER DISEASE

Abnormal Liver Tests

Liver diseases can be divided into distinct patterns based on LFT results:

- **Hepatocellular injury:** ↑↑ **AST and ALT** +/– ↑ bilirubin and alkaline phosphatase.
- **Cholestasis:** ↑↑ **alkaline phosphatase and bilirubin** +/– ↑ aminotransferases.
- **Isolated hyperbilirubinemia:** ↑↑ **bilirubin;** normal aminotransferases and alkaline phosphatase.

Jaundice, which can be seen in any of the patterns outlined above, is a clinical sign that arises when excess bilirubin (> 2.5 mg/dL) is circulating in the blood. Figures 2.6-10 and 2.6-11 summarize the clinical approaches toward cholestasis and isolated hyperbilirubinemia. Hepatocellular injury is described in the section that follows.

Hepatitis

Inflammation of the liver → liver cell injury and necrosis. The causes of **acute** hepatitis include **viruses** (e.g., HAV, HBV, HCV, HDV, HEV) and **drug-induced** disease (e.g., alcohol, acetaminophen, INH, methyldopa). The causes of **chronic** hepatitis include viruses (e.g., HBV, HCV, HDV), **alcoholic** hepatitis, **autoimmune** hepatitis, ischemic hepatitis, and **hereditary** etiologies (e.g., Wilson's disease, hemochromatosis, α_1-antitrypsin deficiency).

HISTORY/PE

- Acute hepatitis often starts with a viral prodrome of nonspecific symptoms (e.g., **malaise,** fever, joint pain, fatigue, URI symptoms, **nausea, vomiting,** changes in bowel habits) followed by **jaundice** and RUQ tenderness.

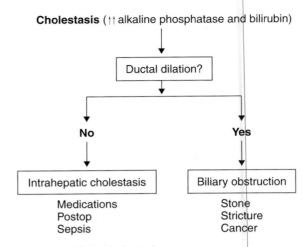

Cholestasis (↑↑ alkaline phosphatase and bilirubin)

↓

Ductal dilation?

No — Intrahepatic cholestasis
  Medications
  Postop
  Sepsis

Yes — Biliary obstruction
  Stone
  Stricture
  Cancer

FIGURE 2.6-10. **Approach to cholestasis.**

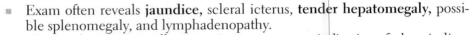

An AST/ALT ratio > 2 suggests alcoholic hepatitis.

Some 80% of patients with HCV infection will develop chronic hepatitis.

- Exam often reveals **jaundice,** scleral icterus, **tender hepatomegaly,** possible splenomegaly, and lymphadenopathy.
- Chronic hepatitis usually gives rise to symptoms indicative of chronic liver disease (jaundice, fatigue, hepatosplenomegaly). At least 80% of those infected with HCV and 10% of those with HBV will develop chronic hepatitis.

DIAGNOSIS

- Dramatically ↑ **ALT and AST** and ↑ bilirubin/alkaline phosphatase are present in the acute form.
- In chronic hepatitis, ALT and AST are ↑ for > 6 months with a concurrent ↑ in alkaline phosphatase/bilirubin and hypoalbuminemia. In severe cases, PT will be prolonged, as all clotting factors except factor VIII are produced by the liver.
- The diagnosis of viral hepatitis is made by **hepatitis serology** (see Table 2.6-7 and Figure 2.6-12 for a description and timing of serologic markers) and by liver biopsy in chronic or severe cases.
- ANA, anti–smooth muscle antibody, and antimitochondrial antibody point to autoimmune hepatitis. Iron saturation (hemochromatosis) and ceruloplasmin (Wilson's disease) can identify other causes.

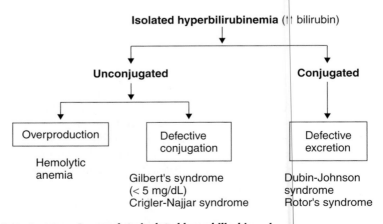

Isolated hyperbilirubinemia (↑↑ bilirubin)

Unconjugated

Overproduction
  Hemolytic anemia

Defective conjugation
  Gilbert's syndrome (< 5 mg/dL)
  Crigler-Najjar syndrome

Conjugated

Defective excretion
  Dubin-Johnson syndrome
  Rotor's syndrome

FIGURE 2.6-11. **Approach to isolated hyperbilirubinemia.**

166

TABLE 2.6-7. **Key Hepatitis Serologic Markers**

SEROLOGIC MARKER	DESCRIPTION
IgM HAVAb	IgM antibody to HAV; best test to detect active hepatitis A.
HBsAg	Antigen found on the surface of HBV; continued presence indicates carrier state.
HBsAb	Antibody to HBsAg; **provides immunity** to HBV.
HBcAg	Antigen associated with core of HBV.
HBcAb	Antibody to HBcAg; ⊕ during **window period.** IgM HBcAb is an indicator of recent disease.
HBeAg	A second, different antigenic determinant in the HBV core. An important indicator of transmissibility. (**BE**ware!)
HBeAb	Antibody to e antigen; indicates low transmissibility.

TREATMENT

- Treatment is etiology specific; monitor for resolution of symptoms over time.
- Steroids for severe alcoholic hepatitis.
- **Immunosuppression** with steroids and other agents (azathioprine) for autoimmune hepatitis.

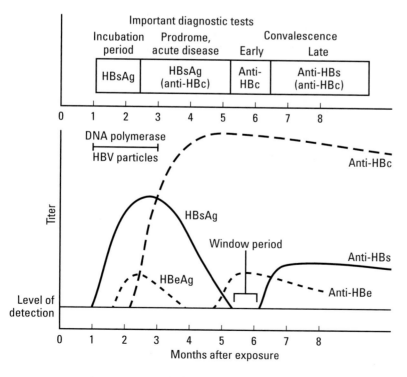

FIGURE 2.6-12. **Time course of hepatitis B with serologic markers.**

The sequelae of chronic hepatitis include cirrhosis, liver failure, and hepatocellular carcinoma.

Alcoholism, chronic hepatitis, and other chronic liver diseases → cirrhosis.

- IFN-α, lamivudine (3TC), or adefovir for chronic HBV infection; peginterferon and ribavirin for chronic HCV infection.
- Liver transplantation is the treatment of choice for patients with end-stage liver failure.
- ICU management and emergent transplant for fulminant hepatic failure.

COMPLICATIONS

Cirrhosis, liver failure, hepatocellular carcinoma (3–5%).

Cirrhosis

Defined as fibrosis and nodular regeneration resulting from hepatocellular injury. Etiologies include causes of chronic hepatitis, biliary tract disease (e.g., 1° biliary cirrhosis, 1° sclerosing cholangitis), right-sided heart failure, constrictive pericarditis, and Budd-Chiari syndrome (hepatic vein thrombosis 2° to hypercoagulability).

HISTORY/PE

- Presents with jaundice, ascites, spontaneous bacterial peritonitis, hepatic encephalopathy (e.g., asterixis, altered mental status), gastroesophageal varices, coagulopathy, and renal dysfunction. Weakness, anorexia, and weight loss are also seen in advanced disease.
- Exam may reveal an enlarged, palpable, or firm liver. Stigmata of portal hypertension and signs of liver failure may be present (see Figures 2.6-13 and 2.6-14).

DIAGNOSIS

- Lab studies show abnormal LFTs: ↓ albumin, ↑ PT/PTT, and ↑ bilirubin. Anemia or thrombocytopenia (2° to hypersplenism) may also be seen.
- Abdominal ultrasound with Doppler can assess liver size, the presence of ascites, and the patency of splenic and hepatic veins. The etiology of ascites

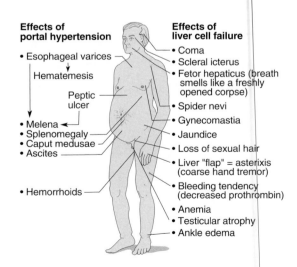

FIGURE 2.6-13.   Presentation of cirrhosis/portal hypertension.

(Adapted, with permission, from Chandrasoma P, Taylor CE. *Concise Pathology*, 3rd ed. Stamford, CT: Appleton & Lange, 1998, p. 654.)

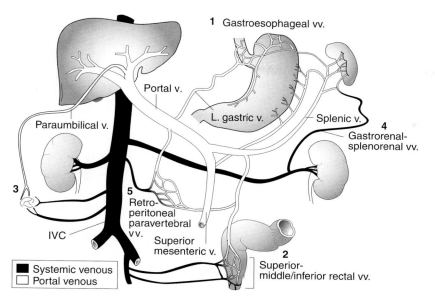

FIGURE 2.6-14. **Portosystemic anastomoses.**

1. Left gastric–azygos → esophageal varices. 2. Superior–middle/inferior rectal → hemor-rhoids. 3. Paraumbilical–inferior epigastric → caput medusae (navel). 4. Gastrorenal-splenore-nal. 5. Retroperitoneal paravertebral.

can be established through measurement of the **serum-ascites albumin gradient** (**SAAG** = ascites albumin − serum albumin); see Table 2.6-8.
- Obtain hepatitis serologies and autoimmune hepatitis studies.
- Serum ferritin, ceruloplasmin, and α_1-antitrypsin may help identify additional causes, such as hemochromatosis, Wilson's disease, and α_1-antitrypsin deficiency, respectively.
- Possible liver biopsy.

TREATMENT

- Aimed at ameliorating the complications of cirrhosis/portal hypertension.
- **Ascites:**
  - Sodium restriction and diuretics (furosemide and spironolactone).
  - Rule out infectious and neoplastic causes; perform paracentesis to obtain SAAG, cell count with differential, and cultures.
  - If possible, treat underlying liver disease.

Gut, butt, and caput—the three anastomoses commonly seen in cirrhosis.

TABLE 2.6-8. **Serum-Ascites Albumin Gradient**

SAAG > 1.1	SAAG < 1.1
Ascites is related to portal hypertension:	Ascites is due to protein leakage:
Presinusoidal: Splenic or portal vein thrombosis, schistosomiasis	Nephrotic syndrome
Sinusoidal: Cirrhosis, massive hepatic metastases	Tuberculosis
Postsinusoidal: Right heart failure, constrictive pericarditis, Budd-Chiari syndrome	Malignancy (e.g., ovarian cancer)

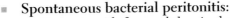

- **Spontaneous bacterial peritonitis:**
  - Presents with fever, abdominal pain, and altered mental status.
  - Check peritoneal fluid if there is a possibility of infection. The fluid is ⊕ if there are > 250 PMNs/mL or > 500 WBCs.
  - Treat with **IV antibiotics** (e.g., third-generation cephalosporin) to cover both gram-⊕ (*Enterococcus*) and gram-⊕ (*E. coli*, *Klebsiella*) organisms until a causative organism is identified.
- **Hepatorenal syndrome:** A diagnosis of exclusion; difficult to treat and often requires dialysis.
- **Hepatic encephalopathy:**
  - Often precipitated by dehydration, infection, electrolyte abnormalities, and GI bleeding.
  - Treat with dietary protein restriction, **lactulose, neomycin,** and/or **metronidazole.**
- **Esophageal varices:** Monitor for GI bleeding; treat medically (β-blockers), endoscopically (band ligation), or surgically (portocaval shunt).
- Consider **liver transplantation** for patients with advanced disease.

Spontaneous bacterial peritonitis is diagnosed by > 250 PMNs/mL or > 500 WBCs in the ascitic fluid.

1° Biliary Cirrhosis

- An **autoimmune** disorder characterized by **destruction of intrahepatic bile ducts.** The disease most commonly presents in **middle-aged women** with other autoimmune conditions.
- **Hx/PE:** Presents with progressive **jaundice, pruritus, fatigue,** xanthomas, xanthelasma, and fat malabsorption.
- **Dx:** Laboratory findings include ↑ **alkaline phosphatase,** ↑ bilirubin, ⊕ **antimitochondrial antibody,** and ↑ cholesterol.
- **Tx:** Ursodeoxycholic acid (slows progression of disease); cholestyramine for pruritus; liver transplantation.

1° biliary cirrhosis is an autoimmune disease that presents with jaundice and pruritus in middle-aged women.

Hepatocellular Carcinoma

One of the most common cancers worldwide despite its relatively low incidence in the United States. 1° risk factors for the development of hepatocellular carcinoma in the United States are **cirrhosis** and **chronic hepatitis** (HCV). In developing countries, **aflatoxins** (in various food sources) and **HBV infection** are also major risk factors.

HISTORY/PE

- Patients commonly present with **RUQ tenderness, abdominal distention,** and signs of chronic liver disease such as **jaundice, easy bruisability,** and **coagulopathy.** Cachexia and weakness may be present.
- Exam may reveal tender **enlargement** of the liver.

DIAGNOSIS

- Often suggested by the presence of a mass on **ultrasound** or **CT** as well as by abnormal LFTs and significantly elevated α-fetoprotein (AFP) levels.
- Liver biopsy for definitive diagnosis.

Complications of hepatocellular carcinoma include GI bleeding, liver failure, and metastasis.

TREATMENT

- For small tumors that are detected early, aggressive tumor resection or **orthotopic liver transplantation** may be successful.
- Chemotherapy and radiation are generally not effective, although they may be used to shrink large tumors prior to surgery (**neoadjuvant therapy**).

- Monitor tumor recurrence with serial AFP levels. Prevent exposure to hepatic carcinogens and vaccinate against hepatitis in high-risk individuals.

Hemochromatosis

Caused by hyperabsorption of iron with parenchymal hemosiderin accumulation in the liver, pancreas, heart, adrenals, testes, pituitary, and kidneys. It is an **autosomal-recessive** disease that usually occurs in males of northern European descent and is rarely recognized before the fifth decade. 2° hemochromatosis may occur with iron overload and is common in patients receiving **chronic transfusion therapy** (e.g., for α-thalassemia) as well as in **alcoholics** (alcohol $\uparrow$ iron absorption).

HISTORY/PE

- Patients may present with abdominal pain or **symptoms of DM, hypogonadism, arthropathy of the MCP joints, heart failure,** or cirrhosis.
- Exam may reveal **bronze skin pigmentation,** pancreatic dysfunction, **cardiac dysfunction** (CHF), hepatomegaly, and testicular atrophy.

DIAGNOSIS

- $\uparrow$ **serum iron,** percent saturation of iron, and ferritin with $\downarrow$ serum transferrin.
- Fasting transferrin saturation (serum iron divided by transferrin level) > 45% is the most sensitive diagnostic test.
- **Glucose intolerance** and mildly elevated AST and alkaline phosphatase can be present.
- Perform a **liver biopsy** (to determine hepatic iron index), hepatic MRI, or *HFE* gene mutation screen.

TREATMENT

- **Weekly phlebotomy;** when serum iron levels $\downarrow$, perform maintenance phlebotomy every 2–4 months.
- **Deferoxamine** can be used for maintenance therapy.

COMPLICATIONS

Cirrhosis, hepatocellular carcinoma, cardiomegaly $\rightarrow$ CHF and/or conduction defects, DM, impotence, arthropathy, hypopituitarism.

Wilson's Disease (Hepatolenticular Degeneration)

- $\downarrow$ ceruloplasmin and **excessive deposition of copper** in the liver and brain due to a deficient copper-transporting protein. Linked to an autosomal-recessive defect on chromosome 13. Usually occurs in patients < 30 years of age; 50% of patients are symptomatic by age 15.
- **Hx:** Patients present with hemolytic anemia, **liver abnormalities** (jaundice 2° to hepatitis/cirrhosis), and neurologic (loss of coordination, **tremor,** dysphagia) as well as **psychiatric** (psychosis, anxiety, mania, depression) **abnormalities.**
- **PE:** May reveal **Kayser-Fleischer rings** in the cornea (green-to-brown deposits of copper in Descemet's membrane) as well as jaundice, hepatomegaly, asterixis, choreiform movements, and rigidity.
- **Dx:** $\downarrow$ serum ceruloplasmin, $\uparrow$ urinary copper excretion, $\uparrow$ hepatic copper.
- **Tx:** **Dietary copper restriction** (avoid shellfish, liver, legumes), **penicillamine** (a copper chelator that $\uparrow$ urinary copper excretion; administer with pyridoxine), and possibly oral zinc ($\uparrow$ fecal excretion).

> *Wilson's disease—*
>
> **ABCD**
>
> **A**sterixis
> **B**asal ganglia deterioration
> **C**eruloplasmin $\downarrow$, **C**irrhosis, **C**opper $\uparrow$, **C**arcinoma (hepatocellular), **C**horeiform movements
> **D**ementia

Pancreatitis

Table 2.6-9 outlines the important features of acute and chronic pancreatitis. Table 2.6-10 lists Ranson's criteria for predicting mortality associated with acute pancreatitis.

TABLE 2.6-9. **Features of Acute and Chronic Pancreatitis**

VARIABLE	ACUTE PANCREATITIS	CHRONIC PANCREATITIS
Pathophysiology	Leakage of pancreatic enzymes into pancreatic and peripancreatic tissue, often 2° to gallstone disease or alcoholism.	Irreversible parenchymal destruction → pancreatic dysfunction.
Time course	Abrupt onset of severe pain.	Persistent, recurrent episodes of severe pain.
Risk factors	**Gallstones, alcoholism,** hypercalcemia, hypertriglyceridemia, trauma, drug side effects (thiazide diuretics), viral infections, post-ERCP, scorpion bites.	**Alcoholism** (90%), gallstones, hyperparathyroidism, congenital malformation (pancreas divisum). May also be idiopathic.
History/PE	**Severe epigastric pain (radiating to the back);** nausea, vomiting, weakness, fever, shock. Flank discoloration **(Grey Turner's sign)** and periumbilical discoloration **(Cullen's sign)** may be evident on exam.	Recurrent episodes of **persistent epigastric pain;** anorexia, nausea, constipation, flatulence, **steatorrhea,** weight loss, DM.
Diagnosis	↑ **amylase,** ↑ **lipase,** ↓ **calcium** if severe; **"sentinel loop"** or **"colon cutoff" sign** on AXR. Abdominal ultrasound or CT may show an enlarged pancreas with stranding, abscess, hemorrhage, necrosis, or pseudocyst.	↑ or normal amylase and lipase, **glycosuria, pancreatic calcifications,** and mild ileus on AXR and CT (**"chain of lakes"**).
Treatment	Removal of offending agent if possible. Standard supportive measures: IV fluids/electrolyte replacement, analgesia, bowel rest, NG suction, nutritional support, O_2, "tincture of time." IV antibiotics, respiratory support, and surgical debridement if necrotizing pancreatitis is present.	Analgesia, exogenous lipase/trypsin and medium-chain fatty-acid diet, avoidance of causative agents (EtOH), celiac nerve block, surgery for intractable pain or structural causes.
Prognosis	Roughly 85–90% are mild and self-limited; 10–15% are severe, requiring ICU admission. Mortality may approach 50% in severe cases.	Can have chronic pain and pancreatic exocrine and endocrine dysfunction.
Complications	**Pancreatic pseudocyst, fistula formation,** hypocalcemia, renal failure, pleural effusion, chronic pancreatitis, sepsis. Mortality 2° to acute pancreatitis can be predicted with Ranson's criteria (see Table 2.6-10).	**Chronic pain,** malnutrition/weight loss, pancreatic cancer.

TABLE 2.6-10. Ranson's Criteria for Acute Pancreatitis[a]

ON ADMISSION	AFTER 48 HOURS
"GA LAW":	**"C HOBBS":**
Glucose > 200 mg/dL	**C**a^{2+} < 8.0 mg/dL
Age > 55 years	**H**ematocrit ↓ by > 10%
LDH > 350 IU/L	Pa**O**$_2$ < 60 mmHg
AST > 250 IU/dL	**B**ase excess > 4 mEq/L
WBC > 16,000/mL	**B**UN ↑ by > 5 mg/dL
	Sequestered fluid > 6 L

[a] The risk of mortality is 20% with 3–4 signs, 40% with 5–6 signs, and 100% with ≥ 7 signs.

Pancreatic Cancer

Roughly 75% are adenocarcinomas in the head of the pancreas. Risk factors include smoking, chronic pancreatitis, a first-degree relative with pancreatic cancer, and a high-fat diet. Most commonly seen in men in their 60s.

HISTORY/PE

- Presents with **abdominal pain** radiating toward the back, as well as with **jaundice,** loss of appetite, nausea, vomiting, **weight loss,** weakness, fatigue, and indigestion.
- Exam may reveal a palpable, nontender gallbladder (**Courvoisier's sign**) or migratory thrombophlebitis (**Trousseau's sign**).

DIAGNOSIS

- Use **CT** to detect a pancreatic mass, dilated pancreatic and bile ducts, the extent of vascular involvement, and metastases.
- If a mass is not visualized, use ERCP or endoscopic ultrasound for better visualization, and consider fine-needle aspiration.

TREATMENT

- Most patients present with metastatic disease, and treatment is palliative.
- Some 10–20% of pancreatic head tumors have no evidence of metastasis and may be resected using the Whipple procedure (pancreaticoduodenectomy).
- Chemotherapy with 5-FU and gemcitabine may improve short-term survival, but long-term prognosis is poor (< 5% survive > 5 years from diagnosis).

The classic presentation of pancreatic cancer is painless, progressive jaundice.

Hematology/Oncology

Coagulation Cascade

Hemostasis requires the interaction of blood vessels, platelets, monocytes, and coagulation factors. This activates the clotting cascade, as shown in Figure 2.7-1.

- **Heparin** ↑ PTT, affects the **intrinsic pathway**, and ↓ fibrinogen levels; safe in pregnancy.
- **Warfarin** ↑ PT, affects the **extrinsic pathway**, and ↓ vitamin K; teratogenic.

Hemophilia

A **deficiency of a clotting factor** that → a bleeding diathesis. There are several types, depending on which factor is lacking (see Table 2.7-1). Although usually hereditary, hemophilia may be **acquired** through the development of an antibody to a clotting factor. This may occur in patients with autoimmune or lymphoproliferative disease, postpartum, or following a blood transfusion. Patients are nearly always male and may have a ⊕ family history.

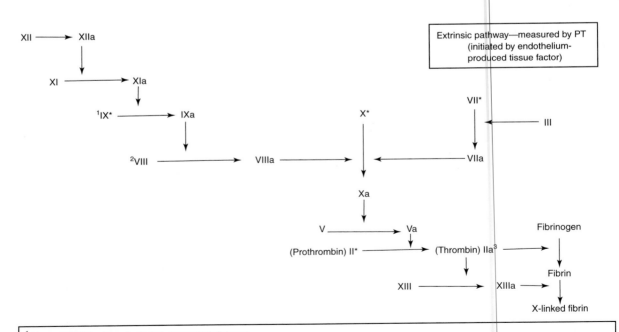

Intrinsic pathway—measured by PTT (initiated by exposure of collagen following vascular trauma)

Extrinsic pathway—measured by PT (initiated by endothelium-produced tissue factor)

[1] Hemophilia B is characterized by factor IX deficiency.
[2] Hemophilia A is characterized by factor VIII deficiency.
[3] Thrombin is inactivated by antithrombin III. The rate of inactivation increases in the presence of heparin.
* Vitamin K–dependent clotting factors (II, VII, IX, X). Their synthesis is inhibited by warfarin.

FIGURE 2.7-1. **Coagulation cascade.**

TABLE 2.7-1. Types of Hemophilia

SUBTYPE	PATHOGENESIS
Hemophilia A (factor VIII deficiency) (90%)	X-linked inheritance; the most common severe congenital clotting deficiency.
Hemophilia B (factor IX deficiency) (9%)	X-linked inheritance.
Hemophilia C (factor XI deficiency) (<1%)	Most common in Ashkenazi Jews.
Factor VII deficiency (<1%)	Presents in a milder, likely heterozygous form.

HISTORY/PE

Presentation varies according to the severity of the disease.
- **Mild deficiencies:**
  - Do not cause spontaneous bleeding.
  - May have major hemorrhage after surgery or trauma.
- **Severe deficiencies:**
  - Present with spontaneous hemorrhage into the tissues and joints that, if left untreated, can → **arthropathy and joint destruction.**
  - May have spontaneous intracerebral hemorrhages, renal and retroperitoneal bleeding, and GI bleeding.

The classic case of hemophilia is the boy (X-linked) from the Imperial Russian family (recessive) who presents with hemarthroses following minimal or no trauma.

DIAGNOSIS

- Patients should be evaluated for suspected clotting factor deficiency as follows:
  - **PT:** Usually normal, but isolated elevations are seen in congenital factor VII deficiency.
  - **aPTT:** Prolonged (the more prolonged, the more severe the hemophilia).
  - **Thrombin time:** Usually normal.
  - **Fibrinogen:** Usually normal.
  - **Bleeding time:** Usually normal.
- The next step is a **mixing study:** mix the patient's plasma with normal plasma; if this corrects the aPTT, a factor deficiency is likely. If the aPTT does not correct, the patient may have a clotting factor inhibitor.
- Specific factor assays should then be performed for factors VII, VIII, IX, XI, and XII. Hemophilia is characterized according to the factor level:
  - **Mild:** > 5% of normal.
  - **Moderate:** 1–3% of normal.
  - **Severe:** ≤ 1% of normal.

TREATMENT

- Bleeding episodes are treated with immediate **transfusion of clotting factors (or cryoprecipitate) to at least 40% of normal concentration.** Factor VIII has a half-life of 12 hours, so patients should be dosed BID to maintain adequate levels. Factor IX has a half-life of 24 hours, so daily transfusion is needed.
- The length of treatment varies with the lesion, extending up to several weeks after orthopedic surgery.
- Mild hemophiliacs may be treated with desmopressin (**DDAVP**); if so, they should be **fluid restricted** to prevent the side effect of **hyponatremia.**

DDAVP helps the body to release extra factor VIII.

- Fifteen percent of patients who are treated for hemophilia A develop neutralizing IgG antibodies to factor VIII, which preclude further treatment with replacement factor.

von Willebrand's Disease (vWD)

The **most common inherited bleeding disorder** (affecting 1% of the population), vWD is an **autosomal-dominant** condition in which patients have deficient or defective von Willebrand's factor (vWF) together with low levels of factor VIII, which is carried by vWF. Symptoms are due to platelet dysfunction and to deficient factor VIII. The disease is milder than hemophilia.

HISTORY/PE

Patients have easy bruising, mucosal bleeding (e.g., epistaxis, oral bleeding), menorrhagia, and postincisional bleeding. Platelet dysfunction is not severe enough to → petechiae. Symptoms worsen with ASA use.

DIAGNOSIS

Ristocetin cofactor assay measures the ability of vWF to agglutinate platelets in vitro in the presence of ristocetin.

- Look for a family history of bleeding disorders.
- Patients have a normal platelet count and a **normal PT** but may have a **prolonged aPTT** resulting from factor VIII deficiency.
- A **ristocetin cofactor assay** of patient plasma can measure the capacity of vWF to agglutinate platelets.

TREATMENT

ASA ↑ the risk of bleeding in patients with von Willebrand's disease.

- Bleeding episodes can be treated with **DDAVP,** and menorrhagia can be controlled with **OCPs.**
- ASA and other inhibitors of platelet function should be avoided.

Hypercoagulable States

Also called **thrombophilias** or **prothrombotic states,** *hypercoagulable states* is a catch-all term describing conditions that ↑ a patient's risk of developing thromboembolic disease. Hypercoagulable states have multiple causes and may be **genetic, acquired, or physiologic** (see Table 2.7-2). Acquired causes are usually 2° to an underlying clinical condition, disease process, or lifestyle. Inherited causes are collectively called *hereditary thrombotic disease,* of which **factor V Leiden** (a polymorphism in factor V, rendering it resistant to inactivity by APC) is the most common.

HISTORY/PE

Suspect pulmonary embolism in a patient with rapid onset of hypoxia, hypocapnia, and an ↑ alveolar-arterial oxygen gradient without another obvious explanation.

- Presents with **recurrent** thrombotic complications, including **DVT, pulmonary embolism, arterial thrombosis, MI, and stroke.** Women may have recurrent miscarriages.
- Although patients may have no recognizable predisposing factors, they usually possess one or more of the causative factors outlined in Table 2.7-2. If the patient's predisposition to thrombosis is hereditary, he or she may also have a ⊕ family history.

DIAGNOSIS

- Under ideal circumstances, patients should be diagnosed before they are symptomatic, but this rarely occurs.

TABLE 2.7-2. **Causes of Hypercoagulable States**

GENETIC	ACQUIRED	PHYSIOLOGIC
Antithrombin III deficiency	Surgery	Age
Protein C deficiency	Trauma	Pregnancy
Protein S deficiency	Malignancy	
Factor V Leiden	Immobilization	
Hyperhomocysteinemia	Smoking	
Dysfibrinogenemia	Obesity	
Plasminogen deficiency	Antiphospholipid syndrome	
Prothrombin G20210A	Nephrotic syndrome	
MTHFR gene mutation	OCPs/HRT	

- Prior to workup for hereditary causes, acquired causes of abnormal coagulation values should be ruled out. **Confirmation of a hereditary abnormality requires two abnormal values that are obtained while the patient is asymptomatic and untreated, with similar values obtained in two other family members.**
- Workup for hypercoagulability varies by age group and includes the following:
  - **< 60 years of age:** Lupus antigen/antiphospholipid syndrome, antithrombin III deficiency, protein C and S deficiencies, APC resistance, homocysteine elevation, prothrombin G20210A.
  - **> 60 years of age:** Lupus antigen/antiphospholipid syndrome, APC resistance, homocysteine elevation, prothrombin G20210A.

TREATMENT

- Treatment should address the type of thrombotic event as well as the area of thrombosis.
- DVT and pulmonary embolism are treated with heparin (unfractionated or LMWH) followed by 3–6 months of oral warfarin anticoagulation for the first event, 6–12 months for the second, and lifelong anticoagulation for subsequent events.
- It is important to use heparin as a bridge to warfarin therapy in order to prevent the complications of paradoxical hypercoagulability (from warfarin's impairment of proteins C and S prior to its inactivation of factors II, VII, IX, and X) and skin necrosis. **INR should be maintained between 2.0 and 3.0.**

Disseminated Intravascular Coagulation (DIC)

A common disease in the hospitalized population, second only to liver disease as a cause of acquired coagulopathy. Caused by **deposition of fibrin in small blood vessels** → thrombosis and end-organ damage. **Depletion of clotting factors and platelets** → a bleeding diathesis. May be associated with almost any severe illness.

HISTORY/PE

- Disorders commonly associated with DIC include obstetric complications, infections with septicemia, neoplasms, acute promyelocytic leukemia,

DIC is characterized by both thrombosis and hemorrhage.

HIGH-YIELD FACTS

HEMATOLOGY/ONCOLOGY

*Petechiae suggest **P**latelet deficiency.*

*Bleeding into body **C**avities or joints suggests **C**lotting factor deficiency.*

pancreatitis, intravascular hemolysis, vascular disorders (e.g., aortic aneurysm), massive tissue injury and trauma, drug reactions, acidosis, and ARDS.

- Presentation varies according to whether the disease is acute or chronic:
  - **Acute:** Presents with generalized bleeding out of venipuncture sites into organs, with ecchymoses and petechiae. Patients who are in shock may have acral cyanosis.
  - **Chronic:** Presents with bruising and mucosal bleeding, thrombophlebitis, renal dysfunction, and transient neurologic syndromes.

DIAGNOSIS

- Diagnosed as outlined in Table 2.7-3.
- DIC may be confused with severe liver disease, but **unlike liver disease, factor VIII is depressed.**

TREATMENT

Treatment of the underlying illness often → spontaneous reversal. Patients often require RBC transfusion and shock management. Platelets should be transfused in the event of hemorrhage with a platelet count < 20,000.

Thrombotic Thrombocytopenic Purpura (TTP)

Part of a spectrum of diseases that includes hemolytic-uremic syndrome (HUS) and HELLP syndrome (**H**emolytic anemia with **E**levated **L**iver enzymes and **L**ow **P**latelets); thought to be due to **platelet microthrombi** that block off small blood vessels → end-organ ischemia and dysfunction. **RBCs are fragmented** by contact with the microthrombi → hemolysis (i.e., microangiopathic hemolytic anemia). The events that → initial microthrombus formation are unknown and may be infectious (bacterial toxins), drug related, autoimmune, or idiopathic.

HISTORY/PE

- A **clinical syndrome** characterized by **five signs/symptoms:** low platelet count, microangiopathic hemolytic anemia (MAHA), neurologic changes (delirium, seizure, stroke), impaired renal function, and fever.
- In many cases, not all of these signs are present, but evidence of hemolytic anemia with schistocytes (broken RBCs) on peripheral smear, along with low platelets and rising creatinine, is highly suggestive.
- Lab findings relating to hemolytic anemia include elevated indirect bilirubin, LDH, and AST along with low haptoglobin. **Coagulation factors are normal.**

TABLE 2.7-3. Laboratory Values in DIC

	PT	aPTT	THROMBIN TIME	PLATELETS	FDPs + D-DIMER	CLOTTING FACTORS
Acute	↑	↑	↑	↓	↑	↓
Chronic	↑	↑	↑	Normal	↑	Normal

DIAGNOSIS

- Diagnosis is largely clinical.
- Overlapping conditions are HUS, HELLP syndrome, and DIC.
  - **HUS:** Characterized by renal failure, hemolytic anemia, and low platelets. **Severe elevations in creatinine are more typical of HUS than of TTP.**
  - **HELLP syndrome:** Affects pregnant women, often occurring in conjunction with preeclampsia.
  - **DIC:** Distinguished from TTP by prolonged PT and aPTT.

TREATMENT

Treat with **steroids** to ↓ formation of microthrombi along with plasma replacement and plasmapheresis. Platelet transfusions are contraindicated.

Idiopathic Thrombocytopenic Purpura (ITP)

A relatively common cause of thrombocytopenia. **IgG antibodies** are formed against the patient's platelets, thereby destroying them. Bone marrow production of platelets is ↑, with ↑ megakaryocytes in the marrow. The **most common immunologic disorder in women of childbearing age.** May be acute or chronic.

HISTORY/PE

- Patients often feel well and present with no systemic symptoms. They may have minor bleeding, easy bruising, petechiae, hematuria, hematemesis, or melena. Bleeding is mucocutaneous. Patients usually do not have splenomegaly.
- ITP is associated with a range of conditions, including lymphoma, leukemia, SLE, HIV, and HCV.
- The clinical presentation is as follows:
  - **Acute:** Presents with abrupt onset of hemorrhagic complications following a viral illness. Commonly affects children 2–6 years of age, with males and females affected equally.
  - **Chronic:** Has an insidious onset that is unrelated to infection. Most often affects adults 20–40 years of age; women are three times more likely to be affected than men.

DIAGNOSIS

- A **diagnosis of exclusion,** as the test for platelet-associated antibodies is a poor one.
- Once other causes of thrombocytopenia have been ruled out, a diagnosis can be made on the basis of the history and physical, a CBC, and a peripheral blood smear showing normal RBC morphology. Most patients do not require bone marrow biopsy, which would show ↑ megakaryocytes as the only abnormality.

TREATMENT

- Most patients with acute childhood ITP spontaneously remit, but this is rarely the case in chronic ITP.
- Patients with platelet counts > 20,000 generally do not require treatment.

The three causes of microangiopathic hemolytic anemia are HUS, TTP, and DIC.

Anti-D (Rh)-Ig and rituximab are emerging therapies for ITP.

- The main therapies are **corticosteroids, high-dose gamma globulin (IVIG), and splenectomy.** Most patients respond to steroids, but if they cannot be tapered after 3–6 months, splenectomy should be considered.
- In **pregnant patients, severe thrombocytopenia may occur in the fetus.**

Figure 2.7-2 shows the various blood cell categories and lineages.

Anemias

Anemia is a disorder of **low hematocrit and hemoglobin.** There are several subtypes, which are classified according to red cell morphology (MCV, RDW, color, shape) and reticulocyte count (see Figure 2.7-3).

IRON DEFICIENCY ANEMIA

Iron deficiency anemia in an elderly patient is colorectal cancer until proven otherwise.

A condition in which iron loss exceeds intake. This may occur when **dietary intake is insufficient** for the patient's needs (e.g., when needs are ↑ by growth or pregnancy) or in the setting of **chronic blood loss,** usually 2° to menstruation or GI bleeding. **Toddlers, adolescent girls, and women of childbearing age** are most commonly affected, but the disease may also occur in men and postmenopausal women.

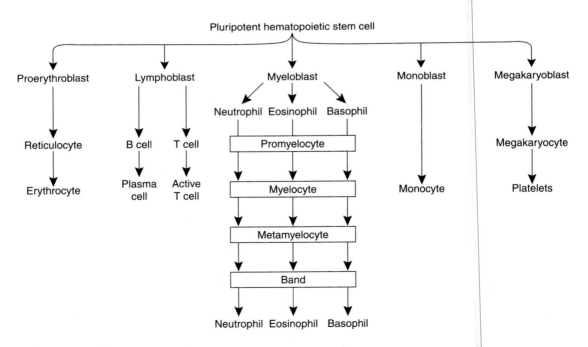

FIGURE 2.7-2. **Blood cell differentiation.**

HIGH-YIELD FACTS

HEMATOLOGY/ONCOLOGY

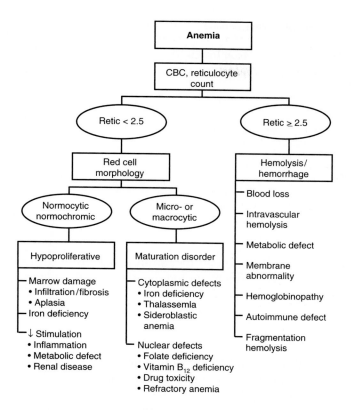

FIGURE 2.7-3. Anemia algorithm.

HISTORY/PE

- Symptoms include **fatigue, weakness, brittle nails, and pica.** If the anemia develops slowly, patients are generally asymptomatic.
- Physical findings include **glossitis, angular cheilitis, and koilonychias ("spoon nails").**
- Peripheral blood smear shows **hypochromic and microcytic RBCs** with a **low reticulocyte count.**
- Low serum ferritin reflects low body stores of iron and clinches the diagnosis. However, ferritin is also an acute-phase reactant and may thus obscure evidence of iron deficiency.

DIAGNOSIS

- Bone marrow biopsy looking for evidence of iron stores is the gold standard but is seldom performed.
- Iron deficiency is often confused with **anemia of chronic disease,** in which iron use by the body is impaired. Labs can help differentiate the two conditions (see Table 2.7-4).

TREATMENT

- Treat with **replacement iron for 4–6 months.** Oral iron sulfate may → nausea, constipation, diarrhea, and abdominal pain. Antacids may interfere with iron absorption.

- *Serum iron = iron available for heme production.*
- *TIBC = amount of protein not bound to iron.*
- *Serum ferritin = iron-protein complex that regulates iron stores and transport.*

Causes of microcytic anemia—

TICS

Thalassemia
Iron deficiency
Chronic disease
Sideroblastic anemia

TABLE 2.7-4. Iron Deficiency Anemia vs. Anemia of Chronic Disease

	IRON DEFICIENCY	CHRONIC DISEASE	BOTH
Serum iron	↓	↓	↓
TIBC or transferrin	↑	↓	Normal / ↑
Ferritin	↓	↑	Normal / ↓
Serum transferrin receptor	↑	Normal	Normal /↑

- If necessary, IV iron dextran can be administered but is associated with a 10% risk of serious side effects, including anaphylaxis. Hence, this is usually done only by a hematologist.

Most macrocytic anemias are caused by processes that interfere with normal DNA synthesis and replication.

MEGALOBLASTIC ANEMIA

Vitamin B$_{12}$ (cobalamin) and **folate deficiency** cause problems with DNA synthesis and → a delay in blood cell maturation. Cobalamin deficiency is due to malabsorption, usually from **pernicious anemia** (destruction of parietal cells, which produce the intrinsic factor needed for cobalamin absorption). Folate deficiency results from insufficient dietary folate, malabsorption, alcoholism, or use of certain drugs. **Drugs that interfere with DNA synthesis,** including many chemotherapeutic agents, may → megaloblastic anemia.

HISTORY/PE

- Presents with **fatigue, pallor, diarrhea, loss of appetite, headaches,** and **tingling/numbness of the hands and feet.**
- Cobalamin deficiency affects the nervous system, so patients lacking that vitamin may develop a **demyelinating disorder** and may present with symptoms of motor, sensory, autonomic, and/or neuropsychiatric dysfunction, known as **subacute combined degeneration of the cord.**

DIAGNOSIS

- Peripheral smear shows RBCs with an **elevated MCV.**
- Bone marrow sample reveals **giant neutrophils** and **hypersegmented mature granulocytes.**
- The **Schilling test** (ingestion of radiolabeled cobalamin both with and without added intrinsic factor) is classic for measuring absorption of cobalamin but is rarely performed.
- Serum vitamin levels are poorly diagnostic of deficiencies, so they are supplemented with methylmalonic acid (MMA) and homocysteine levels:
    - **B$_{12}$ deficiency:** Elevated MMA and homocysteine.
    - **Folate deficiency:** Normal MMA; elevated homocysteine.

TREATMENT

Address the cause of the anemia.

HEMOLYTIC ANEMIA

Occurs when bone marrow production is unable to compensate for ↑ destruction of circulating blood cells. Etiologies include the following:

- **G6PD deficiency:** An X-linked recessive disease that ↑ RBC sensitivity to oxidative stress.
- **Paroxysmal nocturnal hemoglobinuria:** A disorder in which blood cell sensitivity to complement activation is ↑.
- **Hereditary spherocytosis:** An abnormality of the RBC membrane.
- **Autoimmune RBC destruction:** Occurs 2° to EBV infection, mycoplasma, CLL, rheumatoid disease, or medications.
- **Sickle cell disease:** A recessive, β-globin mutation.
- **Microangiopathic hemolytic anemia:** TTP, HUS, DIC.
- **Mechanical hemolysis:** Associated with mechanical heart valves.
- **Other:** Malaria, hypersplenism.

Causes of oxidative stress in G6PD deficiency include infection, metabolic acidosis, fava beans, antimalarials, dapsone, sulfonamides, and nitrofurantoin.

HISTORY/PE

- Presents with **pallor, fatigue, tachycardia, and tachypnea.**
- Patients are typically **jaundiced,** with elevated indirect bilirubin and LDH. Urine is dark with **hemoglobinuria,** and there is ↑ excretion of urinary and fecal urobilinogen. **Reticulocyte count is elevated.**

The classic case of G6PD deficiency is an African-American male soldier in Vietnam who took quinine.

DIAGNOSIS

History and clinical presentation. Obtain a reticulocyte count, indirect bilirubin, LDH, and haptoglobin. **Coombs' test** is used to detect autoimmune hemolysis.

TREATMENT

Treatment varies with the cause of hemolysis but typically includes **steroids** to address immunologic causes and **iron supplementation** to replace urinary losses. Splenectomy may be helpful, and transfusion may be necessary to treat severe anemia.

Indirect Coombs' tests detect antibodies to RBCs in the patient's serum. Direct Coombs' tests detect sensitized erythrocytes.

APLASTIC ANEMIA

A rare condition caused by failure of blood cell production due to **destruction of bone marrow cells.** It may be hereditary, as in **Fanconi's anemia;** may have an **autoimmune** or a **viral** etiology (e.g., HIV, parvovirus B19); or may result from exposure to **toxins** (e.g., drugs, cleaning solvents) or **radiation.**

HISTORY/PE

- Patients are typically **pancytopenic,** with symptoms resulting from a lack of RBCs, WBCs, and platelets—e.g., **pallor, weakness, tendency to infection, petechiae, bruising, and bleeding.**
- The disease may be of sudden or sustained onset and may be of variable severity, depending on the patient's blood counts.

Patients with Fanconi's anemia may be identified on physical exam by café-au-lait spots, short stature, and radial/thumb hypoplasia/aplasia.

DIAGNOSIS

- Diagnosed by clinical presentation and CBC; **verified by a bone marrow biopsy** revealing hypocellularity and space occupied by fat.
- The differential includes megaloblastic anemia, as both diseases feature an elevated MCV.

TREATMENT

Blood transfusion and stem cell transplantation to replace absent cells; immunosuppression with cyclosporin A and Thymoglobulin to prevent autoimmune destruction of marrow. **Infections** are a major cause of mortality and should be treated aggressively.

Sickle Cell Disease (SCD)

SCD represents a qualitative defect in the β-globin chain.

An **autosomal-recessive** disease caused by a mutation of adult hemoglobin (the β chain has glu replaced by val). Signs and symptoms are due to ↓ **red cell survival** and a tendency of sickled cells to → **vaso-occlusion.**

HISTORY/PE

Patients with SCD classically get osteomyelitis with Salmonella. They are also at increased risk of avascular necrosis of the hip.

- Patients are asymptomatic during the first year or two of life and may first present with dactylitis in childhood. Later, hemolysis → **anemia, jaundice, cholelithiasis,** ↑ **cardiac output (murmur and cardiomegaly), and delayed growth.**
- Vaso-occlusion → ischemic organ damage, especially **splenic infarction,** which predisposes to pneumococcal sepsis, and acute chest syndrome (i.e., pneumonia and/or pulmonary infarction). Patients also experience painful crises of unknown etiology.
- Other potential complications include splenic sequestration, which occurs in patients who have not infarcted their spleens, and aplastic crisis, which is usually 2° to infection with parvovirus B19.

DIAGNOSIS

The sickle cell screen is based on a blood smear with sickle cells and target cells. The gold standard is quantitative hemoglobin electrophoresis.

TREATMENT

Treat with **hydroxyurea,** which stimulates the production of fetal hemoglobin. Crises are managed symptomatically with hydration, oxygen, and analgesia. Cholelithiasis is treated with cholecystectomy.

Thalassemias

Thalassemia involves a ↓ quantity of an α or β chain.

Hereditary disorders involving ↓ or absent production of normal globin chains of hemoglobin. α-thalassemia is caused by a mutation of one or more of the four genes for α-hemoglobin; β-thalassemia results from a mutation of one or both of the two genes for β-hemoglobin.

HISTORY/PE

Although patients may be of any ethnic background, thalassemia is most common among people of **African, Middle Eastern, and Asian descent.** Disease presentation and prognosis vary with the number of genes missing (see Table 2.7-5).

DIAGNOSIS

Hemoglobin electrophoresis evaluation (but note that this is normal in α-thalassemia) and DNA studies.

TABLE 2.7-5.   Differential Diagnosis of Thalassemias

SUBTYPE	NUMBER OF GENES PRESENT	CLINICAL FEATURES
β-thalassemia major	0/2 β	Patients develop severe microcytic anemia in the first year of life and need chronic transfusions or marrow transplant to survive.
β-thalassemia minor	1/2 β	Patients are asymptomatic, but their cells are microcytic and hypochromic on peripheral smear.
Hydrops fetalis	0/4 α	Patients die in utero.
Hemoglobin H disease	1/4 α	Patients have severe hypochromic, microcytic anemia with chronic hemolysis, splenomegaly, jaundice, and cholelithiasis. The reticulocyte count elevates to compensate, and one-third of patients have skeletal changes due to expanded erythropoiesis.
α-thalassemia trait	2/4 α	Patients have low MCV but are usually asymptomatic.
Silent carrier	3/4 α	Patients have no signs or symptoms of disease.

TREATMENT

Most patients do not require treatment, but those with β-thalassemia major and hemoglobin H disease are commonly transfusion dependent and should be given iron chelators (desferrioxamine) to prevent overload.

Polycythemias

Erythrocytosis (abnormal elevation of hematocrit) may be either 1° (due to ↑ RBC production) or 2° (due to ↓ plasma volume and hemoconcentration).

HISTORY/PE

- Characterized by ↑ hematocrit, ↓ tissue blood flow and oxygenation, and ↑ cardiac work.
- Patients present with signs and symptoms of **"hyperviscosity syndrome"** (easy bleeding/bruising, blurred vision, neurologic abnormalities, plethora, pruritus [especially after a warm bath], hepatomegaly, splenomegaly, CHF).
- 1° erythrocytosis is associated with hypoxia (from lung disease, smoking, high altitudes, or a poor intrauterine environment) or neoplasia (erythropoietin-producing tumors, or **polycythemia vera [PCV]**, in which there is clonal proliferation of a pluripotent marrow stem cell).
- 2° erythrocytosis is associated with excessive diuresis, severe gastroenteritis, and burns.

True polycythemia vera is characterized by high red cell mass.

DIAGNOSIS

- Erythrocytosis is diagnosed clinically and by cell counts, with ABGs used to assess hypoxia or imaging to demonstrate neoplasia.
- Patients with PCV have an excess of RBCs, WBCs, and platelets. **Levels of erythropoietin** may be useful in distinguishing PCV, in which levels are low, from other causes of polycythemia.

TREATMENT

- **Phlebotomy** relieves symptoms of erythrocytosis, but treatment should also attempt to address the underlying cause.
- PCV can be treated with **cytoreductive drugs** such as hydroxyurea or interferon. Because PCV is prothrombotic, **ASA** should also be used. With treatment, survival is 7–10 years.

Transfusion Reactions

Blood transfusion is generally safe but may result in a variety of adverse reactions (see Table 2.7-8). Nonhemolytic febrile reactions and minor allergic reactions are the most common, each occurring in 3–4% of all transfusions. Etiologies are as follows:

- **Nonhemolytic febrile reactions:** Involve cytokine formation during the storage of blood, and WBC antibodies.
- **Minor allergic reactions:** Involve antibody formation (usually IgA) against donor proteins. Usually occur following transfusion of plasma-containing product.
- **Hemolytic transfusion reactions:** Entail the development of antibodies against donor erythrocytes. Usually result from ABO incompatibility or from antibody against minor antigens.

Hemoglobinuria in hemolytic transfusion reaction may → acute tubular necrosis and subsequent renal failure.

HISTORY/PE

- **Nonhemolytic febrile reactions:** Present with fever, chills, rigors, and malaise. Symptom onset is 1–6 hours following transfusion.
- **Minor allergic reactions:** Characterized by urticaria.
- **Hemolytic transfusion reactions:** Present with fever, chills, nausea, flushing, apprehension, back pain, burning at the IV site, tachycardia, tachypnea, and hypotension. Symptoms begin following the transfusion of only a small amount of blood.

DIAGNOSIS

Clinical impression.

TREATMENT

- **Nonhemolytic febrile reactions:** Stop the transfusion and control fever with acetaminophen. Rule out infection.
- **Minor allergic reactions:** Administer antihistamines. In the setting of a severe reaction, stop the transfusion and give epinephrine +/– steroids.
- **Hemolytic transfusion reactions:** Stop the transfusion immediately. Replace donor blood with normal saline; administer vigorous IV fluids; and maintain good urine output (diuretics and pressors may be used to ↑ renal blood flow).

Porphyria

The porphyrias are a group of inherited disorders that include acute intermittent porphyria, porphyria cutanea tarda, and erythropoietic porphyria. Some porphyrias are **autosomal dominant** (e.g., acute intermittent porphyria) and others **autosomal recessive** (e.g., erythropoietic porphyria). All involve **abnormalities of heme production** → an accumulation of porphyrins.

HISTORY/PE

- Signs and symptoms vary with the type of porphyria. In general, however, porphyrias are characterized by a combination of **photodermatitis, neuropsychiatric complaints,** and **visceral complaints** that typically take the form of a **colicky abdominal pain and seizures.**
- Physical exam reveals **tachycardia, skin erythema and blisters, areflexia,** and a **nonspecific abdominal exam.**
- Patients with the erythropoietic form present with **hemolytic anemia.** Acute attacks are associated with stimulants of ↑ heme synthesis such as fasting or chemical exposures; well-known triggers are alcohol, barbiturates, and OCPs. Urine may appear red or brown after an acute attack. Patients may have a ⊕ family history.

DIAGNOSIS

Diagnosed by a combination of the history and physical along with labs showing elevated blood, urine, and stool porphyrins. Enzyme assays may also be helpful.

TREATMENT

Avoidance of triggers of acute attacks; symptomatic treatment during acute episodes. High doses of **glucose** may be administered to ↓ heme synthesis during mild attacks, and **IV hematin** (provides negative feedback to the heme synthetic pathway) can be given for severe attacks.

Heme is necessary for the production of hemoglobin, myoglobin, and cytochrome molecules.

The classic case of porphyria involves a college student who consumes alcohol and barbiturates at a party, and then has an acute episode of abdominal pain and brown urine the next day.

WHITE BLOOD CELL DISORDERS

Leukemias

Malignant proliferations of hematopoietic cells, categorized by the type of cell involved and their level of differentiation. Leukemias may be acute or chronic, lymphocytic or myelogenous.

ACUTE LEUKEMIAS

Acute myelogenous and lymphocytic leukemias are clonal disorders of early hematopoietic stem cells. They are characterized by rapid growth of immature blood cells (blasts), which overwhelm the ability of bone marrow to produce normal cells.

HISTORY/PE

- Acute myelogenous leukemia (AML) and acute lymphocytic leukemia (ALL) affect children as well as adults. ALL is the **most common childhood malignancy.**

- Disease onset and progression are rapid, and patients present with signs and symptoms of anemia (pallor, fatigue) and thrombocytopenia (**petechiae, purpura, bleeding**). Medullary expansion and periosteal involvement may → **bone pain** (common in ALL).
- The WBC count is usually elevated, but the cells are dysfunctional, and patients may be neutropenic with a **history of frequent infection.** If the WBC is very high (> 100,000), there is a risk of **leukostasis** (blasts occluding the microcirculation → pulmonary edema, CNS symptoms, ischemic injury, and DIC).
- On exam, patients may have **hepatosplenomegaly** and **swollen/bleeding gums** from leukemic infiltration. Leukemic cells also infiltrate the skin and CNS.

DIAGNOSIS

- Based on examination of the patient's bone marrow, obtained by **biopsy and aspiration.** Marrow that is infiltrated with blast cells (i.e., > 20–30%) is consistent with a leukemic process. **In AML, the leukemic cells are myeloblasts; in ALL they are lymphoblasts.** These cells may be distinguished by examination of morphology, cytogenetics, cytochemistry, and immunophenotyping (see Table 2.7-6).
- The type of acute leukemia is further classified according to the **FAB system** (ALL: L1–L3; AML: M0–M7) and karyotype analysis. Prognosis varies with leukemic cytogenetics.

TREATMENT

- ALL and AML are treated primarily with chemotherapeutic agents, although transfusions, antibiotics, and colony-stimulating factors are also used. Patients with unfavorable genetics or those who do not achieve remission may require bone marrow transplantation.
- Prior to therapy, patients should be well hydrated and should be started on **allopurinol** to prevent hyperuricemia and renal insufficiency resulting from blast lysis (**tumor lysis syndrome**).
- Leukostasis syndrome may be treated with hydroxyurea +/– leukapheresis to rapidly ↓ WBC count.
- Indicators of poor prognosis are as follows:
  - **ALL:** Age < 1 year or > 10 years; increasing WBC count to > 50,000; the presence of the Philadelphia chromosome t(9,22) (associated with

Eighty-five percent of children with ALL achieve complete remission with chemotherapy.

TABLE 2.7-6. **Myeloblasts vs. Lymphoblasts**

	MYELOBLAST	**LYMPHOBLAST**
Size	Larger (2–4 times RBC)	Smaller (1.5–3.0 times RBC)
Amount of cytoplasm	More	Less
Nucleoli	Conspicuous	Inconspicuous
Granules	Common, fine	Uncommon, coarse
Auer rods	Present in 50% of cases	Absent
Myeloperoxidase	⊕	⊖

B-cell cancer), CNS involvement at diagnosis, and L3 morphology (associated with Burkitt's lymphoma).
- **AML:** Age > 60 years, CD34+ or MDR1+ phenotype, elevated LDH, mutations in chromosomes 5 or 7, t(6,9), trisomy 8 or a more complex karyotype, FLT3 gene mutation, and FAB M7 (acute megakaryocytic variant).
- AML type (FAB) **M3—acute promyelocytic leukemia (APL)**—has a good prognosis because it is responsive to **all-*trans*-retinoic acid (ATRA) therapy,** which is less toxic than conventional chemotherapy.

CHRONIC LYMPHOCYTIC LEUKEMIA (CLL)

A malignant, clonal proliferation of functionally incompetent lymphocytes that accumulate in the bone marrow, peripheral blood, lymph nodes, spleen, and liver. Constitutes the most common type of leukemia. A rare form of T-cell CLL exists, but almost all cases involve **well-differentiated B lymphocytes.** The etiology is unknown, although there is some genetic contribution, as first-degree relatives of patients with CLL are three times more likely than others to develop a lymphoid malignancy. Primarily affects **older adults** (median age 65), and the male-to-female ratio is 2:1.

HISTORY/PE

- Patients are often asymptomatic, but many present with **fatigue, malaise, and infection.** Common physical findings are **lymphadenopathy and splenomegaly.**
- CBC shows lymphocytosis (lymphocyte count > 5,000) with an abundance of small, normal-appearing lymphocytes and ruptured **smudge cells** on peripheral smear. **Granulocytopenia, anemia, and thrombocytopenia** are common owing to marrow infiltration with leukemic cells. Abnormal function by the leukemic cells → **hypogammaglobulinemia.**

DIAGNOSIS

Diagnosed by the clinical picture; may be confirmed by **flow cytometry** demonstrating the presence of CD5—which is usually found only on T cells—on leukemic cells with the characteristic B-cell antigens CD20 and CD21. Bone marrow biopsy is rarely required for diagnosis or staging but may provide prognostic information and may help assess response to therapy.

TREATMENT

- The clinical stage correlates with expected survival (see Table 2.7-7).
- Treatment is palliative. The degree of peripheral lymphocytosis does not correlate with prognosis, nor does it dictate when treatment should be initiated. **Treatment is often withheld until patients are symptomatic**—e.g., when they present with recurrent infection, severe lymphadenopathy or splenomegaly, anemia, and thrombocytopenia.
- Treatment consists primarily of **chemotherapy,** especially with alkylating agents, although radiation may be useful for localized lymphadenopathy.
- Although CLL is **not curable,** long disease-free intervals may be achieved with adequate treatment of symptoms.

CHRONIC MYELOGENOUS LEUKEMIA (CML)

Involves clonal expansion of myeloid progenitor cells → leukocytosis with excess granulocytes and basophils and sometimes ↑ erythrocytes and platelets as

CLL may be complicated by autoimmune hemolytic anemia.

TABLE 2.7-7. **Clinical Staging of CLL (Rai Staging)**

STAGE	FINDINGS	MEDIAN SURVIVAL
0	Lymphocytosis ($> 15 \times 10^9$)	> 150 months
I	Lymphocytosis + lymphadenopathy	101 months
II	Lymphocytosis + splenomegaly	71 months
III	Lymphocytosis + anemia	19 months
IV	Lymphocytosis + thrombocytopenia	19 months

The Philadelphia chromosome is a balanced translocation between chromosomes 9 and 22. The resulting fusion gene, bcr-abl, produces an abnormal tyrosine kinase, which may suppress apoptosis and induce cell growth and proliferation independent of extracellular growth factors.

well. The **Philadelphia chromosome t(9,22)** is present in > 90% of patients and is virtually diagnostic. CML primarily affects **middle-aged** patients.

HISTORY/PE

- With routine blood testing, many patients are diagnosed while asymptomatic. However, typical signs and symptoms are those of **anemia.**
- Patients frequently have **splenomegaly** with LUQ pain and early satiety. Hepatomegaly may be present as well. **Constitutional symptoms** of weight loss, anorexia, fever, and chills may also be seen.
- CBC shows a **very high WBC**—often > 100,000 at diagnosis, and sometimes reaching > 500,000. Differential shows granulocytes in all stages of maturation. Rarely, the WBC count will be so elevated as to cause a **hyperviscosity syndrome.**
- **Leukocyte alkaline phosphatase is low; LDH, uric acid, and B$_{12}$ levels are elevated.**
- Patients with CML go through three disease phases:
    - **Chronic:** Without treatment, typically lasts 3.5–5.0 years. Signs and symptoms are as described above. Infection and bleeding complications are rare.
    - **Accelerated:** A transition toward blast crisis, with an ↑ in peripheral and bone marrow blood counts. Should be suspected when the differential shows an abrupt ↑ in basophils and thrombocytopenia < 100,000.
    - **Blast:** Resembles acute leukemia; survival is 3–6 months.

DIAGNOSIS

Diagnosed by the clinical picture, including labs; cytogenetic analysis usually reveals the Philadelphia chromosome.

Imatinib (Gleevec) is a selective inhibitor of the bcr-abl tyrosine kinase.

TREATMENT

Varies with disease phase and is undergoing rapid change, particularly since the introduction of targeted therapies:

- **Chronic:** Imatinib. Younger patients can be treated with allogeneic stem cell transplantation if a suitable matched sibling donor is available.
- **Blast:** Therapy as for acute leukemia or dasatinib + hematopoietic stem cell transplant or clinical trial.

HAIRY CELL LEUKEMIA (HCL)

A malignant disorder of well-differentiated B lymphocytes with an unclear cause. HCL is a **rare** disease accounting for 2% of adult leukemia cases; it most commonly affects **older men.** It is significant in research and drug development.

HISTORY/PE

- Typically presents with pancytopenia, bone marrow infiltration, and splenomegaly.
- Patients complain of weakness, fatigue, petechiae and bruising, infection (especially with atypical mycobacteria such as *Mycobacterium avium–intracellulare*), abdominal pain, early satiety, and weight loss. Symptoms are similar to those of CLL except that patients rarely have lymphadenopathy.
- CBC usually demonstrates **leukopenia** (making the name *leukemia* a misnomer); roughly 85% of the time, peripheral smear shows **hairy cells, or mononuclear cells with abundant pale cytoplasm and cytoplasmic projections.**

DIAGNOSIS

- Diagnosed by the history, physical exam, and labs; confirmed through the identification of hairy cells in the blood, marrow, or spleen.
- **Tartrate-resistant acid phosphatase (TRAP) staining of hairy cells,** electron microscopy, and **flow cytometry** (quantification of fluorescence on cells with fluorescent-labeled monoclonal antibodies bound to cell-specific antigens) are helpful in distinguishing the hairy cells that are pathognomonic.

TREATMENT

- Ten percent of patients have a benign course and never require therapy; the remainder develop progressive pancytopenia and splenomegaly and have a median survival of five years without treatment.
- Treatment begins when patients are symptomatic or extremely cytopenic. **Nucleoside analogs** are currently the initial treatment of choice, and effectively induce remission. Other treatment options include splenectomy, which may improve blood counts, and IFN-α.

Lymphomas

Malignant transformations of lymphoid cells residing primarily in lymphoid tissues, especially the lymph nodes. Classically organized into Hodgkin's and non-Hodgkin's varieties, although other classification systems (by cell type or clinical behavior) are also used.

NON-HODGKIN'S LYMPHOMA (NHL)

NHL represents a progressive clonal expansion of B cells, T cells, and/or natural killer (NK) cells stimulated by chromosomal translocations (most commonly t[14,18]), by the inactivation of tumor suppressor genes, or by the introduction of exogenous genes by oncogenic viruses (e.g., EBV, HTLV-1, HCV). There is a strong association between *H. pylori* infection and MALT gastric lymphoma. **Most NHLs (almost 85%) are of B-cell origin.** NHL is the **most common hematopoietic neoplasm** and is five times more common than Hodgkin's lymphoma.

History/PE

Although the median patient age is **over 50 years,** NHL may be found in children, who tend to have more aggressive, higher-grade disease. Patient presentation varies with disease grade (see Table 2.7-8).

Diagnosis

- **Excisional lymph node biopsy** is necessary for diagnosis; disease may first present at an extranodal site, which should be biopsied for diagnosis as well.
- A CSF exam should be done in patients with HIV, neurologic signs or symptoms, or 1° CNS lymphoma. **Disease staging (Ann Arbor classification) is based on the number of nodes and on whether the disease crosses the diaphragm.**

Treatment

Treatment is based on histopathologic classification, rather than stage. Symptomatic patients are treated with radiation and chemotherapy (CHOP: cyclophosphamide [Cytoxan], Adriamycin, vincristine, and prednisone). The rule of thumb is for **low-grade, indolent NHL** to be treated with a **palliative approach** in symptomatic patients, and for **high-grade, aggressive NHL** to be treated **aggressively** with a **curative approach.**

HODGKIN'S DISEASE (HD)

A **predominantly B-cell malignancy** with an unclear etiology. There is a possible association with EBV. HD has a **bimodal age distribution,** peaking first in the third decade (primarily the nodular sclerosing type) and then in the elderly at around age 60 (mainly the lymphocyte-depleted type). It has a male predominance in childhood.

The treatment of high-grade NHL may be complicated by tumor lysis syndrome, in which rapid cell death releases intracellular contents → hyperkalemia, hyperphosphatemia, hyperuricemia, and hypocalcemia.

TABLE 2.7-8. Presentation of Non-Hodgkin's Lymphoma

GRADE	HISTORY	PHYSICAL
Low	Painless peripheral adenopathy. Cytopenia from bone marrow involvement. Fatigue and weakness.	Peripheral adenopathy, splenomegaly, hepatomegaly.
Intermediate to high	Adenopathy. Extranodal disease (GI, GU, skin, thyroid, CNS). B symptoms (temperature > 38.5°C, night sweats, weight loss). Mass formation (e.g., abdominal mass with bowel obstruction in Burkitt's lymphoma; mediastinal mass and SVC syndrome in lymphoblastic lymphoma).	Bulky adenopathy, splenomegaly, hepatomegaly. Masses (abdominal, testicular, mediastinal). Skin findings.

HISTORY/PE

- HD commonly presents as **cervical adenopathy,** although it may present as a mediastinal mass; it is **usually found above the diaphragm,** with infradiaphragmatic involvement suggesting more widely disseminated disease.
- Patients also have **systemic B symptoms, pruritus, and hepatosplenomegaly. Pel-Ebstein fevers** (1–2 weeks of high fever alternating with 1–2 afebrile weeks) **and alcohol-induced pain** at nodal sites are rare signs that are specific for HD.

DIAGNOSIS

- Diagnosed by **excisional lymph node biopsy,** which is examined for the classic **Reed-Sternberg (RS) cells** (giant abnormal B cells with bilobar nuclei and huge, eosinophilic nucleoli, which create an "owl's-eye" appearance) and abnormal nodal morphology.
- There are several histologic types, including nodular sclerosing, mixed cellularity, lymphocyte predominant, and lymphocyte depleted (in descending order of frequency). Staging is based on the **number of nodes, the presence of B symptoms, and whether the disease crosses the diaphragm;** staging laparotomy is not recommended.

TREATMENT

- Treatment is stage dependent, involving chemotherapy and/or radiation. **Radiation is directed toward the involved lymph node area** plus the next contiguous region. Chemotherapy regimens used include ABVD (Adriamycin, bleomycin, vinblastine, dacarbazine), and MOPP (mechlorethamine, vincristine, procarbazine, prednisone).
- **Five-year survival rates are very good** and are 90% for stage I and II disease (nodal disease limited to one side of the diaphragm), 84% for stage III, and 65% for stage IV.

Chemotherapy and radiation can lead to 2° neoplasms such as AML, NHL, breast and thyroid cancer.

PLASMA CELL DISORDERS

Multiple Myeloma

Clonal proliferation of malignant plasma cells at varying stages of differentiation, with **excessive production of monoclonal immunoglobulins or immunoglobulin fragments** (kappa/lambda light chains). Multiple myeloma is commonly believed to be a disease of the elderly, with a peak incidence in the seventh decade. Risk factors for disease development include radiation; monoclonal gammopathy of undetermined significance (MGUS); and, possibly, petroleum, pesticides, and other chemicals.

The combination of anemia and bone pain must always raise suspicion of multiple myeloma.

HISTORY/PE

Patients present with **anemia, plasmacytosis of the bone marrow, lytic bone lesions, hypercalcemia, and renal abnormalities.** They are prone to **infection** and have **elevated monoclonal (M) proteins** in the serum and/or urine.

DIAGNOSIS

- The classic triad of diagnostic criteria are > 10% plasma cells in the bone marrow and/or histologically proven plasma cell infiltration, M protein in serum or urine, and evidence of lytic bone lesions.

Hypercalcemia manifests in symptoms of polyuria, constipation, confusion, nausea, vomiting, and lethargy.

Because multiple myeloma is an osteoclastic process, a bone scan, which detects osteoblastic activity, may be ⊖.

- The **presence of M proteins alone is insufficient for diagnosis of multiple myeloma;** MGUS is relatively common. Other lymphoproliferative diseases may also result in M proteins, including CLL, lymphoma, Waldenström's macroglobulinemia, and amyloidosis.
- Patients should be evaluated with a skeletal survey, bone marrow biopsy, serum and urine protein electrophoresis, and CBC.

TREATMENT

Treated with **chemotherapy. Common initial treatment** involves a combination of melphalan (an oral alkylating agent) and prednisone and other agents. Myeloma cells tend to become resistant to drugs by an **MDR gene** mechanism, and autologous stem cell transplantation may be used to support more intensive doses of chemotherapy.

Waldenström's Macroglobulinemia

A clonal disorder of B cells → a malignant monoclonal gammopathy. **Elevated levels of IgM** → hyperviscosity syndrome, coagulation abnormalities, cryoglobulinemia, cold agglutinin disease (leading to autoimmune hemolytic anemia), and amyloidosis. Tissue is infiltrated by IgM and neoplastic plasma cells. A **chronic, indolent disease of the elderly.**

HISTORY/PE

- Disease begins with nonspecific symptoms of lethargy and weight loss along with **Raynaud's phenomenon** from cryoglobulinemia. Patients complain of **neurologic problems** ranging from mental status changes to sensorimotor peripheral neuropathy and blurry vision. Organomegaly and organ dysfunction affecting the skin, GI tract, kidneys, and lungs are also seen.
- Labs show elevated ESR, uric acid, LDH, and alkaline phosphatase.
- As with multiple myeloma, **MGUS is a precursor** to disease.

DIAGNOSIS

Bone marrow biopsy and aspirate are required to establish the diagnosis. Marrow contains small numbers of abnormal plasma cells, classically with **Dutcher bodies** (PAS-⊕ IgM deposits around the nucleus). Serum and urine protein electrophoresis and immunofixation are also used.

TREATMENT

Excess immunoglobulin is removed with plasmapheresis; the underlying lymphoma is treated with chemotherapy.

Amyloidosis

A generic term referring to extracellular deposition of protein fibrils. There are many different kinds of amyloidosis involving different types of deposited fibrils with varying etiologies (see Table 2.7-9). It is classically a disease of the **elderly.**

HISTORY/PE

Clinical presentation depends on the type of precursor protein, tissue distribution, and the amount of amyloid deposition. In the two most common forms

TABLE 2.7-9. Types of Amyloidosis

AMYLOID	CAUSE
AL	A plasma cell dyscrasia, with deposition of monoclonal light-chain fragments. Associated with multiple myeloma and Waldenström's macroglobulinemia.
AA	Deposition of the acute-phase reactant serum amyloid A. Associated with chronic inflammatory diseases (e.g., rheumatoid arthritis), infections, and neoplasms.
Dialysis-related	Deposition of β_2 microglobulin, which accumulates in patients on long-term dialysis.
Heritable	Deposition of abnormal gene products (e.g., transthyretin, aka prealbumin). A heterogeneous group of disorders.
Senile-systemic	Deposition of otherwise normal transthyretin.

of systemic amyloidosis, 1° (AL) and 2° (AA), the major sites of clinically important amyloid deposition are in the kidneys, heart, and liver. In some disorders, clinically important amyloid deposition is limited to one organ (**e.g., Alzheimer's disease**).

DIAGNOSIS

Diagnosed by the clinical picture; confirmed by tissue biopsy with **Congo red staining** (showing apple-green birefringence under polarized light).

TREATMENT

1° amyloidosis is treated with experimental chemotherapy to reduce protein burden; in 2° amyloidosis, the underlying condition should be addressed. Transplantation is also used; kidney transplantation may cure dialysis-related amyloid, and liver transplantation may cure heritable amyloid.

NEUTROPENIA

An **absolute neutrophil count (ANC) < 1500.** (ANC = [WBC count] [% bands + % segmented neutrophils] [0.01]). Neutropenia may be due to a combination of ↓ production, sequestration to marginated or tissue pools, and ↑ destruction or utilization. It may be acquired or intrinsic (see Table 2.7-10).

HISTORY/PE

Patients are at ↑ **risk of infection,** which varies inversely with neutrophil count.

- **Acute neutropenia:** Associated with *S. aureus, Pseudomonas, E. coli, Proteus,* and *Klebsiella* sepsis.
- **Chronic and autoimmune neutropenia:** Presents with **recurrent sinusitis, stomatitis, gingivitis, and perirectal infections** rather than sepsis. Some chronic neutropenias are accompanied by splenomegaly (e.g., Felty's syndrome, Gaucher's disease, sarcoidosis).

TABLE 2.7-10. Acquired vs. Intrinsic Neutropenia

Type	Causes
Acquired	Drug induced (e.g., ethanol, antibiotics, NSAIDs), usually by marrow suppression. Marrow-infiltrating disorders. Postinfectious. HIV infection. Benign familial leukopenia (seen in Yemenite Jews, West Indians, and people of African descent; due to genetic variation). Chronic idiopathic neutropenia (occurs in infancy and childhood; thought to be due to production of antineutrophil IgG). Autoimmune neutropenia (isolated or 2° to rheumatoid arthritis or SLE). Nutritional deficiency (B_{12}/folate or thiamine deficiency). Metabolic disease (ketoacidosis, hyperglycinuria, orotic aciduria, MMA, hypothyroidism, Gaucher's disease).
Intrinsic	Dyskeratosis congenita (X-linked, with integument abnormalities and hypocellular marrow). Kostmann's syndrome (aka infantile agranulocytosis). Shwachman-Diamond-Oski syndrome (neutropenia, metaphyseal dysplasia, and pancreatic insufficiency). Chédiak-Higashi syndrome (oculocutaneous albinism, neurologic impairment, and giant granules in cells). Fanconi's anemia.

DIAGNOSIS

- The history and physical exam are the cornerstones of diagnosis.
- CBC with ANC may be used to follow neutropenia. If thrombocytopenia or anemia is present, bone marrow biopsy and aspirate should be performed.
- Serum immunologic evaluation, ANA levels, and a workup for collagen vascular disease may be merited.

TREATMENT

Infection management is most important; patients may not be able to mount an inflammatory response to infection owing to their lack of neutrophils. Fever in the context of neutropenia should be treated immediately with **broad-spectrum antibiotics**. Suspected fungal infections should be treated appropriately as well. Hematopoietic stem cell factors such as **G-CSF** can be used to shorten the duration of neutropenia. In some instances, **IVIG and allogeneic bone marrow transplantation** may be used.

EOSINOPHILIA

Absolute eosinophil count = (WBC) (% eosinophils) (0.01). **Normal levels do not exceed 350.** Eosinophilia can be triggered by the overproduction of one or more of three eosinophilopoietic cytokines (IL-3, IL-5, GM-CSF) or by chemokines that stimulate the migration of eosinophils into peripheral

TABLE 2.7-11. Etiologies of Eosinophilia

TYPE	CAUSES
1°	Hypereosinophilic syndrome—the etiology is unknown. Hereditary eosinophilia—autosomal-dominant inheritance; rare. Eosinophilia-myalgia syndrome—results from abnormal tryptophan metabolism.
2°	Allergic states with elevated serum IgE—the most common cause in the United States. Parasitic diseases—the most common cause worldwide. Coccidioidomycosis infection. Vasculitis (e.g., Churg-Strauss syndrome). Benign or malignant hematologic disorders; also solid tumors. Collagen vascular diseases (e.g., dermatomyositis, PAN). Drug induced (e.g., sulfonamides, iodides, ASA, phenytoin).

blood and tissues. Eosinophilia may be a 1° disorder, but it **usually occurs 2° to another cause** (see Table 2.7-11).

HISTORY/PE

- A **travel, medication, atopic, and diet history** should be elicited along with a history of symptoms relating to lymphoma/leukemia.
- Physical exam findings vary with the cause. Patients with hypereosinophilic syndrome (HES) may present with fever, anemia, and prominent cardiac findings (emboli from mural thrombi, abnormal ECGs, CHF, murmurs). Other affected organs include the lung, liver, spleen, skin, and nervous system (due to eosinophilic infiltration).

Causes of eosinophilia—

NAACP

Neoplasm
Allergies
Asthma
Collagen vascular disease
Parasites

TABLE 2.7-12. Types of Transplant Rejection

	HYPERACUTE	ACUTE	CHRONIC
Timing after transplant	Within minutes.	Five days to three months.	Months to years.
Pathomechanism	Preformed antibodies.	T-cell mediated.	Chronic immune reaction causing fibrosis.
Tissue findings	Vascular thrombi; tissue ischemia.	Laboratory evidence of tissue destruction such as ↑ GGT, alkaline phosphatase, LDH, BUN, or creatinine.	Gradual loss of organ function.
Prevention	Check ABO compatibility.	N/A	N/A
Treatment	Cytotoxic agents.	Confirm with sampling of transplanted tissue; treat with steroids, antilymphocyte antibodies (OKT3), tacrolimus, or mycophenolate mofetil (MMF).	No treatment; biopsy to rule out treatable acute reaction.

HIGH-YIELD FACTS

HEMATOLOGY/ONCOLOGY

DIAGNOSIS

- In addition to a history and physical, a CBC and differential should be obtained, and **CSF should be analyzed for eosinophilia,** which is suggestive of a drug reaction or infection with a coccidioidomycosis or a helminth. Hematuria with eosinophilia may be a sign of schistosomiasis.
- **Imaging of the lungs, abdomen, pelvis, and brain** may demonstrate a focal defect that may be helpful in narrowing down the potential causes.

TREATMENT

Medication should be tailored to the cause of the eosinophilia. HES is treated with corticosteroid and cytotoxic agents to ↓ the eosinophilia.

TABLE 2.7-13. **Disorders Associated with Neoplasms**

CONDITION	NEOPLASM
Down syndrome	ALL ("We will ALL go DOWN together").
Xeroderma pigmentosum	Squamous cell and basal cell carcinomas of the skin.
Chronic atrophic gastritis, pernicious anemia, postsurgical gastric remnants	Gastric adenocarcinoma.
Tuberous sclerosis (facial angiofibroma, seizures, mental retardation)	Astrocytoma and cardiac rhabdomyoma.
Actinic keratosis	Squamous cell carcinoma of the skin.
Barrett's esophagus (chronic GI reflux)	Esophageal adenocarcinoma.
Plummer-Vinson syndrome (atrophic glossitis, esophageal webs, anemia; all due to iron deficiency)	Squamous cell carcinoma of the esophagus.
Cirrhosis (alcoholic, HBV or HCV)	Hepatocellular carcinoma.
Ulcerative colitis	Colonic adenocarcinoma.
Paget's disease of bone	2° osteosarcoma and fibrosarcoma.
Immunodeficiency states	Malignant lymphomas.
AIDS	Aggressive malignant NHLs and Kaposi's sarcoma.
Autoimmune diseases (e.g., myasthenia gravis)	Benign and malignant thymomas.
Acanthosis nigricans (hyperpigmentation and epidermal athickening)	Visceral malignancy (stomach, lung, breast, uterus).
Dysplastic nevus	Malignant melanoma.

- Tissue transplantation is increasingly used to treat a variety of diseases. Types of transplantation include the following:
    - **Autologous:** Transplantation from the patient to him/herself.
    - **Allogeneic:** Transplantation from a donor to a genetically different patient.
    - **Syngeneic:** Transplantation between identical twins (i.e., from a donor to a genetically identical patient).
- With allogeneic donation, efforts are made to ABO and HLA match the donor and recipient. Even with antigenic matching and immunosuppression, however, transplants may be rejected. There are three types of rejection: hyperacute, acute, and chronic (see Table 2.7-12).
- **Graft-versus-host disease** (GVHD) is a complication specific to allogeneic bone marrow transplantation in which donated T cells attack host tissues. It may be acute (occurring < 100 days post-transplant) or chronic (occurring > 100 days afterward).
    - **Minor histocompatibility antigens are thought to be responsible for GVHD,** which typically presents with **skin changes, cholestatic liver dysfunction, obstructive lung disease,** or **GI problems.**
    - Patients are treated with **high-dose steroids.**
- A variant of GVHD is the **graft-versus-leukemia effect,** in which leukemia patients who are treated with an allogeneic bone marrow transplant have significantly lower relapse rates than those treated with an autologous transplant. This difference is thought to be due to a reaction of donated T cells against leukemic cells.

DISEASES ASSOCIATED WITH NEOPLASMS

Table 2.7-13 outlines conditions that are commonly associated with neoplasms.

HIGH-YIELD FACTS

HEMATOLOGY/ONCOLOGY

Infectious Disease

Pneumonia

Some common causes of pneumonia are outlined in Table 2.8-1.

HISTORY/PE

- **Classic symptoms:** Sudden onset, fever, productive cough (purulent yellow-green sputum or hemoptysis), dyspnea, night sweats, pleuritic chest pain.
- **Atypical symptoms:** Gradual onset, dry cough, headaches, myalgias, sore throat.
- Lung exam may show ↓ or bronchial breath sounds, rales, wheezing, dullness to percussion, egophony, and tactile fremitus.
- Elderly patients as well as those with COPD, diabetes, or immunocompromised status may have minimal signs on physical exam.

DIAGNOSIS

- Workup includes physical exam, **CXR,** CBC, sputum Gram stain and culture (see Figures 2.8-1 and 2.8-2), blood culture, and ABG.
- Tests for specific pathogens include the following:
  - **Legionella:** Urine *Legionella* antigen test, sputum staining with direct fluorescent antibody, culture.
  - **Chlamydia pneumoniae:** Serologic testing, culture, PCR.
  - **Mycoplasma:** Usually clinical. Serum cold agglutinins and serum *Mycoplasma* antigen may also be used.

An adequate sputum Gram stain sample has many PMNs (> 25 cells/hpf) and few epithelial cells (< 25 cells/hpf).

TABLE 2.8-1. **Common causes of pneumonia**

CHILDREN (6 WKS–18 YRS)	ADULTS (18–40 YRS)	ADULTS (40–65 YRS)	ELDERLY
Viruses (RSV)	Mycoplasma	S. pneumoniae	S. pneumoniae
Mycoplasma	C. pneumoniae	Haemophilus influenzae	Viruses
Chlamydia pneumoniae	S. pneumoniae	Anaerobes	Anaerobes
Streptococcus pneumoniae		Viruses	H. influenzae
		Mycoplasma	Gram-⊕ rods

Special groups:	
Atypical	Mycoplasma, Legionella, Chlamydia
Nosocomial (hospital acquired)	Staphylococcus, gram-⊕ rods, anaerobes, gram-⊖ rods (GNRs)
Immunocompromised	Staphylococcus, gram-⊕ rods, fungi, viruses, Pneumocystis carinii (with HIV)
Aspiration	Anaerobes
Alcoholics/IV drug users	S. pneumoniae, Klebsiella, Staphylococcus
CF	Pseudomonas, S. aureus
COPD	H. influenzae, Moraxella catarrhalis, S. pneumoniae
Postviral	Staphylococcus, H. influenzae
Neonate	Group B streptococci (GBS), E. coli
Recurrent	Obstruction, bronchogenic carcinoma, lymphoma, Wegener's granulomatosis, immunodeficiency, unusual organisms (e.g., Nocardia, Coxiella burnetii, Aspergillus, Pseudomonas)

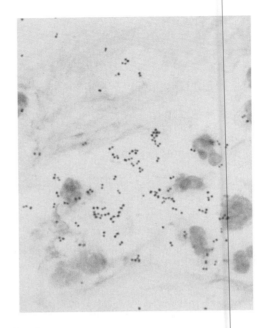

FIGURE 2.8-1. *S. aureus.*

These clusters of gram-⊕ cocci were isolated from the sputum of a patient who developed pneumonia while hospitalized.

TREATMENT

- Table 2.8-2 summarizes the recommended initial treatment for pneumonia.
- Outpatient treatment with oral antibiotics is recommended only in uncomplicated cases.

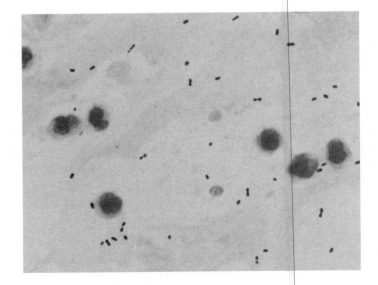

FIGURE 2.8-2. *S. pneumoniae.*

Sputum sample from a patient with pneumonia. Note the characteristic lancet-shaped gram-⊕ diplococci.

TABLE 2.8-2. **Treatment of Pneumonia**

PATIENT TYPE	SUSPECTED PATHOGENS	EMPIRIC COVERAGE
Outpatient community-acquired pneumonia, patients ≤ 65 years of age, otherwise healthy	S. pneumoniae, Mycoplasma pneumoniae, C. pneumoniae, H. influenzae, viral.	Macrolide (azithromycin), doxycycline, or fluoroquinolone.
Patients > 65 years of age or with comorbidity (COPD, heart failure, renal failure, diabetes, liver disease, EtOH abuse)	S. pneumoniae, H. influenzae, aerobic GNRs (E. coli, Enterobacter, Klebsiella), S. aureus, Legionella, viruses.	Macrolide or fluoroquinolone. May need to add a second-generation cephalosporin or β-lactam.
Community-acquired pneumonia requiring hospitalization	S. pneumoniae, H. influenzae, anaerobes, aerobic GNRs, Legionella, Chlamydia.	Extended-spectrum cephalosporin, β-lactam/β-lactamase inhibitor, or fluoroquinolone. Add a macrolide if atypical organisms are suspected.
Community-acquired pneumonia requiring hospitalization (needing ICU care)	S. pneumoniae, H. influenzae, anaerobes, aerobic GNRs, Mycoplasma, Legionella, Pseudomonas.	Fluoroquinolone or extended-spectrum cephalosporin or β-lactam/β-lactamase inhibitor + macrolide.
Institution-/hospital-acquired pneumonia—patients hospitalized > 48 hours or in a long-term care facility > 14 days	GNRs (including Pseudomonas), S. aureus, Legionella, mixed flora.	Extended-spectrum cephalosporin or β-lactam with antipseudomonal activity. Add aminoglycoside or fluoroquinolone for double coverage against Pseudomonas until lab sensitivities identify the best single agent.
Patients who are critically ill or worsening over 24–48 hours on initial antibiotic therapy	Methicillin-resistant S. aureus (MRSA).	Vancomycin or linezolid.

HIGH-YIELD FACTS

INFECTIOUS DISEASE

- **In-hospital treatment with IV antibiotics** is recommended for patients > 65 years of age and in those with comorbidity (alcoholism, COPD, diabetes, malnutrition), immunosuppression, unstable vitals or signs of respiratory failure, altered mental status, and/or multilobar involvement.
- For patients with obstructive diseases (e.g., CF or bronchiectasis), consider adding pseudomonal coverage.

Tuberculosis (TB)

Infection due to *Mycobacterium tuberculosis*. Most symptomatic cases remain confined to the lung and are due to reactivation of old infection rather than to new 1° disease. Risk factors include immunosuppression, alcoholism, preexisting lung disease, diabetes, advancing age, **homelessness,** and crowded liv-

The PORT criteria risk-stratify patients with pneumonia on the basis of age, comorbidity, and presentation. Note: The PORT criteria do not apply to AIDS patients.

TB almost always presents with an extended duration (> 3 weeks) of symptoms.

Drugs for TB—

RIPE

Rifampin
INH
Pyrazinamide
Ethambutol

Rifampin turns body fluids orange. Ethambutol can cause optic neuritis. INH causes peripheral neuritis and hepatitis.

ing conditions (e.g., **prison**). Also at risk are **immigrants** from developing nations, health care workers, and persons with "sick contacts."

HISTORY/PE

Presents with cough, **hemoptysis**, dyspnea, **weight loss, fatigue, night sweats, fever,** cachexia, hypoxia, tachycardia, lymphadenopathy, abnormal lung sounds, and a prolonged (> 3-week) duration of symptoms. TB is a common cause of fever of unknown origin (FUO).

DIAGNOSIS

- Diagnosed by a ⊕ sputum **acid-fast stain** (see Figure 2.8-3). Three A.M. sputum samples are advised. If the results are ⊖ but there is a high degree of clinical suspicion, proceed to bronchoscopy with bronchoalveolar lavage or biopsy.
- CXR may show lower lobe infiltrates (in 1° TB) or apical fibronodular infiltrates with or without cavitation (in reactivated pulmonary TB). Multiple fine nodular densities distributed throughout both lungs are typical of miliary tuberculosis, which represents hematologic or lymphatic dissemination. Especially common in HIV disease.
- A ⊕ PPD test (see Figure 2.8-4) indicates previous exposure (not necessarily active infection). Exposed immunocompromised individuals may not mount a ⊕ PPD (anergy).

TREATMENT

All cases should be reported to local and state health departments. Respiratory isolation should be instituted if TB is suspected. Treatment is as follows:

- Directly observed multidrug therapy with a four-drug regimen (**INH, pyrazinamide, rifampin, ethambutol**) until drug susceptibility tests are finalized. Administer **vitamin B₆** (pyridoxine) with INH to prevent peripheral neuritis.

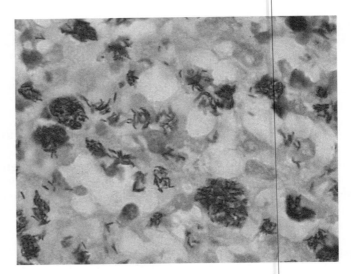

FIGURE 2.8-3. **TB organisms are identified by their red color ("red snappers") on acid-fast staining.**

(Reproduced courtesy of the Pathology Education Instructional Resource Digital Library [http://peir.net] at the University of Alabama, Birmingham.)

PPD is injected intradermally on the volar surface of the forearm. The diameter of induration is measured at 48–72 hours. BCG vaccination typically renders a patient PPD ⊕ but should not preclude prophylaxis as recommended for unvaccinated individuals. The size of induration that indicates a ⊕ test is interpreted as follows:

- **≥ 5 mm:** HIV or risk factors, close TB contacts, CXR evidence of TB.
- **≥ 10 mm:** Indigent/homeless, residents of developing nations, IV drug use, chronic illness, residents of health and correctional institutions, and health care workers.
- **≥ 15 mm:** Everyone else, including those with no known risk factors.

A ⊖ reaction with ⊖ controls implies anergy from immunosuppression, old age, or malnutrition and thus does not rule out TB.

FIGURE 2.8-4. PPD interpretation.

- Therapy on at least rifampin and INH should continue for six months.
- Initiate prophylactic therapy (**INH × 9 months**) for PPD conversion without active symptoms in patients with a CXR suggestive of old TB infection, recent new conversion (< 2 years), or the risk factors mentioned above.

Acute Pharyngitis

Viral causes are more common, but it is important to identify streptococcal pharyngitis (**group A β-hemolytic *Streptococcus pyogenes***). Etiologies are as follows:

- **Bacterial:** Group A streptococci (GAS), *Neisseria gonorrhoeae, Corynebacterium diphtheriae, M. pneumoniae.*
- **Viral:** Rhinovirus, coronavirus, adenovirus, HSV, EBV, CMV, influenza virus, coxsackievirus.

HISTORY/PE

The Centor criteria for identifying streptococcal pharyngitis are erythema, exudate, tender anterior cervical lymphadenopathy, and lack of cough.

- **Typical of streptococcal pharyngitis:** Fever, sore throat, pharyngeal erythema, tonsillar exudate, cervical lymphadenopathy, soft palate petechiae, headache, vomiting, scarlatiniform rash (indicates scarlet fever).
- **Atypical of streptococcal pharyngitis:** Coryza, hoarseness, rhinorrhea, cough, conjunctivitis, anterior stomatitis, ulcerative lesions, GI symptoms.

DIAGNOSIS

Clinical evaluation, rapid GAS antigen detection, and throat culture. With three out of four of the Centor criteria, the sensitivity of rapid antigen testing is > 90%.

TREATMENT

It is important to identify and treat streptococcal pharyngitis to prevent rheumatic fever, but overdiagnosis and overtreatment lead to ↑ cost and antibiotic resistance.

If GAS is suspected, begin empiric antibiotic therapy with penicillin × 10 days. Amoxicillin or azithromycin are alternative options. Symptom relief can be attained with fluids, rest, antipyretics, and salt-water gargles.

COMPLICATIONS

- **Nonsuppurative:** Acute rheumatic fever (see the Cardiology section), poststreptococcal glomerulonephritis.

- **Suppurative:** Cervical lymphadenitis, mastoiditis, sinusitis, otitis media, retropharyngeal or peritonsillar abscess, and, rarely, thrombophlebitis of the jugular vein (**Lemierre's syndrome**) due to *Fusobacterium*, an oral anaerobe.
- **Peritonsillar abscess** may present with odynophagia, trismus ("lockjaw"), muffled voice, unilateral tonsillar enlargement, and erythema, with the uvula and soft palate deviated away from the affected side. Culture abscess fluid and localize the abscess via intraoral ultrasound or CT. Treat with antibiotics and **surgical drainage**.

Sinusitis

Infection of the sinuses due to a collection of pus. The maxillary sinuses are most commonly affected. Subtypes are as follows:

- **Acute sinusitis (symptoms lasting < 1 month):** Most commonly associated with *S. pneumoniae, H. influenzae, M. catarrhalis*, and viral infection.
- **Chronic sinusitis (symptoms persisting > 3 months):** Often due to obstruction of sinus drainage and ongoing low-grade anaerobic infections. In diabetic patients, mucormycosis infection may develop.

HISTORY/PE

- Presents with **fever, facial pain, headache,** nasal congestion, and discharge.
- Exam may reveal tenderness, erythema, and swelling over the affected area.
- High fever, leukocytosis, and purulent nasal discharge are suggestive of acute bacterial sinusitis.

DIAGNOSIS

Always consider occult sinusitis in febrile ICU patients.

- A clinical diagnosis. Culture is generally not required.
- Transillumination shows opacification of the sinuses (low sensitivity).
- CT scan is the test of choice for sinus imaging (see Figure 2.8-5) but is usually necessary only for persistent symptoms after treatment. MRI is useful for differentiating soft tissue (as in a tumor) from mucus.
- Bacterial culture by sinus tap is the gold standard for diagnosis but is not routinely performed because of discomfort. Endoscopically guided cultures from the middle meatus are gaining popularity.

TREATMENT

- Most cases of acute sinusitis are viral and/or self-limited and are treated with symptomatic therapy (decongestants, antihistamines, pain relief).
- For patients with suspected acute bacterial sinusitis, consider amoxicillin/clavulanate 500 mg PO TID × 10 days or clarithromycin, azithromycin, TMP-SMX, or a second-generation cephalosporin × 10 days.

Coccidioidomycosis

Consider coccidioidomycosis in the HIV-⊕, Filipino, black, or pregnant patient from the southwestern United States with respiratory infection.

- A pulmonary fungal infection endemic to the **southwestern United States** (e.g., San Joaquin Valley, California). Can present as a flulike illness or as acute pneumonia, and may involve extrapulmonary sites, including bone, CNS, and skin. The incubation period is 1–4 weeks after exposure. Filipino, black, pregnant, and HIV-⊕ patients are at ↑ risk.

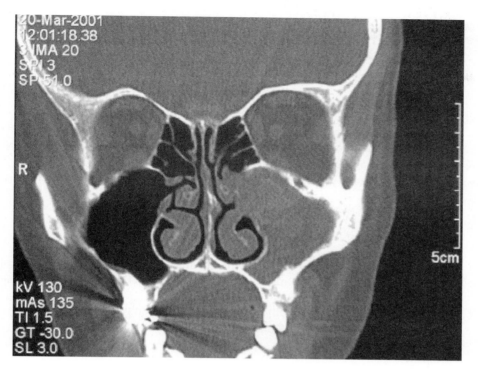

FIGURE 2.8-5. Sinusitis.

Compare the opacified left maxillary sinus and normal air-filled right sinus on this coronal CT scan. (Reproduced, with permission, from Lalwani AK. *Current Diagnosis and Treatment in Otolaryngology: Head and Neck Surgery.* New York, McGraw-Hill, 2004.)

- **Hx/PE:** Patients present with **fever,** anorexia, headache, chest pain, **cough,** dyspnea, arthralgias, and **night sweats.** Disseminated infection can present with meningitis, bone lesions, and soft tissue abscesses.
- **Dx:**
    - Precipitin antibodies (IgM) ↑ within two weeks and disappear after two months; complement fixation antibodies (IgG) ↑ at 1–3 months.
    - Obtain cultures of sputum, wound exudate, and joint aspirate.
    - CXR findings may be normal or may show infiltrates, nodules, cavity, mediastinal or hilar adenopathy, or pleural effusion.
    - Consider bronchoscopy, fine-needle biopsy, open lung biopsy, or pleural biopsy if serology is indeterminate.
- **Tx:** IV therapy is rarely necessary; however, consider IV **amphotericin B** for severe or protracted 1° pulmonary infection and disseminated disease. PO fluconazole or itraconazole may be used for mild infection and long-term suppression.

CNS INFECTIONS

Meningitis

Risk factors include recent ear infection, sinusitis, immunodeficiencies, recent neurosurgical procedures, and sick contacts. Causes are listed in Table 2.8-3.

HISTORY/PE

Patients present with **fever,** malaise, **headache, neck stiffness, photophobia,** altered mental status, **nausea/vomiting,** seizures, or signs of meningeal irritation (⊕ Kernig's and Brudzinski's signs).

TABLE 2.8-3. **Causes of Meningitis**[a,b]

Newborn (0–6 mos)	Children (6 mos–6 yrs)	6–60 yrs	60 yrs +
GBS	*S. pneumoniae*	*N. meningitidis*	*S. pneumoniae*
E. coli/GNRs	*Neisseria meningitidis*	Enteroviruses	GNRs
Listeria	*H. influenzae* B	*S. pneumoniae*	*Listeria*
	Enteroviruses	HSV	*N. meningitidis*

[a] Causes in HIV include *Cryptococcus*, CMV, toxoplasmosis (brain abscess), and JC virus (PML).

[b] Note: The incidence of *H. influenzae* meningitis has ↓ greatly with the introduction of the *H. influenzae* vaccine in the last 10–15 years.

Check for papilledema or focal neurologic deficits before performing an LP!

DIAGNOSIS

- **Blood cultures.**
- **LP** for **CSF Gram stain and culture;** obtain glucose, protein, WBC count plus differential, RBC, and opening pressure (in the absence of papilledema or focal neurologic deficits).
- **CT or MRI** to rule out other diagnoses. CBC may reveal leukocytosis; CSF findings vary (see Table 2.8-4).

TREATMENT

Antibiotics should be administered rapidly (see Table 2.8-5) and may be empirically given up to two hours prior to performing an LP. Viral disease can be treated with supportive care and close follow-up. Close contacts of patients with meningococcal meningitis should receive **rifampin,** ciprofloxacin, or ceftriaxone prophylaxis. **Dexamethasone** may be beneficial in bacterial meningitis if given 15–20 minutes before antibiotics, especially for *S. pneumoniae* or TB meningitis.

If LP is delayed for neuroimaging, begin empiric antibiotic therapy after blood cultures are drawn.

COMPLICATIONS

- **Cerebral edema:** Visible on CT/MRI. Presents with loss of oculocephalic reflex. Treat with IV mannitol.
- **Subdural effusions:** May be seen on CT scan. Occur in 50% of infants with *H. influenzae* meningitis. No treatment is necessary.
- **Ventriculitis/hydrocephalus:** Presents as a worsening clinical picture with improved CSF findings. Requires ventriculostomy and possibly intraventricular antibiotics.
- **Seizures:** Treat with benzodiazepines and phenytoin.
- **Hyponatremia:** Administer fluids and monitor sodium concentration.
- **Subdural empyema:** Presents with intractable seizures. Requires surgical evacuation.
- **Other:** Cranial nerve palsies, sensorineural hearing loss, coma, death.

Although other medications may be used, rifampin is the frequently tested prophylaxis of choice for close contacts of patients with meningococcal meningitis.

Encephalitis

HSV and **arboviruses** are the most common causes of encephalitis. Rarer etiologies include CMV, toxoplasmosis, West Nile virus, VZV, *Borrelia*, *Rickettsia*, *Legionella*, enterovirus, *Mycoplasma*, and cerebral malaria. Children and the elderly are the most vulnerable.

HISTORY/PE

Presents with **altered consciousness, headache, fever, and seizures.** Lethargy, confusion, coma, and focal neurologic deficits (cranial nerve deficits, accen-

TABLE 2.8-4. CSF Profiles

	RBCs (PER mm³)	WBCs (PER mm³)	GLUCOSE (mg/dL)	PROTEIN (mg/dL)	OPENING PRESSURE (cm H₂O)	APPEARANCE	GAMMA GLOBULIN (% PROTEIN)
Normal	< 10	< 5	~2/3 of serum	15–45	10–20	Clear	3–12
Bacterial meningitis	↔	↑ (> 1000 PMN)	↓	↑	↑	Cloudy	↔ or ↑
Viral meningitis	↔	↑ (monos/ lymphs)	↔	↔ or ↑	↔ or ↑	Most often clear	↔ or ↑
Aseptic meningitis	↔	↑	↔	↔ or ↑	↔	Clear	↔
SAH	↑↑	↑	↔	↑	↔ or ↑	Yellow/red	↔ or ↑
Guillain-Barré syndrome	↔	↔	↔ or ↑	↑↑	↔	Clear or yellow (high protein)	↔
MS	↔	↔ or ↑	↔	↔	↔	Clear	↑↑
Pseudotumor cerebri	↔	↔	↔	↔	↑↑↑	Clear	↔

tuated DTRs) may also be present. The differential includes brain abscess or malignancy, toxic-metabolic encephalopathy, subdural hematoma, and SAH.

DIAGNOSIS

- CSF shows lymphocytic pleocytosis and moderately ↑ protein. RBCs without evidence of trauma suggest HSV encephalitis. Glucose level is low in tuberculous, fungal, bacterial, and amebic infections.

The presence of RBCs in CSF without a history of trauma indicates HSV encephalitis.

TABLE 2.8-5. Empiric Treatment of Bacterial Meningitis

AGE	CAUSATIVE ORGANISM	TREATMENT
< 1 month	GBS, *E. coli*/GNRs, *Listeria*.	Ampicillin + cefotaxime or gentamicin.
1–3 months	Pneumococci, meningococci, *H. influenzae*.	Vancomycin IV + ceftriaxone or cefotaxime.
3 months – adulthood	Pneumococci, meningococci.	Vancomycin IV + ceftriaxone or cefotaxime.
> 60 years/alcoholism/ chronic illness	Pneumococci, gram-⊖ bacilli, *Listeria*, meningococci.	Ampicillin + vancomycin + cefotaxime or ceftriaxone.

HIGH-YIELD FACTS

INFECTIOUS DISEASE

- CSF Gram stain (bacteria), acid-fast stain (mycobacteria), India ink (*Cryptococcus*), wet preparation (free-living amebae), and Giemsa stain (trypanosomes). **PCR** for HSV, CMV, EBV, VZV, and enterovirus.
- **MRI** may demonstrate a **contrast-enhancing lesion** in the **temporal** lobe (in HSV).

TREATMENT

HSV encephalitis requires immediate IV acyclovir. CMV encephalitis is treated with IV ganciclovir +/– foscarnet. Administer doxycycline for suspected Rocky Mountain spotted fever, Lyme disease, or ehrlichiosis.

Brain Abscess

- A focal, suppurative infection of the brain parenchyma, usually with a **"ring-enhancing"** appearance due to fibrous capsule. The most common infective organisms are **streptococci, staphylococci,** and **anaerobes; multiple** organisms are often implicated. Etiologies include the following:
  - **Direct spread** due to paranasal sinusitis (10% overall; frequently affects young males, and often due to *Streptococcus milleri*); **otitis media** or **mastoiditis** (33%); or **dental infection** (2%).
  - **Direct inoculation** in patients with a history of head trauma or neurosurgical procedures.
  - **Hematogenous spread** (25% of cases). Often shows an **MCA distribution** with **multiple abscesses** that are poorly encapsulated and located at the **gray-white junction.**
- Hx/PE: **Headache,** drowsiness, inattention, confusion, and **seizures** are early symptoms, followed by signs of **increasing ICP** and then **a focal neurologic deficit. Headache is the most common symptom** and is **often dull, constant, and refractory to treatment.** ↑ ICP → CN III and CN VI deficits.
- Dx: **CT scan** will show a **ring-enhancing lesion** with a low-density core. MRI has higher sensitivity for early abscesses and posterior fossa lesions. **CSF analysis** is not necessary and **may precipitate a herniation syndrome.** Lab values may show peripheral leukocytosis, ↑ ESR, and ↑ CRP.

- Tx:
  - **Initiate broad-spectrum IV antibiotics** and **surgical drainage** (aspiration or excision) if necessary for diagnostic and/or therapeutic purposes. Lesions < 2 cm can often be treated medically.
  - Administer a third-generation cephalosporin + metronidazole +/– vancomycin; give IV therapy for 6–8 weeks followed by 2–3 weeks PO. Obtain serial CT/MRIs to follow resolution.
  - **Dexamethasone** with taper may be used in severe cases to ↓ cerebral edema. **IV mannitol** may be used to ↓ ICP.

HUMAN IMMUNODEFICIENCY VIRUS (HIV)

A retrovirus that targets and destroys CD4+ T lymphocytes. Infection is characterized by a progressively high rate of viral replication → a progressive decline in the CD4+ count.

- **CD4+ count** indicates the **degree of immunosuppression,** guides therapy, and helps determine prognosis.
- **Viral load** indicates the **rate** of disease progression, provides indications for treatment, and gauges response to antiretroviral therapy.
- Figure 2.8-6 illustrates the typical time course of HIV infection.

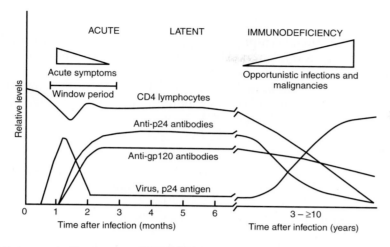

FIGURE 2.8-6. **Time course of HIV infection.**

(Adapted, with permission, from Levinson W, Jawetz E. *Medical Microbiology and Immunology: Examination & Board Review*, 6th ed. New York: McGraw-Hill, 2000, p. 276.)

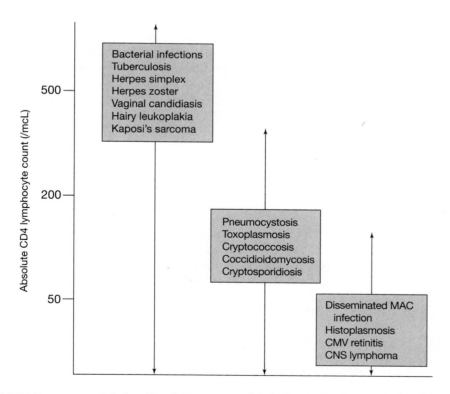

FIGURE 2.8-7. **Relationship of CD4 count to development of opportunistic infections.**

(Reproduced, with permission, from McPhee SJ, Tierney LM. *Current Medical Diagnosis & Treatment: 2007*, 46th ed. New York: McGraw-Hill, 2006.)

HISTORY/PE

- 1° infection is often **asymptomatic;** patients may also present with **flulike symptoms** (e.g., fever, lymphadenopathy, maculopapular rash, pharyngitis, diarrhea, nausea/vomiting, weight loss, headache).
- HIV may later present as night sweats, weight loss, thrush, recurrent infections, or opportunistic infections. Complications are inversely correlated with CD4+ count (see Figure 2.8-7).

DIAGNOSIS

- The **ELISA test** (high sensitivity, moderate specificity) detects anti-HIV antibodies in the bloodstream (can take up to six months to appear after exposure).
- The **Western blot** (low sensitivity, high specificity) is confirmatory.
- **Rapid HIV tests.**
- Baseline evaluation should include HIV RNA PCR (viral load), CD4+ cell count, CXR, PPD skin testing, Pap smear, VDRL/RPR, and serologies for CMV, hepatitis, toxoplasmosis, and VZV.

TREATMENT

- Currently, **antiretroviral therapy** is considered for patients with a CD4+ count < 350 who are committed to therapy or for those with 2° health problems such as metabolic wasting or opportunistic infections.
- The **starting regimen** usually include some combination of **nucleoside/nucleotide reverse transcriptase inhibitors (RTIs), non-nucleoside RTIs,** and **protease inhibitors.** The most important principle is to select multiple medications (usually three) to limit resistance.
- The choice of regimen depends on drug-drug interactions, drug tolerance, and patient adherence. Do not use monotherapy or dual therapy.
- See Table 2.8-6 for an outline of prophylactic measures against opportunistic infections.

OPPORTUNISTIC INFECTIONS

Figure 2.8-8 illustrates the microscopic appearance of some common opportunistic organisms.

Candidal Thrush

- Risk factors include xerostomia, antibiotic use, denture use, and immunosuppressed states (e.g., HIV, leukemias, lymphomas, cancer, diabetes, corticosteroid inhaler use, immunosuppressive treatment).
- **Hx/PE:** Presents with **soft white plaques that can be rubbed off,** with an erythematous base and possible mucosal burning. The differential includes oral hairy leukoplakia (lateral borders of the tongue; not easily rubbed off).
- **Dx:** Usually clinical. KOH or Gram stain shows **budding yeast and/or pseudohyphae.**
- **Tx:** Treat with local therapy (e.g., nystatin suspension or clotrimazole tablets, or a PO azole such as fluconazole).

Cryptococcal Meningitis

- Risk factors include AIDS and exposure to **pigeon droppings.**
- **Hx/PE:** Presents with headache, fever, impaired mentation, and **absent**

TABLE 2.8-6. Prophylaxis for HIV-Related Opportunistic Infections

PATHOGEN	INDICATION FOR PROPHYLAXIS	MEDICATION	COMMENTS
Pneumocystis carinii pneumonia (PCP)	CD4+ < 200/mm³, prior PCP, unexplained fever × 2 weeks, or HIV-related oral candidiasis.	TMP-SMX SS[a] or dapsone +/– pyrimethamine.	Discontinue prophylaxis when CD4+ > 200/mm³ for ≥ 3 months.
Mycobacterium avium complex (MAC)	CD4+ < 50–100/mm³.	Weekly azithromycin or daily clarithromycin.	Discontinue prophylaxis when CD4+ > 100/mm³ for > 6 months.
Toxoplasma gondii	CD4+ < 100/mm³ + ⊕ IgG serologies.	TMP-SMX DS.[a]	–
M. tuberculosis	PPD > 5 mm or "high risk" (see TB section).	**Sensitive:** INH × 9 months (+ pyridoxine) or rifampin +/– pyrazinamide × 2 months.	Include pyridoxine with INH-containing regimens.
Candida	Multiple recurrences.	**Esophagitis:** Fluconazole. **Oral:** Nystatin swish and swallow.	–
HSV	Multiple recurrences.	Acyclovir, famciclovir, or valacyclovir.	–
S. pneumoniae	All patients.	Pneumovax.	Give every five years or when CD4+ > 200.
Influenza	All patients.	Influenza vaccine annually.	–

[a] SS = single strength; DS = double strength.

(Adapted, with permission, from Mandell GL. *Principles and Practice of Infectious Diseases,* 5th ed. London: Churchill Livingstone, 2000:1507; and from Bartlett JG, Gallant JE. *2003 Medical Management of HIV Infection.* Baltimore, MD: Johns Hopkins University Division of Infectious Diseases and AIDS Services, 2003:40–45.)

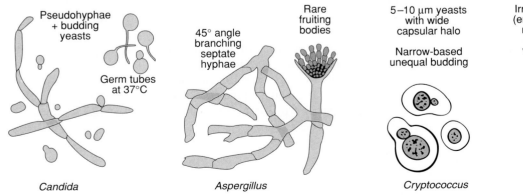
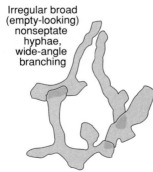

Pseudohyphae + budding yeasts

Germ tubes at 37°C

Candida

45° angle branching septate hyphae

Aspergillus

Rare fruiting bodies

5–10 μm yeasts with wide capsular halo

Narrow-based unequal budding

Cryptococcus

Irregular broad (empty-looking) nonseptate hyphae, wide-angle branching

Mucor

FIGURE 2.8-8. Common opportunistic organisms.

217

meningismus. The differential includes toxoplasmosis, lymphoma, TB meningitis, AIDS dementia complex, PML, HSV encephalitis, and other fungal disease.

- **Dx: LP** ($\downarrow$ CSF glucose; $\uparrow$ protein; $\uparrow$ leukocyte count with monocytic predominance); $\oplus$ **CSF cryptococcal antigen test, India ink stain,** and fungal culture.
- **Tx:**
  - **IV amphotericin B** + flucytosine $\times$ 2 weeks; then give fluconazole 400 mg $\times$ 8 weeks. Lifelong **maintenance therapy** with fluconazole 200 mg QD, or until CD4 > 200 for > 6 months.
  - $\uparrow$ opening pressure may require serial LPs.

The CSF antigen test for cryptococcal meningitis is highly sensitive and specific.

Histoplasmosis

- Risk factors include AIDS, spelunking, and exposure to bird or bat excrement, especially in the **Ohio** and **Mississippi** river valleys.
- **Hx/PE:** 1° exposure is often asymptomatic or causes a flulike illness. Fever, weight loss, hepatosplenomegaly, lymphadenopathy, nonproductive cough, and pancytopenia indicate disseminated infection (often within 14 days and in immunocompromised hosts). The differential includes atypical bacterial pneumonias, blastomycosis, coccidioidomycosis, TB, sarcoidosis, pneumoconiosis, and lymphoma.
- **Dx: CXR** shows diffuse nodular densities, focal infiltrate, cavity, or hilar lymphadenopathy (chronic infection is usually cavitary). The **urine and serum polysaccharide antigen test** is the most sensitive test for making the initial diagnosis, monitoring response to therapy, and diagnosing relapse. Culture is also diagnostic (blood, sputum, bone marrow, CSF). The yeast form is seen with **silver stain** on biopsy (bone marrow, lymph node, liver) or bronchoalveolar lavage.
- **Tx: Amphotericin B** or amphotericin B liposomal $\times$ 3–10 days, followed by itraconazole $\times$ 12 weeks. Maintenance therapy with daily itraconazole. Can be treated supportively in the immunocompetent host in mild cases.

> **AIDS pathogens—**
>
> **The Major Pathogens Concerning Complete T-Cell Collapse**
>
> **T**oxoplasma gondii
> **M**ycobacterium
> avium–intracellulare
> **P**neumocystis carinii
> **C**andida albicans
> **C**ryptococcus
> neoformans
> **T**uberculosis
> **C**MV
> **C**ryptosporidium
> parvum

Pneumocystis carinii Pneumonia (PCP)

- Risk factors include impaired cellular immunity and AIDS.
- **Hx/PE:** Presents with dyspnea on exertion, fever, nonproductive cough, tachypnea, weight loss, fatigue, and impaired oxygenation. CXR shows diffuse, bilateral interstitial infiltrates with a ground-glass appearance, but any presentation is possible. PCP can also present as disseminated disease or local disease in other organ systems. The differential includes TB, histoplasmosis, and coccidioidomycosis.
- **Dx:** Cytology of induced sputum or bronchoscopy specimen with silver stain and immunofluorescence. Obtain an ABG to check PaO_2.
- **Tx:** Treat with TMP-SMX $\times$ 21 days. Prednisone taper should be used in patients with moderate to severe hypoxemia (PaO_2 < 70 mm or A-a gradient > 35). Clindamycin and primaquine constitute an alternative regimen for patients with sulfa allergy.

Suspect PCP in any HIV patient who presents with nonproductive cough and dyspnea.

Cytomegalovirus (CMV)

- Most 1° infections are asymptomatic; serious reactivation occurs in immunocompromised patients. Seventy percent of adults have been infected in the United States.

- Transmission occurs via **sexual contact**, in **breast milk**, via **respiratory droplets** in nursery or day care, and via **blood transfusions**. Risk factors for reactivation include the first 100 days status post tissue or bone marrow transplant and HIV positivity with a CD4 < 100 or a viral load > 10,000.
- **Hx/PE:**
    - Systemic infection may resemble EBV mononucleosis (see the discussion of infectious mononucleosis).
    - **CMV retinitis** has a high rate of retinal detachment (i.e., "pizza pie" retinopathy) and presents with floaters and visual field changes (CD4 < 50).
    - **GI and hepatobiliary** involvement can present with multiple nonspecific GI symptoms. CMV and microsporidia have been implicated in the development of **AIDS cholangiopathy.**
    - **CMV pneumonitis** presents with cough, fever, and sparse sputum production and is associated with a high mortality rate.
    - **CNS involvement** can include **polyradiculopathy, transverse myelitis,** and subacute **encephalitis** (CD4 < 50; periventricular calcifications).
- **Dx:** Virus isolation, culture, **tissue examination**, PCR.
- **Tx: Ganciclovir** or foscarnet. Treat underlying disease if the patient is immunocompromised.

Treat CMV infection with ganciclovir.

Mycobacterium avium Complex (MAC)

- Ubiquitous organisms causing **pulmonary** and **disseminated** infection in several demographic groups. More common than *M. tuberculosis* as a cause of pulmonary disease in the United States.
- The 1° form occurs in **apparently healthy nonsmokers; a 2°** form affects patients with **preexisting pulmonary disease** such as COPD, TB, and CF. Disseminated infection occurs in AIDS patients with a **CD4 < 100.** There is no evidence that behavioral change affects exposure
- **Hx/PE:** Disseminated *M. avium* infection in AIDS is associated with **fever, weakness,** and **weight loss in patients not on HAART or chemoprophylaxis for MAC.** Hepatosplenomegaly and lymphadenopathy are occasionally seen.
- **Dx:** Blood cultures (⊕ in 2–3 weeks). Labs show anemia, hypoalbuminemia, and ↑ **serum alkaline phosphatase and LDH.** Biopsy of bone marrow, intestine, or liver reveals **foamy macrophages** with **acid-fast bacilli.** Typical granulomas may be absent in immunocompromised patients.
- **Tx: Clarithromycin** and **ethambutol +/– rifabutin** and **HAART.** Continue for 10 months and until CD4 > 100 for > 6 months.
- **Prevention: Weekly azithromycin** for those with a CD4 < 50 or AIDS-defining opportunistic infection.

*HIV-⊕ patients with a CD4 < 50 or AIDS-defining illness should be on chemoprophylaxis for MAC with **azithromycin,** which is highly effective for preventing disseminated infection.*

Toxoplasmosis

- Risk factors include ingesting **raw or undercooked meat and changing cat litter.** Worldwide, exposure is highest in **France.**
- **Hx/PE:** 1° infection is usually asymptomatic. Reactivated toxoplasmosis occurs in immunosuppressed patients and may present in specific organs (brain, lung, and eye > heart, skin, GI tract, and liver). Encephalitis is common in seropositive AIDS patients. Classically, CNS lesions present with fever, headache, altered mental status, seizures, and focal neurologic deficits.
- **Dx: Serology, PCR,** tissue examination for histology, isolation of the

*The two most likely differential diagnoses of **ring-enhancing lesions** in AIDS patients are **toxoplasmosis** and **CNS lymphoma.***

organism in mice, or tissue culture. In the setting of CNS involvement, obtain a **CT scan** (can show **multiple, isodense or hypodense, ring-enhancing** mass lesions) or an **MRI** (predilection for **basal ganglia; more sensitive).

- **Tx:** PO pyrimethamine, sulfadiazine, and folate × 4–8 weeks, followed by pyrimethamine, clindamycin, and folate until the disease has resolved clinically and radiographically. TMP-SMX (Bactrim DS) or pyrimethamine + dapsone can be used for prophylaxis in patients with a CD4 < 100 and a ⊕ IgG.

SEXUALLY TRANSMITTED DISEASES (STDs)

Chlamydia

Chlamydia is a common cause of nongonococcal urethritis in men.

Chlamydia species cause arthritis, neonatal conjunctivitis, pneumonia, nongonococcal urethritis/PID, and lymphogranuloma venereum.

- The most common bacterial STD in the United States. Caused by *Chlamydia trachomatis*, which can infect the genital tract, urethra, anus, and eye. Risk factors include **unprotected sexual intercourse, new or multiple partners, and frequent douching.** Often coexists with or mimics *N. gonorrhoeae* infection (known as nongonococcal urethritis when gonorrhea is absent).
- **Hx/PE:** Infection is often asymptomatic but may present with **urethritis, mucopurulent cervicitis,** or **PID.** Exam may reveal cervical/adnexal tenderness in women or penile discharge and testicular tenderness in men. The differential includes gonorrhea, endometriosis, PID, orchitis, vaginitis, and UTI.
- **Dx:** Usually clinical. Urine tests (PCR or ligase chain reaction) are a rapid means of detection, while DNA probes and immunofluorescence (for gonorrhea/chlamydia) take 48–72 hours. **Gram stain** of urethral or genital discharge may show **PMNs but no bacteria (intracellular).**
- **Tx: Doxycycline** 100 mg PO BID × 7 days or azithromycin 1 g PO × 1 day. Use erythromycin in pregnant patients. **Treat sexual partners.** Maintain a low threshold to treat for *N. gonorrhoeae.*
- **Cx:** Chronic infection and pelvic pain, Reiter's syndrome (urethritis, conjunctivitis, arthritis), Fitz-Hugh–Curtis syndrome (perihepatic inflammation and fibrosis). Ectopic pregnancy/infertility can result from PID (in women) and epididymitis (in men).

Gonorrhea

Treat for gonorrhea and chlamydia in light of the high prevalence of coinfection.

- This gram-⊖ intracellular diplococcus can infect almost any site in the female reproductive tract, whereas infection in men tends to be limited to the urethra.
- **Hx/PE:** Presents with a **greenish-yellow discharge,** pelvic or **adnexal pain,** and swollen Bartholin's glands. Men experience **purulent urethral discharge,** dysuria, and erythema of the urethral meatus. The differential includes chlamydia, endometriosis, pharyngitis, PID, vaginitis, UTI, salpingitis, and tubo-ovarian abscess.
- **Dx:** Swab the pharynx, cervix, urethra, or anus as appropriate. Conduct urine and probe tests as with chlamydia. Obtain a Gram stain of cervical discharge. Disseminated disease may present with **monoarticular septic arthritis,** rash, and/or **tenosynovitis.**
- **Tx: Ceftriaxone IM.** Also treat for presumptive chlamydia coinfection (doxycycline × 7 days or macrolide × 1 dose). Condoms are effective prophylaxis. Treat the sexual partner or partners if possible.
- **Cx:** Persistent infection with pain; infertility; tubo-ovarian abscess with rupture; disseminated gonococcal infection (see Figure 2.8-9).

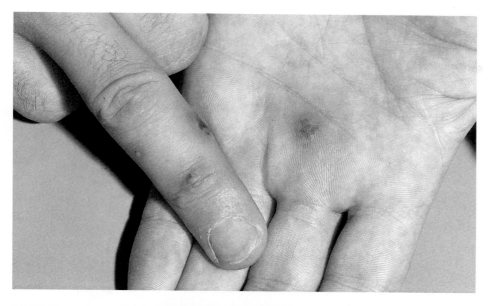

FIGURE 2.8-9.   **Disseminated gonococcal infection.**

Hemorrhagic, painful pustules on erythematous bases. (Reproduced, with permission, from Wolff K, Johnson RA, Suurmond D. *Fitzpatrick's Color Atlas & Synopsis of Clinical Dermatology*, 5th ed. New York: McGraw-Hill, 2005, p. 910.)

Syphilis

Caused by *Treponema pallidum*, a spirochete. AIDS can accelerate the course of disease progression.

HISTORY/PE

- 1° (**10–90 days after infection**): Presents with a **painless ulcer (chancre;** see Figure 2.8-10).
- 2° (**4–8 weeks after chancre**): Low-grade fever, headache, malaise, and generalized lymphadenopathy with a diffuse, symmetric, asymptomatic (non-

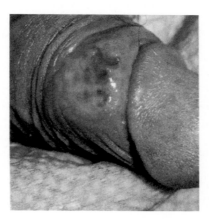

FIGURE 2.8-10.   **1° syphilis.**

The chancre is an ulcerated papule with a smooth, clean base; raised, indurated borders; and scant discharge. (Reproduced, with permission, from Bondi EE. *Dermatology: Diagnosis and Therapy*, 1st ed. Stamford, CT: Appleton & Lange, 1991, p. 394.)

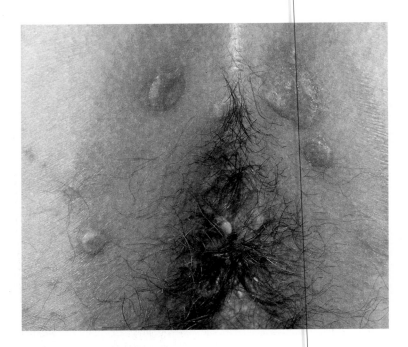

FIGURE 2.8-11. **Condylomata lata.**

Typical appearance of the verrucous heaped-up lesions of condylomata lata. (Reproduced, with permission, from Wolff K, Johnson RA, Suurmond D. *Fitzpatrick's Color Atlas & Synopsis of Clinical Dermatology*, 5th ed. New York: McGraw-Hill, 2005, p. 921.)

pruritic) **maculopapular rash on the soles and palms.** Highly infective 2° eruptions include mucous patches or **condylomata lata** (see Figure 2.8-11). Meningitis, hepatitis, nephropathy, and eye involvement may also be seen.

- **Early latent:** No symptoms; ⊕ serology; first year of infection.
- **Late latent:** No symptoms; ⊕ or ⊖ serology; > 1 year of infection. One-third progress to 3° syphilis.
- **3° (1–20 years after initial infection):** Destructive, granulomatous **gummas.** Neurologic findings include **tabes dorsalis** (posterior column degeneration), meningitis, and **Argyll Robertson pupil** (constricts with accommodation but not reactive to light). Cardiovascular findings include dilated aortic root, aortitis, **aortic root aneurysms,** and aortic regurgitation.

TABLE 2.8-7. **Diagnostic Tests for Syphilis**

Test	Comments
Dark-field microscopy	Identifies motile spirochetes (only 1° and 2° lesions).
VDRL/RPR	Rapid and cheap, but sensitivity is only 60–75% in 1° disease. Many false positives.
FTA-ABS	Sensitive, specific. Used as a 2° diagnostic test.
TPPAa	Similar sensitivity and specificity to FTA-ABS and easier to use. Becoming the 2° test of choice.

aTPPA = *T. pallidum* particle agglutination test.

TABLE 2.8-8. Sexually Transmitted Genital Lesions[a]

	CALYMMATOBACTERIUM GRANULOMATIS (GRANULOMA INGUINALE-DONOVANOSIS)	*HAEMOPHILUS DUCREYI* (CHANCROID)	HSV-1 OR -2[a]	HPV[b]	*TREPONEMA PALLIDUM*
Lesion	Papule becomes a **beefy-red ulcer,** with a characteristic rolled edge of granulation tissue	Papule or pustule (chancroid; see Figure 2.8-12)	Vesicle	Papule (condylomata acuminata; warts)	Papule (chancre)
Appearance	Raised red lesions with a white border	Irregular, deep, well demarcated, necrotic	Regular, red, shallow ulcer	Irregular, pink or white, raised; cauliflower	Regular, red, round, raised
Number	1 or multiple	1–3	Multiple	Multiple	Single
Size	5–10 mm	10–20 mm	1–3 mm	1–5 mm	1 cm
Pain	No	**Yes**	**Yes**	No	No
Concurrent signs and symptoms	Granulomatous ulcers	Inguinal lymphadenopathy	Vulvar pain and pruritus	Pruritus	Regional adenopathy
Diagnosis	Clinical exam, biopsy (Donovan bodies)	Difficult to culture; diagnosis made on clinical grounds	Tzanck smear, viral cultures, DFA or serology	Clinical exam; biopsy for confirmation	Spirochetes seen under dark-field microscopy; *T. pallidum* identified by serum antibody test
Treatment[c]	Doxycycline (100 mg BID) or azithromycin (1 g weekly) × 3 weeks	Doxycycline (100 mg BID) or azithromycin (1 g weekly) × 3 weeks	Acyclovir for 1° infection	Cryotherapy, topical agents such as podophyllin, trichloroacetic acid, or 5-FU cream	Penicillin IM

[a] Some 85% of genital herpes lesions are caused by HSV-2.

[b] HPV serotypes 6 and 11 are associated with genital warts; types 16, 18, and 31 are associated with cervical cancer.

[c] For all, treat sexual partners.

DIAGNOSIS

- See Table 2.8-7. **VDRL false positives** are seen with **V**iruses (mononucleosis, HSV, HIV, hepatitis), **D**rugs/IV drug use, **R**heumatic fever/**R**heumatoid arthritis, and S**LE**/**L**eprosy.

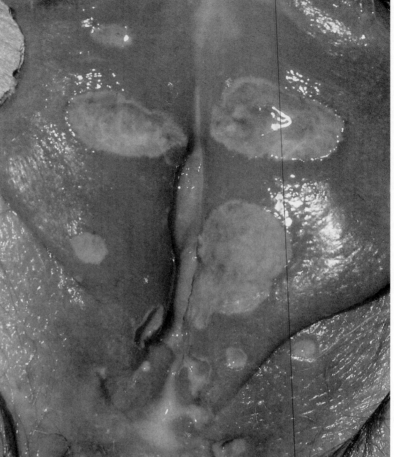

FIGURE 2.8-12. Chancroid.

Multiple, painful ulcers. (Reproduced, with permission, from Wolff K, Johnson RA, Suurmond D. *Fitzpatrick's Color Atlas & Synopsis of Clinical Dermatology,* 5th ed. New York: McGraw-Hill, 2005, p. 927.)

Syphilis is the "great imitator" because the dermatologic findings resemble those of many other diseases.

Remember that treatment of syphilis can result in an acute flulike illness known as the Jarisch-Herxheimer reaction.

- Neurosyphilis should be suspected and ruled out in any AIDS patient with neurologic symptoms and a ⊕ RPR.

TREATMENT

- 1°/2°: **Benzathine penicillin IM.** Tetracycline or doxycycline × 14 days may be used for patients with penicillin allergies.
- Latent infection should be treated with penicillin once weekly × 3 weeks.
- Neurosyphilis should be treated with penicillin IV; penicillin-allergic patients should be desensitized prior to therapy.

Genital Lesions

See Table 2.8-8 for a description of common sexually transmitted genital lesions along with an outline of their diagnosis and treatment.

224

Urinary Tract Infections (UTIs)

Affect women more frequently than men, and ⊕ *E. coli* cultures are obtained in 80% of cases. See the mnemonic **SEEKS PP** for other pathogens. Risk factors include catheters or other urologic instrumentation, anatomic abnormalities (e.g., BPH, vesicoureteral reflux), previous UTIs or pyelonephritis, diabetes mellitus (DM), recent antibiotic use, immunosuppression, and pregnancy.

HISTORY/PE

Present with **dysuria, urgency, frequency,** suprapubic pain, and possibly hematuria. Children may present with **bed-wetting,** poor feeding, recurrent fevers, and foul-smelling urine. The differential includes vaginitis, STDs, urethritis or acute urethral syndrome, and prostatitis.

DIAGNOSIS

- Diagnosed by **clinical symptoms.** In the absence of symptoms, treatment is warranted only for children, those with anatomical GU tract anomalies, pregnant women, those with instrumented urinary tracts, patients scheduled for GU surgery, and renal transplant patients.
- **Urine dipstick/UA:** ↑ **leukocyte esterase** (a marker of WBCs) is 75% sensitive and up to 95% specific (good to rule out UTI). ↑ **nitrites** (a marker of bacteria), ↑ urine pH (*Proteus* infections), and hematuria (seen with cystitis) are also commonly seen.
- **Microscopic analysis: Pyuria** (> 5 WBCs/hpf) and **bacteriuria** (1 organism/hpf = 10^6 organisms/mL) are suggestive.
- **Urine culture** (gold standard: > 10^5 **CFU/mL**).

TREATMENT

- Treat healthy young females on an outpatient basis with oral **TMP-SMX** or a **fluoroquinolone** × 3 days, but note that resistance to TMP-SMX has been increasing.
- Treat with fluoroquinolone or TMP-SMX for at least 7–10 days in high-risk patients (immunosuppressed, DM, pregnancy) and in cases of complicated UTI (urinary obstruction, men, renal transplant, catheters, instrumentation).
- Patients with urosepsis should be hospitalized and initially treated with **IV antibiotics** (ciprofloxacin or ampicillin/sulbactam + gentamicin to cover enterococcus).
- Prophylactic antibiotics may be given to women with uncomplicated recurrent UTIs. Check for prostatitis in men.
- In pregnancy, treat UTI with TMP-SMX, nitrofurantoin, or cephalexin × 3 days. Document with urine culture 10 days after treatment. If infection recurs, place on prophylactic antibiotics for the remainder of the pregnancy.

Pyelonephritis

- Nearly 85% of community-acquired cases result from the same pathogens that cause cystitis. Cystitis and pyelonephritis have similar risk factors.
- **Hx/PE: Flank pain, fever/chills,** nausea/vomiting. Dysuria, frequency, and urgency are possible.
- **Dx:**
    - **UA and culture:** Similar to cystitis plus **WBC casts.**

> ### *Common UTI bugs—*
> ### SEEKS PP
>
> **S**erratia
> **E**. coli
> **E**nterobacter
> **K**lebsiella pneumoniae
> **S**. saprophyticus
> **P**seudomonas
> **P**roteus mirabilis

HIGH-YIELD FACTS

INFECTIOUS DISEASE

Pyelonephritis is the most common serious medical complication of pregnancy. Twenty to thirty percent of patients with untreated bacteriuria will develop pyelonephritis.

- **CBC:** Leukocytosis.
- In general, imaging is not necessary. **Ultrasound** can be used to rule out obstruction and calculi and can often confirm the diagnosis non-invasively, but **CT scan** is becoming the **test of choice** in patients with adequate renal function who are not responding to therapy. In recurrent cases, IVP may demonstrate renal scarring.
- **Tx:**
  - For mild cases, patients may be treated on an outpatient basis for 10–14 days. **Fluoroquinolone** is first line. Encourage ↑ PO fluids and monitor closely.
  - Admit and administer IV antibiotics for patients who have serious medical complications, are **pregnant,** present with severe **nausea and vomiting,** or have suspected bacteremia.

HEMATOLOGIC INFECTIONS

Sepsis

Systemic inflammatory response syndrome **(SIRS)** with a **documented infection,** induced by microbial invasion or toxins in the bloodstream. **Septic shock** refers to sepsis-induced hypotension and organ dysfunction due to poor perfusion. Etiologies include the following:

- **Gram-⊕ shock** (e.g., staphylococci and streptococci) 2° to fluid loss caused by exotoxins.
- **Gram-⊖ shock** (e.g., *E. coli, Klebsiella, Proteus,* and *Pseudomonas*) 2° to vasodilation caused by endotoxins (lipopolysaccharide).
- **Neonates:** GBS, *E. coli, Listeria monocytogenes, H. influenzae.*
- **Children:** *H. influenzae,* pneumococcus, meningococcus.
- **Adults:** Gram-⊕ cocci, aerobic gram-⊖ bacilli, anaerobes (dependent on the presumed site of infection).
- **IV drug users/indwelling lines:** *S. aureus,* coagulase-⊖ *Staphylococcus* spp.
- **Asplenic patients:** Pneumococcus, *H. influenzae,* meningococcus (encapsulated organisms).

History/PE

- Presents with abrupt onset of fever and chills, altered mental status, tachycardia, and tachypnea. **Hypotension** and shock occur in severe cases.
- Septic shock is typically a warm shock with **warm skin and extremities.** Cold shock with **cool skin and extremities** is possible with other underlying factors (e.g., CHF).
- Petechiae or ecchymoses suggest DIC (2–3% of cases).

Diagnosis

- A clinical diagnosis.
- Labs show leukocytosis or leukopenia with ↑ bands, thrombocytopenia (50% of cases), and evidence of ↓ tissue perfusion (↑ creatinine, ↑ LFTs). Blood, sputum, and urine cultures may be ⊕ (sepsis may also result from toxins in the bloodstream); CXR may show an infiltrate. Obtain coagulation studies and consider a DIC panel (fibrinogen, fibrin split products, D-dimer).

Treatment

- May require ICU admission. Treat aggressively with IV fluids, pressors, and empiric antibiotics (based on the likely source of infection).
- Treat underlying factors (e.g., remove Foley catheter or infected lines).
- The 1° goal is to **maintain BP and perfusion** to end organs.

Malaria

A protozoal disease caused by four strains of the genus *Plasmodium* (*P. falciparum*, *P. vivax*, *P. ovale*, and *P. malariae*) and transmitted by the bite of an infected female *Anopheles* mosquito. **P. falciparum** has the highest morbidity and causes the largest number of deaths, occasionally within 24 hours of symptom onset. There are 300–500 million new infections and 1–3 million deaths per year worldwide, although the disease has been largely eliminated in North America, Europe, and Russia. Recent outbreaks have occurred in parts of the southern and eastern United States and in Europe, mainly through the arrival of infected travelers and immigrants from endemic areas. Travelers to endemic areas should take chemoprophylaxis and use mosquito repellent and bed nets to minimize exposure.

HISTORY/PE

- Patients have a history of exposure in a malaria-endemic area with **periodic** attacks of sequential **chills, fever (> 41°C)**, and **diaphoresis** occurring over 4–6 hours. Associated symptoms include malaise, headache, dizziness, GI symptoms (anorexia, nausea, vomiting, mild diarrhea), myalgias, arthralgia, backache, and dry cough. **Splenomegaly** often appears four or more days after onset of symptoms. Often asymptomatic between attacks, which recur every 2–3 days, depending on the *Plasmodium* strain.
- The severely ill patient may present with hyperpyrexia, prostration, impaired consciousness, agitation, hyperventilation, and bleeding. The presence of rash, lymphadenopathy, neck stiffness, or photophobia suggests a different or additional diagnosis.
- The differential includes influenza, typhoid fever, infectious mononucleosis, viral gastroenteritis, community-acquired pneumonia, dengue fever, visceral leishmaniasis, amebic liver abscess, babesiosis, leptospirosis, and relapsing fever.

DIAGNOSIS

- Timely diagnosis of the correct strain is essential because *P. falciparum* can be fatal and is often resistant to standard chloroquine treatment.
- **Giemsa-** or **Wright-**stained **thick and thin blood films** should be sent for expert microscopic evaluation. Specimens should be obtained at eight-hour intervals for three days, including during and between febrile periods.
- CBC usually demonstrates normochromic, normocytic anemia with reticulocytosis.
- If resources allow, more sensitive serologic tests are available, including rapid antigen detection methods, fluorescent antibody methods, and PCR.

TREATMENT

- Uncomplicated malarial infection can be treated orally, with the choice of medication determined by the *Plasmodium* strain. **Chloroquine** has been the standard antimalarial medication used in many parts of the world, but increasing resistance has led to the use of other medications, including quinine, atovaquone, mefloquine, artesunate, and halofantrine.
- The life cycle of *P. vivax* and *P. ovale* strains include dormant liver hypnozoite forms, which are resistant to treatment with **chloroquine**. Thus, in cases of *P. vivax*, *P. ovale*, or an unknown strain, **primaquine** is added to eradicate the hypnozoites in the liver.
- Severe infections can be treated with parenteral antimalarial medications with transition to oral regimens as tolerated. Newer combinations such as **proguanil/atovaquone (Malarone)** eliminate the need for multiple medications. Symptoms can be treated with supportive care.

Malaria should be considered in the differential for any patient who has emigrated from or recently traveled to tropical locations and presents with fever.

P. vivax, P. ovale, and P. malariae can all cause symptoms months to years after initial infection.

COMPLICATIONS

- **Cerebral malaria:** Headache, change in mental status, neurologic signs, retinal hemorrhages, convulsions, delirium, **coma.**
- **Severe hemolytic anemia:** Usually associated with *P. falciparum* infection.
- **Acute tubular necrosis and renal failure:** Associated with **blackwater fever** (dark urine due to hemoglobinuria).
- **Noncardiogenic pulmonary edema:** Often precipitated by overly rapid rehydration.
- Other complications include gram-⊖ bacteremia, acute hepatopathy, hypoglycemia, cardiac dysrhythmias, secretory diarrhea, lactic acidosis, DIC, and a low birth rate in children of infected mothers.

Infectious Mononucleosis

Most commonly occurs in **young adult** patients. Usually due to acute EBV infection. Transmission most often occurs through exchange of body fluids, including saliva.

HISTORY/PE

- Presents with **fever** and **pharyngitis. Fatigue** invariably accompanies initial illness and may persist for 3–6 months. Exam may reveal low-grade fever, generalized lymphadenopathy (especially **posterior cervical**), tonsillar exudate and enlargement, palatal petechiae, a generalized maculopapular rash, splenomegaly, and **bilateral upper eyelid edema.**
- Patients who present with pharyngitis as their 1° symptom may be misdiagnosed as having streptococcal pharyngitis (30% of patients with infectious mononucleosis are asymptomatic carriers of group A strep in their oropharynx).
- **Treatment of patients with ampicillin (i.e., for streptococcal pharyngitis) during acute EBV infection can cause a prolonged, pruritic, drug-related maculopapular rash.** This rash does not portend future sensitivity to β-lactams and will remit with discontinuation of ampicillin.
- The differential also includes CMV, toxoplasmosis, HIV, HHV-6, other causes of viral hepatitis, and lymphoma.

DIAGNOSIS

- Diagnosed by the **heterophile antibody (Monospot) test** (may be ⊖ in the first few weeks after symptoms begin). The EBV-infected proliferating B cells produce a characteristic antibody that agglutinates the horse and sheep RBCs that are the basis for the Monospot test.
- **EBV-specific antibody** can be ordered in patients with suspected mononucleosis and a ⊖ Monospot test. Heterophile ⊖ and EBV-antibody ⊖ infectious mononucleosis is most often due to CMV infection.
- CBC with differential often reveals mild **thrombocytopenia** with relative **lymphocytosis** and > 10% **atypical T lymphocytes.**
- CMP usually reveals mildly elevated transaminases, alkaline phosphatase, and total bilirubin.

TREATMENT

Treatment is mostly supportive, as there is no effective antiviral therapy. Steroids are indicated for airway compromise due to tonsillar enlargement, severe thrombocytopenia, or severe autoimmune hemolytic anemia.

Obtain a finger stick in a patient with malaria and mental status changes to rule out hypoglycemia.

*A young adult who presents with the triad of **fever, sore throat,** and **lymphadenopathy** may have infectious mononucleosis.*

The lymphocytosis in EBV infection is predominantly due to B-cell proliferation, but the atypical cells are T lymphocytes.

About one-third of patients with infectious mononucleosis have coexisting streptococcal pharyngitis requiring treatment.

- **CNS infection:** Can present as aseptic meningitis, encephalitis, meningoencephalitis, CN palsies (particularly CN VII), optic and peripheral neuritis, transverse myelitis, or Guillain-Barré syndrome.
- **Splenic rupture:** Occurs in < 0.5% of cases. More common in males and presents with abdominal pain, referred shoulder pain, or hemodynamic compromise.
- **Upper airway obstruction:** Treat with steroids.
- **Bacterial superinfection:** Ten percent of patients develop streptococcal pharyngitis secondarily.
- **Fulminant hepatic necrosis:** More common in men; the most common cause of death in affected males.
- **Autoimmune hemolytic anemia:** Occurs in 2% of patients during the first two weeks. Coombs ⊕. Mild anemia lasts 1–2 months. Treat with steroids if severe.
- Other rare complications associated with acute EBV infection include hepatitis (which can be fulminant), myocarditis or pericarditis with electrocardiographic changes, pneumonia with pleural effusion, interstitial nephritis, genital ulcerations, and vasculitis.

FEVER

Fever of Unknown Origin (FUO)

- A temperature of > 38.3°C of at least three weeks' duration that remains undiagnosed following three outpatient visits or three days of hospitalization. In adults, infections and cancer account for > 60% of cases of FUO, while autoimmune diseases account for approximately 15%.
- **Hx/PE:** Fever, headache, myalgia, malaise. The differential includes the following:
    - **Infectious:** TB, endocarditis (e.g., HACEK organisms; see the discussion of infective endocarditis), occult abscess, osteomyelitis, catheter infections.
    - **Neoplastic:** Lymphomas, leukemias, hepatic and renal cell carcinomas.
    - **Autoimmune:** Still's disease, SLE, cryoglobulinemia, polyarteritis nodosa, connective tissue disease, granulomatous disease (including sarcoidosis).
    - **Miscellaneous:** Pulmonary emboli, alcoholic hepatitis, drug fever, familial Mediterranean fever, factitious fever.
    - Undiagnosed (10–15%).
- **Dx:**
    - Confirm fever and take a detailed history (including family, social, occupational, dietary, exposures, and travel); obtain CXR, CBC with differential, ESR, multiple blood cultures, sputum Gram stain and culture, UA, and PPD. Specific tests (ANA, RF, viral cultures, viral serologies/antigen tests) can be obtained if an infectious or autoimmune etiology is suspected.
    - CT of the chest and abdomen should be done early in the workup of a true FUO. Rule out drug fever. Invasive testing (marrow/liver biopsy) is generally low yield. Laparoscopy and colonoscopy are higher yield as second-line tests (after CT).
- **Tx: Stop unnecessary medications.** Give empiric antibiotics to severely ill patients until the etiology has been determined. Stop antibiotics if there is no response.

FUO patients without other symptoms do not require empiric antibiotic therapy.

Overall, infections and cancer account for the majority of cases of FUO. In the elderly, rheumatic diseases account for one-third of cases.

HIGH-YIELD FACTS

INFECTIOUS DISEASE

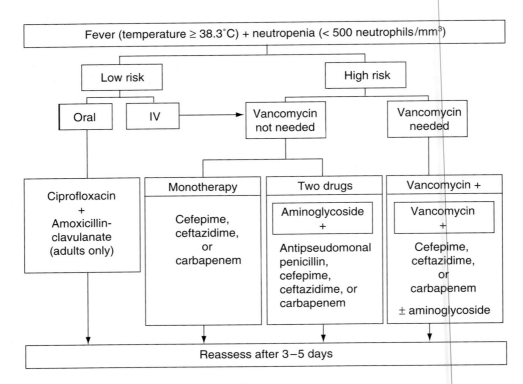

FIGURE 2.8-13. **Empiric treatment algorithm for a neutropenic fever patient.**

(Reproduced, with permission, from Hughes WT. 2002 guidelines for the use of antimicrobial agents in neutropenic patients with cancer. *Clin Infec Dis* 34:730–751, 2002.)

Neutropenic Fever

Avoid doing a rectal exam on a neutropenic patient.

- Defined as a single oral temperature of ≥ 38.3°C (101°F) or a temperature of ≥ 38.0°C (100.4°F) for ≥ 1 hour in a neutropenic patient (i.e., a neutrophil count of < 500 cells/mm^3).
- **Hx/PE:** Common in cancer patients undergoing chemotherapy (neutropenic nadir 7–10 days postchemotherapy). Inflammation may be minimal or absent.
- **Dx:** Thorough physical examination, but **avoid rectal examination** because of the bleeding risk. CBC with differential, serum creatinine, BUN, and transaminases; blood, urine, lesion, and stool cultures. CXR for patients with respiratory symptoms; CT scan to evaluate for abscess.
- **Tx:** Empiric antibiotic therapy (see Figure 2.8-13). Routine use of colony-stimulating factors is not indicated. If fevers persist after 72 hours despite antibiotic therapy, start antifungal treatment.

TICK-BORNE INFECTIONS

Lyme Disease

Lyme disease is the most common vector-borne disease in North America.

- A tick-borne disease caused by the spirochete *Borrelia burgdorferi*. Usually seen during the **summer months** and carried by *Ixodes* ticks on white-tailed deer and white-footed mice. Endemic to the **Northeast,** northern Midwest, and Pacific coast.
- **Hx/PE:** Onset of rash with fever, malaise, fatigue, headache, myalgias, and/or arthralgias. Infection usually occurs after a tick feeds for > 18 hours.

- **1°: Erythema migrans** begins as a small erythematous macule or papule that is found at the tick-feeding site and expands slowly over days to weeks. The border may be macular or raised, often with central clearing ("bull's eye").
- **2°:** Presents with migratory polyarthropathies, neurologic phenomena (e.g., Bell's palsy), meningitis and/or myocarditis, and conduction abnormalities (third-degree heart block).
- **3°:** Arthritis and subacute encephalitis (memory loss and mood change).
- **Dx—erythema migrans:**
  - **ELISA** and **Western blot.** Use the Western blot to confirm a ⊕ or indeterminate ELISA. A ⊕ ELISA denotes **exposure** but is not specific for active disease.
  - Tissue culture/PCR.
- **Tx:** Treat early disease with **doxycycline** and more advanced disease (e.g., CNS or arthritic disease) with **ceftriaxone.** Consider empiric therapy for patients with the characteristic rash, arthralgias, or a tick bite acquired in an endemic area. Prevent with tick bite avoidance.

Lyme arthritis can be very subtle and minimally inflammatory and can wax and wane.

Rocky Mountain Spotted Fever

- A disease caused by ***Rickettsia rickettsii*** and carried by the American dog tick (*Dermacentor variabilis*). The organism invades the endothelial lining of capillaries and causes **small vessel vasculitis.**
- **Hx/PE:** Headache, fever, malaise, rash. The characteristic rash is initially macular (beginning on the wrists and ankles) but becomes petechial/purpuric as it spreads centrally (see Figure 2.8-14). Altered mental status or DIC may develop in severe cases.

Rocky Mountain spotted fever starts on the wrists and ankles and then spreads centrally.

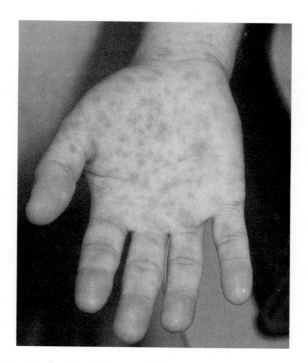

FIGURE 2.8-14. **Rocky Mountain spotted fever.**

These erythematous macular lesions will evolve into a petechial rash that will spread centrally. (Courtesy of Daniel Noltkamper, MD.)

- **Dx:** Clinical diagnosis should be confirmed with indirect immunofluorescence of rash biopsy.
- **Tx: Doxycycline** or chloramphenicol (for multidrug-resistant organisms). The condition can be rapidly fatal if left untreated. Prevent by avoiding tick bites.

CONGENITAL INFECTIONS

Pregnant women should not change the cat's litterbox. First-trimester toxoplasmosis infection is less common and more severe. Third-trimester infection is more common and less severe.

May occur at any time during pregnancy, labor, and delivery. Common sequelae include **premature delivery, CNS abnormalities,** anemia, **jaundice,** hepatosplenomegaly, and growth retardation. The most common pathogens can be remembered through use of the mnemonic **TORCHeS** (see also Table 2.8-9):

- **T**oxoplasmosis: Transplacental transmission, with 1° infection occurring via consumption of **raw meat** or contact with **cat feces.** Specific findings include hydrocephalus, **intracranial calcifications,** chorioretinitis, and **ring-enhancing lesions** on head CT. See the discussion of toxoplasmosis in this chapter.
- **O**ther: **HIV,** parvovirus, varicella, *Listeria,* TB, malaria, fungi.
- **R**ubella: Transplacental transmission in the first trimester. Specific findings include a purpuric **"blueberry muffin" rash,** cataracts, mental retardation, hearing loss, and **PDA.**
- **C**MV: The **most common congenital infection,** primarily transmitted transplacentally. Specific findings include petechial rash (similar to "blueberry muffin" rash) and **periventricular calcifications.** See the discussion of CMV in this chapter.

TABLE 2.8-9. Diagnosis and Treatment of Common Congenital Infections

DISEASE	DIAGNOSIS	TREATMENT	PREVENTION
Toxoplasmosis	Serologic testing.	Pyrimethamine + sulfadiazine; spiramycin prophylaxis (for pregnant women).	Avoid exposure to cats and cat feces (e.g., changing litter or gardening) during pregnancy. Treat the mother during the third trimester.
Rubella	Serologic testing.		Immunize before pregnancy; otherwise, consider abortion if infected or exposed (≤ 20 weeks' gestation). Vaccinate the mother after delivery if serologic titers remain ⊖.
CMV	Urine culture, PCR of amniotic fluid.	Postpartum ganciclovir.	
HSV	Serologic testing.	Acyclovir.	Perform a C-section if lesions are present at delivery.
HIV	ELISA, Western blot.		AZT or nevirapine in pregnant women with HIV; perform a C-section if viral load > 1000; treat infants with prophylactic AZT; avoid breast-feeding.
Syphilis	Dark-field microscopy, VDRL/RPR, FTA-ABS.	Penicillin.	Penicillin in pregnant women who test ⊕.

- Herpes: Intrapartum transmission if the mother has **active lesions**. Can cause skin, eye, and mouth infections or life-threatening CNS/systemic infection.
- Syphilis: Primarily intrapartum transmission. Specific findings include a **maculopapular skin rash**, lymphadenopathy, hepatomegaly, "snuffles" (mucopurulent rhinitis), and osteitis. In childhood, late congenital syphilis is characterized by saber shins, saddle nose, CNS involvement, and Hutchinson's triad: **peg-shaped upper central incisors, deafness**, and **interstitial keratitis** (photophobia, lacrimation). See the discussion of syphilis in this chapter.

Infectious Conjunctivitis

A common complaint in the emergency room setting, inflammation of the conjunctiva is most often bacterial or viral but can be fungal, parasitic, allergic, or chemical. It is essential to differentiate potentially vision-threatening infectious etiologies from allergic or other causes of conjunctivitis, as well as to identify other vision-threatening conditions that may mimic conjunctivitis. See Table 2.8-10 for the common etiologies of infectious conjunctivitis.

Neisseria *conjunctivitis is an ocular emergency often requiring inpatient parenteral antibiotic therapy.*

TABLE 2.8-10. Common Causes of Infectious Conjunctivitis

TYPE	PATHOGEN	CHARACTERISTIC	DIAGNOSIS	TREATMENT
Bacterial	Staphylococci, streptococci, *Haemophilus*, *Pseudomonas, Moraxella*	Foreign body sensation, purulent discharge.	Gram stain and culture if severe.	Antibiotic drops/ointment.
	N. gonorrhoeae	**An emergency!** Corneal involvement can lead to perforation and blindness.	Gram stain shows gram-$\ominus$ intracellular diplococci.	IM ceftriaxone, PO ciprofloxacin or ofloxacin. **Inpatient** treatment if complicated.
	C. trachomatis A–C	**Recurrent epithelial keratitis** in childhood, trichiasis, corneal scarring, and entropion. **The leading cause of preventable blindness worldwide.**	Giemsa stain, chlamydial cultures.	Azithromycin, tetracycline, or erythromycin for 3–4 weeks.
Viral	**Adenovirus** (most common)	Copious **watery discharge,** severe ocular irritation, preauricular lymphadenopathy. Occurs in epidemics.		**Contagious,** self-limited. Topical corticosteroids with supervision of an ophthalmologist.

Orbital Cellulitis

- Commonly due to infection of the **paranasal sinuses;** can lead to endophthalmitis and blindness. Usually caused by **streptococci, staphylococci,** and **H. influenzae** (in children). In diabetic and immunocompromised patients, **mucormycosis and *Rhizopus*** are in the differential.
- **Hx/PE:** Presents with **acute-onset fever, proptosis, ↓ EOM,** ocular pain, and ↓ visual acuity. Look for a **history of ocular trauma or sinusitis.** Palatal or nasal mucosal ulceration with coexisting maxillary and/or ethmoid sinusitis suggests mucormycosis or *Rhizopus.*
- **Dx: Mostly clinical.** Blood and tissue fluid culture; CT scan (to rule out orbital abscess and intracranial involvement).
- **Tx: Admit. Immediate IV antibiotics;** request an **ophthalmologic/ENT** consult. Abscess formation may necessitate surgery. **In the diabetic and immunocompromised,** treat with **amphotericin B** and **surgical debridement** (often associated with **cavernous sinus thrombosis**) if *Mucor* or *Rhizopus* is diagnosed.

Otitis Externa

- An inflammation of the external auditory canal, also known as "swimmer's ear." *Pseudomonas* (from poorly chlorinated pools) and Enterobacteriaceae are the most common etiologic agents. Both grow in the presence of excess moisture.
- **Hx/PE:** Presents with pain, pruritus, and possible purulent discharge. Exam reveals **pain with movement of the tragus/pinna** (unlike otitis media) and an edematous and erythematous ear canal.
- **Dx:** A clinical diagnosis. Gram stain and culture are helpful if a fungal etiology is suspected. CT scan if the patient is toxic appearing.
- **Tx: Antibiotic** and **steroid** eardrops. Use systemic antibiotics in patients with severe disease. Diabetics are at risk for malignant otitis externa and osteomyelitis of the skull base and thus require hospitalization and IV antibiotics.

MISCELLANEOUS INFECTIONS

Infective Endocarditis

Infection of the endocardium, usually 2° to bacterial or other infectious causes. Most commonly affects the heart valves, especially the mitral valve. Risk factors include rheumatic, congenital, or valvular heart disease; prosthetic heart valves; IV drug abuse; and immunosuppression. Etiologies are as follows:

- ***S. aureus*** is the causative agent in > 80% of cases of acute bacterial endocarditis in patients with a history of IV drug abuse.
- **Viridans streptococci** are the most common pathogens for left-sided subacute bacterial endocarditis.
- Coagulase ⊖ *Staphylococcus* is the most common infecting organism in prosthetic valve endocarditis.
- *Streptococcus bovis* endocarditis is associated with coexisting GI malignancy.
- *Candida* and *Aspergillus* species account for most cases of fungal endocarditis. Predisposing factors include long-term indwelling IV catheters, malignancy, AIDS, organ transplantation, and IV drug use. Table 2.8-11 lists the causes of endocarditis.

TABLE 2.8-11. Causes of Endocarditis

ACUTE	SUBACUTE
S. aureus (IV drug abuse)	Viridans streptococci
S. pneumoniae	Enterococcus
N. gonorrhoeae	Staphylococcus epidermidis
	Fungi

MARANTIC	HACEK (CULTURE-NEGATIVE)	SLE
Cancer (poor prognosis). Mets seed valves; emboli can cause cerebral infarcts.	Haemophilus parainfluenzae Actinobacillus Cardiobacterium Eikenella Kingella	Libman-Sacks (autoantibody to valve)

HISTORY/PE

- Fever, chills, weakness, dyspnea, sweats, anorexia, skin lesions, IV drug use, FUO.
- Exam reveals **heart murmur.** Affects the mitral valve more than the aortic valve in non–IV drug users; more right-sided involvement is found in IV drug users (tricuspid valve > mitral valve > aortic valve).
- **Osler's nodes** (small, tender nodules on the finger and toe pads), **Janeway lesions** (small peripheral hemorrhages; see Figure 2.8-15), **splinter hem-**

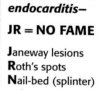

Presentation of endocarditis—

JR = NO FAME

Janeway lesions
Roth's spots
Nail-bed (splinter)
  hemorrhage
Osler's nodes
Fever
Anemia
Murmur
Emboli

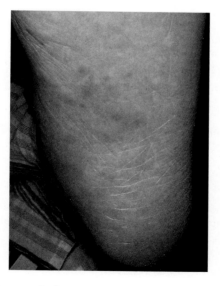

FIGURE 2.8-15. Janeway lesions.

Peripheral embolization to the sole → a cluster of erythematous macules known as Janeway lesions. (Courtesy of the Department of Dermatology, Wilford Hall USAF Medical Center and Brooke Army Medical Center, San Antonio, TX.)

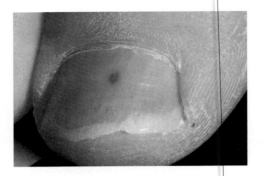

FIGURE 2.8-16. **Splinter hemorrhages.**

Note the splinter hemorrhages along the distal aspect of the nail plate, due to emboli from subacute bacterial endocarditis. (Courtesy of the Armed Forces Institute of Pathology, Bethesda, MD.)

orrhages (subungual petechiae; see Figure 2.8-16), **Roth's spots** (retinal hemorrhages), and other embolic phenomena are also seen.

DIAGNOSIS

- Diagnosis is guided by risk factors, clinical symptoms, and the **Duke criteria** (see Table 2.8-12).
- **CBC** with leukocytosis and left shift; ↑ **ESR** and CRP.

TREATMENT

Early empiric IV antibiotic treatment includes vancomycin or ceftriaxone + gentamicin. Acute valve replacement is sometimes necessary. The prognosis for prosthetic valve endocarditis is poor. See the mnemonic **PUS RIVER** for indications for surgery. Give antibiotic prophylaxis before dental work in patients with valvular disease.

Anthrax

Caused by the spore-forming gram-⊕ bacterium *Bacillus anthracis*. Its natural incidence is rare, but infection is an occupational hazard for veterinarians,

> ***Endocarditis: indications for surgery—***
>
> **PUS RIVER**
>
> **P**rosthetic valve endocarditis (most cases)
> **U**ncontrolled infection
> **S**uppurative local complications with conduction abnormalities
> **R**esection of mycotic aneurysm
> **I**neffective antimicrobial therapy (e.g., vs. fungi)
> **V**alvular damage (significant)
> **E**mbolization (repeated systemic)
> **R**efractory CHF (or sudden onset)

TABLE 2.8-12. **Duke Criteria for the Diagnosis of Endocarditis**

CRITERIA	COMPONENTS
Major	1. At least two separate ⊕ blood cultures for a typical organism, persistent bacteremia with any organism, or single ⊕ culture of *Coxiella burnetii*.
	2. Evidence of endocardial involvement (via transesophageal echocardiography [TEE] or new murmur).
Minor	1. Predisposing risk factors.
	2. Fever ≥ 38.3°C.
	3. **Vascular phenomena:** Septic emboli, septic infarcts, mycotic aneurysm, Janeway lesions.
	4. **Immunologic phenomena:** Glomerulonephritis, Osler's nodes, Roth's spots.
	5. Microbiological evidence that does not meet major criteria.

farmers, and individuals who handle **animal wool, hair, hides, or bone meal products.** Also a biological weapon. *B. anthracis* can cause cutaneous (most common), inhalation (most deadly), or GI anthrax.

HISTORY/PE

- **Cutaneous:** Presents 1–7 days after skin exposure and penetration of spores. The lesion begins as a **pruritic papule** that enlarges to form an ulcer surrounded by a satellite bulbus/lesion with an edematous halo and a round, regular, and raised edge. **Regional lymphadenopathy** is also characteristic. The lesion evolves into a **black eschar** within 7–10 days.
- **Inhalational:** Fever, dyspnea, hypoxia, hypotension, or symptoms of pneumonia (1–3 days after exposure), classically due to hemorrhagic mediastinitis.
- **GI:** Occurs after the ingestion of poorly cooked, contaminated meat; can present with dysphagia, nausea/vomiting, bloody diarrhea, and abdominal pain.

The anthrax-associated *pruritic papule* forms an ulcer with an edematous halo and then a *black eschar.*

DIAGNOSIS

CXR is the most sensitive test for inhalational disease (widened mediastinum, pleural effusions, infiltrates). Aerobic culture and Gram stain of ulcer exudate show nonmotile short chains of bacilli. Antibody tests are also useful in confirming the diagnosis.

TREATMENT

Ciprofloxacin or doxycycline plus one or two additional antibiotics for at least 14 days are first line for inhalational disease or cutaneous disease of the face, head, or neck. Many strains express β-lactamases that confer resistance to penicillin; therefore, penicillin and amoxicillin are no longer recommended as single agents for inhalational disease. For cutaneous disease, treat for 7–10 days. Postexposure prophylaxis (**ciprofloxacin**) to prevent inhalation anthrax should be continued for 60 days.

Penicillin and amoxicillin are no longer recommended as single agents for the treatment of disseminated anthrax. Treat with ciprofloxacin plus one or two other antibiotics.

Osteomyelitis

- Bone marrow infection 2° to **direct spread** from a soft tissue infection (80% of cases) is most common in adults, whereas infection due to **hematogenous seeding** (20% of cases) is more common in children (metaphyses of the long bones) and IV drug users (**vertebral bodies**). Common pathogens are outlined in Table 2.8-13.
- **Hx/PE:** Localized **bone pain and tenderness;** warmth, swelling, erythema, and limited motion of the adjacent joint. Systemic symptoms (fevers, chills) and purulent drainage may be present.
- **Dx:**
  - ↑ WBC count, **ESR** (> 100), and **CRP** levels. Blood cultures may be ⊕.
  - X-rays are often ⊖ initially but may show **periosteal elevation** within 10–14 days. Bone scans are sensitive for osteomyelitis but lack specificity.
  - **MRI** (test of choice) will show ↑ signal in the bone marrow and associated soft tissue infection.
  - Definitive diagnosis is made by bone aspiration with Gram stain and culture. Clinical diagnosis made by probing through the soft tissue to bone is usually sufficient, as aspiration carries a risk of infection.

Osteomyelitis is associated with peripheral vascular disease, diabetes, penetrating soft tissue injuries, and IV drug abuse.

TABLE 2.8-13. Common Pathogens in Osteomyelitis

IF	THINK
Most people	*S. aureus*
IV drug user	*S. aureus* or *Pseudomonas*
Sickle cell disease	*Salmonella*
Hip replacement	*S. epidermidis*
Foot puncture wound	*Pseudomonas*
Chronic	*S. aureus, Pseudomonas,* Enterobacteriaceae
Diabetic	Polymicrobial, *Pseudomonas, S. aureus,* streptococci, anaerobes

Diabetic osteomyelitis should be treated with antibiotics targeting gram-⊕ organisms and anaerobes.

- **Tx:** Treat with **surgical debridement** of necrotic, infected bone and then with **IV antibiotics** × 4–6 weeks. Empiric antibiotic selection is based on the suspected organism and Gram stain. Consider clindamycin + ciprofloxacin, ampicillin/sulbactam, or oxacillin/nafcillin (for methicillin-resistant *S. aureus*); vancomycin (for MRSA); or ceftriaxone or ciprofloxacin (for gram-⊖ bacteria).
- **Complications:** Chronic osteomyelitis, sepsis, septic arthritis. Long-standing chronic osteomyelitis with a draining sinus tract may eventually → **squamous cell carcinoma** (Marjolin's ulcer).

Musculoskeletal

Volkmann's contracture of the wrist and fingers is caused by compartment syndrome due to supracondylar fractures.

The 6 P's of compartment syndrome:

Pain
Pallor
Paresthesias
Poikilothermia
Paralysis
Pulselessness

Phalen maneuver—place wrists in flexion resulting in aching and numbness in > 60 seconds.

Tinel's sign—tapping over median nerve at the wrist reproduces symptoms.

COMPARTMENT SYNDROME

- ↑ **pressure** within a confined space that compromises nerve, muscle, and soft tissue perfusion. Occurs primarily in the anterior compartment of the lower leg and forearm 2° to trauma (fracture or muscle injury) to the affected compartment.
- **Hx/PE:** Presents with pain out of proportion to physical findings; **pain with passive motion** of the fingers and toes; and paresthesias, pallor, poikilothermia, pulselessness, and paralysis. Pulselessness occurs late.
- **Dx:** Measure compartment pressures (usually ≥ 30 mmHg); measure delta pressures (diastolic pressure − compartment pressure).
- **Tx: Immediate fasciotomy** to ↓ pressures and ↑ tissue perfusion.

CARPAL TUNNEL SYNDROME (CTS)

Entrapment of the **median nerve at the wrist** caused by ↓ size or space of the carpal tunnel → paresthesias, pain, and occasionally paralysis. Can be precipitated by overuse of wrist flexors, DM, or thyroid dysfunction. Commonly occurs in pregnant and middle-aged women.

HISTORY/PE

- Presents with aching over the **thenar area of the hand** and proximal forearm. Pain may extend to the shoulder.
- Paresthesia or numbness is seen in a median nerve distribution.
- Symptoms **worsen at night** or when the wrists are held in flexion or extension.
- Patients may report frequently dropping objects or inability to open jars.
- Examination shows thenar atrophy (if CTS is long-standing).
- **Phalen's maneuver** and **Tinel's sign** are ⊕.

DIAGNOSIS

A clinical diagnosis, although EMG testing can be used to confirm the diagnosis.

TREATMENT

- Splint the wrist in a neutral position at night and during the day if possible. Administer NSAIDs.
- If conservative treatment fails, consider corticosteroid injection of the carpal canal.
- Work-related CTS may benefit from ergonomic aids.
- CTS of pregnancy usually resolves after delivery.
- Surgical treatment is reserved for fixed sensory loss, thenar weakness, or intolerable symptoms.

COMPLICATIONS

Permanent loss of sensation, hand strength, and fine motor skills.

BURSITIS

Inflammation of the bursa by **repetitive use, trauma, infection, or systemic inflammatory disease.** A bursa is a flattened sac filled with a small amount of synovial fluid that serves as a protective buffer between bones and overlapping muscles. Common sites of bursitis include subacromial, olecranon, trochanteric, prepatellar, and infrapatellar bursae. Septic bursitis is more common in superficial bursae (olecranon, prepatellar, and infrapatellar bursae).

HISTORY/PE

- Presents with localized tenderness, ↓ range of motion (ROM), edema, and erythema.
- Patients may have a history of trauma or inflammatory disease.

DIAGNOSIS

- Aspiration is indicated if septic bursitis is suspected.
- No labs or imaging is needed.

TREATMENT

- Conservative treatment includes rest, heat and ice, elevation, and NSAIDs.
- Intrabursal steroid injection can be considered (**contraindicated if septic bursitis** is suspected).
- Septic bursitis should be treated with 7–10 days of antibiotics.

TENDONITIS

An **inflammatory condition** characterized by pain at tendinous insertions into bone associated with swelling or impaired function. Commonly occurs in the supraspinatus, **biceps,** wrist extensor, **patellar,** iliotibial band, posterior tibial, and **Achilles tendons.** Overuse is the most common cause and includes work-related activities or an ↑ in activity level.

Oral fluoroquinolones are associated with ↑ risk of tendon rupture and tendonitis.

HISTORY/PE

- Presents with pain at a tendinous insertion that worsens with **repetitive stress** and **resisted strength testing** of the affected muscle group.
- Wrist flexor tendonitis (lateral epicondylitis, or tennis elbow) worsens with resisted dorsiflexion of the wrist.

DIAGNOSIS

A clinical diagnosis. Consider a radiograph if there is a history of trauma.

TREATMENT

- Rest, NSAIDs; ice for the first 24–48 hours.
- Consider splinting or immobilization.
- Begin strengthening exercises once pain has subsided.
- If conservative treatment fails, consider peritendinous injection of lidocaine and corticosteroids. **Never inject the Achilles tendon** in view of the ↑ risk of rupture. Avoid repetitive injection.

LOW BACK PAIN (LBP)

May arise from paraspinous muscles, ligaments, facet joints, disks, or nerve roots (see Table 2.9-1); typically resolves within four weeks. Prolonged bed rest is contraindicated. Risk factors for malignancy include age > 50, a previous history of cancer, pain not relieved by lying down, symptoms lasting > 1 month, pain that worsens at night, and constitutional symptoms.

TABLE 2.9-1.   Motor and Sensory Deficits in Back Pain

| NERVE ROOT | ASSOCIATED DEFICIT | | |
	MOTOR	REFLEX	SENSORY
L4	Foot dorsiflexion (tibialis anterior).	Patellar	Medial aspect of the lower leg.
L5	Big toe dorsiflexion (extensor hallucis longus), foot eversion (peroneus muscles).	None	Dorsum of the foot and lateral aspect of the lower leg.
S1	Plantar flexion (gastrocnemius/soleus), gluteus maximus (hip extension).	Achilles	Plantar and lateral aspects of the foot.

Herniated Disk

Causes include degenerative changes, trauma, or neck/back strain or sprain. Most common (95%) in the lumbar region, especially at **L4–L5** and **L5–S1**.

HISTORY/PE

- Presents with sudden onset of severe, electricity-like LBP, usually preceded by several months of aching, "discogenic" pain.
- Common among middle-aged and older men.
- Exacerbated by ↑ intra-abdominal pressure or Valsalva (e.g., coughing).
- Associated with **sciatica,** paresthesias, muscle weakness, atrophy, contractions, or spasms.
- A **passive straight leg raise ↑ pain** (highly sensitive but not specific).
- A crossed straight leg raise ↑ pain (highly specific but not sensitive). Large midline herniations can cause **cauda equina syndrome.**

Bowel or bladder dysfunction (unrinary overflow incontinence), impotence, and saddle-area anesthesia are consistent with cauda equina syndrome, which is a surgical emergency.

DIAGNOSIS

- Obtain an ESR and a plain radiograph if other causes of back pain are suspected (e.g., infection, trauma, compression fracture).
- Order a stat MRI for cauda equina syndrome or for a severe or rapidly progressing neurologic deficit.
- Order an MRI if symptoms are refractory to conservative management. May show disk herniation (see Figure 2.9-1).

TREATMENT

- NSAIDs in scheduled doses, physical therapy, and local heat → resolution within four weeks in 80% of cases.
- Epidural or nerve block may be of benefit.
- Severe or rapidly evolving neurologic deficits and cauda equina syndrome are indications for discectomy.

Lung, breast, and prostate cancer can metastasize to the vertebrae and cause back pain.

Spinal Stenosis

Narrowing of the lumbar or cervical spinal canal → compression of the nerve roots. Most commonly due to degenerative joint disease; typically occurs in middle-aged or elderly patients.

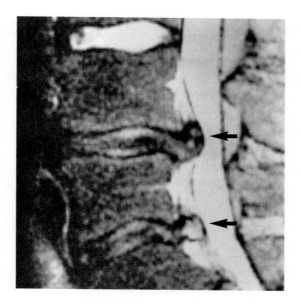

FIGURE 2.9-1. **Disk herniation.**

MRI reveals herniations of L4–L5 and L5–S1 (arrows). (Reproduced, with permission, from Skinner HB. *Current Diagnosis & Treatment in Orthopedics*, 1st ed. Stamford, CT: Appleton & Lange, 1995, p. 186.)

HISTORY/PE

- Presents with neck pain; back pain that radiates to the buttocks and legs; and leg numbness and weakness.
- Leg cramping is worse **at rest, with standing,** and **with walking (pseudo- or neurogenic claudication).**
- Symptoms **improve** with **flexion at the hips** and bending forward.

DIAGNOSIS

- Radiographs show degenerative changes that include disk space narrowing, facet hypertrophy, and spondylolisthesis → a narrowed spinal canal.
- MRI or CT shows spinal stenosis.

TREATMENT

- **Mild to moderate:** NSAIDs and abdominal muscle strengthening.
- **Advanced:** Epidural steroid injections can provide relief.
- **Refractory:** Surgical laminectomy may achieve significant short-term success, but many patients will have a recurrence of symptoms.

COMMON ADULT ORTHOPEDIC INJURIES

Table 2.9-2 outlines the presentation and treatment of orthopedic injuries that commonly affect adults.

TABLE 2.9-2. Common Adult Orthopedic Injuries

INJURY	MECHANICS	TREATMENT
Shoulder dislocation	**Anterior dislocation:** Most common; the axillary artery and nerve are at risk. Patients hold the arm in external rotation. **Posterior dislocation:** Associated with seizure and electrocutions; can injure the radial artery. Patients hold the arm in internal rotation.	Reduction followed by a sling and swath. Recurrent dislocations may need surgical repair.
Hip dislocation	**Posterior dislocation:** Most common (> 90%); occurs via a posteriorly directed force on an internally rotated, flexed, adducted hip ("dashboard injury"). Associated with a risk of sciatic nerve injury and avascular necrosis (AVN). **Anterior dislocation:** Can injure the obturator nerve.	Closed reduction followed by abduction pillow/bracing. Evaluate with CT scan after reduction.
Colles' fracture	Involves the distal radius. Often results from a fall onto an outstretched hand → a dorsally displaced, dorsally angulated fracture. Commonly seen in the elderly (osteoporosis) and children.	Closed reduction followed by application of a long-arm cast; open reduction if the fracture is intra-articular.
Scaphoid (carpal navicular) fracture	The **most commonly fractured carpal bone.** May take two weeks for radiographs to show the fracture. Assume a fracture if there is tenderness in the anatomical snuff box.	Thumb spica cast. If displacement or navicular nonunion is present, treat with open reduction. With proximal third scaphoid fractures, AVN may result from disruption of blood flow.
Boxer's fracture	Fracture of the fifth metacarpal neck. Due to forward trauma of a closed fist (e.g., punching a wall).	Closed reduction and ulnar gutter splint; percutaneous pinning if the fracture is excessively angulated. If skin is broken, assume infection by human oral pathogens → surgical irrigation, debridement, and IV antibiotics (covering *Eikenella*).
Humerus fracture	Direct trauma. May have radial nerve palsy → wrist drop and loss of thumb abduction (see Figure 2.9-2).	Hanging-arm cast vs. coaptation splint and sling. Functional bracing.
"Nightstick fracture"	Ulnar shaft fracture resulting from self-defense with the arm against a blunt object.	Open reduction and internal fixation (ORIF) if significantly displaced.
Monteggia's fracture	Diaphyseal fracture of the proximal ulna with subluxation of the radial head.	ORIF of the shaft fracture (due to poor fracture diaphyseal blood supply) and closed reduction of the radial head.
Galeazzi's fracture	Diaphyseal fracture of the radius with dislocation of the distal radioulnar joint. Results from a direct blow to the radius.	ORIF of the radius and casting of the fracture forearm in supination to reduce the distal radioulnar joint.

TABLE 2.9-2.   Common Adult Orthopedic Injuries (continued)

INJURY	MECHANICS	TREATMENT
Hip fracture	↑ risk with osteoporosis. Presents with a shortened and externally rotated leg. **Displaced femoral neck fractures:** Associated with an ↑ risk of AVN, nonunion, and DVTs.	ORIF with parallel pinning of the femoral neck. Displaced fractures in elderly patients may require a hip hemiarthroplasty. Anticoagulate to ↓ the likelihood of DVTs.
Femoral fracture	Direct trauma. Beware of fat emboli, which present with fever, change in mental status, dyspnea, hypoxia, petechiae, and ↓ platelets.	Intramedullary nailing of the femur. Irrigate and debride open fractures.
Tibial fracture	Direct trauma. Watch for compartment syndrome.	Casting vs. intramedullary nailing.
Open fractures	An orthopedic emergency; patients must be taken to the OR in < 6 hours owing to ↑ infection risk.	OR emergently to repair fracture. Treat with antibiotics and tetanus prophylaxis.
Achilles tendon rupture	Presents with a sudden "pop" like a rifle shot. More likely with ↓ physical conditioning. Exam shows limited plantar flexion and a ⊕ Thompson's test (pressure on the gastrocnemius → absent foot plantar flexion).	Treat surgically followed by long leg cast for six weeks.
Knee injuries	Present with knee instability, edema, and hematoma. **ACL:** ▪ Results from noncontact twisting mechanism, forced hyperextension, or impact to an extended knee. ▪ ⊕ anterior drawer and Lachman tests. ▪ Rule out a meniscal or MCL injury. **PCL:** ▪ Results from forced hyperextension. ▪ ⊕ posterior drawer test. **Meniscal tears:** ▪ Results from acute twisting injury or a degenerative tear in elderly patients. ▪ Clicking or locking may be present. ▪ Exam shows joint line tenderness and a ⊕ McMurray's test.	Treatment of MCL/LCL and meniscal tears is usually conservative. Treatment of ACL injuries is generally surgical with graft from the patellar or hamstring tendons. Operative PCL repair is reserved for highly competitive athletes. Operative meniscal repair is for younger patients with significant tears or older patients whose symptoms did not respond to conservative treatment.

HIGH-YIELD FACTS

MUSCULOSKELETAL

Table 2.9-3 outlines the presentation and treatment of common pediatric orthopedic injuries.

TABLE 2.9-3. Orthopedic Injuries in Children

INJURY	MECHANICS	TREATMENT
Clavicular fracture	The most commonly fractured long bone in children. May be birth related (especially in large infants) and can be associated with brachial nerve palsies. Usually involves the middle third of the clavicle, with the proximal fracture end displaced superiorly owing to the pull of the sternocleidomastoid.	Figure-of-eight sling vs. arm sling.
Greenstick fracture	Incomplete fracture involving the cortex of only one side of the bone.	Reduction with casting. Order films at 10–14 days.
Nursemaid's elbow	Radial head subluxation that typically occurs as a result of being pulled or lifted by the hand. Presents with pain and refusal to bend the elbow.	Manual reduction by gentle supination of the elbow at 90 degrees of flexion. No immobilization.
Torus fracture	Buckling of the cortex of a long bone 2° to trauma. Usually occurs in the distal radius or ulna.	Cast immobilization for 3–5 weeks.
Supracondylar humerus fracture	Tends to occur at 5–8 years of age. Proximity to the brachial artery ↑ the risk of Volkmann's contracture (results from compartment syndrome of the forearm).	Cast immobilization; closed reduction with percutaneous pinning if significantly displaced.
Osgood-Schlatter disease	Overuse apophysitis of the tibial tubercle. Causes localized pain, especially with quadriceps contraction, in active young boys.	↓ activity for 2–3 months or until asymptomatic. A neoprene brace may provide symptomatic relief.
Salter-Harris fracture	Fractures of the growth plate in children. Classified by fracture location: ▪ **I:** Physis (growth plate). ▪ **II:** Metaphysis and physis. ▪ **III:** Epiphysis and physis. ▪ **IV:** Epiphysis, metaphysis, and physis. ▪ **V:** Crush injury of the physis.	**Types I and II:** Conservative. **Types III–V:** Surgical repair to prevent complications such as leg length inequality.

DUCHENNE MUSCULAR DYSTROPHY (DMD)

An **X-linked recessive disorder** resulting from a deficiency of **dystrophin**, a cytoskeletal protein. Onset is usually at 3–5 years of age.

HISTORY/PE

- Affects axial and proximal muscles more than distal muscles.
- May present with progressive **clumsiness, fatigability,** difficulty standing or walking, difficulty walking on toes (gastrocnemius shortening), **Gowers' maneuver** (using the hands to push off the thighs when rising from the floor), and waddling gait.
- **Pseudohypertrophy of the gastrocnemius muscles** is also seen.
- Mental retardation is common.
- Table 2.9-4 outlines the differential diagnosis of DMD and Becker muscular dystrophy.

DIAGNOSIS

- $\ominus$ dystrophin immunostain; ↑ CK.
- EMG shows polyphasic potentials and ↑ recruitment.
- **Muscle biopsy** shows necrotic muscle fibers from degeneration and variation in fiber size with fibrosis from regeneration.

TREATMENT

- Physical therapy is necessary to maintain ambulation and to prevent contractures.
- Liberal use of tendon release surgery may prolong ambulation.

COMPLICATIONS

Mortality is due to pulmonary congestion caused by high-output cardiac failure; cardiac fibrosis → arrhythmias and weak skeletal muscles → cardiopulmonary complications → pneumonia and respiratory failure.

DEVELOPMENTAL DYSPLASIA OF THE HIP

Also called congenital hip dislocation; can result in subluxed, dislocatable, or dislocated femoral heads → early degenerative joint disease of the hips. Dislocations result from poor development of the acetabulum and hip due to lax musculature and **excessive uterine packing** in the flexed and adducted

TABLE 2.9-4. **DMD vs. Becker Muscular Dystrophy**

	DMD	BECKER MUSCULAR DYSTROPHY
Onset	3–5 years.	5–15 years and beyond.
Life expectancy	Teens.	30s–40s.
Mental retardation	Common.	Uncommon.
Western blot	Dystrophin is markedly ↓ or absent.	Dystrophin levels are normal, but protein is abnormal.

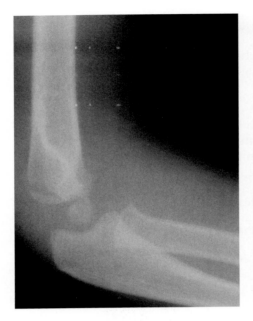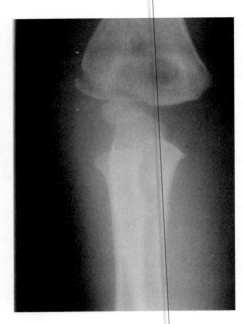

FIGURE 2.9-2. Lateral condyle fracture of the humerus.

(Reproduced, with permission, from Skinner HB. *Current Diagnosis & Treatment in Orthopedics*, 2nd ed. Stamford, CT: Appleton & Lange, 2000, p. 572.)

position (e.g., breech presentation) → excessive stretching of the posterior hip capsule and adductor muscle contracture.

HISTORY/PE

- Most commonly found in **first-born females** born in the **breech position.**
- **Barlow's maneuver:** Pressure is placed on the inner aspect of the abducted thigh, and the hip is then adducted → an audible "clunk" as the femoral head dislocates posteriorly.
- **Ortolani's maneuver:** The thighs are gently abducted from the midline with anterior pressure on the greater trochanter. A **soft click** signifies reduction of the femoral head into the acetabulum.
- **Allis' (Galeazzi's) sign:** The knees are at unequal heights when the hips and knees are flexed (the dislocated side is lower).
- **Asymmetric skin folds** and limited abduction of the affected hip are also seen.

DIAGNOSIS

- **Early detection is critical** to allow for proper hip development.
- Ultrasound may be helpful, especially after 10 weeks of age.
- Radiographs are unreliable until patients are > 4 months of age because of the radiolucency of the neonatal femoral head.

TREATMENT

Begin treatment early.

- **< 6 months:** Splint with a **Pavlik harness** (maintains the hip flexed and abducted). Do not flex the hips > 60 degrees to prevent AVN.
- **6–15 months:** Spica cast.
- **15–24 months:** Open reduction followed by spica cast.

COMPLICATIONS

- Joint contractures and AVN of the femoral head.
- Without treatment, a significant defect is likely in patients < 2 years of age.

One of the most common musculoskeletal disorders of childhood. There are multiple etiologies, but trauma remains the most common cause.

HISTORY/PE

- Presents with abnormal gait (e.g., Trendelenburg, antalgic gaits) and pain.
- **Trauma-associated limp:** Characterized by point tenderness.
- **Infection:** Consider septic joint, osteomyelitis, toxic synovitis, or infection acquired during contact with TB-⊕ patients. Presents with fever, erythema, edema, and limited ROM.
- Look for neurologic involvement (e.g., reflexes, muscle atrophy, changes in sensation, bowel and bladder function).
- Young children and toddlers are more likely to have an infected joint.
- Adolescents are more likely to develop JRA, slipped capital femoral epiphyses (SCFEs), and Legg-Calvé-Perthes disease.
- The **STARTSS HOTT** mnemonic summarizes the differential for limp.

DIAGNOSIS

- Obtain a thorough H&P.
- Radiograph the affected joint as well as the joint above and that below.
- CBC, ESR, and CRP may reveal inflammation.
- Additional tests include bone scan, CT scan, MRI, nerve conduction studies, and joint aspiration and culture.

TREATMENT

Depends on the etiology. Immediate treatment for emergent causes (e.g., septic joint).

Legg-Calvé-Perthes Disease

Idiopathic AVN of the femoral head (see Figure 2.9-3). Most commonly found in boys 4–10 years of age. Usually a self-limited disease, with symptoms lasting < 18 months.

HISTORY/PE

- Usually asymptomatic at first, but patients can develop a painless limp.
- If pain is present, it can be in the groin or anterior thigh, or it may be referred to the knee.
- **Limited abduction and internal rotation;** atrophy of the affected leg.
- Usually unilateral (85–90%).

TREATMENT

- **Observation** if there is limited femoral head involvement or if full ROM is present.
- If extensive or if there is ↓ ROM, consider bracing, hip abduction with a Petrie cast, or an osteotomy.
- The prognosis is good if the patient is < 5 years of age and has full ROM, ↓ femoral head involvement, and a stable joint.

> *Differential diagnosis of limp—*
>
> **STARTSS HOTT**
>
> **S**eptic joint
> **T**umor
> **A**vascular necrosis (Legg-Calvé-Perthes)
> **R**heumatoid arthritis/JRA
> **T**uberculosis
> **S**ickle cell disease
> **S**CFE
> **H**enoch-Schönlein purpura
> **O**steomyelitis
> **T**rauma
> **T**oxic synovitis

HIGH-YIELD FACTS

MUSCULOSKELETAL

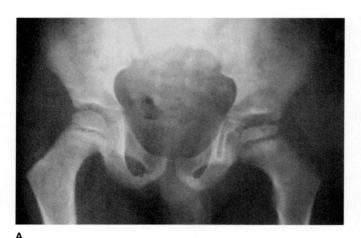

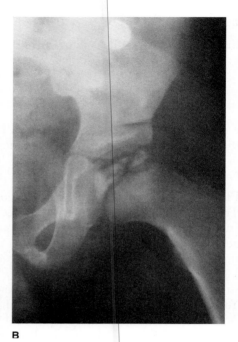

A
B

FIGURE 2.9-3. **Legg-Calvé-Perthes disease.**

AVN of the femoral head. (Reproduced, with permission, from Skinner HB. *Current Diagnosis & Treatment in Orthopedics*, 2nd ed. Stamford, CT: Appleton & Lange, 2000, p. 543.)

Slipped Capital Femoral Epiphysis (SCFE)

Separation of the proximal femoral epiphysis through the growth plate → medial and posterior displacement of the femoral head (relative to the femoral neck). May be due to an imbalance between growth hormone and sex hormones. Risk factors include obesity, age 11–13, male gender, and African-American ethnicity. Associated with hypothyroidism and other endocrinopathies.

HISTORY/PE

- Typically presents with acute or insidious **thigh** or **knee pain** and a **painful limp.**
- Acute cases present with restricted ROM and, commonly, **inability to bear weight.**
- Bilateral in 40–50% of cases.
- Characterized by limited internal rotation and abduction of the hip. Flexion of the hip → an obligatory external rotation 2° to physical displacement that is observed as further loss of internal rotation with hip flexion.

DIAGNOSIS

- Radiographs of **both** hips in **AP and frog-leg lateral views** reveal **posterior and medial displacement** of the femoral head (see Figure 2.9-4).
- Rule out hypothyroidism with TSH.

TREATMENT

- The disease is progressive, so treatment should begin promptly.

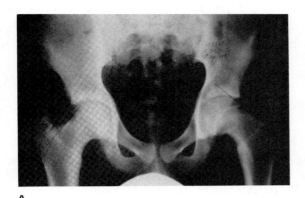

A

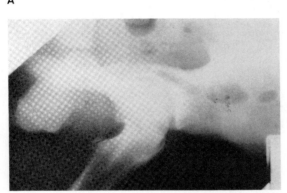

B

FIGURE 2.9-4. **Slipped capital femoral epiphysis.**

(A) AP x-ray. The medial displacement of the left femoral epiphysis is best seen with a line drawn up the lateral femoral neck. The abnormal epiphysis does not protrude beyond this line. (B) Frog-leg lateral x-ray. Posterior displacement of the femoral epiphysis is characteristic. (Reproduced, with permission, from Skinner HB. *Current Diagnosis & Treatment in Orthopedics,* 2nd ed. Stamford, CT: Appleton & Lange, 2000, p. 546.)

- **No weight bearing** should be allowed until the defect is surgically stabilized.
- **Gentle closed reduction** is appropriate only in acute slips.

COMPLICATIONS

Chondrolysis, AVN of the femoral head, and premature hip osteoarthritis → hip arthroplasty.

OSTEOSARCOMA

The second most common 1° malignant tumor of bone (after multiple myeloma). Tends to occur in the **metaphyseal** regions of the **distal femur, proximal tibia,** and proximal humerus; often metastasizes to the lungs. Some cases are preceded by Paget's disease. Risk factors include male gender and age 20–30.

HISTORY/PE

- Presents as progressive and eventually intractable **pain that is worse at night.**
- Constitutional symptoms such as fever, weight loss, and night sweats may be present.
- Erythema and enlargement over the site of the tumor may be seen.

DIAGNOSIS

- Radiographs show **Codman's triangle** (periosteal new bone formation at the diaphyseal end of the lesion) or a **"sunburst pattern"** of the osteosarcoma (see Figure 2.9-5)—in contrast to multilayered **"onion skinning,"** which is classic for Ewing's sarcoma.
- MRI and CT for staging (soft tissue and bony invasion) and to plan for surgery.

TREATMENT

- Limb-sparing surgical procedures and pre- and postoperative chemotherapy (e.g., methotrexate, doxorubicin, cisplatin, ifosfamide).
- Amputation may be necessary.

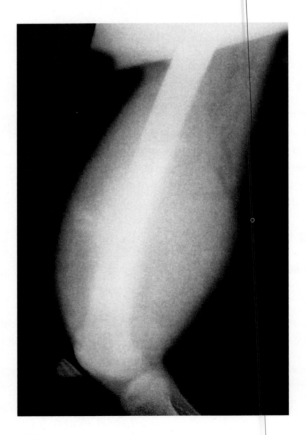

FIGURE 2.9-5.   Osteosarcoma.

"Sunburst" appearance of neoplastic bone formation in the femur of a 15-year-old girl. Amputation was required owing to the size of the tumor. (Reproduced, with permission, from Skinner HB. *Current Diagnosis & Treatment in Orthopedics*, 2nd ed. Stamford, CT: Appleton & Lange, 2000, p. 272.)

A **lateral curvature of the spine of** > 10 degrees occurring in the thoracic and/or lumbar spine and associated with rotation of the vertebrae and some-times excessive kyphosis or lordosis. **Most commonly idiopathic,** developing in early adolescence. Other etiologies are congenital or associated with neuro-muscular, vertebral, or spinal cord disease. The male-to-female ratio is 1:7 for curves that progress and require treatment.

HISTORY/PE

- Idiopathic disease is usually identified during school physical screening.
- Vertebral and rib rotation deformities are accentuated by a forward bend-ing test.

DIAGNOSIS

Radiographs of the spine (posterior, anterior, and full-length views).

TREATMENT

- Regular observation for < 20 degrees of curvature.
- Spinal bracing for 20–45 degrees of curvature. **Curvature may progress even with bracing.**
- Surgical correction for > 50 degrees of curvature.

COMPLICATIONS

Hypokyphosis ↑ the risk of restrictive pulmonary disorder.

OSTEOARTHRITIS (OA)

A common, chronic, noninflammatory arthritis of the synovial joints (e.g., **DIP** joints). Characterized by deterioration of the articular cartilage and os-teophyte and subchondral bone formation at the joint surfaces. Risk factors in-clude a ⊕ family history, **obesity,** and a **history of joint trauma.**

HISTORY/PE

Presents with **crepitus;** ↓ ROM; and initially **pain that worsens with activity and weight bearing but improves with rest.** Morning stiffness **lasts** for < 30 minutes. Stiffness is also experienced after periods of rest ("gelling").

DIAGNOSIS

- Radiographs show **joint space narrowing,** osteophytes, subchondral sclero-sis, and subchondral bone cysts. Radiograph severity does not correlate with symptomatology.
- Synovial fluid shows straw-colored fluid, normal viscosity, and a WBC count < 2000 cells/μL.

TREATMENT

Physical therapy, **weight reduction, NSAIDs.** Intra-articular corticosteroid in-jections may provide temporary relief. **Consider joint replacement** (e.g., total hip/knee arthroplasty) in advanced cases.

REFLEX SYMPATHETIC DYSTROPHY

A **pain syndrome** accompanied by **loss of function and autonomic dysfunction,** usually occurring after trauma. The disease has three phases: acute sympathetic denervation and underactivity → dystrophic phase → atrophic phase.

HISTORY/PE

- **Diffuse pain occurs,** often in a **nonanatomic** distribution, and out of proportion to the initial injury.
- Pain can occur at any time relative to the initial injury.
- **Loss of function** of the affected limb is seen.
- **Sympathetic dysfunction** occurs and may be documented by skin, soft tissue, or blood flow changes.
- Skin temperature, hair growth, and nail growth may ↑ or ↓. Edema may be present.

DIAGNOSIS

A clinical diagnosis, but objective evidence of changes in skin temperature, hair growth, or nail growth may be present.

TREATMENT

- Medications include NSAIDs, corticosteroids, low-dose TCAs, gabapentin, pregabalin, and calcitonin. (Note: No oral medications are consistently effective.)
- Physical therapy modalities such as heat, ice, desensitization techniques, and gentle ROM exercises may be helpful.
- **Chemical sympathetic blockade** may relieve symptoms.
- Referral to a chronic pain specialist is appropriate for complicated cases.

FIBROMYALGIA

- A chronic disorder characterized by myalgias, weakness, and fatigability of soft tissues. Joints are spared. Inflammation is notably absent.
- Hx/PE: Most common in **women 30–50 years of age;** associated with depression, anxiety, sleep disorders, IBS, and cognitive disorders ("fibro fog").
- Dx: Multiple (≥ 11 of 18), diffuse tender points all four body quadrants and the axial skeleton must be present (see Figure 2.9-6). The presence of < 11 of 18 tender points or non-fibromyalgia-associated tender points is known as **myofascial pain syndrome.**
- Tx: Antidepressants (TCAs have proven efficacy), **physical therapy,** stretching, heat application, hydrotherapy, transcutaneous electrical nerve stimulation (TENS).

GOUT

Gout crystals appear yeLLow when paraLLel to the condenser.

Recurrent attacks of **acute monoarticular arthritis** resulting from intra-articular deposition of **monosodium urate crystals** due to disorders of urate metabolism. Risk factors include male gender, obesity, and postmenopausal status in females.

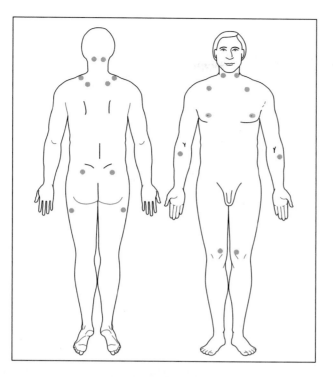

FIGURE 2.9-6.   Tender points characteristic of fibromyalgia.

HISTORY/PE

- Presents with excruciating joint pain of sudden onset that can awaken the patient from sleep.
- Most commonly affects the **first MTP joint** (podagra) and the midfoot, knees, ankles, and wrists; the hips and shoulders are generally spared.
- Joints are erythematous, swollen, and exquisitely tender.
- **Tophi** (urate crystal deposits in soft tissue) may be seen with chronic disease.

DIAGNOSIS

- Joint fluid aspirate shows **needle-shaped, negatively birefringent crystals** (see Table 2.9-5 and Clinical Images).
- An elevated WBC count in the joint aspirate or peripheral blood may be seen during flares.
- Serum uric acid is usually ↑ (≥ 7.5), but some patients have normal levels.
- Punched-out erosions with overhanging cortical bone (**"rat-bite" erosions**) are seen in advanced gout.

TABLE 2.9-5.   Gout vs. Pseudogout

DISORDER	CRYSTAL SHAPE	CRYSTAL BIREFRINGENCE
Gout	Needle shaped	⊖
Pseudogout	Rhomboid	⊕

Colchicine inhibits chemotaxis and is most effective when used early during a gout flare (use is limited by a narrow therapeutic window).

Causes of hyperuricemia:

↑ cell turnover (hemolysis, blast crisis, tumor lysis, myelodysplasia, psoriasis)
Cyclosporine
Dehydration
Diabetes insipidus
Diet (e.g., ↑ red meat, alcohol)
Diuretics
Lead poisoning
Lesch-Nyhan syndrome
Salicylates (low dose)
Starvation

TREATMENT

- **Acute attacks:** High-dose **NSAIDs** (e.g., indomethacin), colchicine, and/or **steroids.**
- **Maintenance therapy: Allopurinol** for overproducers, those with contraindications to probenecid treatment (tophi, renal stones, chronic renal failure), and refractory cases; **probenecid** for undersecretors.
- Weight loss and avoidance of triggers of hyperuricemia will prevent recurrent attacks in many patients.

ANKYLOSING SPONDYLITIS

A chronic inflammatory disease of the spine and pelvis that causes sacroiliitis and, eventually, fusion of the affected joints. Strongly associated with **HLA-B27.** Risk factors include male gender and a ⊕ family history.

HISTORY/PE

- Typical onset is in the late teens and early 20s. Presents with fatigue, intermittent hip pain, and LBP that **worsens with inactivity and in the mornings.**
- ↓ spine flexion (⊕ Schober test), loss of lumbar lordosis, hip pain and stiffness, and ↓ chest expansion are seen as the disease progresses.
- Anterior **uveitis** and **heart block** may occur.
- Other forms of seronegative spondyloarthropathy must be ruled out, including the following:
  - **Reactive arthritis** (formerly known as **Reiter's syndrome**): A disease of young men. The characteristic arthritis, uveitis, conjunctivitis, and urethritis usually follow an infection with *Campylobacter*, *Shigella*, *Salmonella*, *Chlamydia*, or *Ureaplasma*.
  - **Psoriatic arthritis:** An oligoarthritis that can include the **DIP joints.** Associated with psoriatic skin changes and **sausage-shaped digits** (dactylitis).

DIAGNOSIS

- ⊕ **HLA-B27** in 85–95% of cases.
- Radiographs may show **fused sacroiliac joints,** squaring of the lumbar vertebrae, development of vertical syndesmophytes, and bamboo spine.
- ESR or CRP is ↑ in 75% of cases.
- ⊖ **RF;** ⊖ ANA.

TREATMENT

- **NSAIDs** (e.g., indomethacin) for pain; exercise to improve posture and breathing.
- **Tumor necrosis factor (TNF) inhibitors** or sulfasalazine can be used in refractory cases.

POLYMYOSITIS AND DERMATOMYOSITIS

Polymyositis is a progressive, systemic connective tissue disease characterized by immune-mediated striated muscle inflammation. **Dermatomyositis** presents with symptoms of polymyositis plus cutaneous involvement, although the pathogenesis is different. Most often affect patients 50–70 years of age; the male-to-female ratio is 1:2. African-Americans are affected more often than Caucasians.

HISTORY/PE

- Distinguished as follows:
  - **Polymyositis:** Presents with **symmetric,** progressive **proximal** muscle weakness; pain; and difficulty breathing or swallowing (advanced disease).
  - **Dermatomyositis:** Patients may have **heliotrope rash** (a violaceous periorbital rash), **"shawl sign"** (a rash involving the shoulders, upper chest, and back), and/or **Gottron's papules** (a papular rash with scales located on the dorsa of the hands, over bony prominences).
- Patients may also develop myocarditis, cardiac conduction deficits.
- Can be associated with an underlying malignancy, especially lung and breast carcinoma.

DIAGNOSIS

- ↑ **serum CK, aldolase,** AST, and ALT.
- **EMG** shows fibrillations.
- **Muscle biopsy** reveals inflammation and muscle fibers in varying stages of necrosis and regeneration.

TREATMENT

- High-dose corticosteroids with taper after 4–6 weeks to ↓ the maintenance dose.
- Azathioprine and/or methotrexate can be used as an adjunct.

RHEUMATOID ARTHRITIS (RA)

A systemic autoimmune disorder characterized by chronic, destructive, inflammatory arthritis with **symmetric** involvement of both large and small joints → synovial hypertrophy and pannus formation → erosion of adjacent cartilage, bone, and tendons. Risk factors include female gender, age 35–50, and **HLA-DR4.**

HISTORY/PE

- Presents with **insidious onset of morning stiffness** for > 1 hour along with painful, warm swelling of multiple symmetric joints (**wrists, MCP** and **PIP joints,** ankles, knees, shoulders, hips, elbows, and cervical spine) for > 6 weeks.
- Fever, fatigue, malaise, anorexia, and weight loss may also be seen.
- Ulnar deviation of the fingers is seen with MCP joint hypertrophy (see Figure 2.9-7).
- Also presents with ligament and tendon deformations (e.g., swan-neck and boutonnière deformities), **Baker's cysts,** vasculitis, atlantoaxial subluxation, carpal tunnel syndrome, rheumatoid nodules, keratoconjunctivitis sicca, pulmonary nodules, inflammatory endocarditis, and Felty's syndrome (triad of spenomegaly, leukopenia, and cutaneous manifestations).

DIAGNOSIS

- **Labs:**
  - ↑ **RF** (IgM antibodies against Fc IgG) is seen in > 75% of cases.
  - ↑ ESR may also be seen.
  - Anemia of chronic disease.
- Synovial fluid aspirate shows turbid fluid, ↓ viscosity, and an ↑ WBC count (3000–50,000 cells/μL).

Felty's syndrome is characterized by RA, splenomegaly, and neutropenia.

257

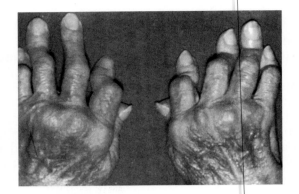

FIGURE 2.9-7. Rheumatoid arthritis.

Note the boutonnière deformities of the digits, ulnar deviation of the fingers, MCP joint hypertrophy, and severe involvement of the PIP joints. (Reproduced, with permission, from Chandrasoma P. *Concise Pathology*, 3rd ed. Stamford, CT: Appleton & Lange, 1998, p. 978.)

- **Radiographs:**
  - **Early:** Soft tissue swelling and juxta-articular demineralization.
  - **Late:** Joint space narrowing and erosions.

TREATMENT

- **NSAIDs** (can be reduced or discontinued following successful treatment with **disease-modifying antirheumatic drugs [DMARDs]**).
- DMARDs should be started early. First-line drugs are hydroxychloroquine, sulfasalazine, methotrexate, and azathioprine. Second-line agents include rituximab (anti-CD20), and leflunomide.

JUVENILE RHEUMATOID ARTHRITIS (JRA)`

A nonmigratory, nonsuppurative mono- and polyarthritis with bony destruction that occurs in patients ≤ 16 years of age and lasts > 6 weeks. Approximately 95% of cases resolve by puberty. More common in girls than boys.

HISTORY/PE

- Can be accompanied by **fever, nodules, erythematous rashes, pericarditis,** and **fatigue.**
- Subtypes are as follows:
  - **Pauciarticular:** An asymmetric arthritis that involves weight-bearing joints. Associated with an ↑ risk of **iridocyclitis** that → blindness if left untreated.
  - **Polyarticular:** Resembles RA with symmetric involvement of multiple (≥ 5) small joints. Systemic features are less prominent; carries a ↓ risk of iridocyclitis.
  - **Acute febrile:** The least common subtype; manifests as arthritis with **daily high, spiking fevers** and a maculopapular, **evanescent, salmon-colored rash.** Hepatosplenomegaly and serositis may also be seen. No iridocyclitis is present; remission may occur within one year. Occurs equally in girls and boys.

DIAGNOSIS

- There is **no diagnostic test for JRA.**
- **Labs:**
  - ⊕ RF in 15% of cases.
  - ANA may be ⊕, especially in the pauciarticular subtype.
  - ↑ ESR, WBC count, and platelets.
- **Imaging:** Soft tissue swelling and osteoporosis may be seen.

TREATMENT

- **NSAIDs** or corticosteroids; methotrexate is second-line therapy.
- ROM and strengthening exercises.

SCLERODERMA

Also called systemic sclerosis; characterized by inflammation → progressive tissue fibrosis by excessive deposition of type I and type III collagen. Commonly manifests as **CREST syndrome,** but can also occur in a diffuse form involving the skin as well as the GI, GU, renal, pulmonary, and cardiovascular systems. Risk factors include female gender and age 35–50.

CREST *syndrome:*

Calcinosis
Raynaud's phenomenon
Esophageal dysmotility
Sclerodactyly
Telangiectasias

HISTORY/PE

- Exam may reveal symmetric thickening of the skin of face and/or distal extremities.
- **CREST syndrome** involves **C**alcinosis, **R**aynaud's phenomenon, **E**sophageal dysmotility, **S**clerodactyly, and **T**elangiectasias.
- The diffuse form can → **pulmonary fibrosis,** cor pulmonale, acute renal failure, and malignant hypertension.

DIAGNOSIS

- RF and ANA may be ⊕.
- **Anticentromere antibodies** are specific for CREST syndrome.
- **Anti-Scl-70** (antitopoisomerase 1) **antibodies** are associated with a poor prognosis.
- Eosinophilia may be seen.

TREATMENT

- Steroids for acute flares; penicillamine can be used for skin changes.
- **Calcium channel blockers** for Raynaud's.
- ACEIs for renal disease and malignant hypertension.

COMPLICATIONS

Mortality is due to pulmonary hypertension and complications of pulmonary hypertension.

SYSTEMIC LUPUS ERYTHEMATOSUS (SLE)

A multisystem autoimmune disorder related to antibody-mediated cellular attack and deposition of antigen-antibody complexes. African-American women are at highest risk. Usually affects women of childbearing age.

HISTORY/PE

- Presents with nonspecific symptoms such as fever, anorexia, weight loss, and symmetric joint pain.
- The mnemonic **DOPAMINE RASH** summarizes the criteria for diagnosing SLE (see also Figure 2.9-8 and Clinical Images). Patients with four of the criteria are likely to have SLE (96% sensitive and specific).

DIAGNOSIS

- A ⊕ ANA is highly sensitive.
- **Anti-dsDNA** and **anti-Sm antibodies** are highly specific but not as sensitive.
- **Drug-induced SLE:** ⊕ antihistone antibodies are seen **in 100% of cases** but are nonspecific.
- **Neonatal SLE:** ⊕ anti-Ro antibodies.
- The following may also be seen:
  - Antiphospholipid antibodies.
  - Anemia, leukopenia, and/or thrombocytopenia.
  - Proteinuria and/or casts.

TREATMENT

- **NSAIDs** for mild joint symptoms.
- **Steroids** for **acute exacerbations.**
- Steroids, hydroxychloroquine, cyclophosphamide, and azathioprine for progressive or refractory cases.

TEMPORAL ARTERITIS (TA)

Also called giant cell arteritis; due to subacute granulomatous inflammation of the large vessels, including the aorta, external carotid (especially the **tem-**

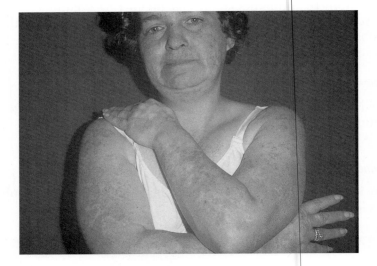

FIGURE 2.9-8. Systemic lupus erythematosus.

Erythematous patches and plaques of SLE, predominantly in sun-exposed areas. Note the malar rash across the bridge of the nose. (Reproduced, with permission, from Hurwitz RM. *Pathology of the Skin: Atlas of Clinical-Pathological Correlation,* 2nd ed. Stamford, CT: Appleton & Lange, 1998, p. 39.)

poral branch), and vertebral arteries. The most feared manifestation is **blindness** 2° to occlusion of the **central retinal artery** (a branch of the internal carotid artery). Risk factors include polymyalgia rheumatica (affects almost half of TA patients), age > 50, and female gender.

HISTORY/PE

- Presents with new headache (unilateral or bilateral); scalp pain and **temporal tenderness; and jaw claudication.**
- Fever, transient or permanent **monocular blindness,** weight loss, and myalgias/arthralgias (especially of the shoulders and hips) are also seen.

DIAGNOSIS

- **ESR > 50** (usually > 100).
- Ophthalmologic evaluation.
- **Temporal artery biopsy:** Look for thrombosis; necrosis of the media; and lymphocytes, plasma cells, and giant cells.

TREATMENT

High-dose prednisone for 1–2 months before tapering. Obtain a biopsy, but do not delay treatment; follow-up eye exam.

POLYMYALGIA RHEUMATICA

- Risk factors include female gender and age > 50.
- Hx/PE:
  - **Pain and stiffness of the shoulder and pelvic girdle** areas with difficulty getting out of a chair or lifting the arms above the head.
  - Other symptoms include **fever,** malaise, and weight loss. Weakness is generally not appreciated on exam.
- Dx: Markedly ↑ **ESR, often associated with anemia.**
- Tx: **Low-dose prednisone** (10–20 mg/day).

HIGH-YIELD FACTS IN

Neurology

Tables 2.10-1 through 2.10-5 and Figure 2.10-1 outline critical aspects of clinical neuroanatomy, including cranial nerve functions; the clinical presentation of common facial nerve lesions; spinal cord anatomy and functions; UMN and LMN signs; and pertinent clinical reflexes.

VASCULAR DISORDERS

Stroke

Acute onset of focal neurologic deficits resulting from disruption of cerebral circulation. **Nonmodifiable risk factors** include **age, male** gender, genetics (family history of MI or stroke), and ethnicity (African-American, Hispanic, Asian). **Modifiable risk factors** include **hypertension, DM, obesity, smoking, hypercholesterolemia, CAD,** age > 60 years, carotid stenosis, heavy alcohol intake, cocaine use, IV drug use, and **atrial fibrillation (AF).**

TABLE 2.10-1.   Cranial Nerve Functions

Nerve	CN	Function	Type	Mnemonic
Olfactory	I	Smell	**S**ensory	**S**ome
Optic	II	Sight	**S**ensory	**S**ay
Oculomotor	III	Eye movement, pupil constriction, accommodation, eyelid opening	**M**otor	**M**arry
Trochlear	IV	Eye movement	**M**otor	**M**oney
Trigeminal	V	Mastication, facial sensation	**B**oth	**B**ut
Abducens	VI	Eye movement	**M**otor	**M**y
Facial	VII	Facial movement, taste from the anterior two-thirds of the tongue, lacrimation, salivation (submaxillary and sublingual glands), eyelid closing	**B**oth	**B**rother
Vestibulocochlear	VIII	Hearing, balance	**S**ensory	**S**ays
Glossopharyngeal	IX	Taste from the posterior third of the tongue, swallowing, salivation (parotid gland), monitoring carotid body and sinus chemo- and baroreceptors	**B**oth	**B**ig
Vagus	X	Taste from the epiglottic region, swallowing, palate elevation, talking, thoracoabdominal viscera, monitoring aortic arch chemo- and baroreceptors	**B**oth	**B**rains
Accessory	XI	Head turning, shoulder shrugging	**M**otor	**M**atter
Hypoglossal	XII	Tongue movement	**M**otor	**M**ost

Reproduced, with permission, from Bhushan V et al. *First Aid for the USMLE Step 1 2006.* New York: McGraw-Hill, 2006, p. 342.

TABLE 2.10-2. Facial Nerve Lesions

TYPE	DESCRIPTION	COMMENTS
UMN lesion	Lesion of the motor cortex or the connection between the cortex and the facial nucleus. Contralateral paralysis of the lower face only.	**AL**exander **Bell** with **STD**: **A**IDS, **L**yme, **S**arcoid, **T**umors, **D**iabetes.
LMN lesion	Ipsilateral paralysis of the upper and lower face.	
Bell's palsy	Complete destruction of the facial nucleus itself or its branchial efferent fibers (facial nerve proper). Peripheral ipsilateral facial paralysis with inability to close the eye on the involved side. Can occur idiopathically; gradual recovery is seen in most cases. Seen as a complication in **A**IDS, **L**yme disease, **S**arcoidosis, **T**umors, and **D**iabetes.	

Reproduced, with permission, from Bhushan V et al. *First Aid for the USMLE Step 1 2006.* New York: McGraw-Hill, 2006, p. 356.

Stroke is the third most common cause of death and the leading cause of disability in the United States.

Many classifications exist, but the most common comparison involves ischemic (80%) vs. hemorrhagic (20%). Etiologies are as follows:

- **Atherosclerosis** of the extracranial vessels (internal/common carotid, basilar, and vertebral arteries).
- **Lacunar infarcts** in regions supplied by perforating vessels (result from hypertension, atherosclerosis, or diabetes).
- **Cardiac:** e.g., emboli from mural thrombi, diseased or prosthetic valves, arrhythmias, or endocarditis.

TABLE 2.10-3. Spinal Tract Functions

TRACT	FUNCTION	DECUSSATION	ORIGIN
Lateral corticospinal	Movement of contralateral limbs	Pyramidal, at the medulla	1° motor cortex
Dorsal column medial lemniscus	Tactile, vibration, sensation	Arcuate fibers at the medulla	Pacini's and Meissner's tactile disks, muscle spindles, and Golgi tendon organs
Spinothalamic	Pain, temperature	Ventral white commissure at spinal cord level	Free nerve endings, pain fibers

Reproduced, with permission, from Bhushan V et al. *First Aid for the USMLE Step 1 2005.* New York: McGraw-Hill, 2005, p. 105.

TABLE 2.10-4. **LMN vs. UMN Signs**

CLINICAL FEATURES	UMN	LMN
Pattern of weakness	Pyramidal (arm extensors, leg flexors)	Variable
Tone	Spastic (↑; initially flaccid)	Flaccid (↓)
DTRs	↑ (initially ↓)	↓
Miscellaneous signs	Babinski's, other CNS signs	Atrophy, fasciculations

- **Fibromuscular dysplasia** (young females), inflammatory diseases, arterial dissection, migraine, venous thrombosis, and sickle cell anemia.
- **Hypercoagulable states** such as those associated with malignancy, pregnancy, venous stasis, smoking, and OCPs. Also arguably associated with hypercoagulable states (e.g., antiphospholipid antibody) and elevated homocysteine.

HISTORY/PE

Symptoms are dependent on the vascular territory affected:

- **Middle cerebral artery (MCA):** Aphasia (dominant hemisphere), neglect (nondominant hemisphere), contralateral paresis and sensory loss in the face and arm, gaze preference toward the side of the lesion, homonymous hemianopia.
- **Anterior cerebral artery (ACA):** Contralateral paresis and sensory loss in the leg, amnesia, personality changes, foot drop, gait dysfunction, cognitive changes.
- **Posterior cerebral artery (PCA):** Homonymous hemianopia, memory deficits, dyslexia/alexia.
- **Basilar artery:** Coma, "locked-in" syndrome, cranial nerve palsies (e.g., diplopia), apnea, visual symptoms, drop attacks, dysphagia, dysarthria, vertigo, "crossed" weakness and sensory loss affecting the ipsilateral face and contralateral body.

> The 4 "deadly D's" of posterior circulation strokes—
>
> **D**iplopia
> **D**izziness
> **D**ysphagia
> **D**ysarthria

TABLE 2.10-5. **Clinical Reflexes**

DISTRIBUTION	LOCATION	COMMENTS
C5, 6 / C7, 8 / L3, 4 / S1, 2	Biceps = C5 nerve root.	Reflexes count up in order.
	Triceps = C7 nerve root.	S1, 2
	Patella = L4 nerve root.	L3, 4
	Achilles = S1 nerve root.	C5, 6
	Babinski––dorsiflexion of the big toe and fanning of other toes; sign of UMN lesion, but normal reflex in the first year of life.	C7, 8

Reproduced, with permission, from Bhushan V et al. *First Aid for the USMLE Step 1 2006.* New York: McGraw-Hill, 2006, p. 341.

Poliomyelitis and Werdnig-Hoffmann disease: lower motor neuron lesions only, due to destruction of anterior horns; flaccid paralysis

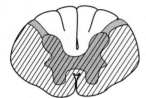

Multiple sclerosis: mostly white matter of cervical region; random and asymmetric lesions, due to demyelination; scanning speech, intention tremor, nystagmus

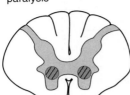

ALS: combined upper and lower motor neuron deficits with no sensory deficit; both upper and lower motor neuron signs

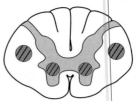

Complete occlusion of ventral artery; spares dorsal columns and tract of Lissauer

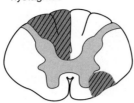

Tabes dorsalis (3° syphilis): degeneration of dorsal roots and dorsal columns; impaired proprioception, locomotor ataxia

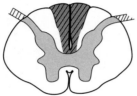

Syringomyelia: crossing fibers of corticospinal tract damaged; bilateral loss of pain and temperature sensation

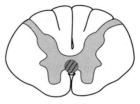

Vitamin B$_{12}$ neuropathy and Friedreich´s ataxia: demyelination of dorsal columns, lateral corticospinal tracts, and spinocerebellar tracts; ataxic gait, hyperreflexia, impaired position and vibration sense

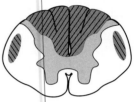

FIGURE 2.10-1.   Spinal cord lesions.

Reproduced, with permission, from Bhushan V et al. *First Aid for the USMLE Step 1 2006.* New York: McGraw-Hill, 2006, p. 353.

- **Lacunar stroke:** Pure motor or sensory stroke, dysarthria–clumsy hand syndrome, ataxic hemiparesis.
- **TIA:** A transient neurologic deficit that lasts < 24 hours (most last < 1 hour).

DIAGNOSIS

- **Emergent head CT without contrast** (see Figure 2.10-2) to differentiate ischemic from hemorrhagic stroke and to identify potential candidates for thrombolytic therapy.
- **MRI** to identify early ischemic changes (e.g., diffusion-weighted MRI is specific for acute stroke).
- **ECG** and an **echocardiogram** if embolic stroke is suspected.
- **Vascular studies** of intracranial and extracranial disease include carotid ultrasound, transcranial Doppler, MRA, and angiography (see Figure 2.10-3).
- **Screen for hypercoagulable states** with a history of bleeding, in the setting of a first stroke, or in patients < 50 years of age.

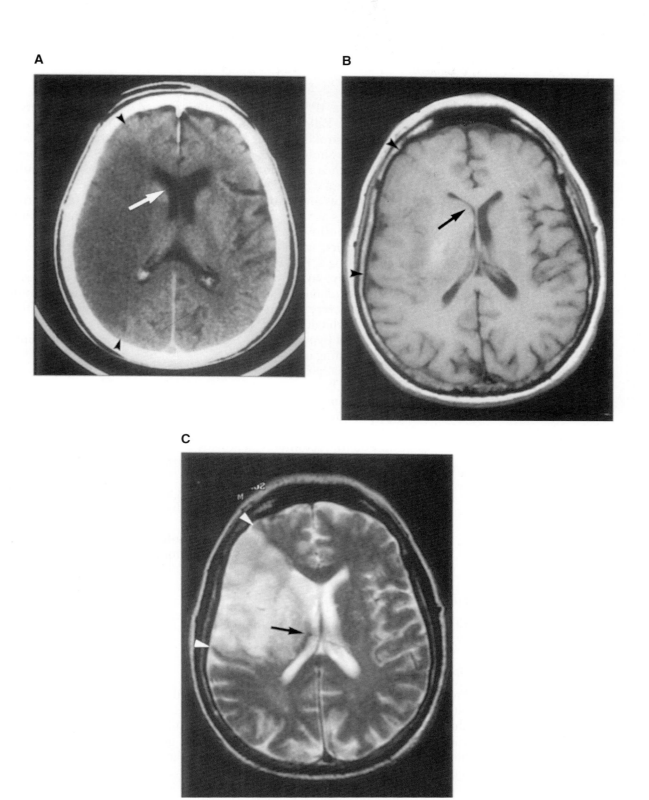

FIGURE 2.10-2. **CT/MRI findings in ischemic stroke in the right MCA territory.**

(A) CT shows low density and effacement of cortical sulci (between arrowheads) and compression of the anterior horn of the lateral ventricle (arrow). (B) T1-weighted MRI shows loss of sulcal markings (between arrowheads) and compression of the anterior horn of the lateral ventricle (arrow). (C) T2-weighted MRI scan shows increased signal intensity (between arrowheads) and ventricular compression (arrow). (Reproduced, with permission, from Aminoff MJ. *Clinical Neurology*, 3rd ed. Stamford, CT: Appleton & Lange, 1996, p. 275.)

Contraindications to tPA
therapy:

- *Systolic BP >185 or*
  diastolic BP >110
- *Prior intracranial*
  hemorrhage
- *Stroke or head trauma*
  within the last three
  months
- *Recent MI*
- *Current anticoagulation*
  with INR > 1.7 or
  prolonged PTT
- *A platelet count <*
  100,000/mm³
- *Major surgery in the past*
  14 days
- *GI or urinary bleeding in*
  the past 21 days
- *Seizures present at the*
  onset of stroke
- *Blood glucose < 50 or >*
  400 mg/dL
- *Age <18*
- *Mild symptoms or rapid*
  improvement of
  symptoms (e.g., TIA)

SAH will give the patient "the
worst headache of my life."

TREATMENT

- **Acute:**
    - **Ischemic stroke:** tPA is indicated if administered within **three hours** of symptom onset. Patients must first be screened for contraindications.
    - **Hemorrhagic stroke:** See the discussion of parenchymal hemorrhage.
    - ICU admission should be considered, especially for comatose patients or for those who are unable to protect their airways for possible intubation.
    - Monitor for signs and symptoms of brain swelling, ↑ ICP, and herniation. Serial CTs are helpful in the evaluation of deteriorating patients. Treat with **mannitol** and **hyperventilation**.
    - **ASA** is associated with ↓ morbidity and mortality in acute ischemic stroke presenting ≤ 48 hours from onset.
    - **Allow permissive hypertension and hypoxemia** to maintain perfusion of ischemic cerebral tissue. Treat with **labetalol** or IV hydralazine in the setting of **severe hypertension** (systolic BP > 220 or diastolic BP > 120) or **hemorrhagic stroke**.
    - **Treat fever and hyperglycemia,** as both are associated with worse prognoses in the setting of acute stroke.
    - Prevent and treat post-stroke complications such as aspiration pneumonia, UTI, and DVT.
- **Prevention and long-term treatment:**
    - **ASA, clopidogrel:** If stroke is 2° to small vessel disease or thrombosis, or if anticoagulation is contraindicated.
    - **Carotid endarterectomy:** If stenosis is > 70% in symptomatic patients or > 60% in asymptomatic patients (contraindicated in 100% occlusion).
    - **Anticoagulation:** In new AF or hypercoagulable states, the target INR is 2–3. In cases involving a prosthetic valve, the target INR is 3–4 or add an antiplatelet agent.
    - **Management of hypertension, hypercholesterolemia,** and **diabetes** (hypertension is the single greatest risk factor for stroke).

Subarachnoid Hemorrhage (SAH)

Etiologies include **trauma, berry aneurysms,** AVM, or trauma to the circle of Willis (often at the MCA).

HISTORY/PE

Presents with an **acute-onset, intensely painful "thunderclap" headache,** often followed by **neck stiffness** and other signs of meningeal irritation, including fever, photophobia, nausea/vomiting, and a fluctuating level of consciousness. More than one-third of patients will give a history of a **"sentinel bleed"** days to weeks earlier marked by headache, neck stiffness, and nausea/vomiting 2° to a leaking aneurysm.

DIAGNOSIS

- Immediate head **CT without contrast** (see Figure 2.10-4) to look for blood in the subarachnoid space.
- Immediate **LP if CT is** ⊖ to look for **RBCs, xanthochromia** (yellowish CSF due to breakdown of RBCs), ↑ protein (from the RBCs), and ↑ ICP.
- **Four-vessel angiography** should be performed once SAH is confirmed.
- Call neurosurgery.

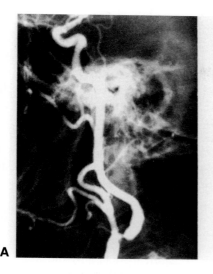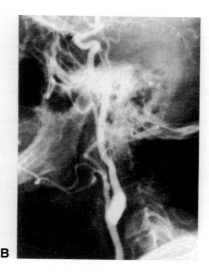

FIGURE 2.10-3. Pre- and postendarterectomy.

(A) Carotid arteriogram showing stenosis of the proximal internal carotid artery. (B) Postoperative arteriogram with restoration of the normal luminal size following endarterectomy. (Reproduced, with permission, from Way LW. *Current Surgical Diagnosis & Treatment*, 10th ed. Stamford, CT: Appleton & Lange, 1994, p. 763.)

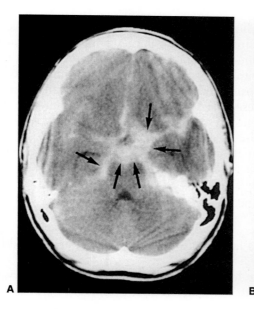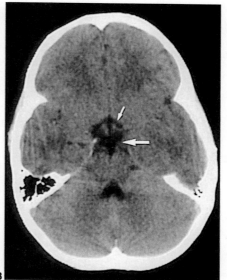

FIGURE 2.10-4. Subarachnoid hemorrhage.

(A) CT scan without contrast reveals blood in the subarachnoid space at the base of the brain (arrows). (B) A normal CT scan without contrast shows no density in this region (arrows). (Reproduced, with permission, from Aminoff MJ. *Clinical Neurology*, 3rd ed. Stamford, CT: Appleton & Lange, 1996, p. 78.)

TREATMENT

- **Prevent rebleeding** (most likely to occur in the first 48 hours) by maintaining systolic BP < 150 until the aneurysm is clipped or coiled.
- **Prevent vasospasm and associated neurologic deterioration** (most likely to occur 5–7 days after SAH) by administering calcium channel blockers (CCBs), IV fluids, and pressors to maintain BP. Give phenytoin for seizure prophylaxis.
- ↓ **ICP** by raising the head of the bed and instituting hyperventilation.
- **Treat hydrocephalus** through a lumbar drain or serial LPs.
- **Surgical clipping** is the **definitive treatment for aneurysms.** Endovascular coiling is an option for poor surgical candidates.

Intracerebral Hemorrhage

- Risk factors include hypertension, tumor, amyloid angiopathy (in the elderly), anticoagulation, and vascular malformations (AVMs, cavernous hemangiomas).
- **Hx/PE:** Presents with **lethargy and severe headache with sudden onset; nausea and vomiting;** and **focal motor and sensory deficits.** Seizures or obtundation may also be seen.
- **Dx:** Immediate noncontrast head CT (see Figure 2.10-5). Look for mass effect or edema that may predict herniation.
- **Tx:** Similar to that of SAH. Elevate the head of the bed and institute anti-seizure prophylaxis. Surgical evacuation may be necessary if mass effect is present. Several types of herniation may occur, including central, **uncal,** subfalcine, and tonsillar (see Figure 2.10-6 and Table 2.10-6).

Subdural Hematoma

- Typically occurs following head trauma (usually falls or assaults) → rupture of **bridging veins** and accumulation of blood between the dura and arachnoid membranes. Common in the **elderly** and **alcoholics.**
- **Hx/PE:** Presents with **headache, changes in mental status, contralateral hemiparesis,** and **ipsilateral pupillary dilation.** Changes may be subacute or chronic. May present as dementia in the elderly.
- **Dx:** CT demonstrates a **crescent-shaped, concave hyperdensity** that does **not cross the midline** (see Figure 2.10-7A).
- **Tx:** Surgical evacuation if symptomatic. Subdural blood may regress spontaneously if it is chronic.

Epidural Hematoma

- Usually a result of a **lateral skull fracture** → tear of the **middle meningeal artery.**
- **Hx/PE: Immediate loss of consciousness** → a **lucid interval (minutes to hours)** → **coma** with hemiparesis and, ultimately, a **"blown pupil"** (fixed and dilated ipsilateral pupil).
- **Dx:** CT shows a **lens-shaped, convex hyperdensity** limited by the sutures (see Figure 2.10-7B).
- **Tx:** Emergent neurosurgical evacuation. May quickly evolve to brain herniation and death 2° to the arterial source of bleeding.

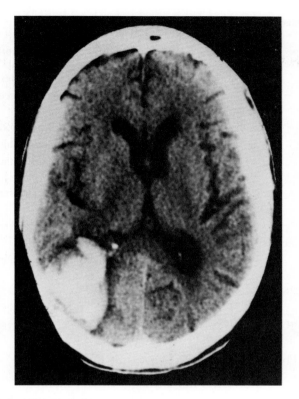

FIGURE 2.10-5. Intraparenchymal hematoma.

Head CT without contrast reveals the irregularly shaped hyperdensity with midline shift of the choroid plexus. (Reproduced, with permission, from Saunders CE. *Current Emergency Diagnosis & Treatment*, 4th ed. Stamford, CT: Appleton & Lange, 1992, p. 248.)

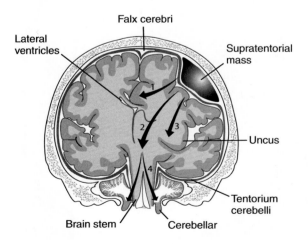

1. Cingulate herniation under falx cerebri
2. Downward transtentorial (central) herniation
3. Uncal herniation
4. Cerebellar tonsillar herniation into the foramen magnum

Coma and death result when these herniations compress the brain stem

FIGURE 2.10-6. Sites of herniation syndromes.

(Adapted, with permission, from Simon RP et al. *Clinical Neurology*, 4th ed. Stamford, CT: Appleton & Lange, 1999, p. 314.)

TABLE 2.10-6. Clinical Presentation of Herniation Syndromes

TYPE OF HERNIATION	PRESENTATION
Cingulate herniation	Occurs 2° to mass lesions of the frontal lobes. No specific signs or symptoms; frequently seen on head CT.
Downward transtentorial (central) herniation	Occurs when large supratentorial mass lesions push the midbrain inferiorly. Presents with a rapid change in mental status; bilaterally small and reactive pupils; Cheyne-Stokes respirations; and flexor or extensor posturing.
Uncal herniation	Occurs 2° to mass lesions of the middle fossa. CN III becomes entrapped → a fixed and dilated ipsilateral pupil.
Cerebellar tonsillar herniation into the foramen magnum	Occurs 2° to posterior fossa mass lesions. Tonsillar herniation → medullary compression → respiratory arrest. Usually rapidly fatal.

HEADACHES

The causes of headache include the following:

- **Acute:** SAH, hemorrhagic stroke, meningitis, seizure, acutely ↑ ICP, hypertensive encephalopathy, post-LP, ocular disease (glaucoma, iritis), new migraine, cerebral venous thrombosis, cavernous sinus thrombosis.

A

B

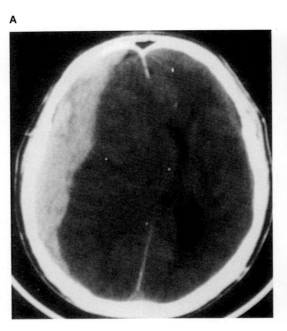
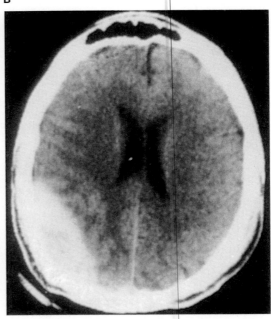

FIGURE 2.10-7. Subdural vs. epidural hematoma.

(A) Subdural hematoma. Note the crescent shape and the mass effect with midline shift. (B) Epidural hematoma with classic biconvex lens shape. (Reproduced, with permission, from Aminoff MJ. *Clinical Neurology*, 3rd ed. Stamford, CT: Appleton & Lange, 1996, p. 296.)

- **Subacute:** Temporal arteritis, intracranial tumor, subdural hematoma, pseudotumor cerebri, trigeminal/glossopharyngeal neuralgia, postherpetic neuralgia, hypertension.
- **Chronic/episodic:** Migraine, cluster headache, tension headache, rebound headaches from NSAID or caffeine use, sinusitis, dental disease, neck pain, caffeine withdrawal.

HISTORY/PE

- Conduct full general and neurologic exams, including a **fundic** exam.
- Evaluate the following:
    - **Is the headache new or old?** Recent or sudden-onset, severe headaches (e.g., those that awaken the patient from sleep) warrant immediate workup (e.g., for tumor, temporal arteritis, SAH, and meningitis).
    - **What are its characteristics?** Assess intensity, quality, location, and duration.
    - **Are there associated symptoms?** Look for associated jaw claudication, fever, nausea, vomiting, tongue biting, and weight loss.
    - **Are there neurologic symptoms?** Look for paresthesias, numbness, ataxia, visual disturbances, photophobia, and neck stiffness. Focal neurologic deficits and papilledema warrant immediate workup for more serious causes.

DIAGNOSIS

- **If SAH is suspected,** obtain a **head CT without contrast.**
- **If CT is ⊖, LP is mandatory.**
- Obtain a CBC.
- If temporal arteritis is suspected, obtain ESR.
- CT/MRI for suspected SAH, ↑ ICP, or focal neurologic findings. Use **CT without contrast** to evaluate acute hemorrhage.

Migraine Headache

- Affects **women** more often than men; may be familial. Associated with **vascular** and brain neurotransmitter (**serotonin**) abnormalities. Onset usually occurs by the **early 20s.**
- **Triggers** include certain foods (e.g., chocolate), fasting, stress, menses, OCPs, bright light, and disruptions in normal sleep patterns.
- Hx/PE:
    - Presents with a throbbing headache (> 2 hours but usually < 24 hours in duration) that is associated with **nausea, vomiting, photophobia, and noise sensitivity.** Headache is usually relieved by **sleep and darkness.**
    - **Classic migraines** are often **unilateral** and are preceded by a visual **aura** in the form of either scintillating scotomas (bright or flashing lights) or visual field cuts. **Common migraines** may be **bilateral** and periorbital **without preceding auras.**
- **Dx:** Based on history.
- **Tx:**
    - **Avoid known triggers.**
    - **Abortive therapy** includes **triptans** (e.g., sumatriptan), which are first line, and metoclopramide. Consider symptomatic treatment for nausea.
    - **Prophylaxis** for frequent or severe migraines includes β-blockers (propranolol), **TCAs** (amitriptyline), CCBs, and valproic acid.

Recent-onset headaches warrant immediate workup! If headache is associated with focal neurologic deficits, rule out more serious etiologies with CT or MRI. Also rule out meningitis or SAH with an LP if symptoms are acute in onset.

Cluster Headache

- **Men** are affected more often than women; average age of onset is 25. Risk factors include recent alcohol use or vasodilating drugs. Generally responds well to treatment.
- **Hx/PE:** Presents as a brief, **excruciating, unilateral periorbital headache** that lasts 30 minutes to three hours, during which the patient tends to be extremely restless. Attacks tend to occur in **clusters**, affecting the same part of the head at the same time of day (commonly during sleep) and in a certain season of the year. Associated symptoms include **ipsilateral lacrimation** of the eye, injected conjunctiva, Horner's syndrome, and nasal stuffiness.
- **Dx:** Classic presentations require no evaluation.
- **Tx:**
    - **Acute therapy:** High-flow O_2 (100% nonrebreather), ergots, sumatriptan, intranasal lidocaine, corticosteroids.
    - **Prophylactic therapy:** Ergots, CCBs, prednisone, lithium, valproic acid, topiramate.

Tension Headache

Tension headaches are the most common type of headache diagnosed in adults.

- Now considered a mild type of migraine headache. More common in women than in men.
- **Hx/PE:** Presents with **tight, bandlike pain** that is exacerbated by noise, bright lights, fatigue, and stress. Nonspecific symptoms (e.g., anxiety, poor concentration, difficulty sleeping) may also be seen. May be generalized or most intense in the **frontal, occipital, and neck regions.** Usually occurs at the end of the day.
- **Dx:** A diagnosis of exclusion. There are no focal neurologic signs.
- **Tx:** Relaxation, massage, hot baths, and **avoidance of exacerbating factors.** **NSAIDs** are first-line abortive therapy, but triptans and ergots may also be considered.

Cavernous Sinus Thrombosis

The usual etiology involves a **suppurative process** of the orbit, nasal sinuses, or central face that → **septic thrombosis** of the cavernous sinus. Nonseptic thrombosis is rare; *S. aureus* is the most common causative agent. Current antibiotics have greatly ↓ the incidence and mortality of cavernous sinus thrombosis.

History/PE

- **Headache is the most common presenting symptom.**
- Patients may present with orbital pain, edema, diplopia (2° to oculomotor nerve impairment), or visual disturbances and may describe a recent history of sinusitis or facial infection. On exam, they typically appear ill and have a **fever.**
- Exophthalmos, ophthalmoplegia, or diminished pupillary responses may also be seen.
- Changes in mental status such as confusion, drowsiness, or coma suggest spread to the CNS or sepsis. Late findings include meningismus or systemic signs of sepsis.

Diagnosis

- Lab studies show an ↑ WBC count.
- Blood cultures reveal the causative agent in up to 50% of cases.

- CSF exam may reveal ↑ pressure consistent with an aseptic meningeal reaction unless there is frank meningitis.
- CT, MRI, and MR venography are also important in establishing the diagnosis.

TREATMENT

- Treat with **aggressive empiric antibiotic therapy** with a penicillinase-resistant penicillin plus a third- or fourth-generation cephalosporin to provide broad-spectrum coverage pending blood culture results.
- IV antibiotics are recommended for at least 3–4 weeks.

SEIZURE DISORDERS

Paroxysmal events associated with aberrant electrical activity in the brain detectable by EEG → changes in neurologic perception or behavior. An aura is experienced by 50–60% patients with epilepsy. See Table 2.10-7 for common etiologies by age.

DIAGNOSIS

Assess the following:

- **Was the seizure associated with epilepsy?** Determine whether the patient has a history of epilepsy (i.e., a history of unprovoked and recurrent seizures). Other seizures may be self-limited and may resolve once an underlying medical condition has been treated. ↑ serum prolactin levels are consistent with an epileptic seizure in the immediate postictal period.
- **Was the seizure provoked by a systemic process?** Non-neurologic etiologies include **hypoglycemia, hyponatremia, hypocalcemia, hyperosmolar states, hepatic encephalopathy,** uremia, porphyria, **drug overdose** (cocaine, antidepressants, neuroleptics, methylxanthines, lidocaine), **drug withdrawal** (alcohol and other sedatives), eclampsia, hyperthermia, hypertensive encephalopathy, head trauma, and cerebral hypoperfusion.
- **Was the seizure caused by an underlying neurologic disorder?** Seizures with focal onset (or focal postictal deficit) suggest focal CNS pathology. They may be the presenting sign of a tumor, stroke, AVM, infection, hemorrhage, or developmental abnormality.
- **Is anticonvulsant therapy indicated?** First seizures that resolve after a single episode are frequently left untreated when the underlying cause is unknown.

TABLE 2.10-7. **Causes of Seizure by Age Group**

INFANTS	CHILDREN (2–10)	ADOLESCENTS	ADULTS (18–35)	ADULTS (35+)
Perinatal injury	Idiopathic	Idiopathic	Trauma	Trauma
Infection	Infection	Trauma	Alcoholism	Stroke
Metabolic	Trauma	Drug withdrawal	Brain tumor	Metabolic disorder
Congenital	Febrile seizure	AVM		Alcoholism
				Brain tumor

Partial Seizures

- Arise from a **discrete region,** or an "epileptogenic focus," in one cerebral hemisphere and **do not → loss of consciousness** unless they secondarily generalize.
- Hx/PE:
    - **Simple partial seizures** may include motor features (e.g., jacksonian march, or the progressive jerking of successive body regions) as well as sensory, autonomic, or psychic features (e.g., fear, déjà vu, hallucinations) **without alteration of consciousness.** A postictal focal neurologic deficit (e.g., hemiplegia/hemiparesis, or Todd's paralysis) is possible and usually resolves within 24 hours. Often confused with acute stroke (ruled out by MRI).
    - **Complex partial seizures** typically involve the temporal lobe (70-80%) with bilateral spread of the aberrant electrical discharge and are characterized by an **impaired level of consciousness,** auditory or visual hallucinations, déjà vu, automatisms (e.g., lip smacking, chewing, or even walking), and postictal confusion/disorientation and amnesia.
- Dx:
    - Obtain an **EEG.**
    - Rule out systemic causes with CBC, electrolytes, calcium, fasting glucose, LFTs, a renal panel, RPR, ESR, and a toxicology screen.
    - A focal seizure implies a focal brain lesion. Rule out a mass by MRI or CT with contrast.
- Tx:
    - **Treat the underlying cause.**
    - **Recurrent partial seizures:** Phenytoin, oxcarbazepine, carbamazepine (Tegretol), phenobarbital, and valproic acid can be administered as monotherapy. In **children, phenobarbital** is the first-line anticonvulsant.
    - **Intractable temporal lobe seizures:** Consider **anterior temporal lobectomy.**

Both simple partial and complex partial seizures may evolve into 2° generalized tonic-clonic (grand mal) seizures.

Tonic-Clonic (Grand Mal) Seizures

- Primarily idiopathic. Partial seizures can evolve into secondarily generalized tonic-clonic seizures.
- Hx/PE: Sudden onset of loss of consciousness with tonic extension of the back and extremities, continuing with 1–2 minutes of repetitive, symmetric clonic movements. Marked by **incontinence** and **tongue biting.** Patients may appear **cyanotic** during the ictal period. Consciousness is slowly regained in the postictal period, but patients are confused and may prefer to sleep; muscle aches and headaches may be present.
- Dx: EEG typically shows 10-Hz activity during the tonic phase and slow waves during the clonic phase.
- Tx:
    - **Protect the airway.**
    - Treat the underlying cause if known.
    - **1° generalized tonic-clonic seizures: Phenytoin,** fosphenytoin, or valproate constitutes first-line therapy. Lamotrigine or topiramate may be used as adjunctive therapy.
    - **Secondarily generalized tonic-clonic seizures:** Treatment is the same as that for partial seizures.

Absence (Petit Mal) Seizures

- Begin in **childhood**; subside before adulthood. Often **familial.**
- **Hx/PE:** Present with brief (**5- to 10-second**), often unnoticeable episodes of **impaired consciousness** occurring up to hundreds of times per day. Patients are **amnestic** during and immediately after seizures and may appear to be **daydreaming** or **staring.** Eye fluttering or lip smacking is common.
- **Dx: EEG** shows classic three-per-second spike-and-wave discharges.
- **Tx:** Ethosuximide is the first-line agent.

Status Epilepticus

- A **medical emergency** consisting of prolonged (**> 10-minute**) or repetitive seizures that occur without a return to baseline consciousness. May be either convulsive (the more medically urgent form) or nonconvulsive.
- Common causes include anticonvulsant withdrawal/noncompliance, anoxic brain injury, EtOH/sedative withdrawal or other drug intoxication, metabolic disturbances (e.g., hyponatremia), head trauma, and infection.
- Death usually results from an underlying medical condition. However, death may occur in 10% of cases of status epilepticus.
- **Dx:**
  - Determine the underlying cause with pulse oximetry, CBC, electrolytes, calcium, glucose, ABGs, LFTs, BUN/creatinine, ESR, antiepileptic drug levels, and a toxicology screen.
  - **Obtain an EEG and brain imaging, but defer testing until the patient is stabilized.**
  - **Obtain a stat head CT** to evaluate for intracranial hemorrhage.
  - Obtain a LP in the setting of fever or meningeal signs, but only after having done a CT scan to assess the safety of the LP.
- **Tx:**
  - Maintain **ABCs;** consider rapid intubation for airway protection.
  - Administer **thiamine, glucose, and naloxone** to presumptively treat potential etiologies.
  - Give **IV benzodiazepine** (lorazepam or diazepam) plus a loading dose of **fosphenytoin.**
  - If seizures continue, intubate and load with **phenobarbital.** Consider an IV sedative (midazolam or pentobarbital) and initiate continuous EEG monitoring.
  - Initiate a meticulous search for the underlying cause.

Infantile Spasms (West Syndrome)

- A form of **generalized epilepsy** that typically begins within six months of birth. May be idiopathic or 2° to a variety of conditions, including PKU, perinatal infections, hypoxic-ischemic injury, and tuberous sclerosis.
- Affects males more often than females; associated with a ⊕ family history.
- **Hx/PE:** Presents with tonic, bilateral, symmetric **jerks of the head, trunk, and extremities** that tend to occur in clusters of 5–10; **arrest of psychomotor development** occurs at the age of seizure onset. The majority of patients have mental retardation.
- **Dx:** An **abnormal interictal EEG** characterized by **hypsarrhythmia.**
- **Tx:** Hormonal therapy with **ACTH,** prednisone, and clonazepam or valproic acid. Medications may treat the spasms but have little impact on patients' long-term prognosis.

Benign Paroxysmal Positional Vertigo (BPPV)

- A common cause of recurrent **peripheral vertigo** resulting from a **dislodged otolith** that → disturbances in the semicircular canals.
- **Hx/PE:** Patients present with **transient, episodic vertigo (lasting < 1 minute)** and **torsional nystagmus triggered by changes in head position** (classically while turning in bed, getting out of bed, or reaching overhead), together with nausea and vomiting.
- **Dx:** Have the patient go from a sitting to a supine position while quickly turning his/her head to the side **(Dix-Hallpike maneuver)**. If vertigo and/or nystagmus is reproduced, BPPV is the likely diagnosis.
- **Tx:** Usually subsides spontaneously in weeks to months. Repositioning exercises or the Epley maneuver (the reverse of Dix-Hallpike) may be of benefit.

Acute Labyrinthitis

- Typically a **diagnosis of exclusion** once the more serious causes of vertigo are ruled out.
- **Hx/PE:**
  - Presents with **acute onset of severe vertigo** accompanied by **nausea, vomiting, and nystagmus,** usually **following a viral illness.** Symptoms typically last no longer than two weeks.
  - Patients may feel unsteady on their feet or have unilateral hearing loss, tinnitus, or ear fullness.
- **Dx:** Consider caloric testing.
- **Tx:** Usually subsides spontaneously within weeks to months. Cautious engagement in normal physical activities should be encouraged.

Ménière's Disease

- A cause of recurrent **vertigo** that affects at least 1 in 500 in the United States. More common in women; thought to be 2° to water retention.
- **Hx/PE:** Presents with **recurrent episodes of severe vertigo, hearing loss, tinnitus, or ear fullness** lasting hours to days. Nausea, vomiting, and diaphoresis may be seen. Patients progressively lose low-frequency hearing and may become deaf on the affected side.
- **Dx: The diagnosis is made clinically** and is based on a thorough history and physical exam. **Two episodes** with remission of symptoms between episodes are needed to make the diagnosis. A brain MRI and carotid and transcranial Doppler ultrasounds are indicated to assess potential intracranial pathology as well as cerebrovascular disease.
- **Tx:** A low-sodium diet and diuretic therapy are first-line treatment. A variety of other treatments (e.g., surgery, introduction of gentamicin into the middle ear) have been used with varying success.

Syncope

- One of the **most common causes** of partial or complete loss of consciousness **2° to an abrupt drop in cerebral perfusion.** Etiologies include cardiac arrhythmias and structural problems, vasovagal syncope, orthostatic hypotension, micturition-related syncope, TIAs, migraines, and idiopathic causes. Commonly **confused with seizures.**

- **Hx/PE:**
  - Patients may report a **trigger** (e.g., standing for long period of time, Valsalva maneuver).
  - Follows a typical course of **lightheadedness, malaise, apprehension, profuse diaphoresis** → **loss of consciousness and muscle tone for < 30 seconds,** and **recovery within seconds.**
- **Dx:** Place the patient on telemetry or Holter monitoring to evaluate cardiac causes. Obtain an EEG to rule out seizures. Evaluate for underlying causes of syncope with an ECG, an echocardiogram, a tilt-table test, a head CT or MRI, and carotid or intracerebral artery vascular studies.
- **Tx:** Treat the underlying cause; avoid triggers.

DISORDERS OF THE NEUROMUSCULAR JUNCTION

Myasthenia Gravis

An **autoimmune disease** caused by antibodies that bind to **postsynaptic acetylcholine (ACh) receptors** located at the neuromuscular junction. Most often affects young adult women, and can be associated with **thyrotoxicosis, thymoma,** and other autoimmune disorders.

HISTORY/PE

- Presents with fluctuating **fatigable ptosis or double vision,** bulbar symptoms (e.g., dysarthria, dysphagia), and **proximal muscle** weakness. **Symptoms typically worsen as the day progresses.**
- Patients may report difficulty climbing stairs, rising from a chair, brushing their hair, and swallowing.
- Respiratory compromise and aspiration are rare but potentially lethal complications and are termed **myasthenic crisis.**

DIAGNOSIS

- **Edrophonium (Tensilon test):** Anticholinesterase → **rapid** amelioration of symptoms.
- **Ice test:** Place a pack of ice on one eye for five minutes; ptosis resolves transiently.
- An abnormal **single-fiber EMG** and/or a **decremental response to repetitive nerve stimulation** can yield additional confirmation.
- ACh antibodies are ⊕ in 80% of patients; anti-muscle-specific kinase (anti-MuSK) antibodies are ⊕ in 5%.
- Chest CT is used to evaluate for thymoma. Eighty-five percent of patients with thymoma have ⊕ antibodies against striated muscle.
- Follow serial FVCs to determine the need to intubate.

TREATMENT

- Anticholinesterase drugs (**neostigmine,** pyridostigmine) are used for symptomatic treatment.
- **Prednisone** and other immunosuppressants are the mainstays of treatment.
- In severe cases, plasmapheresis or IVIG may provide temporary relief (days to weeks).

- **Resection of thymoma** can be curative.
- **Avoid certain antibiotics** (e.g. aminoglycosides) **and drugs** (β-blockers) in patients with myasthenia gravis.

Lambert-Eaton Myasthenic Syndrome

- Small cell lung carcinoma is a risk factor (60% of cases).
- **Hx/PE:** Presents with weakness and fatigability of proximal muscles along with depressed or absent DTRs. Extraocular, respiratory, and bulbar muscles are typically spared.
- **Dx: Repetitive nerve stimulation** reveals the characteristic incremental response. Also diagnosed by autoantibodies to presynaptic calcium channels and a chest CT indicative of a lung neoplasm.
- **Tx:** Treat small cell lung carcinoma; tumor resection may reverse symptoms. Guanidine hydrochloride is the mainstay of treatment. Anticholinesterases may also improve symptoms.

Multiple Sclerosis (MS)

Although the pathogenesis of MS is unclear, there is evidence of an autoimmune etiology in genetically susceptible individuals who are exposed to environmental triggers such as viral infections. Such potential etiologies are thought to be **T-cell mediated.** The female-to-male ratio is 3:2, and onset is typically between 20 and 40 years of age. MS is more common as one moves farther away from the equator. Subtypes are **relapsing/remitting,** 2° progressive, and 1° progressive.

Pregnancy is often associated with a ↓ frequency of MS.

The classic triad in MS is scanning speech, intranuclear ophthalmoplegia, and nystagmus.

MS treatment—

as easy as **ABC**

Avonex/Rebif
Betaseron
Copaxone

HISTORY/PE

- Presents with **multiple neurologic complaints that are separated in time and space and are not explained by a single lesion.** As the disease progresses, permanent deficits may accumulate.
- Limb weakness, **optic neuritis,** paresthesias, diplopia, nystagmus, urinary retention, vertigo, sexual and bowel dysfunction, depression, and cognitive impairment are also seen. Symptoms classically worsen with hot showers.
- Attacks are unpredictable but on average occur every 1.5 years, lasting for 6–8 weeks.
- Neurologic symptoms can wax and wane or be progressive. The prognosis is best with a relapsing and remitting history.
- Lhermitte's sign may be present, consisting of sharp pain traveling up or down the neck with flexion.

DIAGNOSIS

- MRI shows **multiple, asymmetric,** often **periventricular** white matter lesions (Dawson's fingers), especially in the **corpus callosum.** Active lesions enhance with gadolinium.
- CSF reveals mononuclear pleocytosis (> 5 cells/μL), ↑ IgG index, or oligoclonal bands (nonspecific).
- Abnormal somatosensory or visual evoked potentials may also be present.

TREATMENT

- **Steroids** should be given during acute exacerbations.
- Immunomodulators alter relapse rates in relapsing/remitting MS and include interferon-α_{1a} (**A**vonex/Rebif), interferon-α_{1b} (**B**etaseron), and copolymer-1 (**C**opaxone).

- Mitoxantrone can be given for worsening relapsing/remitting or progressive MS.
- Alternative treatments include cyclophosphamide, IVIG, and plasmapheresis.
- **Symptomatic therapy** is crucial and includes baclofen for spasticity; cholinergics for urinary retention; anticholinergics for urinary incontinence; carbamazepine or amitriptyline for painful paresthesias; and antidepressants for depression.

Guillain-Barré Syndrome (GBS)

Also known as acute inflammatory demyelinating polyneuropathy. An **acute, rapidly progressive,** acquired demyelinating autoimmune disorder of the peripheral nerves → weakness. Associated with recent *Campylobacter jejuni* infection, viral infection, or influenza vaccination. Approximately 85% of patients make a complete or near-complete recovery (may take up to one year). The mortality rate is < 5%.

HISTORY/PE

- Presents with rapidly progressive, symmetric, **ascending paralysis** (distal → proximal) involving the trunk, diaphragm, and cranial nerves.
- Autonomic dysregulation, areflexia, and dysesthesias may be present.

DIAGNOSIS

- Evidence of diffuse demyelination is seen on **EMG** and **nerve conduction studies,** which show ↓ nerve conduction velocity.
- Supported by a **CSF protein level > 55 mg/dL** with little or no pleocytosis (albuminocytologic dissociation).

TREATMENT

- Admit to the ICU for impending **respiratory failure.**
- **Plasmapheresis** and **IVIG** are first-line treatments. Steroids are **not indicated.**
- Aggressive physical rehabilitation is imperative.

> **The 5 A's of GBS:**
>
> **A**cute inflammatory demyelinating polyradiculopathy
> **A**scending paralysis
> **A**utonomic neuropathy
> **A**rrhythmias
> **A**lbuminocytologic dissociation

Amyotrophic Lateral Sclerosis (ALS)

A **chronic, progressive degenerative disease** of unknown etiology characterized by loss of **upper and lower motor neurons** (UMNs/LMNs). Also known as **Lou Gehrig's disease,** ALS has an unrelenting course and almost always progresses to respiratory failure and death, usually within five years of diagnosis. Males are more commonly affected than females, and onset is generally between ages 40 and 80.

HISTORY/PE

- Presents with asymmetric, slowly progressive weakness affecting the arms, legs, diaphragm, and cranial nerves. Some patients initially present with fasciculations. Weight loss is common.
- Associated with **UMN signs** and/or **LMN signs** (see Table 2.10-4). Eye movements and sphincter tone are generally spared. Tongue atrophy and fasciculation may be apparent.
- Emotional lability is a common feature.

DIAGNOSIS

- The clinical presentation is usually diagnostic.
- **EMG/nerve conduction studies** reveal widespread denervation and fibrillation potentials.
- CT/MRI of the cervical spine is done to exclude structural lesions.

TREATMENT

Supportive measures and patient education.

DEMENTIA

A chronic, progressive, global decline in multiple cognitive areas (see the mnemonic **the 5 A's of dementia**). Alzheimer's disease accounts for 70–80% of cases. The differential diagnosis is described in the mnemonic **DEMENTIAS**. Take care not to confuse delirium and dementia (see the Psychiatry section).

Alzheimer's Disease (AD)

Risk factors include **age,** female gender, a **family history, Down syndrome,** and low educational status. Pathology involves **neurofibrillary tangles, neuritic plaques** with **amyloid** deposition, amyloid angiopathy, and neuronal loss.

HISTORY/PE

- **Amnesia** for newly acquired information is usually the first presenting sign, followed by language deficits, acalculia, depression, agitation, psychosis, and apraxia (inability to perform skilled movements).
- Mild cognitive impairment may precede AD by 10 years. **Survival is 5–10 years** from the onset of symptoms, with death usually occurring 2° to **aspiration pneumonia** or other infections. Except for the mental state, the physical exam is generally normal.

DIAGNOSIS

- A **diagnosis of exclusion** that can be **definitively diagnosed only on autopsy;** suggested by clinical features and by an insidiously progressive course.
- MRI or CT may show atrophy and can rule out other causes; PET imaging shows nonspecific bilateral temporoparietal hypometabolism. CSF is normal.
- Neuropsychological testing can help distinguish dementia from depression. Hypothyroidism and subdural hematoma should also be ruled out.

TREATMENT

- **Prevention of associated symptoms:**
  - Provide supportive therapy for the patient and family.
  - Treat depression, agitation, sleep disorders, hallucinations, and delusions.
- **Prevention of disease progression: Cholinesterase inhibitors** (donepezil, rivastigmine, and galantamine, an NMDA receptor antagonist) are first-line therapy.
- **Prophylaxis:** Vitamin E (α-tocopherol) may slow cognitive decline.

The 5 A's of dementia:

Aphasia
Amnesia
Agnosia
Apraxia
Disturbances in **A**bstract thought

Differential diagnosis—

DEMENTIAS

Neuro**D**egenerative diseases
Endocrine
Metabolic
Exogenous
Neoplasm
Trauma
Infection
Affective disorders
Stroke/Structural

Vascular Dementia

Dementia associated with a history of stroke and cerebrovascular disease is the second most common type of dementia. **Risk factors** include **age, hypertension, diabetes,** embolic sources, and a history of **stroke.**

DIAGNOSIS

Criteria for the diagnosis of vascular dementia include the presence of dementia and two or more of the following:

- Focal neurologic signs on exam.
- Symptom onset that was abrupt, stepwise, or related to stroke.
- Brain imaging showing evidence of old infarctions or extensive deep white matter changes 2° to chronic ischemia.

TREATMENT

The prevention and treatment of vascular dementia are the same as those for stroke.

Frontotemporal Dementia (Pick's Disease)

A **rare,** progressive form of dementia characterized by **atrophy of the frontal and temporal lobes.** Round intraneuronal inclusions known as **Pick bodies** are the classic pathologic finding.

HISTORY/PE

Patients present with **significant changes in personality early in the disease.** Other symptoms include speech disturbance, alteration of social behavior, inattentiveness, and occasionally extrapyramidal signs.

DIAGNOSIS

The diagnosis is suggested by clinical features and by evidence of circumscribed frontotemporal atrophy revealed by MRI or CT.

TREATMENT

Symptomatic treatment only; no curative therapy has yet been made available.

Normal Pressure Hydrocephalus (NPH)

A **potentially treatable** form of dementia that is thought to arise from impaired CSF outflow in the brain.

HISTORY/PE

Symptoms include the **classic triad of dementia, gait apraxia, and urinary incontinence.** Headaches and signs of ↑ ICP typically do not occur.

DIAGNOSIS

- The diagnosis is suggested by clinical features.
- LP reveals elevated pressure and may → clinically significant improvement of the patient's symptoms.
- CT or MRI shows ventricular enlargement out of proportion to sulcal atrophy.

TREATMENT

Surgical CSF shunting is the treatment of choice.

Creutzfeldt-Jakob Disease (CJD)

Although it is the most common **prion disease,** CJD remains an extremely rare form of dementia. CJD is a member of the transmissible spongiform encephalopathies, all of which are characterized by spongy degeneration, neuronal loss, and astrocytic proliferation. In CJD, an abnormal protease-resistant prion protein accumulates in the brain.

HISTORY/PE

- CJD causes a **subacute dementia** with significant clinical decline that is noted weeks to months after symptom onset.
- Additional symptoms include **pyramidal signs, myoclonus, and periodic sharp waves on EEG.** Most patients die within one year of symptom onset.

DIAGNOSIS

- Suggested by clinical features.
- MRI with diffusion-weighted imaging may show evolving cortical and basal ganglia abnormalities during the course of the disease.
- CSF is usually normal, but the presence of protein 14-3-3 may be associated with CJD.
- Definitive diagnosis can be made only by brain biopsy or autopsy.

TREATMENT

Currently, there is no treatment.

MOVEMENT DISORDERS

Huntington's Disease (HD)

A rare, **hyperkinetic, autosomal-dominant** disease involving multiple **abnormal CAG triplet repeats** (< 29 is normal) within the HD gene on chromosome 4. The number of repeats typically expands in subsequent generations → earlier expression and more severe disease (**anticipation**). Life expectancy is 20 years from the time of diagnosis.

HISTORY/PE

Presents at 30–50 years of age with gradual onset of **chorea** (sudden onset of purposeless, involuntary dance-like movements), **altered behavior,** and **dementia** (begins as irritability, clumsiness, fidgetiness, moodiness, and antisocial behavior). Weight loss and depression may also be seen.

DIAGNOSIS

- **A clinical diagnosis.**
- CT/MRI show cerebral atrophy (especially of the **caudate** and putamen). Molecular genetic testing is conducted to determine the number of CAG repeats.

TREATMENT

- There is no cure, and disease progression cannot be halted. Symptomatic treatment only.
- Haloperidol can be used for psychosis; reserpine can be given to minimize unwanted movements; give antidepressants for depression.
- Genetic counseling should be offered to offspring.

Parkinson's Disease

An **idiopathic hypokinetic** disorder that usually begins after age 50–60 and is attributable to **dopamine depletion** in the **substantia nigra.** It is characterized by **Lewy bodies,** which are intraneuronal eosinophilic inclusions. Etiologies include **postencephalitic, toxic** (e.g., carbon disulfide, manganese, MPTP, "designer drugs"), bihemispheric, ischemic, traumatic, and iatrogenic (especially neuroleptic) insults.

HISTORY/PE

- The "**Parkinson's tetrad**" consists of the following:
  - **Resting tremor** (e.g., "pill rolling").
  - **Rigidity:** "Cogwheeling" due to the combined effects of rigidity and tremor.
  - **Bradykinesia:** Slowed movements and difficulty initiating movements. Festinating gait (wide leg stance with short accelerating steps) without arm swing is also seen.
  - **Postural instability:** Stooped posture, impaired righting reflexes, freezing, falls.
- Other manifestations include masked facies, memory loss, and micrographia.

TREATMENT

- Dopamine agonists (ropinirole or pramipexole) are first-line treatment for early disease.
- **Levodopa** and **carbidopa** are the mainstays of therapy.
- Selegiline (an MAO-B inhibitor) may be neuroprotective and may ↓ the need for levodopa.
- Catechol-O-methyltransferase (COMT) inhibitors (e.g., entacapone) ↑ the availability of levodopa to the brain and may ↓ motor fluctuations.
- If medical therapy fails, **surgical pallidotomy** or chronic **deep brain stimulation** may be attempted.

A side effect associated with pramipexole is uncontrolled gambling.

NEOPLASMS

Intracranial neoplasms may be 1° (30%) or **metastatic (70%).**

- Of all 1° brain tumors, 40% are benign, and these rarely spread beyond the CNS.
- Metastatic tumors are most often from 1° **lung, breast, kidney, and GI tract neoplasms** and **melanoma.** They occur at the **gray-white junction; may be multiple discrete nodules;** and are characterized by rapid growth, invasiveness, necrosis, and neovascularization.
- More common in males than in females, except for meningiomas.

Most CNS tumors are metastatic. The most common 1° CNS tumors in adults are glioblastoma multiforme and meningioma. The most common 1° CNS tumors in children are medulloblastomas and astrocytomas.

Signs of ↑ ICP:

- *Nausea*
- *Vomiting*
- *Headache that is worse in the morning*

History/PE

- Symptoms depend on tumor type and location (see Table 2.10-8), local growth and **resulting mass effect,** cerebral edema, ↑ ICP, and ventricular obstruction.
- Symptoms develop gradually and include nausea and vomiting, headache, and focal neurologic deficits.
- Personality changes, lethargy, intellectual decline, aphasias, seizures, and mood swings may also be seen.
- Metastases that tend to present with intracranial hemorrhage include renal cell carcinoma, thyroid cancer, choriocarcinoma, and melanoma.

Diagnosis

- Contrast CT and MRI with and without gadolinium to localize and determine the extent of the lesion.
- Histologic diagnosis via CT-guided biopsy or surgical tumor debulking.

TABLE 2.10-8. Common 1° Neoplasms

TUMOR	PRESENTATION	TREATMENT
Astrocytoma	Presents with headache and ↑ ICP. May cause unilateral paralysis in CN V–VII and CN X. Has a slow, **protracted course.** The prognosis is much better than that of glioblastoma multiforme (GBM; see below).	Resection if possible; radiation.
GBM (grade IV astrocytoma)	The most common 1° brain tumor. Often presents with headache and ↑ ICP. Progresses rapidly. Has a poor prognosis (< 1 year from the time of prognosis).	Surgical removal/resection. Radiation and chemotherapy have variable results.
Meningioma	Originates from the **dura mater or arachnoid.** Has a good prognosis. Incidence ↑ with age. Imaging may reveal **dural tails.**	Surgical resection; radiation for unresectable tumors.
Acoustic neuroma (schwannoma)	Presents with ipsilateral hearing loss, tinnitus, vertigo, and signs of cerebellar dysfunction. Derived from **Schwann cells.**	Surgical removal.
Medulloblastoma	A primitive neuroectodermal tumor. **Common in children.** Arises from the fourth ventricle and → ↑ ICP. **Highly malignant;** may seed the subarachnoid space.	Surgical resection coupled with radiation and chemotherapy.
Ependymoma	Common in children. May arise from the ependyma of a ventricle (commonly the fourth) or the spinal cord; may → obstructive hydrocephalus.	Surgical resection; radiation.

TREATMENT

- **Resection** (if possible), **radiation,** and **chemotherapy.**
- Therapy is highly dependent on tumor type, histology, progression, and site (see Table 2.10-8).
- **Corticosteroids** can be used to ↓ vasogenic edema and ↓ ICP. Management is often palliative.
- Seizure prophylaxis in patients who have had a seizure.

NEUROCUTANEOUS DISORDERS

Neurofibromatosis (NF)

The most common neurocutaneous disorder. There are **two major types:** neurofibromatosis 1 (NF1, or von Recklinghausen's syndrome) and neurofibromatosis 2 (NF2). Both obey **autosomal-dominant inheritance.** The NF genes are located on **chromosome 17 and 22,** respectively, for NF1 and NF2.

HISTORY/PE

- Diagnostic criteria for **NF1** include two or more of the following:
    - Six **café-au-lait spots** (each ≥ 5 mm in children or ≥ 15 mm in adults).
    - Two neurofibromas of any type.
    - **Freckling in the axillary or inguinal area.**
    - **Optic glioma.**
    - **Two Lisch nodules (pigmented iris hamartomas).**
    - Bone abnormality (e.g., kyphoscoliosis).
    - A **first-degree relative** with NF1.
- Diagnostic criteria for **NF2** are as follows:
    - **Bilateral acoustic neuromas or** a first-degree relative with NF2 and **either** unilateral acoustic neuromas or two of any of the following: neurofibromas, meningiomas, gliomas, or schwannoma.
    - Other features include seizures, skin nodules, and café-au-lait spots.

DIAGNOSIS

- **MRI of the brain, brain stem, and spine.**
- Obtain a complete dermatologic exam, ophthalmologic exam, and family history. Auditory testing is recommended.

TREATMENT

- There is no cure; treatment is symptomatic (e.g., surgery for kyphoscoliosis).
- Acoustic neuromas and optic gliomas can be treated with surgery or radiosurgery.

Tuberous Sclerosis

Affects many organ systems, including the CNS, skin, heart, retina, and kidneys. Obeys **autosomal-dominant** inheritance.

HISTORY/PE

- Presents with **convulsive seizures** (infantile spasms in infants),"**ash-leaf**" **hypopigmented lesions** on the trunk and extremities, and **mental retardation** (↑ likelihood with early age of onset).

Two-thirds of 1° brain tumors in adults are supratentorial. One-third of those in children are supratentorial.

NF1 and NF2 are clinically evident by ages 15 and 20, respectively.

- Other skin manifestations include **sebaceous adenomas** (small red nodules on the nose and cheeks in the shape of a butterfly) and a **shagreen patch** (a rough papule in the lumbosacral region with an orange-peel consistency).
- Two retinal lesions are recognized: (1) mulberry tumors, which arise from the nerve head; and (2) phakomas, which are round, flat, gray lesions located peripherally in the retina.
- Symptoms are 2° to small benign tumors that grow on the face, eyes, brain, kidney, and other organs.
- Mental retardation and CHF from cardiac rhabdomyoma may also be seen.
- Renal involvement may include hamartomas, angiomyolipomas, or, rarely, renal cell carcinoma.

DIAGNOSIS

- Diagnosis is usually clinical.
- **Head CT:** Reveals calcified tubers within the cerebrum in the periventricular area. Lesions may on rare occasion transform into malignant astrocytomas.
- Skin lesions are enhanced by a Wood's UV lamp.
- **ECG:** Evaluate for rhabdomyoma of the heart, especially in the apex of the left ventricle (affects > 50% of patients).
- **Renal ultrasound:** May reveal renal hamartomas, masses, or polycystic disease.
- **Renal CT:** May show angiomyolipomas (causing cystic or fibrous pulmonary changes).
- **CXR:** May reveal pulmonary lesions or cardiomegaly 2° to rhabdomyoma.

TREATMENT

- Treatment should be based on symptoms (e.g., cosmetic surgery for adenoma sebaceum).
- Maintain seizure control with clonazepam or valproic acid. Treat infantile spasms with ACTH.
- Surgical intervention may be indicated in the setting of ↑ ICP or for seizures associated with an epileptogenic focus or severe developmental delay.

APHASIA

A general term for speech and language disorders. Usually result from insults (e.g., strokes, tumors, abscesses) to the "dominant hemisphere" (the left hemisphere in > 95% of people).

Broca's Aphasia

- **A disorder of language production, including writing,** with **intact comprehension.** Due to an insult to Broca's area in the **posterior inferior frontal gyrus.** Often 2° to a left superior **MCA stroke.** Also known as **motor aphasia.**
- **Hx/PE:** Presents with **impaired repetition, frustration** with awareness of deficits, arm and face **hemiparesis,** hemisensory loss, and apraxia of the oral muscles.
- **Tx: Speech therapy** (varying outcomes with intermediate prognosis).

> **B**roca's is **B**roken speech.
> **W**ernicke's is **W**ordy but makes no sense.

Broca's aphasia is also known as expressive or nonfluent aphasia.

Wernicke's Aphasia

- A **disorder of language comprehension** with **intact yet nonsensical production**. Also known as **sensory aphasia**.
- Due to an insult to Wernicke's area in the left posterior superior temporal (perisylvian) lobe. Often 2° to left **inferior/posterior MCA** embolic stroke.
- Hx/PE: Presents with **preserved fluency** of language with impaired repetition and comprehension → "**word salad**." Patients are unable to follow commands; make frequent use of **neologisms** (made-up words) and paraphasic errors (word substitutions); show **lack of awareness** of deficits; and exhibit right upper homonymous quadrantanopia 2° to involvement of Meyer's loop.
- Tx: Treat the underlying etiology and institute speech therapy.

Wernicke's aphasia is also known as fluent or receptive aphasia.

COMA

A state of unconsciousness marked by a profound suppression of responses to external and internal stimuli. Due to either catastrophic structural CNS injury or diffuse metabolic dysfunction. Causes include **brain herniation; hemorrhage; infarction;** abscesses; tumors; endogenous electrolyte disturbances; endocrine or metabolic dysfunction; **exogenous toxins** (medications, EtOH, other drugs); infectious or inflammatory disease; and generalized seizure activity or postictal states.

HISTORY/PE

- Obtain a complete medical history, including current medications (e.g., **sedative medications**).
- Conduct thorough medical and neurologic exams, including assessments of mental status, motor responses, muscular tone, breathing pattern, pupillary response, eye movements (including doll's-eye maneuver), cold-water caloric testing, and response to noxious stimuli.

DIAGNOSIS

- Typically made by a history and physical and by exclusion of other etiologies.
- Check glucose, electrolytes, calcium, a renal panel, LFTs, ABG, a toxicology screen, and blood and CSF cultures. Other metabolic tests (e.g., TSH) may be performed based on the clinical index of suspicion.
- Obtain a **head CT without contrast before** other imaging to evaluate for hemorrhage or structural changes. Imaging should **precede LP** in light of the risk of herniation.
- Obtain an MRI to exclude structural changes and ischemia. **EEG** can be both diagnostic and prognostic (alpha, spindle, and theta coma).
- Rule out catatonia, hysterical or conversion unresponsiveness, "**locked-in syndrome**," or **persistent vegetative state**, all of which be confused with true coma.
  - In "**locked-in**" syndrome, patients are awake and alert but can move only their eyes and eyelids. Associated with central pontine myelinolysis, brain stem stroke, and advanced ALS.
  - **Persistent vegetative state** is characterized by normal wake-sleep cycles but lack of awareness of self or the environment. The most common causes are trauma with diffuse cortical injury or hypoxic ischemic injury.

TREATMENT

Initial treatment should consist of the following measures:

- **Stabilize the patient:** Attend to **ABCs.**
- **Reverse the reversible:** Administer **DONT**—Dextrose, Oxygen, Naloxone, and Thiamine.
- **Identify and treat the underlying cause** and associated complications.
- **Prevent further damage.**

NUTRITIONAL DEFICIENCIES

Table 2.10-9 describes the neurologic symptoms commonly associated with nutritional deficiencies.

TABLE 2.10-9. Neurologic Syndromes Associated with Nutritional Deficiencies

VITAMIN	SYNDROME	SIGNS/SYMPTOMS	CLASSIC PATIENTS	TREATMENT
Thiamine (vitamin B$_1$)	Wernicke's encephalopathy	The classic triad consists of **encephalopathy** (disorientation, inattentiveness, confusion), **ophthalmoplegia** (nystagmus, lateral rectus palsy, conjugate-gaze palsy), and **ataxia** (polyneuropathy, cerebellar and vestibular dysfunction → problems standing or walking).	**Alcoholics, hyperemesis, starvation, renal dialysis,** AIDS. **Can be elicited by high-dose glucose administration.**	Reversible almost immediately with thiamine administration. Always give thiamine before glucose.
	Korsakoff's dementia	Above, plus anterograde and retrograde amnesia, horizontal nystagmus, and confabulations.	Same as above.	Irreversible.
Cyanocobalamin (vitamin B$_{12}$)[a]	Combined system disease (CSD) *or* subacute combined degeneration of the posterior and lateral columns of the spinal cord (see the discussion of clinical neuroanatomy)	Gradual, progressive onset. Symmetric paresthesias, stocking-glove sensory neuropathy, leg stiffness, spasticity, paraplegia, bowel and bladder dysfunction, sore tongue. Dementia.	Patients with pernicious anemia; strict vegetarians; status post gastric or ileal resection.	B$_{12}$ injections or large oral doses.
Folate[a]	Folate deficiency	Irritability; personality changes without the neurologic symptoms of CSD.	Alcoholics; patients with pernicious anemia.	Reversible if corrected early.

[a] Associated with ↑ homocysteine and ↑ risk of vascular events.

Visual Field Defects

Figure 2.10-8 illustrates common visual field defects and the anatomic areas with which they are associated.

Closed-Angle Glaucoma

- Risk factors include older age, Asian ethnicity, **pupillary dilation** (prolonged time in a darkened area, stress, medications), anterior uveitis, and lens dislocation.
- **Hx/PE:** Presents with extreme pain and blurred vision; nausea and vomiting may also be seen.
- **Dx:** Hard, red eye is seen (from acute closure of a narrow anterior chamber angle); the pupil is dilated and nonreactive to light. Intraocular pressure is ↑.
- **Tx:** This is a **medical emergency** that may → blindness. ↓ **intraocular pressure** with acetazolamide and then pilocarpine. **Laser iridotomy** is curative.

Open-Angle Glaucoma

- Risk factors include age > 40 years, **African-American ethnicity**, diabetes, and myopia.
- **Hx/PE:** Initially asymptomatic. Should be suspected in patients > 35 years of age who need **frequent lens changes** and have mild headaches, visual disturbances, and impaired adaptation to darkness. The earliest visual defect is seen in the peripheral nasal fields. **Cupping** of the optic disk is seen on funduscopic exam.
- **Dx:** Tonometry, ophthalmoscopic visualization of the optic nerve, and visual field testing are most important. A diseased trabecular meshwork that obstructs proper drainage of the eye → gradually ↑ pressure and progressive vision loss.

Open-angle glaucoma is much more common than closed-angle glaucoma and is almost always bilateral (closed angle is usually unilateral).

1. Right anopia
2. Bitemporal hemianopia
3. Left homonymous hemianopia
4. Left upper quadrantic anopia (right temporal lesion)
5. Left lower quadrantic anopia (right parietal lesion)
6. Left hemianopia with macular sparing

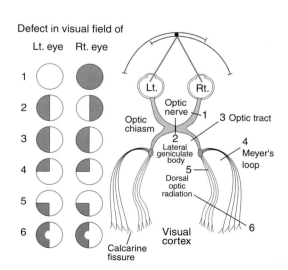

FIGURE 2.10-8. Visual field defects.

- **Tx:** Prevention (ophthalmology exam every 3–5 years for all people > 40 years of age). Treat with topical β-blockers (timolol, betaxolol) to ↓ aqueous humor production or with pilocarpine to ↑ aqueous outflow. Carbonic anhydrase inhibitors may also be used. If medication fails, laser trabeculoplasty can improve aqueous drainage.

Macular Degeneration

In the United States, macular degeneration is the leading cause of permanent bilateral visual loss in the elderly.

- More common among Caucasians, females, smokers, and those with a ⊕ family history.
- **Hx/PE:** Presents with **painless loss of central vision.**
    - **Atrophic macular degeneration:** Causes gradual vision loss.
    - **Exudative macular degeneration:** Associated with more rapid and severe vision damage.
- **Dx:** Funduscopy by an ophthalmologist reveals pigmented or hemorrhagic disturbance in the macular region.
- **Tx:** Options are limited. Laser photocoagulation may delay loss of central vision in exudative macular disease.

Retinal Occlusion

- Occurs in **elderly patients** and is often idiopathic.
- **Hx/PE:**
    - **Central retinal artery occlusion:** Sudden, painless, **unilateral blindness.** The pupil accommodates but is sluggishly reactive to direct light. Patients present with a **cherry-red spot** on the fovea, retinal swelling, and retinal arteries that may appear bloodless.
    - **Central retinal vein occlusion:** Rapid, painless vision loss. Retinal hemorrhage, cotton-wool spots, and edema of the fundus may be seen on funduscopic exam.
- **Tx:**
    - **Central retinal artery occlusion: Thrombolysis** of the ophthalmic artery within **eight** hours of onset of symptoms. ↓ intraocular pressure through drainage of the anterior chamber. IV acetazolamide may improve retinal perfusion. If treatment is not instituted immediately, retinal infarction and permanent blindness may result.
    - **Central retinal vein occlusion:** Laser photocoagulation has variable results.

The Basics of Pregnancy

The following terms and concepts are central to an understanding of the physiologic processes of pregnancy.

- **Gravity:** The number of times a woman has been pregnant.
- **Parity:** The number of pregnancies that led to a birth beyond 20 weeks' gestational age or an infant weighing > 500 g.
- **Developmental age (DA):** The number of weeks and days since fertilization.
- **Gestational age (GA):** The number of weeks and days measured from the last menstrual period (LMP). GA can be determined by:
    - LMP
    - Fundal height
    - Quickening (at 17–18 weeks)
    - Fetal heart tones (at 10 weeks via Doppler)
    - Ultrasound (fetal crown-rump length at 5–12 weeks; biparietal diameter at 13 weeks until delivery, although less reliable as the pregnancy progresses)
- **Nägele's rule** for calculating the estimated date of delivery is to add 9 months + 7 days to the LMP.
- **Pregnancy tests:** Over-the-counter and laboratory serum assays test for the beta subunit of the human chorionic gonadotropin (β-hCG). This hormone is produced by the placenta and peaks at 100,000 mIU/mL by 10 weeks of gestation, ↓ throughout the second trimester, and levels off in the third trimester. **Levels of hCG double approximately every 48 hours during early pregnancy.**

Table 2.11-1 outlines normal physiologic changes associated with pregnancy.

Nägele's rule: due date = last menstrual period (LMP) + nine months + seven days.

TABLE 2.11-1. Normal Physiologic Changes During Pregnancy

ORGAN/SYSTEM	PHYSIOLOGIC CHANGE
Cervix	Softening and cyanosis at approximately four weeks (Goodell's sign). Thick mucus plug in the cervical os expelled at or near labor (**"bloody show"**). Mucus appears granular microscopically due to progesterone.
Uterus	Softening of the uterus after six weeks (Ladin's sign). Palpated above the pubic symphysis at **12 weeks.**
Vagina	Thick acidic secretions; violet colorations (Chadwick's sign) from ↑ blood flow.
Cardiovascular	↑ **cardiac output** (30–50%), **heart rate** (by 10–15 bpm), and **stroke volume.** ↓ systemic vascular resistance (progesterone → smooth muscle relaxation). ↓ **BP in the first trimester** (SBP = 5–10 mmHg; DBP = 10–15 mmHg); reaches a nadir at 24 weeks and normalizes by 40 weeks. Systolic murmur and an audible S3 are normal; a **new diastolic murmur is not.** The heart is displaced by the uterus upward and to the left → cardiomegaly on CXR.

TABLE 2.11-1. Normal Physiologic Changes During Pregnancy (continued)

ORGAN/SYSTEM	PHYSIOLOGIC CHANGE
Endocrine	**Thyroid hormone:** ↑ estrogen levels → ↑ thyroid-binding globulin. Total and bound T_3/T_4 ↑ (hCG is a thyroid stimulator), but active unbound hormone is unchanged. **Human placental lactogen (HPL):** ↑ lipolysis → ↑ free fatty acids. Acts as an insulin antagonist to maintain fetal glucose levels → postprandial **hyperglycemia,** fasting **hyperinsulinemia/hypertriglyceridemia,** and exaggerated starvation **ketosis** response. Change can → or worsen gestational diabetes. **Cortisol:** ↑ total and free cortisol (produced by the fetal adrenal gland and the placenta).
GI	**Nausea and vomiting** (affects 70–85% of women); resolves by 14–16 weeks after the hCG rise plateaus. ↑ **acid reflux** from ↓ gastroesophageal junction sphincter tone. **Constipation** from ↓ large bowel motility and ↑ water resorption. ↑ biliary cholesterol saturation predisposes to gallstone formation.
Hematologic	**Physiologic anemia:** Unequal ↑ in **plasma volume (50%)** and RBC mass (20–30%) → ↓ hemoglobin and hematocrit. However, a **hemoglobin < 11.0 mg/dL is never normal** and is likely due to iron deficiency. **WBC count:** ↑ throughout pregnancy to a mean of 10.5 million/mL, but can ↑ during labor to > 20 million/mL. **Hypercoagulable state:** DVT risk is highest in the puerperium. **The leading nonobstetric cause of postpartum death is thromboembolic disease (pulmonary embolism).**
Musculoskeletal	↑ motility of sacroiliac, sacrococcygeal, and pubic joints.
Pulmonary	↑ in **tidal volume (V_T)** of 30–40%; ↓ in total lung capacity, residual volume, and expiratory reserve volume. **Respiratory rate (RR) is unchanged.** ↑ minute ventilation of 30–40% ($V_T \times RR$) → ↑ alveolar and arterial P_{O_2} and ↓ alveolar and arterial P_{CO_2}. **"Dyspnea of pregnancy"** is common and likely caused by ↑ V_T and ↓ P_{CO_2}.
Renal	Kidneys dilate, leading to physiologic hydronephrosis caused by uterine compression of the ureter. ↑ risk of pyelonephritis from asymptomatic bacteruria. **GFR ↑ by 50%;** renal plasma flow ↑ by 30%; BUN and creatinine ↓ by roughly 25%. ↑ estrogen and progesterone stimulate the renin-angiotensin system. ↑ **aldosterone** contributes to water retention and ↑ plasma volume.
Skin	↑ estrogen may → changes that resemble cirrhotic disease, such as **striae** (on the abdomen, breast, and thighs), **spider angiomas,** and **palmar erythema.** **Hyperpigmentation** over the abdominal midline **(linea nigra),** face (chloasma/melasma), nipples, and perineum is due to ↑ α-melanocyte-stimulating hormone and steroids. **Diastasis recti:** Rectus muscles may separate in the midline, leaving part of the anterior uterus covered only by skin, fascia, and peritoneum.

PRENATAL CARE AND NUTRITION

The goal of prenatal care is to prevent, diagnose, and treat conditions that → adverse outcomes in pregnancy (see Table 2.11-2).

TABLE 2.11-2. Standard Prenatal Care

CATEGORY	RECOMMENDATIONS
Weight gain	Approximately 25–35 lbs for an average-weight woman with a BMI of 19.8–26.0 (less for obese women and more for thin women). An **additional 100–300 kcal/day** is needed during pregnancy and 500 kcal/day during breast-feeding.
Nutrition	Requirements for important vitamins/minerals in pregnancy are as follows: <ul><li>**Folic acid: 0.4 mg daily;** required to ↓ neural tube defects, especially three months prior to conception.</li><li>**Iron:** Demand is ↑ by fetal needs and by expanding maternal blood supply. Supplement with **30 mg/day elemental iron (which is equivalent to 325 mg iron sulfate)** in the latter half of pregnancy.</li><li>**Vitamin A:** Routine supplementation of vitamin A is not recommended because excessive vitamin A (> 10,000 IU/day) is associated with fetal malformation.</li><li>Patients are advised to take prenatal vitamins, but most needs can be met through diet.</li></ul>
Exercise	Thirty minutes of moderate exercise daily is recommended.
Prenatal visits	Recommendations: <ul><li>Weeks 0–28: Every four weeks.</li><li>Weeks 29–36: Every two weeks.</li><li>Weeks 36–birth: Every week.</li></ul>
Prenatal labs Initial visit	**Heme:** CBC, blood type, Rh factor, and antibody screen. **Infectious disease:** UA and culture, rubella antibody titer, HBV surface antigen test, syphilis screen (RPR/VDRL), cervical gonorrhea and chlamydia PCR or culture, PPD, HIV (in high-risk groups). **Other:** Pap smear, glucose challenge test if patient has a family history of diabetes, sickle prep.
15–20 weeks	Maternal serum α-fetoprotein (MSAFP) or **quad screen (MSAFP, estriol, β-hCG and inhibin A).** Offer amniocentesis to patients > 35 years of age at the time of delivery.
18–20 weeks	Ultrasound to determine GA (if unknown or uncertain) and to survey fetal anatomy, amniotic fluid volume, and placental location.
26–28 weeks	Glucose challenge test.
32–36 weeks	Cervical chlamydia and gonorrhea cultures, HIV, RPR in high-risk patients; repeat hematocrit. **Screen for group B streptococcus (GBS). If ⊕, give penicillin during labor** to prevent transmission to the infant.

PRENATAL DIAGNOSTIC TESTING

α-Fetoprotein (AFP)

- Produced by the fetus and found primarily in amniotic fluid. Small amounts cross the placenta and enter the maternal circulation.
- **MSAFP (15–20 weeks' gestation):** Results are reported as multiples of the median (MoMs) and depend on accurate gestational dating.
  - Causes of elevated MSAFP (> 2.5 MoMs) include open neural tube defects (anencephaly, spina bifida), abdominal wall defects (gastroschisis, omphalocele), multiple gestation, incorrect gestational dating, fetal death, and placental abnormalities (e.g., placental abruption).
  - Abnormally low MSAFP levels (< 0.5 MoM) warrant amniocentesis and karyotyping to rule out chromosomal abnormalities.

- **Quad screen:** Sensitivity for detecting chromosomal abnormalities is ↑ by adding inhibin A to estriol, β-hCG, and MSAFP.
    - **Trisomy 18:** All four are ↓.
    - **Trisomy 21:** AFP and estriol are ↓; β-hCG and inhibin A are ↑.

Amniocentesis

- Consists of transabdominal aspiration of amniotic fluid using an ultrasound-guided needle and evaluation of fetal cells for genetic studies.
- There is ample fluid in **weeks 15–17** to perform the test. Risks are fetal-maternal hemorrhage (1–2%) and fetal loss (0.5%). Amniocentesis is indicated for the following:
    - In women who will be > **35 years of age at the time of delivery.**
    - In conjunction with an abnormal quad screen.
    - In Rh-sensitized pregnancy to obtain fetal blood type or to detect fetal hemolysis.
    - To evaluate fetal lung maturity via a lecithin-sphingomyelin ratio ≥ 2.5 or to detect the presence of phosphatidylglycerol (done during the third trimester).

Chorionic Villus Sampling

- Transcervical or transabdominal aspiration of placental (chorionic villi) tissue.
    - **Advantages:** Has a diagnostic accuracy comparable to that of amniocentesis; availability at **10–12 weeks' gestation.**
    - **Disadvantages: Risk of fetal loss and inability to diagnose neural tube defects is 0.5–1.0% higher than with amniocentesis.**
- Limb defects have been associated with chorionic villus sampling performed at ≤ 9 weeks.

Percutaneous Umbilical Blood Sampling (PUBS)

- Transabdominal phlebotomy of the umbilical cord. Performed in the second and third trimesters, when umbilical cord vessels are large enough to puncture safely.
- Amniocentesis and chorionic villus sampling are now used preferentially for prenatal diagnosis.
- PUBS is used to diagnose fetal hemolytic disease and fetal infection.

TERATOLOGY

Major defects are apparent in about 3% of births and in roughly 4.5% of children by five years of age. Table 2.11-3 lists FDA risk classifications of pharmaceutical products for use during pregnancy. See Tables 2.11-4 and 2.11-5 for a list of common teratogenic agents and pathogens.

NORMAL LABOR AND DELIVERY

Stages of Labor

Table 2.11-6 and Figure 2.11-1 depict the normal stages of labor.

Obstetric Examination

- Leopold's maneuvers are used to determine fetal lie (longitudinal or transverse) and fetal presentation (breech or cephalic) if possible.

TABLE 2.11-3   FDA Risk Classification of Pharmaceutical Products for Use During Pregnancy

CATEGORY	DESCRIPTION	EXAMPLE
Category A	Adequate and well-controlled studies in women fail to demonstrate a risk to the fetus in the first trimester (and there is no risk in later trimesters). The possibility of fetal harm seems remote.	Vitamin C (when use does not exceed the recommended daily allowance)
Category B	Either animal reproduction studies have not demonstrated risk to the fetus but no adequate and well-controlled studies in pregnant women have been reported, or animal reproduction studies have shown an adverse effect that was not confirmed in controlled studies in women in the first trimester (and there is no evidence of risk in later trimesters).	Ampicillin
Category C	Either studies in animals have revealed adverse effects on the fetus but no controlled studies in women have been reported, or studies in women and animals are not available. Drugs should be given only if the potential benefit justifies the potential risk to the fetus.	Zidovudine
Category D	Positive evidence of human fetal risk exists, but the benefits from use in pregnant women may be acceptable despite the risk.	Phenytoin
Category X	Studies in animals or humans have demonstrated fetal abnormalities, or evidence exists of fetal risk based on human experience, or both, and the risk in pregnant women clearly outweighs any possible benefit.	Isotretinoin

TABLE 2.11-4.   Common Teratogenic Agents and Their Associated Defects

DRUGS AND CHEMICALS	DEFECTS
Alcohol	Fetal alcohol syndrome (growth restriction before and after birth, mental retardation, midfacial hypoplasia, renal and cardiac defects). Fetuses of women who ingest six drinks per day have a 40% risk of developing features of fetal alcohol syndrome.
Androgens and testosterone derivatives	Virilization of females; advanced genital development in males.
ACEIs	Fetal renal tubular dysplasia and neonatal renal failure, oligohydramnios, intrauterine growth restriction (IUGR), lack of cranial ossification.
Coumadin derivatives	Nasal hypoplasia and stippled bone epiphyses, developmental delay, IUGR, ophthalmologic abnormalities.
Carbamazepine	Neural tube defects, fingernail hypoplasia, microcephaly, developmental delay, IUGR.
Folic acid antagonists (e.g., methotrexate, aminopterin)	↑ spontaneous abortion (SAB) rate.
Cocaine	Bowel atresias; congenital malformations of the heart, limbs, face and genitourinary tract; microcephaly; IUGR; cerebral infarctions.

DRUGS AND CHEMICALS	DEFECTS
Diethylstilbestrol (DES)	Clear cell adenocarcinoma of the vagina or cervix, vaginal adenosis, abnormalities of the cervix and uterus or testes, possible infertility.
Lead	↑ SAB rate; stillbirths.
Lithium	Congenital heart disease (Ebstein's anomaly).
Organic mercury	Cerebral atrophy, microcephaly, mental retardation, spasticity, seizures, blindness.
Phenytoin	IUGR, mental retardation, microcephaly, dysmorphic craniofacial features, cardiac defects, fingernail hypoplasia.
Radiation	Microcephaly, mental retardation. Medical diagnostic radiation delivering < 0.05 Gy to the fetus has no teratogenic risk.
Streptomycin and kanamycin	Hearing loss; CN VIII damage.
Tetracycline	Permanent yellow-brown discoloration of deciduous teeth, hypoplasia of tooth enamel.
Thalidomide	Bilateral limb deficiencies, anotia and microtia, cardiac and GI anomalies.
Trimethadione and paramethadione	Cleft lip or cleft palate, cardiac defects, microcephaly, mental retardation.
Valproic acid	Neural tube defects (spina bifida), minor craniofacial defects.
Vitamin A and derivatives	↑ SAB rate, microtia, thymic agenesis, cardiovascular defects, craniofacial dysmorphism, microphthalmia, cleft lip or cleft palate, mental retardation.

- Cervical examination:
  - Evaluate dilation, effacement, station, cervical position, and cervical consistency (five aspects of the **Bishop score**). A Bishop score > 8 is consistent with a cervix favorable for both spontaneous and induced labor.
  - Confirm or determine fetal presentation.
  - Determine fetal position in the vertex presentation by palpation of the fetal sutures and fontanelles.
- Conduct a **sterile speculum exam if rupture of membranes (ROM) is suspected.**

TABLE 2.11-5. Infections with Teratogenic Potential

PATHOGEN	DEFECTS	COMMENTS
CMV	Microcephaly, hydrocephaly, chorioretinitis, cerebral calcifications, IUGR, microphthalmos, mental retardation, hearing loss.	The most common congenital infection.
Rubella	Microcephaly, mental retardation, cataracts, hearing loss, congenital heart disease.	Immunization is not recommended during pregnancy, although the live attenuated vaccine has not been shown to cause the malformations of congenital rubella syndrome.
Syphilis	Fetal hydrops (severe); abnormalities of the skin, teeth, and bones (mild).	
Toxoplasmosis	Microcephaly, hydrocephaly, cerebral calcifications, chorioretinitis.	*Toxoplasma gondii* is transmitted to humans by raw meat or through exposure to infected cat feces.
Varicella	Skin scarring, chorioretinitis, cataracts, microcephaly, hypoplasia of the hands and feet, muscle atrophy.	

Fetal Heart Rate (FHR) Monitoring

The most common obstetric procedure. Used in 85% of live births in the United States. Recommendations are as follows (see also Table 2.11-7 and Figure 2.11-2):

- **Patients without complications:** FHR tracing reviewed every 30 minutes in the first stage of labor and every 15 minutes in the second stage of labor.
- **Patients with complications:** FHR tracing reviewed every 15 minutes in the first stage of labor and every 5 minutes in the second stage of labor.

> *Factors affecting the active phase—*
>
> *The 3 P's:*
>
> **P**ower
> **P**assenger
> **P**elvis

TABLE 2.11-6. Stages of Labor

STAGE	STARTS/ENDS	DURATION Primi[a]	Multi[b]	COMMENTS
First		**Primi[a]**	**Multi[b]**	
Latent	Onset of labor to 3–4 cm dilation	6–11 hrs	4–8 hrs	Prolongation seen with excessive sedation and hypertonic uterine contractions.
Active	4 cm to complete cervical dilation (10 cm)	4–6 hrs (1.2 cm/hr)	2–3 hrs (1.5 cm/hr)	Prolongation seen with **cephalopelvic disproportion.**
Second	Complete cervical dilation to delivery of infant	0.5–3.0 hrs	5–30 min	Baby goes through all cardinal movements of labor (see the **3 P's** mnemonic).
Third	Delivery of infant to delivery of placenta	0–0.5 hr	0–0.5 hr	Placenta separates and uterus contracts to establish hemostasis.

[a] Primiparous (first-time mother).

[b] Multiparous (prior pregnancy and delivery).

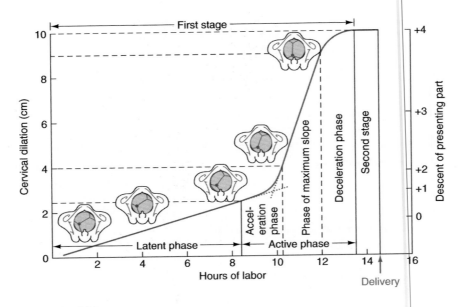

FIGURE 2.11-1. Stages of labor.

Cervical dilation, level of descent, and orientation of occipitoanterior presentation during various stages of labor. (Reproduced, with permission, from DeCherney AH. *Current Obstetric & Gynecologic Diagnosis & Treatment*, 8th ed. Stamford, CT: Appleton & Lange, 1994, p. 211.)

TABLE 2.11-7. Fetal Heart Rate Patterns[a]

TYPE	DESCRIPTION	COMMON CAUSES
Acceleration	A visually apparent increase (onset to peak in < 30 sec) in FHR from the most recent baseline.	Fetal movements.
Early deceleration	A visually apparent, gradual (onset to nadir in > 30 sec) decrease in FHR with return to baseline that mirrors the uterine contraction.	Head compression from the uterine contraction (normal).
Late deceleration	A visually apparent, gradual (onset to nadir in > 30 sec) decrease in FHR with return to baseline whose onset, nadir, and recovery occur after the beginning, peak, and end of uterine contraction, respectively.	Uteroplacental insufficiency and fetal hypoxemia.
Variable deceleration	An abrupt (onset to nadir in < 30 sec), visually apparent decrease in FHR below baseline lasting ≥ 15 sec but < 2 min.	Umbilical cord compression (most often 2° to oligohydramnios).
Bradycardia baseline	FHR < 110 bpm.	Congenital heart malformations, severe hypoxia (2° to uterine hyperstimulation, cord prolapse, rapid fetal descent).
Tachycardia	Baseline FHR > 160 bpm.	Hypoxia, maternal fever, anemia.

[a]Baseline FHR is rounded to increments of 5 bpm during a 10-minute period and must be present for a minimum of 2 minutes; baseline variability is quantitated by the amplitude of fluctuations in the FHR and is described as absent, minimal, moderate (normal), or marked.

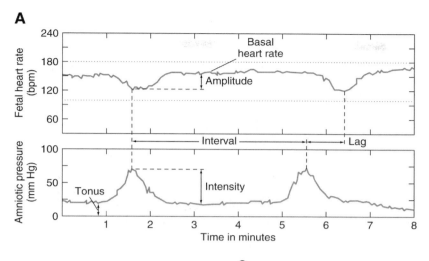

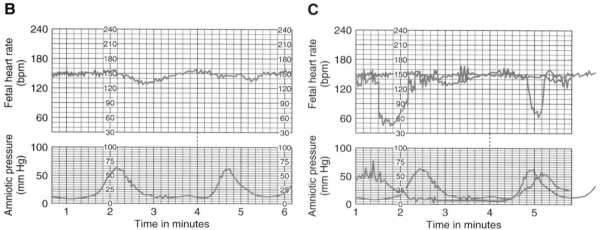

FIGURE 2.11-2. **Fetal heart tracings.**

(A) Schematic tracing. (B) Late deceleration. (C) Variable deceleration. (Reproduced, with permission, from DeCherney AH. *Current Obstetric & Gynecologic Diagnosis & Treatment*, 8th ed. Stamford, CT: Appleton & Lange, 1994, p. 301.)

Antepartum Fetal Surveillance

In general, antepartum fetal surveillance is used in pregnancies in which the risk of antepartum fetal demise is ↑. Testing is initiated in most at-risk patients at 32–34 weeks (or 26–28 weeks if there are multiple worrisome risk factors present). These tests do not predict the risk of stillbirth related to acute changes in status.

- **Fetal movement assessment:** Assessed by the mother as the number of fetal movements over one hour. Average time to obtain 10 movements is 20 minutes. Maternal reports of ↓ fetal movements should be evaluated by means of the tests described below.
- **Nonstress test (NST):** Performed with the mother resting in the lateral tilt position (to prevent supine hypotension). FHR is monitored externally by Doppler along with a tocodynamometer to detect uterine contractions. Acoustic stimulation may be used.
  - **"Reactive" (normal response):** Two accelerations of ≥ 15 bpm above baseline for at least 15 seconds over a 20-minute period.

- ■ "Nonreactive": Fewer than two accelerations over a 20-minute period. Perform further tests (e.g., a biophysical profile). Lack of FHR accelerations may occur with any of the following: GA < 32 weeks, fetal sleeping, fetal CNS anomalies, and maternal sedative or narcotic administration.
- ■ **Contraction stress test (CST):** Performed in the lateral recumbent position. FHR is monitored during spontaneous or induced (via nipple stimulation or oxytocin) contractions. Reactivity is determined from fetal heart monitoring, as with the NST. Contraindicated in women with preterm membrane rupture or known placenta previa, women with a history of uterine surgery, and women who are at high risk for preterm labor.
  - ■ A "positive" CST is defined by late decelerations following 50% or more of contractions in a 10-minute window, and raises concerns about fetal jeopardy. Delivery is usually warranted.
  - ■ A "negative" CST is defined as no late or significant variable decelerations within 10 minutes and at least three contractions. It is highly predictive of fetal well-being in conjunction with a normal NST.
  - ■ An "equivocal" CST is defined by intermittent late decelerations or significant variable decelerations.
- ■ **Biophysical profile (BPP):** Real-time ultrasound is used to assign a score of 2 (normal) or 0 (abnormal) to five parameters: fetal tone, breathing, movement, amniotic fluid volume, and NST.
  - ■ A score of 8–10 is reassuring for fetal well-being.
  - ■ A score of 6 is considered equivocal. Term pregnancies are usually delivered with this profile.
  - ■ A score of 0–4 is extremely worrisome for fetal asphyxia, and strong consideration should be given to immediate delivery if no nonhypoxic explanation is found.
- ■ **Modified biophysical profile (mBPP):** Combines the NST with the amniotic fluid index (AFI, sum of the measurements of the deepest cord-free amniotic fluid in each of the abdominal quadrants). The test is considered normal with a reactive NST and an AFI > 5 cm.
- ■ **Umbilical artery Doppler velocimetry:** With IUGR, there is reduction and even reversal of umbilical artery diastolic flow. The test is of benefit only when IUGR is suspected.
- ■ **Oligohydramnios (AFI < 5 cm) always warrants further workup.**

> *When performing a BPP, remember to—*
>
> **Test the Baby, MAN!**
>
> Fetal **T**one
> Fetal **B**reathing
> Fetal **M**ovement
> **A**mniotic fluid volume
> **N**onstress test

Obstetric Analgesia and Anesthesia

Uterine contractions and cervical dilation result in visceral pain (T10–L1). Descent of the fetal head and pressure on the vagina and perineum result in somatic pain (pudendal nerve, S2–S4). In the absence of a medical contraindication, maternal request is a sufficient medical indication for pain relief during labor. Absolute contraindications to regional anesthesia (epidural, spinal, or combination) include the following (see also Table 2.11-8):

- ■ Refractory maternal hypotension
- ■ Maternal coagulopathy
- ■ Maternal use of a once-daily dose of low-molecular-weight heparin (LMWH) within 12 hours
- ■ Untreated maternal bacteremia
- ■ Skin infection over the site of needle placement
- ■ ↑ ICP caused by a mass lesion

TABLE 2.11-8. Available Methods of Anesthesia and Analgesia

AVAILABLE METHODS	DISADVANTAGES	ADVANTAGES
Parenteral (opioid agonists and agonist-antagonists)	Produces a limited analgesic effect in labor (primarily acts through sedation); increases the risk of neonatal naloxone administration and five-minute Apgar scores < 7 (due to significant transplacental passage of these drugs); decreases FHR variability.	Provides an adequate level of pain relief for some women without the risks associated with regional anesthesia.
Epidural	Can result in pruritus, fever, **hypotension,** and **transient FHR deceleration.**	Provides the most effective form of pain relief; can also be used for cesarean delivery or postpartum tubal ligation.
Spinal	Acts for a limited duration; puts patients at risk for **hypotension, postdural puncture headache,** and transient neurologic symptoms.	Rapid-onset analgesia that provides excellent pain relief for procedures of limited duration (30–250 minutes).
Combined spinal epidural	Carries the risks of both procedures; may increase the risk of bradycardia and emergent cesarean delivery over epidural analgesia alone.	Offers the rapid onset of spinal analgesia combined with the ability to prolong the duration of analgesia with continuous epidural infusion.
General	Requires airway control; carries a significant risk of **maternal aspiration** and **neonatal depression** (inhaled anesthetic agents readily cross the placenta); associated with higher maternal morbidity rates than epidural anesthesia.	Used in emergent cesarean delivery and indicated in some cases of FHR abnormality; can be useful in cases where regional anesthesia is absolutely contraindicated (see below).
Local (e.g., lidocaine, 2-chloroprocaine)	In rare circumstances, can cause seizures, hypotension, and cardiac arrhythmias.	Provides anesthesia (20- to 40-minute duration) before episiotomy and during repair of lacerations; can be used to perform a pudendal block.

HIGH-YIELD FACTS

OBSTETRICS

For both elective and indicated cesarean delivery, sodium citrate should be used to ↓ gastric acidity and prevent acid aspiration syndrome.

MEDICAL COMPLICATIONS OF PREGNANCY

Hyperemesis Gravidarum

Persistent vomiting not related to other causes, **acute starvation** (usually large ketonuria), and weight loss (usually at least a 5% decrease from pre-pregnancy weight). Occurs in 0.5–2.0% of pregnancies. More common in nulliparas, multiple gestations, and molar pregnancies. ↑ β-hCG and ↑ estradiol have been implicated in the pathophysiology.

HISTORY/PE

Differentiate from "morning sickness," acid reflux, gastroenteritis, hyperthyroidism, and neurologic conditions.

DIAGNOSIS

Evaluate for ketonemia, ketonuria, hyponatremia, and hypokalemic-hypochloremic metabolic alkalosis. Measure liver enzymes, serum bilirubin, and serum amylase/lipase. Check β-hCG level.

TREATMENT

Vitamin B_6 +/– doxylamine for nausea and vomiting of pregnancy. Can also consider most antiemetics. Ginger, IV hydration, hospitalization (when severe), and parenteral nutrition (for persistent weight loss) may also be used.

Gestational Diabetes Mellitus

Carbohydrate intolerance of variable severity that is first diagnosed during pregnancy. Occurs in **3–5% of all pregnancies, usually in late pregnancy.** Hyperglycemia at < 20 weeks' gestation usually suggests preexisting undiagnosed diabetes and should be managed as pregestational diabetes. May result from insulin antagonist hormones from the placenta (e.g., HPL, cortisol). Risk factors include obesity, a family or personal history of diabetes, recurrent abortions, stillbirths, maternal age > 25 years, a prior macrosomic infant (> 4000–4500 g) or an infant with congenital anomalies, and prior polyhydramnios.

HISTORY/PE

Typically asymptomatic. Edema, polyhydramnios, or a **large-for-GA infant (> 90th percentile) may be warning signs.**

DIAGNOSIS

- UA reveals glycosuria.
- Diagnosis requires an **abnormal glucose challenge test,** routinely performed at 24–28 weeks' gestation. If > 140, confirm with a three-hour (100-g) glucose tolerance test showing any two of the following: fasting > 95 mg/dL; one hour > 180; two hours > 155; three hours > 140.

TREATMENT

- **Mother:**
  - Start with the **ADA diet,** regular exercise, and strict glucose monitoring (four times a day). Tight maternal glucose control improves outcomes.
  - **Add insulin** if dietary control is insufficient.
  - Give intrapartum insulin and dextrose to maintain tight control during delivery.
- **Fetus:**
  - Obtain periodic ultrasound and NSTs to assess fetal growth and well-being.
  - It may be necessary to induce labor at 39–40 weeks.

COMPLICATIONS

More than 50% of patients go on to **develop glucose intolerance and/or type 2 DM** later in life.

Hyperglycemia in the first trimester suggests preexisting diabetes.

A fetus that is large for GA may indicate occult diabetes.

Pregestational Diabetes and Pregnancy

Observed in 1% of all pregnancies. Insulin requirements may ↑ as much as threefold. Poorly controlled DM ($HbA_{1C} > 8\%$) is associated with an ↑ **risk of congenital malformations** and ↑ maternal/fetal morbidity during labor and delivery.

TREATMENT

- **Mother:**
    - Routine prenatal screening/care and nutritional counseling.
    - Renal, ophthalmologic, and cardiac evaluation to assess for end-organ damage.
    - Strict glucose control (with diet, exercise, insulin therapy, and frequent self-monitoring for type 1 and type 2 DM) to minimize fetal defects.
        - **Fasting morning:** ≤ 90 mg/dL.
        - **Two-hour postprandial:** < 120 mg/dL.
- **Fetus:**
    - **18–20 weeks:** Ultrasound to determine fetal age and growth; evaluate for cardiac anomalies and polyhydramnios; quad screen to screen for developmental anomalies.
    - **32–34 weeks:** Close fetal surveillance (e.g., NST, CST, BPP). Admit if maternal DM has been poorly controlled or fetal parameters are a concern. May require serial ultrasounds for growth.
- **Delivery and postpartum:**
    - Maintain normoglycemia (80–100 mg/dL) during labor with an IV insulin drip and hourly readings of glucose levels.
    - Consider early delivery if there is poor maternal glucose control, preeclampsia, macrosomia, or evidence of fetal lung maturity.
    - Cesarean delivery should be considered for an estimated fetal weight (EFW) > 4500 g.
    - Encourage breast-feeding with an appropriate ↑ in caloric intake.
    - Continue glucose monitoring postpartum. Insulin needs rapidly ↓ after delivery.

COMPLICATIONS

See Table 2.11-9.

TABLE 2.11-9. Complications of Pregestational Diabetes Mellitus

MATERNAL COMPLICATIONS	FETAL COMPLICATIONS
DKA (type 1) or HHNK (type 2)	Macrosomia
Preeclampsia/eclampsia	Cardiac and renal defects
Cephalopelvic disproportion (from macrosomia) and need for C-section	Neural tube defects (e.g., sacral agenesis)
	Hypocalcemia
Preterm labor	Polycythemia
Infection	Hyperbilirubinemia
Polyhydramnios	Intrauterine growth restriction (IUGR)
Postpartum hemorrhage	Hypoglycemia from hyperinsulinemia
Maternal mortality	Respiratory distress syndrome (RDS)
	Birth injury (e.g., shoulder dystocia)
	Perinatal mortality

Gestational and Chronic Hypertension

- **Gestational hypertension** (formerly known as pregnancy-induced hypertension) is idiopathic hypertension without significant proteinuria (< 300 mg/L) that develops at > 20 weeks' gestation. As many as 25% of patients may go on to develop preeclampsia.
- **Chronic hypertension** is present before conception and at < 20 weeks' gestation or may persist for > 12 weeks postpartum. Up to one-third of patients may develop superimposed preeclampsia.
- **Tx:** Monitor BP closely and treat with appropriate antihypertensives (e.g., methyldopa, labetalol, nifedipine). **Do not give ACEIs or diuretics,** as ACEIs are known to → uterine ischemia and diuretics can aggravate low plasma volume to the point of uterine ischemia. Complications are similar to those of preeclampsia.

Preeclampsia and Eclampsia

Signs of severe preeclampsia are persistent headache or other cerebral or visual disturbances, persistent epigastric pain, and hyperreactive reflexes.

- **Preeclampsia** is defined as **new-onset hypertension** (SBP ≥ 140 mmHg or DBP ≥ 90 mmHg) **and proteinuria** (> 300 mg of protein in a 24-hour period) occurring at **> 20 weeks' gestation.**
- **Eclampsia** is defined as new-onset **grand mal seizures** in women with preeclampsia.
- **HELLP syndrome** is a variant of preeclampsia with a poor prognosis (see the mnemonic).
    - The etiology is unknown, but clinical manifestations are explained by vasospasm → hemorrhage and organ necrosis.
    - Risk factors include nulliparity, black ethnicity, extremes of age (< 20 or > 35), multiple gestation, molar pregnancy, renal disease (due to SLE or type 1 DM), a family history of preeclampsia, and chronic hypertension.
- **Hx/PE:** See Table 2.11-10 for the signs and symptoms of preeclampsia and eclampsia.
- **Dx:** Modalities include UA, 24-hour urine protein, CBC, electrolytes, BUN/creatinine, uric acid, precise measurement of fetal age, **amniocentesis** (to assess **fetal lung maturity**), LFTs, PT/PTT, fibrinogen and fibrin split products (for DIC), urine toxicology screen, ultrasound, and NST/CST/BPP (as indicated).
- **Tx: The only cure for preeclampsia/eclampsia is delivery of the fetus.** See Table 2.11-10 for management.

Antepartum Hemorrhage

Any bleeding after 20 weeks' gestation. Complicates 3–5% of pregnancies (prior to 20 weeks, bleeding is referred to as threatened abortion). The most common causes are **placental abruption** and **placenta previa** (see Table 2.11-11 and Figure 2.11-3). Other causes include other forms of abnormal placentation (e.g., placenta accreta), ruptured uterus, genital tract lesions, and trauma.

OBSTETRIC COMPLICATIONS OF PREGNANCY

Table 2.11-12 lists fetal complications of pregnancy.

TABLE 2.11-10. Signs, Symptoms, and Management of Preeclampsia and Eclampsia

	SIGNS AND SYMPTOMS	MANAGEMENT	COMPLICATIONS
Mild preeclampsia	BP ≥ **140/90** on two occasions > 6 hours apart. Proteinuria (> 300 mg/24 hrs or 1–2 ⊕ urine dipsticks).	If the patient is close to term or preeclampsia worsens, induce delivery with IV oxytocin, prostaglandins, or amniotomy. If the patient is far from term, treat with modified bed rest and **expectant management.**	Prematurity, fetal distress, stillbirth, placental abruption, seizure, DIC, cerebral hemorrhage, serous retinal detachment, fetal/maternal death.
Severe preeclampsia	BP > **160/110** on two occasions > 6 hours apart. **Renal:** Proteinuria (> 5 g/24 hrs or 3–4 ⊕ urine dipsticks) or oliguria (< 500 mL/24 hrs). **Cerebral changes:** Headache, somnolence. **Visual changes:** Blurred vision, scotomata. **Hyperactive reflexes/clonus.** **Hemolysis, elevated liver enzymes, thrombocytopenia (HELLP syndrome).**	**Control BP** with labetalol and/or hydralazine (goal < 160/110 with a diastolic BP of 90–100 to maintain fetal blood flow). Deliver by induction or C-section if the mother is stable. **Prevent seizures with continuous magnesium sulfate (MgSO$_4$) drip.** Watch for signs of Mg^{2+} toxicity (loss DTRs, respiratory paralysis, coma). **Continue seizure prophylaxis for 24 hours postpartum.** Treat Mg^{2+} toxicity with IV Ca^{2+} gluconate.	Same as above.
Eclampsia	The most common signs preceding an eclamptic attack are **headache, visual changes,** and **RUQ/epigastric pain.** **Seizures** are severe if not controlled with anticonvulsant therapy.	ABCs with supplemental O$_2$. Seizure control/prophylaxis with **MgSO$_4$**. If seizures recur, give IV diazepam. Control BP (labetalol and/or hydralazine). Limit fluids; Foley for strict I/Os. Monitor Mg^{2+} blood levels and Mg^{2+} toxicity; monitor fetal status. Initiate delivery if the patient is stable and convulsions are controlled. Postpartum management is the same as that for preeclampsia. Seizures may occur antepartum (25%), intrapartum (50%), and postpartum (25%); most occur within 48 hours after delivery.	Cerebral hemorrhage, aspiration pneumonia, hypoxic encephalopathy, thromboembolic events, fetal/maternal death.

HIGH-YIELD FACTS

OBSTETRICS

TABLE 2.11-11. Placental Abruption vs. Placenta Previa

	PLACENTAL ABRUPTION	PLACENTA PREVIA
Pathophysiology	**Premature** (before onset of labor) **separation** of normally implanted placenta.	**Abnormal placental implantation:** ▪ **Total:** Placenta covers the cervical os. ▪ **Marginal:** Placenta extends to the margin of the os. ▪ **Low-lying:** Placenta is in close proximity to the os.
Incidence	1 in 100.	1 in 200.
Risk factors	Hypertension, abdominal/pelvic trauma, tobacco or cocaine use, previous abruption, rapid decompression of overdistended uterus.	Prior C-sections, grand multiparous, advanced maternal age, multiple gestation, prior placenta previa.
Symptoms	**Painful, dark** vaginal bleeding that does not spontaneously cease. Abdominal pain, uterine hypertonicity. Fetal distress.	**Painless, bright red** bleeding that often ceases in 1–2 hours with or without uterine contractions. Usually no fetal distress.
Diagnosis	**Primarily clinical.** Transabdominal/transvaginal ultrasound sensitivity is only 50%; look for retroplacental clot; most useful for ruling out previa.	**Transabdominal/transvaginal ultrasound sensitivity is > 95%;** look for abnormally positioned placenta.
Management	Stabilize patients with mild abruption and a premature fetus; **manage expectantly** (hospitalize; start IV and fetal monitoring; type and cross blood; bed rest). **Moderate to severe abruption:** Immediate delivery (vaginal delivery with amniotomy if mother and fetus are stable; C-section for maternal or fetal distress).	**NO vaginal exam!** **Stabilize patients with a premature fetus;** manage expectantly. Give tocolytics. Serial ultrasound to assess fetal growth; resolution of partial previa. Give betamethasone to help with fetal lung maturity **Deliver by C-section. Indications for delivery include labor, life-threatening bleeding, fetal distress, documented fetal lung maturity, and 36 weeks' GA.**
Complications	Hemorrhagic shock. Coagulopathy: **DIC** in 10%. Recurrence risk is 5–16% and rises to 25% after two previous abruptions. Fetal hypoxia.	↑ risk of placenta accreta. Vasa previa (fetal vessels crossing the internal os). Preterm delivery, premature rupture of membranes (PROM), IUGR, congenital anomalies. Recurrence risk is 4–8%.

ABNORMAL LABOR AND DELIVERY

Dystocia

Slow, abnormal progression of labor. The leading indication for cesarean delivery in the United States. Risk factors include chorioamnionitis, occiput posterior position, nulliparity, and elevated birth weight.

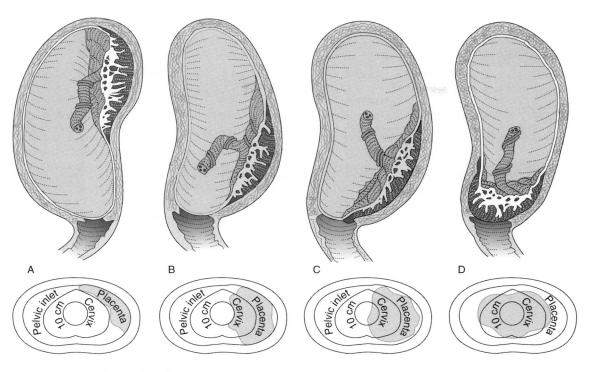

FIGURE 2.11-3. Placental implantation.

(A) Normal placenta. (B) Low implantation. (C) Partial placenta previa. (D) Complete placenta previa. (Adapted, with permission, from DeCherney AH. *Current Obstetric & Gynecologic Diagnosis & Treatment*, 8th ed. Stamford, CT: Appleton & Lange, 1994, p. 404.)

TABLE 2.11-12. Obstetric Complications of Pregnancy

PROBLEM	DEFINITION	HISTORY /PE	DIAGNOSIS	TREATMENT	COMPLICATIONS
Ectopic pregnancy	Most often tubal, but can be abdominal, ovarian, or cervical.	Presents with abdominal pain and vaginal spotting/bleeding; some patients are asymptomatic. +/– pregnancy test. Associated with a **history of PID.**	Serial hCG testing in conjunction with transvaginal ultrasound.	Medical treatment (methotrexate) for small, unruptured tubal pregnancies; surgical options for salpingectomy (laparoscopy vs. laparotomy).	Tubal rupture and hemoperitoneum (an obstetric emergency).
Intrauterine growth restriction (IUGR)	EFW < 10th percentile for GA.	Affected infants are commonly born to women with systemic diseases that → uteroplacental insufficiency (intrauterine infection, hypertension, anemia). Other risk factors include maternal substance abuse, placenta previa, and multiple gestations.	Serial fundal height measurements confirmed by ultrasound.	Explore the underlying etiology and correct if possible; administer steroids (e.g., betamethasone) to accelerate fetal lung maturity. Fetal monitoring with NST, CST, BPP, and umbilical artery Doppler velocimetry. A nonreassuring status near term may prompt delivery.	↑ perinatal morbidity and mortality.

TABLE 2.11-12. **Obstetric Complications of Pregnancy** (continued)

PROBLEM	DEFINITION	HISTORY /PE	DIAGNOSIS	TREATMENT	COMPLICATIONS
Fetal macrosomia	Birth weight > 90th percentile.	A common sequela of gestational diabetes.	Weighing the newborn at birth (prenatal diagnosis is imprecise).	Planned cesarean delivery may be considered for an EFW > 5000 g in women without diabetes and for an EFW > 4500 g in women with diabetes.	↑ risk of shoulder dystocia (→ brachial plexus injury and Erb-Duchenne palsy) as birth weight ↑.
Oligohydramnios	AFI < 5 cm on ultrasound.	Usually asymptomatic, but IUGR or fetal distress may be present. Etiologies include fetal urinary tract abnormalities (e.g., renal agenesis, GU obstruction), chronic uteroplacental insufficiency, and ROM.	The sum of the deepest amniotic fluid pocket in all four abdominal quadrants. Rule out inaccurate gestational dates.	Treat the underlying cause if possible.	Associated with a 40-fold ↑ in perinatal mortality. Other complications include musculoskeletal abnormalities (e.g., clubfoot, facial distortion), pulmonary hypoplasia, umbilical cord compression, and IUGR.
Polyhydramnios	AFI > 20 on ultrasound. May be present in normal pregnancies, but fetal chromosomal or developmental abnormalities are common.	Usually asymptomatic, or exam may reveal a fundal height greater than expected. Etiologies include maternal DM, multiple gestation, isoimmunization, pulmonary abnormalities (e.g., cystic lung malformations), fetal anomalies (e.g., duodenal atresia, tracheo-esophageal fistula, anencephaly), and twin-twin transfusion syndrome.	Evaluation includes ultrasound for fetal anomalies, glucose testing for DM, and Rh screen.	Etiology specific.	Preterm labor, fetal malpresentation, cord prolapse.

TABLE 2.11-12. Obstetric Complications of Pregnancy (continued)

PROBLEM	DEFINITION	HISTORY /PE	DIAGNOSIS	TREATMENT	COMPLICATIONS
Rh isoimmunization	Fetal RBCs leak into the maternal circulation; maternal anti-Rh IgG antibodies form that can cross the placenta → hemolysis of fetal Rh RBCs **(erythroblastosis fetalis).**		Sensitized Rh-⊖ mothers with titers > 1:16 should be closely monitored with serial ultrasound and amniocentesis for evidence of fetal hemolysis.	In severe cases, initiate preterm delivery when fetal lungs are mature. Prior to delivery, intrauterine blood transfusions may be given to correct a low fetal hematocrit. Prevention: • If the mother is Rh ⊖ at 28 weeks and the father is Rh ⊕ or unknown, give **RhoGAM** (Rh immune globulin). • If the baby is Rh ⊕, give RhoGAM postpartum. • Give RhoGAM to Rh-⊖ mothers who undergo abortion or who have had an ectopic pregnancy, amniocentesis, vaginal bleeding, or placenta previa/placental abruption.	**Hydrops fetalis** occurs when hemoglobin drops to < 7 g/dL. Other complications include fetal hypoxia and acidosis, kernicterus, prematurity, and death.
Gestational trophoblastic disease (GTD)	A range of proliferative trophoblastic abnormalities that can be benign or malignant. • **Complete moles:** Usually result from sperm fertilization of an empty ovum; **46,XX** (paternally derived).	Presents with first-trimester **uterine bleeding** (most common), hyperemesis gravidarum, preeclampsia/ eclampsia at < 24 weeks, and uterine size greater than dates. No fetal heartbeat is detected; pelvic	Markedly ↑ serum **β-hCG (usually > 100,000 mIU/mL)** and a "snowstorm" appearance on pelvic ultrasound with no gestational sac or fetus present. CXR may show lung metastases; D&C reveals **"cluster-of-grapes"** tissue.	Type and screen is critical; follow β-hCG closely and prevent pregnancy for one year. Treat malignant disease with chemotherapy (methotrexate or dactinomycin) and residual uterine disease	**Molar pregnancy may progress to malignant GTD,** including invasive moles (10–15%) and choriocarcinoma (2–5%) with pulmonary or CNS metastases. Trophoblastic pulmonary

TABLE 2.11-12. **Obstetric Complications of Pregnancy (continued)**

PROBLEM	DEFINITION	HISTORY /PE	DIAGNOSIS	TREATMENT	COMPLICATIONS
Gestational trophoblastic disease (GTD) (continued)	• **Incomplete (partial) moles:** Occur when a normal ovum is fertilized by two sperm (or a haploid sperm that duplicates its chromosomes); usually **69,XXY** and contain fetal tissue.	exam may reveal enlarged ovaries (bilateral theca-lutein cysts) or expulsion of **grapelike molar clusters** into the vagina. Risk factors include extremes of age (< 20 or > 40), a diet deficient in folate or β-carotene, and blood group.		with hysterectomy; chemotherapy and irradiation are highly successful for metastases.	emboli may also be seen.
Multiple gestations	Affect 3% of all live births. Since 1980, there has been a 65% ↑ in the frequency of twins and a 500% ↑ in triplet and high-order births (most due to the advent of assisted reproductive technology).	Characterized by rapid uterine growth, excessive maternal weight gain, and palpation of three or more large fetal parts on Leopold's maneuvers.	Ultrasound; hCG, HPL, and MSAFP are elevated for GA.	Multifetal reduction and selective fetal termination; antepartum fetal surveillance for IUGR. Management by a high-risk specialist is recommended.	**Maternal:** Patients are six times more likely to be hospitalized with complications (e.g., for preeclampsia, preterm labor, PPROM, placental abruption, pyelonephritis, and postpartum hemorrhage). **Fetal:** Complications include twin-to-twin transfusion syndrome, IUGR, preterm labor, and an ↑ risk for a major long-term handicap such as cerebral palsy (patients have a nearly threefold greater risk of cerebral palsy).

DIAGNOSIS

- Cannot be diagnosed until an adequate trial of labor has been achieved.
- **First stage, protraction, or arrest:** Labor that fails to produce adequate rates of progressive cervical change.
- **Second-stage arrest:**
    - **Nulliparous:** More than three hours with regional anesthesia; more than two hours without.

- **Multiparous:** More than two hours with regional anesthesia; more than one hour without.

TREATMENT

See Table 2.11-13.

COMPLICATIONS

Chorioamnionitis → fetal infection, pneumonia, bacteremia.

Premature Rupture of Membranes (PROM)

Defined as spontaneous ROM > 1 hour before onset of labor. May be precipitated by vaginal or cervical infections, abnormal membrane physiology, or cervical incompetence. Preterm PROM (PPROM) occurs at < 37 weeks' gestation. Prolonged ROM is defined as rupture > 18 hours prior to delivery. Risk factors include low socioeconomic status (SES), young maternal age, smoking, and STIs.

HISTORY/PE

Patients often report a **"gush" of clear or blood-tinged amniotic fluid.** Uterine contractions may be present.

DIAGNOSIS

- **Sterile speculum exam** reveals **pooling** of amniotic fluid in the vaginal vault, a ⊕ **Nitrazine paper test** (paper turns blue in alkaline amniotic fluid), and a ⊕ **fern test** (a ferning pattern is seen under a microscope after amniotic fluid dries on a glass slide).
- Ultrasound-guided transabdominal instillation of indigo carmine dye to check for leakage (unequivocal test).
- Ultrasound to assess amniotic fluid volume.
- Obtain cultures or smears to rule out infections. Minimize infection risk; **do not** perform digital vaginal exams in women who are not in labor or for whom labor is not planned immediately.
- Check fetal heart tracing, maternal temperature, WBC count, and uterine tenderness for evidence of chorioamnionitis.

TABLE 2.11-13. Failure to Progress

STAGE		DEFINITION	TREATMENT[a]
First			
	Latent	Failure to have progressive cervical change:	Therapeutic rest via parenteral analgesia; oxytocin; amniotomy; cervical ripening.
		■ **Prima:** > 20 hours	
		■ **Multi:** > 14 hours	
	Active	Failure to have progressive cervical change after reaching 3–4 cm.	Amniotomy; oxytocin; C-section if the previous interventions are ineffective.
Second		Arrest of fetal descent:	Close observation with a ↓ in epidural rate and continued oxytocin.
		■ **Prima:** > 3 hours	
		■ **Multi:** > 2 hours	Assisted vaginal delivery (forceps or vacuum).
			C-section.

[a]Augmentation with oxytocin should be considered when contraction frequency is < 3 in a 10-minute period, or intensity of contraction is < 25 mmHg above baseline.

TREATMENT

- **Depends on GA and fetal lung maturity.**
  - **Term:** Check GBS status and fetal presentation; labor may be induced or the patient can be observed for 24–72 hours.
  - **> 34–36 weeks' gestation:** Labor induction may be considered.
  - **< 32 weeks' gestation:** Expectant management with bed rest and pelvic rest.
- **Antibiotics** are given to prevent infection and to prolong the latency period in the absence of infection.
- **Antenatal corticosteroids** (e.g., betamethasone or dexamethasone × 48 hours) can be given to promote fetal lung maturity in the absence of intra-amniotic infection prior to 32 weeks' GA.
- If signs of infection or fetal distress develop, give antibiotics (ampicillin and gentamicin) and induce labor.

COMPLICATIONS

Preterm labor and delivery, chorioamnionitis, placental abruption, cord prolapse.

Preterm Labor

Defined as onset of labor between **20 and 37 weeks' gestation.** Occurs in > 10% of all U.S. pregnancies and is the 1° cause of neonatal morbidity and mortality. Risk factors include multiple gestation, infection, PROM, uterine anomalies, previous preterm labor or delivery, polyhydramnios, placental abruption, poor maternal nutrition, and low SES. **Most patients have no identifiable risk factors.**

HISTORY/PE

Patients may have menstrual-like cramps, onset of low back pain, pelvic pressure, and new vaginal discharge or bleeding.

DIAGNOSIS

- Requires **regular uterine contractions** (≥ 3 contractions of 30 seconds each over a 30-minute period) and **concurrent cervical change** at < 37 weeks' gestation.
- **Assess for contraindications to tocolysis** (e.g., infection, nonreassuring fetal testing, placental abruption).
- Perform a **sterile speculum exam** to rule out PROM.
- Obtain an **ultrasound** to rule out fetal or uterine anomalies, verify GA, and assess fetal presentation and amniotic fluid volume.
- Obtain cultures for chlamydia, gonorrhea, and GBS. Obtain a UA and urine culture.

TREATMENT

- Hydration and bed rest.
- Unless contraindicated, begin **tocolytic therapy** (β-mimetics, $MgSO_4$, Ca^{2+} channel blockers, PGIs) and give **steroids** to accelerate fetal lung maturation. Give **penicillin or ampicillin for GBS prophylaxis** if preterm delivery is likely.

COMPLICATIONS

RDS, intraventricular hemorrhage, PDA, necrotizing enterocolitis, retinopathy of prematurity, bronchopulmonary dysplasia, death.

Fetal Malpresentation

Defined as any presentation other than vertex (i.e., head closest to birth canal, chin to chest, occiput anterior). Risk factors include **prematurity,** prior breech delivery, uterine anomalies, poly- or oligohydramnios, multiple gestations, PPROM, hydrocephalus, anencephaly, and placenta previa. **Breech presentations** are the most common (3% of all deliveries) and involve presentation of the fetal lower extremities or buttocks into the maternal pelvis (see Figure 2.11-4). Subtypes include the following:

- **Frank breech (50–75%):** Thighs are flexed and knees are extended.
- **Footling breech (20%):** One or both legs are extended below the buttocks.
- **Complete breech (5–10%):** Thighs and knees are flexed.

DIAGNOSIS

See the discussion above on the obstetric examination.

Breech presentation is the most common fetal malpresentation.

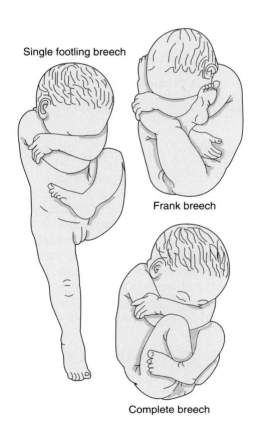

Single footling breech

Frank breech

Complete breech

FIGURE 2.11-4. Types of breech presentations.

(Reproduced, with permission, from DeCherney AH. *Current Obstetric & Gynecologic Diagnosis & Treatment*, 8th ed. Stamford, CT: Appleton & Lange, 1994, p. 411.)

HIGH-YIELD FACTS

OBSTETRICS

TABLE 2.11-14. **Indications for Cesarean Section**

MATERNAL FACTORS	FETAL AND MATERNAL FACTORS	FETAL FACTORS
Prior classical C-section (vertical incision predisposes to uterine rupture with vaginal delivery) Active genital herpes infection Cervical carcinoma Maternal trauma/demise	Cephalopelvic disproportion (most common cause of 1° C-section) Placenta previa/placental abruption Failed operative vaginal delivery Post-term pregnancy (relative indication)	Fetal malposition (e.g., posterior chin, transverse lie, shoulder presentation) Fetal distress Cord compression Erythroblastosis fetalis (Rh incompatibility)

TREATMENT

- **Follow:** Up to 75% spontaneously change to vertex by week 38.
- **External version:** If the fetus has not reverted spontaneously, apply pressure to the maternal abdomen to turn the infant to vertex. The success rate is roughly 50%. Risks are placental abruption and cord compression, so be prepared for an emergency C-section if needed.
- **Trial of breech vaginal delivery:** Attempt **only if delivery is imminent;** otherwise contraindicated. Complications include cord prolapse and/or head entrapment.
- **Elective C-section:** The standard of care in many hospitals, but it has not been shown to improve outcome.

Indications for Cesarean Section

See Table 2.11-14 for indications.

Episiotomy

- Surgical extension of the vaginal opening into the perineum. Performed in 30–35% of vaginal births in the United States.
- There are two types: **median** (midline) and **mediolateral.**
- Complications include extension to the anal sphincter (third degree) or rectum (fourth degree), which is more common with midline episiotomy, as well as bleeding, infection, dyspareunia, and, in rare cases, rectovaginal fistula formation or maternal death.
- Routine episiotomy has not been shown to influence the risk of pelvic floor damage, dyspareunia, or shoulder dystocia during delivery. **Evidence suggests that routine use of episiotomy should not be employed.**

PUERPERIUM

Postpartum Hemorrhage

- Defined as a loss of > 500 mL of blood for vaginal delivery or > 1000 mL for C-section occurring before, during, or after delivery of the placenta. Table 2.11-15 summarizes common causes.
- Complications include acute blood loss (potentially fatal), anemia due to chronic blood loss (predisposes to puerperal infection), and **Sheehan's syndrome** (pituitary ischemia and necrosis; the 1° cause of anterior pitu-

TABLE 2.11-15. **Common Causes of Postpartum Hemorrhage**

	UTERINE ATONY	GENITAL TRACT TRAUMA	RETAINED PLACENTAL TISSUE
Risk factors	Uterine overdistention (multiple gestation, macrosomia, polyhydramnios). Exhausted myometrium (rapid or prolonged labor, oxytocin stimulation). Uterine infection. Conditions interfering with contractions (anesthesia, myomas, $MgSO_4$).	Precipitous labor. Operative vaginal delivery (forceps, vacuum extraction). Large infant. Inadequate episiotomy repair.	Placenta accreta/increta/percreta. Placenta previa. Uterine leiomyomas. Preterm delivery. Previous C-section/curettage.
Diagnosis	Palpation of a soft, enlarged, "boggy" uterus. **The most common cause of postpartum hemorrhage (90%).**	Manual and visual inspection of the lower genital tract for any laceration > 2 cm long.	Manual and visual inspection of the placenta and uterine cavity for missing cotyledons. Ultrasound may also be used to inspect the uterus.
Treatment[a]	Bimanual **uterine massage** (usually successful). **Oxytocin** infusion. **Methergine** (methylergonovine) if not hypertensive. **Prostin** ($PGF_{2\alpha}$) if not asthmatic.	Surgical repair of the physical defect.	Manual removal of remaining placental tissue. Curettage with suctioning (take care not to perforate the uterine fundus).

[a] For all uterine causes, when bleeding persists after conventional therapy, uterine/internal iliac artery ligation or hysterectomy can be lifesaving.

itary insufficiency in adult females, most commonly presenting as **failure to lactate**).

Postpartum Infections

- Genital tract infection with a temperature ≥ 38°C for **at least two of the first ten postpartum days (not including the first 24 hours)**. Endometrial infection is most common.
- Risk factors include emergent C-section, PROM, prolonged labor, multiple intrapartum vaginal exams, and intrauterine manipulations.
- For endometritis, hospitalize and give **broad-spectrum empiric IV antibiotics** (e.g., clindamycin and gentamicin) **until patients have been afebrile for 48 hours** for endometritis (24 hours for chorioamnionitis). Add ampicillin for complicated cases.

Sheehan's Syndrome (Postpartum Pituitary Necrosis)

- Defined as pituitary ischemia and necrosis → anterior pituitary insufficiency 2° to massive obstetric hemorrhage and shock.

> **The 7 W's of postpartum fever:**
>
> **W**omb (endomyometritis)
> **W**ind (atelectasis, pneumonia)
> **W**ater (UTI)
> **W**alk (DVT, pulmonary embolism)
> **W**ound (incision, episiotomy)
> **W**eaning (breast engorgement, abscess, mastitis)
> **W**onder drugs (drug fever)

HIGH-YIELD FACTS

OBSTETRICS

- The 1° cause of anterior pituitary insufficiency in adult females. The **most common presenting syndrome is failure to lactate** (due to ↓ prolactin levels).
- Other symptoms include weakness, lethargy, cold insensitivity, genital atrophy, and menstrual disorders.

Lactation and Breast-Feeding

Breast-feeding is contraindicated in maternal HIV infection, active hepatitis, and use of certain medications.

- During pregnancy, ↑ estrogen and progesterone → breast hypertrophy and inhibition of prolactin release. After delivery of the placenta, hormone levels ↓ markedly and prolactin is released, stimulating milk production. Periodic infant suckling → further release of **prolactin** and **oxytocin,** which stimulate myoepithelial cell contraction and milk ejection ("let-down reflex").
- Colostrum ("early breast milk") contains protein, fat, **secretory IgA,** and minerals. Within one week postpartum, mature milk with protein, fat, lactose, and water is produced.
    - High IgA levels in colostrum provide passive immunity for the infant and protect against enteric bacteria.
    - Other benefits include ↓ incidence of allergies, facilitation of mother-child bonding, and maternal weight loss.
    - Contraindications to breast-feeding include HIV infection, active HBV and HCV, and use of certain medications (e.g., tetracycline, chloramphenicol, warfarin).

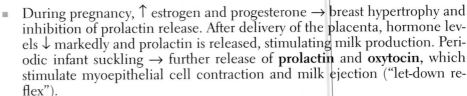

SPONTANEOUS AND ELECTIVE TERMINATION OF PREGNANCY

Spontaneous Abortion (SAB)

Loss of the fetus prior to the 20th week of pregnancy. Some 75% of cases occur before the 16th week, with 75% of these occurring before the eighth week. Approximately 20% of clinically recognized pregnancies terminate in SAB. ↑ risk is associated with a history of incompetent cervix, cervical conization or loop electrosurgical excision procedure (LEEP), cervical injury, DES exposure, and anatomical abnormalities of the cervix. Additional risk factors are as follows:

- **First trimester: Fetal factors (chromosomal abnormalities).**
- **Second trimester:** Maternal factors (cervical incompetence, infection, hypercoagulable states); maternal trauma, infection, dietary deficiency, DM, hypothyroidism, or anatomic malformation.

HISTORY/PE

See Table 2.11-16 for types of SAB.

DIAGNOSIS

- ↓ levels of hCG.
- **Ultrasound:**
    - Can identify the gestational sac 5–6 weeks from the LMP, a fetal pole at six weeks, and fetal cardiac activity at 6–7 weeks.
    - With accurate dating, a small, irregular intrauterine sac without a fetal pole on transvaginal ultrasound is diagnostic of an abnormal pregnancy.

TABLE 2.11-16. **Types of Spontaneous Abortion**

TYPE	DESCRIPTION	DIAGNOSIS	TREATMENT
Complete	All products of conception (POC) expelled; pain ceases, but spotting may persist.	Os is closed; ultrasound shows an empty uterus. POC is submitted to pathology to confirm fetal tissue.	D&C if ↑ likelihood that abortion was incomplete.
Incomplete	Mild cramping and bleeding; some POC expelled. Visible tissue in the vagina or endocervical canal.	Os is open; ultrasound reveals retained fetal tissue.	D&C to remove remaining POC and to control bleeding. Hemodynamic stabilization for heavy bleeding.
Threatened	No POC expelled; membranes remain intact. Uterine bleeding is present; abdominal pain may be present. The fetus is still viable.	Os is closed; ultrasound is normal.	Avoid heavy activity. Pelvic rest for 24–48 hours with gradual resumption of activities, but abstinence from coitus and douching.
Inevitable	No POC expelled, but considered inevitable. Uterine bleeding and cramps.	Os is open +/− ROM.	D&C or expectant management. Surgical evacuation of uterine contents. Prostaglandin suppositories are an alternative.
Missed	Pregnancy has ceased to develop. No POC is expelled; fetal tissue is retained. No uterine bleeding; symptoms of pregnancy disappear. Brownish vaginal discharge.	Os is closed; ultrasound reveals **no fetal cardiac activity. Fetal tissue is retained.**	D&C; prostaglandin suppositories are an alternative. DIC is a serious but rare complication whose risk ↑ with ↑ GA.
Septic	Infection with abortion. Endometritis → septicemia. Maternal mortality is 10–15%.	Hypotension, hypothermia, oliguria, respiratory distress if in shock; ↑ WBC.	Complete uterine evacuation, D&C; IV antibiotics.
Recurrent	Two or more consecutive SABs or a total of three SABs in one year. If early, often due to chromosomal abnormalities → karyotyping of both parents. Incompetent cervix should be suspected with a history of painless dilation of the cervix and delivery of a normal fetus between 18 and 32 weeks.	**Evaluate for uterine abnormalities.** Cervical cultures for gonococcus, chlamydia, and GBS should be obtained before the procedure.	Surgical cerclage procedures to suture the cervix closed until labor or ROM occurs with subsequent removal prior to delivery. Restriction of activities.
Intrauterine fetal demise	Absence of fetal cardiac activity.	Uterus small for GA; no fetal heart tones or movement on ultrasound.	Induce labor and evacuate the uterus to avoid DIC at GA > 16 weeks.

HIGH-YIELD FACTS

OBSTETRICS

TABLE 2.11-17. **Elective Termination of Pregnancy**

	PROCEDURE	TIMING	COMMENTS
First trimester (90% of elective abortions)	Medical management: ■ Oral mifepristone (low dose) + oral/vaginal misoprostol ■ IM/oral methotrexate + oral/vaginal misoprostol ■ Vaginal misoprostol (high dose), repeated up to 3 times Surgical management: ■ Manual aspiration ■ D&C with vacuum aspiration	Up to: 49 days' GA 49 days' GA 56 days' GA Up to 13 weeks' GA	FDA approved. Faster expulsion; fewer side effects.
Second trimester	Obstetric management: ■ Induction of labor (typically cervical ripening agent, amniotomy, and oxytocin) Surgical management: ■ D&E	13–24 weeks' GA (depending on state laws) Same as above	Can be a multiday procedure; delivery of an intact fetus is possible. Outpatient procedure.

■ Maternal Rh type should be determined and RhoGAM given if the type is Rh ⊖.

Elective Termination of Pregnancy

In the United States, it is estimated that 50% of all pregnancies are unintended. Twenty-five percent of pregnancies end in elective abortion. Options for elective abortion (see Table 2.11-17) depend on gestational age and patient preferences.

Gynecology

Mastitis

Cellulitis of the periglandular tissue caused by nipple trauma from breast-feeding coupled with the introduction of bacteria (often S. *aureus*) from the infant's pharynx into the nipple ducts.

The treatment of mastitis includes antibiotics and continued breast-feeding.

HISTORY/PE

Symptoms often begin 2–4 weeks postpartum. Patients complain of significant fever, chills, and malaise. Breast symptoms are **usually unilateral** and include breast tenderness, erythema, edema, warmth, and possible purulent nipple drainage.

DIAGNOSIS

Differentiate from simple breast swelling. Infection is suggested by focal symptoms, a ⊕ breast milk culture, ↑ WBC count, and fever.

TREATMENT

Continued breast-feeding to prevent the accumulation of infected material (or use of a breast pump in patients who are no longer breast-feeding) and PO penicillinase-resistant antibiotics (e.g., dicloxacillin). Incision and drainage of breast abscess if present.

Fibrocystic Change

The most common of all benign breast conditions. Involves exaggerated stromal tissue response to hormones and growth factors. Microscopic findings include cysts (gross and microscopic), papillomatosis, adenosis, fibrosis, and ductal epithelial hyperplasia. Primarily affects women 30–50 years of age; rarely found in postmenopausal woman. Associated with trauma and caffeine use.

The differential diagnosis of a breast mass includes fibrocystic disease, fibroadenoma, mastitis/abscess, fat necrosis, and breast cancer.

HISTORY/PE

- Presents with cyclic bilateral mastalgia and swelling, with symptoms most prominent just before menstruation.
- Rapid **fluctuation** in the size of the masses is common.
- Other symptoms include an irregular, bumpy consistency to the breast tissue ("oatmeal with raisins").

DIAGNOSIS

- See Figure 2.12-1 for an algorithm of a breast mass workup.
- Mammography is of limited use. Ultrasound can help differentiate a cystic from a solid mass.
- Fine-needle aspiration (FNA) of a discrete mass that is suggestive of a cyst is indicated to alleviate pain as well as to confirm the cystic nature of the mass.
    - Perform an excisional biopsy if no fluid is obtained or if the fluid is bloody on aspiration.
    - There is an ↑ risk of **breast cancer** if ductal epithelial hyperplasia or cellular atypia is present.

Intraductal papilloma is a common cause of bloody nipple discharge.

TREATMENT

- Dietary modifications (e.g., caffeine restriction).

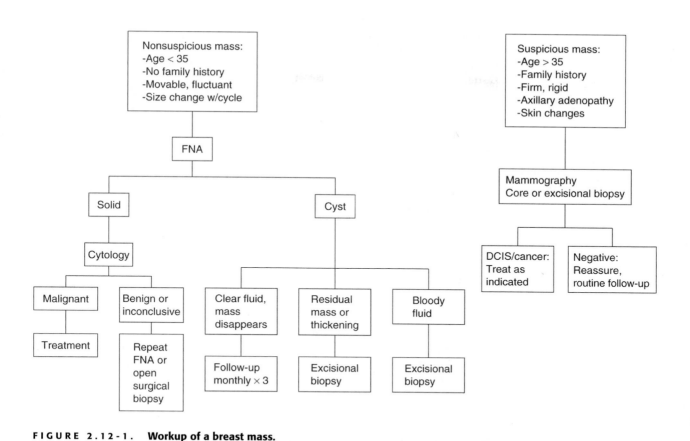

FIGURE 2.12-1.   Workup of a breast mass.

- Danazol may be given for severe pain but is rarely used owing to its side effects (acne, hirsutism, edema).
- Consider use of OCPs, which would ↓ hormonal fluctuations.

Fibroadenoma

A benign, slow-growing breast tumor with epithelial and stromal components. **The most common breast lesion in women < 30 years of age.** Cystosarcoma phyllodes is a large fibroadenoma.

HISTORY/PE

- Presents as a round or ovoid, rubbery, discrete, relatively mobile, non-tender mass 1–3 cm in diameter.
- Usually solitary, although up to 20% of patients develop multiple fibroadenomas.
- Tumors do not change during the menstrual cycle.
- Does not occur after menopause unless the patient is on HRT.

DIAGNOSIS

- **Breast ultrasound** can differentiate cystic from solid masses.
- **Needle biopsy or FNA.**
- Excision with pathologic exam if the diagnosis remains uncertain.

TREATMENT

Excision is curative, but recurrence is common.

↑ exposure to estrogen (early menarche, late menopause, nulliparity) ↑ the risk of breast cancer.

Breast cancer stages:

Stage I: Tumor size < 2 cm

Stage II: Tumor size 2–5 cm

Stage III: Axillary node involvement

Stage IV: Distant metastasis

Breast Cancer

The most common cancer (affects one in eight women) and the second most common cause of cancer death in women (after lung cancer). **Forty-five percent occur in the upper outer quadrant.** Risk factors include the following:

- Female gender, older age.
- A personal history of breast cancer.
- Breast cancer in a first-degree relative.
- BRCA1 and BRCA2 mutations (associated with early onset).
- **A high-fat and low-fiber diet.**
- A history of fibrocystic change with cellular atypia.
- **↑ exposure to estrogen (nulliparity, early menarche, late menopause).**
- First full-term pregnancy after age 35.

HISTORY/PE

Ninety percent of breast cancers are found by the patient. Clinical manifestations are as follows:

- **Early findings:** May present as a single, nontender, firm-to-hard mass with ill-defined margins or as mammographic abnormalities with no palpable mass.
- **Later findings:** Skin or nipple retraction, axillary lymphadenopathy, breast enlargement, redness, edema, pain, fixation of the mass to the skin or chest wall.
- **Late findings:**
  - Ulceration; supraclavicular lymphadenopathy; edema of the arm; metastases to the bone, lung, and liver.
  - Prolonged unilateral scaling erosion of the nipple with or without discharge (Paget's disease of the nipple).
- **Metastatic disease:**
  - Back or bone pain, jaundice, weight loss.
  - A firm or hard axillary node > 1 cm.
  - Axillary nodes that are matted or fixed to the skin (stage III); ipsilateral supraclavicular or infraclavicular nodes (stage IV).

DIAGNOSIS

Diagnostic measures are as follows (see also Figure 2.12-1):

- **Mammography:** Look for ↑ density with microcalcifications and irregular borders. Mammography can detect lesions roughly two years before they become clinically palpable.
- **Ultrasound:** To distinguish a solid mass from a benign cyst.
- **Tumor markers for recurrent breast cancer: CEA and CA 15-3 or CA 27-29.**
- **Receptor status of tumor:** Determine estrogen receptor (ER), progesterone receptor (PR), and HER2/neu status.
- **Metastatic disease:**
  - **Labs:** ↑ ESR, ↑ alkaline phosphatase (liver and bone metastases), ↑ calcium.
  - **Imaging:** CXR; CT of the chest, abdomen, pelvis, and brain; and bone scan.

TREATMENT

- **Pharmacologic:**
  - **All hormone receptor–⊕ patients should receive tamoxifen.**
  - **ER-⊖ patients should receive chemotherapy.**

- **Trastuzumab,** a monoclonal antibody that binds to HER2/neu receptors on the cancer cell, is highly effective in HER2/neu-expressive cancers.
- **Surgical options** include the following:
  - Partial mastectomy plus axillary dissection followed by radiation therapy.
  - Modified radical mastectomy (total mastectomy plus axillary dissection).
  - **Contraindications to breast-conserving therapy** include large tumor size, subareolar location, multifocal tumors, fixation to the chest wall, or involvement of the nipple or overlying skin.
- **Stage IV:** Treat with radiotherapy and hormonal therapy; mastectomy may be required for local symptom control.
- **TNM staging (I–IV) is the most reliable indicator of prognosis.**
  - ER- and PR-⊕ status is associated with a favorable course.
  - Cancer localized to the breast has a 75–90% cure rate. With spread to the axilla, the five-year survival is 40–50%.
  - Aneuploidy is associated with a poor prognosis.

COMPLICATIONS

Pleural effusion occurs in 50% of patients with metastatic breast cancer; edema of the arm is common.

CONTRACEPTION

- The relative advantages and disadvantages of common contraceptive methods are outlined in Table 2.12-1.
- **Absolute contraindications to OCPs** are as follows:
  - Pregnancy.
  - A history of stroke, CAD, or DVT.
  - Breast cancer.
  - Undiagnosed abnormal vaginal bleeding.
  - Estrogen-dependent cancer.
  - A benign or malignant tumor of the liver.
  - Cigarette smoking and age > 35.
- **Absolute contraindications to IUD use** include the following:
  - Pregnancy.
  - A history of PID.
  - Acute cervical, uterine, or salpingeal infection.
  - Suspected gynecologic malignancy.
  - Undiagnosed abnormal vaginal bleeding.
  - More than one sexual partner.
  - Prior ectopic pregnancy.

ABNORMALITIES OF THE MENSTRUAL CYCLE

Amenorrhea

May be 1° or 2°. Menarche typically occurs between 11 and 15 years of age. Etiologies are outlined in Table 2.12-2.

HISTORY/PE

- **1° amenorrhea:** No menses by age 16 with 2° sexual development present; no sexual characteristics by age 14.
- **2° amenorrhea:** Absence of menses for six consecutive months in women who have passed menarche.

TABLE 2.12-1. **Contraceptive Methods**

METHOD	DESCRIPTION/ADVANTAGES	DISADVANTAGES
Behavioral methods		
Rhythm	Uses body temperature and cervical mucus consistency to predict time of fertility.	Unreliable compared to other methods.
Coitus interruptus	Withdrawal of the penis before ejaculation.	High failure rate.
Barrier methods		
Diaphragm/cervical cap	A dome-shaped sheet of rubber or latex placed over the cervix after contraceptive jelly or a cream that contains spermicide has been applied to the device. Must be fitted by a physician and remain in the vagina 6–8 hours after intercourse.	Possible allergy to latex or spermicides; risk of UTI and toxic shock syndrome (TSS).
Condoms	A latex sheath covers the penis or the vagina and cervix during intercourse.	Possible allergy to latex or spermicides.
Intrauterine devices (IUDs)		
Copper-releasing (ParaGard)	Renders the intrauterine environment hostile via a foreign-body inflammatory response. Copper enhances the inflammatory response and exerts a spermicidal effect on cervical mucus. Has up to a 10-year life span.	Increased vaginal bleeding and menstrual pain in 5–10% of users; uterine perforation; risk of insertional infection. Contraindicated for women with multiple sex partners.
Progesterone-releasing (Mirena)	Renders the intrauterine environment hostile via a foreign-body inflammatory response. Progesterone enhances contraception via thickening of the cervical mucus and decidualization of the endometrium. Has at least a five-year life span.	Uterine perforation; risk of insertional infection. Contraindicated for women with multiple sex partners.
Hormonal methods		
OCPs (combination estrogen and progestin)	Suppress ovulation by inhibiting FSH/LH; change the consistency of cervical mucus, making the endometrium unsuitable for implantation. Highly reliable, with a failure rate of < 1% if used properly. Protect against endometrial and ovarian cancer; associated with a ↓ incidence of pelvic infections and ectopic pregnancy. Menses are more predictable, lighter, and less painful.	Require daily compliance; no STD protection; 10–30% have breakthrough bleeding; ↑ risk of thromboembolism (pulmonary embolism, DVT). Side effects of estrogen include bloating, weight gain, breast tenderness, nausea, and headache. Side effects of progestin include depression, acne, and hypertensive crisis.
Progestin-only "minipills"	Act primarily by thickening cervical mucus and making the endometrium hostile to implantation. Lactating women can start immediately postpartum.	Higher failure rate than OCPs (ovulation continues in 40%); require strict compliance (taking pill at the same time each day).

TABLE 2.12-1.   Contraceptive Methods (continued)

METHOD	DESCRIPTION/ADVANTAGES	DISADVANTAGES
Hormonal methods (continued)		
Depo-Provera (medroxyprogesterone)	IM injection every three months for a maximum of two years. Eliminates noncompliance with daily OCPs; can be used by lactating women.	Irregular vaginal bleeding; reversible decreases in bone mineral density (of concern in patients at risk for osteoporosis); 50% of patients are infertile for 10 months after last injection.
Postcoital "morning-after pill"	Progesterone +/− estrogen taken within 72 hours of unprotected sex to suppress ovulation or inhibit implantation.	Nausea, vomiting, fatigue, headache, dizziness, breast tenderness.
Surgical sterilization		
Tubal litigation, vasectomy, Essure	Tubes are ligated, cauterized, or mechanically occluded.	Essentially irreversible; associated with bleeding, infection, failure, and ectopic pregnancy.

TABLE 2.12-2.   Causes of Amenorrhea

CAUSE/LABS	1° AMENORRHEA	2° AMENORRHEA
Anatomic abnormalities		
Normal FSH	Müllerian anomalies, vaginal agenesis, imperforate hymen.	Asherman's syndrome,[a] cervical stenosis.
↑ LH	Testicular feminization.	
Ovarian or uterine dysfunction		
↑ FSH	Ovarian failure, gonadotropin-resistant ovary syndrome (Savage's syndrome), gonadal dysgenesis (Turner's syndrome, X-chromosome long-arm deletion).	Premature ovarian failure; 1° hypogonadism before age 40; menopause; chemotherapy with alkylating agents.
↓ or normal FSH	Steroidogenic enzyme defects, constitutional developmental delay.	PCOS.
↑ β-hCG		Pregnancy.
Central regulatory disorders		
↓ or normal FSH	Hypothalamic dysfunction (Kallmann's syndrome, anorexia, excess exercise, weight loss, stress, tumor, infection); 1° pituitary dysfunction (rate).	Hypothalamic dysfunction (anorexia, excess exercise, weight loss, stress); pituitary dysfunction (Sheehan's syndrome, neoplasms, panhypopituitarism); hyperprolactinemia (prolactinoma, hypothyroidism).

[a] Asherman's syndrome is associated with endometritis, scarring after delivery, or D&C. It is the most common anatomic cause of amenorrhea.

HIGH-YIELD FACTS

GYNECOLOGY

DIAGNOSIS

Workup is as follows (see also Figures 2.12-2 and 2.12-3):

- **Pregnancy test: Pregnancy is the most common cause of 2° amenorrhea.**
- Ultrasound to determine the presence of the uterus. If the uterus is absent, consider karyotyping.
- If β-hCG is ⊖:
    - Obtain FSH, LH, prolactin, TSH, and free T_4.
        - ↑ FSH indicates ovarian failure.
        - ↑ prolactin (which inhibits the release of LH and FSH) points to thyroid pathology. Order an MRI of the pituitary to rule out tumor.
        - ↑↑ prolactin points to a prolactin-secreting pituitary adenoma.
    - Obtain potassium, creatinine, and liver enzymes.
    - Assess testosterone levels (in hirsute or virilized women). If testosterone is ↑, rule out hyperandrogenism and adrenal hyperplasia, PCOS, and ovarian tumor.
    - Conduct a 1-mg overnight dexamethasone suppression test to look for signs of hypercortisolism.
    - Obtain a Pap smear and vaginal smear to assess estrogen effect.
- **Progestin withdrawal test:** In nonpregnant women with a normal pelvic exam and normal labs, give a 10-day course of progestin.
    - Absence of withdrawal menses points to a possible pregnancy, uterine abnormality, or estrogen deficiency.

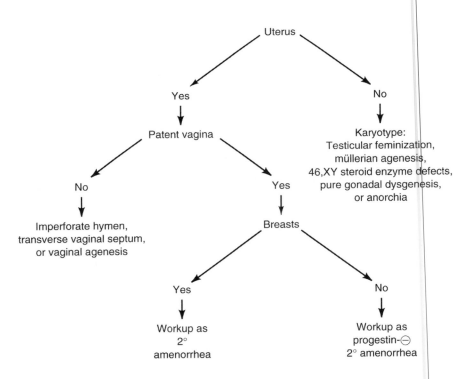

FIGURE 2.12-2. **Workup for patients with 1° amenorrhea.**

(Reproduced, with permission, from DeCherney AH. *Current Obstetric & Gynecologic Diagnosis & Treatment*, 8th ed. Stamford, CT: Appleton & Lange, 1994, p. 1010.)

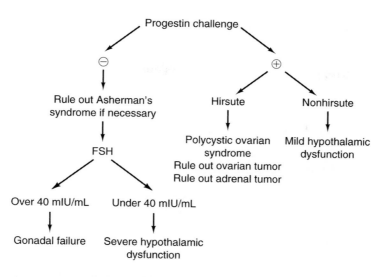

FIGURE 2.12-3. Workup for patients with 2° amenorrhea without hyperprolactinemia.

(Reproduced, with permission, from DeCherney AH. *Current Obstetric & Gynecologic Diagnosis & Treatment*, 8th ed. Stamford, CT: Appleton & Lange, 1994, p. 1012.)

- Occurrence of withdrawal bleeding indicates anovulation that is likely due to noncyclic gonadotropin secretion, pointing to PCOS or idiopathic anovulation.

TREATMENT

- **Hypothalamic:** Reverse the underlying cause and induce ovulation with gonadotropins.
- **Tumors:** Excision; medical therapy for prolactinomas (e.g., bromocriptine, cabergoline).
- **Premature ovarian failure (age < 40 years):**
  - **Uterus present:** Estrogen + progestin replacement therapy.
  - **Uterus absent:** Estrogen replacement therapy.

1° Dysmenorrhea

- Menstrual pain associated with ovulatory cycles in the **absence of pathologic findings.** Caused by uterine vasoconstriction, anoxia, and sustained contractions mediated by an excess of prostaglandin ($PGF_2\alpha$). Onset is within 1–2 years of menarche; may become more severe with time. The frequency of cases ↑ up to age 20 and then ↓ with age.
- **Hx/PE:**
  - Presents with low, midline, spasmodic, colicky pelvic pain that often radiates to the back or inner thighs.
  - Cramps occur in the first 1–3 days of menstruation and may be associated with nausea, diarrhea, headache, and flushing.
  - **No pathologic findings on pelvic exam.**
- **Dx:** A diagnosis of exclusion. 2° dysmenorrhea must be ruled out.
- **Tx:** NSAIDs; topical heat therapy; combined OCPs.

2° Dysmenorrhea

- Menstrual pain for which an organic cause exists. Common causes include endometriosis and adenomyosis, tumors, fibroids, adhesions, polyps, and PID.
- **Hx/PE:** Although symptoms are more noticeable during menstruation, symptoms that continue between menstrual periods strongly suggest a 1° source of pain. Onset is after menarche, sometimes in the 30–40s.
- **Tx:** Treatment is etiology specific.

Abnormal Uterine Bleeding

Normal menstrual bleeding lasts an average of four days (range is 2–7 days) and → a mean blood loss of 40 mL.

History/PE

- Vaginal bleeding that occurs **six or more months** following the cessation of menstrual function is **cancer-related** until proven otherwise.
- Assess the duration and amount of flow, related pain, and relationship to last menstrual period.
- Look for clots and assess the degree of inconvenience caused by the bleeding.
- Assess the extent of the bleeding:
    - **Menorrhagia:** ↑ amount of flow (> 80 mL of blood loss per cycle) or prolonged bleeding (flow lasting > 8 days); may → anemia.
    - **Oligomenorrhea:** ↑ length of time between menses (35–90 days between cycles).
    - **Polymenorrhea:** Frequent menstruation (< 21-day cycle); anovular.
    - **Metrorrhagia:** Bleeding between periods.
    - **Menometrorrhagia:** Excessive and irregular bleeding.
- Assess the nature of the bleeding:
    - **Anovulatory bleeding:** Dysfunctional uterine bleeding; overgrowth of endometrium due to estrogen stimulation without adequate progesterone to stabilize growth.
    - **Ovulation bleeding:** A single episode of spotting between regular menses (common).
- **Pelvic exam:** Look for pregnancy, uterine myomas, adnexal masses, or infections.

Diagnosis

- **Labs:** β-hCG, CBC, ESR.
- If bleeding is **ovulatory** (associated with regular menses), further workup is indicated to rule out pathology.
    - Obtain platelet count, bleeding time, and PT/PTT.
    - Check for cervical masses and polyps.
    - Perform a D&C or hysteroscopy and obtain a biopsy if necessary.
- If bleeding is **anovulatory** (irregular, excessive bleeding with no organic causes):
    - Obtain cervical smears as needed for cytologic and culture studies.
    - Order TFTs.
    - **Ultrasound:** Evaluate endometrial thickness; look for intrauterine or ectopic pregnancy or adnexal masses. If thickness is **> 4 mm in a postmenopausal woman,** perform endocervical curettage and endometrial aspiration.
    - Endometrial biopsy (age > 35 years, obese, PCOS) to rule out hyperplasia.

Pregnancy is the most common cause of abnormal uterine bleeding and amenorrhea. Always check a pregnancy test!

- **Anovulatory bleeding:** Give progestins (medroxyprogesterone acetate or norethindrone × 14 days) to stimulate withdrawal bleeding (to convert proliferative endometrium to secretory endometrium).
- **Heavy bleeding:**
  - Estrogen 25 mg IV q 6 h × 4 doses stabilizes the endometrial lining and stops bleeding within one hour.
  - Danazol for intractable bleeding.
  - GnRH agonists (leuprolide or nafarelin).
  - OCPs if the patient is hemodynamically stable to thicken the endometrium and control the bleeding.
- **Ovulatory bleeding:**
  - NSAIDs to ↓ blood loss.
  - Prolonged use of progestin can → intermittent bleeding.

COMPLICATIONS

Anemia; endometrial hyperplasia +/– carcinoma.

Endometriosis and Adenomyosis

An aberrant growth of endometrium outside the uterus, particularly in the dependent parts of the pelvis and ovaries. Has a 2% prevalence among fertile women. Adenomyosis is endometrial tissue in the myometrium that makes the uterus symmetrically enlarged and globular.

HISTORY/PE

- Pain does not correlate with the extent of disease.
- Cyclic pain begins 2–7 days before the onset of menses and becomes increasingly severe until flow slackens.
- **2° dysmenorrhea** occurs twice as often in women with endometriosis.
- May present with **dyspareunia** (painful intercourse), infertility, intermenstrual bleeding, pelvic pain, and rectal pain with bleeding.
- **Pelvic exam:**
  - Tenderness is best detected at the time of menses.
  - Nodularity of the uterosacral ligaments and cul-de-sac may be found.
  - The uterus may be fixed and retroverted due to adhesions.

DIAGNOSIS

- Establishing the diagnosis requires direct visualization by laparoscopy or, on occasion, laparotomy.
- Classic lesions have a **blue-black ("raspberry") or dark brown ("powder-burned") appearance.** Ovaries may have endometriomas, the characteristic "chocolate cyst."

TREATMENT

- Depends on the extent and location of disease as well as on symptom severity and the desire for future fertility.
- **Pharmacologic: Inhibit ovulation** for 4–9 months to prevent cyclic stimulation of endometrial implants. Options are as follows:
  - **GnRH analogs:** Nafarelin or leuprolide.

- **Danazol:** Suppresses menstruation by inhibiting midcycle FSH and LH surges.
        - Combination OCPs.
    - **Surgery** is indicated for moderate to extensive endometriosis.
        - **Conservative:** Excision, cauterization, or ablation of the lesions and lysis of adhesions. Some 20% of patients can become pregnant.
        - **Extirpative:** For patients finished with reproduction and for those disabled by pain refractory to other forms of conservative therapy, TAH/BSO plus lysis of adhesions may be necessary.

ENDOCRINOLOGY

Late-Onset Congenital Adrenal Hyperplasia

A 21-hydroxylase deficiency that can present in its most severe, classic form as a newly born female infant with ambiguous genitalia and life-threatening salt wasting. Milder forms present later in life. (11β-hydroxylase is a less common cause of adrenal hyperplasia.)

Hypertrichosis is excessive nonsexual hair; the etiology may be drug related or hereditary.

HISTORY/PE

Presents with excessive hirsutism (terminal body hair in a male pattern of distribution) as well as with acne, amenorrhea and/or abnormal uterine bleeding, and infertility.

DIAGNOSIS

- ↑ **androgens** (testosterone > 2 ng; DHEAS > 7 µg/mL): Rule out adrenal or ovarian neoplasm.
    - ↑ **serum testosterone:** Suspect an ovarian tumor.
    - ↑ **DHEAS:** Suspect an adrenal source (adrenal tumor, Cushing's syndrome, congenital adrenal hyperplasia).
- ↑ 17-OH progesterone levels (either basally or in response to ACTH stimulation).
- See Table 2.12-3 for further diagnostic measures.

TREATMENT

Supplemental glucocorticoids (e.g., prednisone). Medical therapy for adrenal and ovarian disorders prevents new terminal hair growth but does not resolve

TABLE 2.12-3. Workup of Hirsutism and Virilization

TESTOSTERONE	DHEAS	DISEASE	WORKUP
> 200 ng/dL	Normal	Ovarian neoplasm.	Adrenal CT, pelvic ultrasound.
Variable	> 7 µg/mL	Adrenal tumor, Cushing's syndrome.	Adrenal CT, dexamethasone suppression test.
> 70 ng/dL	↑ but < 7 µg/mL	PCOS, late-onset adrenal hyperplasia, Cushing's syndrome.	No further workup; rule out congenital adrenal hyperplasia and Cushing's syndrome.
Normal	Normal	↓ end-organ sensitivity.	Free testosterone, androstenediol glucuronide.

hirsutism. Laser ablation, electrolysis, or conventional hair removal techniques must be used to remove unwanted hair.

Polycystic Ovarian Syndrome (PCOS)

Hyperandrogenism and chronic anovulation in cases where 2° causes have been excluded. One of the most common endocrine disorders in reproductive woman; also known as Stein-Leventhal syndrome. The etiology is thought to be selective insulin resistance. Compensatory hyperinsulinemia → ↑ sex hormone–binding globulin (SHBG) and acts as a trophic stimulus to the adrenals and ovaries.

HISTORY/PE

- Presents with **hirsutism** (40–50%), obesity (40%), and virilization (20%).
- Amenorrhea and/or abnormal uterine bleeding is frequently seen.
- **Infertility** is common.
- Acanthosis nigricans may be present.
- **HAIR-AN syndrome** is a variant of PCOS that → hyperandrogenism, insulin resistance, and acanthosis nigricans.

DIAGNOSIS

- **Labs:**
  - ↑ **LH/FSH ratio** (> 2:1).
  - ↑ **testosterone** (total +/– free).
  - ↑ androstenedione, ↑ DHEAS, ↓ glucose/insulin ratio.
- **Ultrasound:** Polycystic ovaries typically show multiple, 2- to 8-mm, subcapsular preantral follicles forming a black **"pearl necklace" sign** (see Figure 2.12-4).
- All women with PCOS should be screened for glucose intolerance (with a two-hour glucose level after a 75-g fasting glucose challenge) and for dyslipidemia.

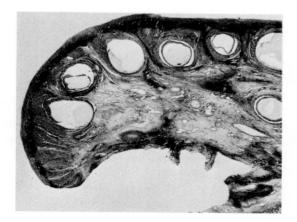

FIGURE 2.12-4. Polycystic ovary with prominent multiple cysts.

(Reproduced, with permission, from DeCherney AH. *Current Obstetric & Gynecologic Diagnosis & Treatment*, 8th ed. Stamford, CT: Appleton & Lange, 1994, p. 747.)

TREATMENT

- **Maintenance:** Combination OCPs, progestin, insulin-sensitizing agents.
- **Hirsutism:** Antiandrogens.
- **Infertility:**
  - Clomiphene +/– dexamethasone or other drugs for ovulatory stimulation (80% of women with PCOS will ovulate with clomiphene and 50% will become pregnant).
  - If clomiphene fails, metformin, thiazolidinediones, and gonadotropin therapy may be tried.
  - If the above treatment fails, IVF may be tried.
- OCP or progestin to ↓ the risk of endometrial hyperplasia/carcinoma.
- Address cardiovascular risk factors and lipid levels.
- Diet, weight loss, and exercise are important for diabetes and cardiovascular disease control.

COMPLICATIONS

↑ risk of early-onset type 2 DM; ↑ long-term risk of breast and endometrial cancer owing to unopposed estrogen secretion.

Menopause

Cessation of menses for a minimum of 12 months due to cessation of follicular development. Average age of onset is 51. "Premature menopause" is ovarian failure and menstrual cessation before age 40.

HISTORY/PE

- See the mnemonic HAVOC.
- Other symptoms include insomnia, anxiety/irritability, vaginal bleeding, poor concentration, mood changes, dyspareunia, and loss of libido.

Menopause wreaks HAVOC:

Hot flashes (vasomotor instability)
Atrophy of the
Vagina
Osteoporosis
Coronary artery disease

DIAGNOSIS

- ↑ FSH and ↑ LH.
- Vaginal cytologic exam shows low estrogen effect with parabasal cells.
- DEXA scan for osteoporosis.
- Lipid profile (↑ total cholesterol, ↓ HDL).

TREATMENT

- **Vasomotor symptoms:**
  - HRT; combination estrogen and progestin.
  - Posthysterectomy patients do not need progestin.
  - Clinicians should review the risks and benefits of HRT with their patients. Long-term HRT for symptom prevention is no longer indicated.
  - Contraindications to HRT include vaginal bleeding, suspected or known breast cancer, endometrial cancer, a history of thromboembolism, chronic liver disease, and hypertriglyceridemia.
  - Venlafaxine and, less commonly, clonidine to ↓ the frequency of hot flashes.
- **Vaginal atrophy:**
  - **Long term:** Estradiol vaginal ring.
  - **Short term:** Estrogen vaginal cream will relieve symptoms.
- **Osteoporosis:** Daily calcium supplementation and exercise, and possible need for bisphosphonates.

TABLE 2.12-4. Infertility Workup

	MALE	**FEMALE**
History/PE	Testicular injury or infection. Medications (steroids, cimetidine, spironolactone). Thyroid or liver disease → abnormalities of spermatogenesis. Signs of hypogonadism, ⊕ varicocele on physical exam.	Age (incidence ↑ with age). Previous STDs. Abortions, pregnancies, and menstrual cycle characteristics (length, duration, premenstrual symptoms).
Diagnosis	Semen analysis: ↓ sperm count and motility (accounts for **40% of infertility cases**). ↑ FSH, ↑ LH, ↓ testosterone = 1° testicular failure (hypergonadotropic hypogonadism). ↓ FSH, ↓ LH, ↓ testosterone = 2° testicular failure (hypogonadotropic hypogonadism). Check prolactin.	**Basal body temperature** to evaluate ovulation (↓ temperature at time of menses, then an ↑ two days after LH surge at the time of progesterone rise). Hysterosalpingogram, endometrial biopsy, postcoital test, antisperm antibodies, luteal progesterone levels, urinary LH levels.
Treatment	Intrauterine insemination, donor insemination, IVF, ICSI.	Induction of ovulation with **clomiphene;** tubal or uterine surgery; GnRH analogs (for fibroids and endometriosis); IVF, ICSI.

COMPLICATIONS

Dyspareunia from vaginal atrophy and ↓ vaginal lubrication.

Infertility

- Etiologies include abnormal spermatogenesis (40%), anovulation (30%), and female anatomic defects (20%). Ten percent of cases are of unknown etiology.
- Defined as inability to conceive after 12 months of normal, regular, unprotected sexual activity (see Table 2.12-4).

GYNECOLOGIC INFECTIONS

External Anogenital Lesions

Table 2.12-5 outlines the clinical presentation, diagnosis, and treatment of common external anogenital lesions.

Vaginitis

A spectrum of conditions that cause vulvovaginal symptoms such as itching, burning, irritation, and abnormal discharge. The most common causes are bacterial vaginosis, vulvovaginal candidiasis, and trichomoniasis (see Table 2.12-6). Lactobacilli are the predominant bacteria in the vaginal tract and produce lactic acid that maintains the normal vaginal pH of 3.8–4.5 and inhibits the adherence of other bacteria to the vaginal wall. Estrogen improves the colonization of lactobacilli by enhancing vaginal epithelial cell production of glycogen, which acts as a substrate for the lactobacilli. Other bacteria present in the vagina include streptococcal species, gram-negative bacteria, *Gardnerella vaginalis*, and anaerobes.

Table 2.12-5. External Anogenital Lesions

DISEASE/LESION	PRESENTATION	PATHOGEN	DIAGNOSIS	TREATMENT
Syphilis	■ **1° (10–60 days postexposure):** Presents with a chancre—a painless red ulcer roughly 1 cm in diameter with raised edges. ■ **2° (4–8 weeks after appearance of chancre):** Maculopapular rash (palms and soles); condylomata lata. ■ **3° (1–10 years after infection):** Granulomas (gummas) of the skin and bones, aortitis, neurosyphilis with meningovascular disease, paresis, and tabes dorsalis.	*Treponema pallidum*	Usually diagnosed by serologic testing (RPR or VDRL).	Penicillin G. Alternatives for 1° and 2° syphilis include tetracycline and doxycycline. There are no alternatives for 3° syphilis; patients with penicillin allergies are desensitized.
Herpes genitalis	■ **1 °infection:** Presents with malaise, myalgias, and fever with vulvar burning/pruritus (2–5 days postexposure) followed by vesicular genital lesions (3–7 days postexposure) that progress to shallow, painful ulcers with a red border. ■ **Recurrent infections (occur in 30% of patients):** Similar in nature to 1° infection, but lesions are generally milder in severity and shorter in duration.	HSV-2 (85% of genital infections), HSV-1.	**Tzanck smear** shows the presence of multinucleated giant cells with eosinophilic inclusions. Viral culture is the most sensitive method.	Sitz baths followed by drying with a heat lamp or a hair dryer. Acyclovir, famciclovir, or valacyclovir for 1° infection or for suppressive treatment if frequent recurrences (usually > 6 episodes).
Chancroid	Painful, nonindurated, purulent, hemorrhagic ulcer(s) with painful inguinal lymphadenopathy.	*Haemophilus ducreyi*	A diagnosis of exclusion; culture is difficult.	Ceftriaxone, azithromycin, erythromycin, ciprofloxacin.
Lymphogranuloma venereum	■ **1°:** Presents with a painless, transient papule or shallow ulcer that can often go unnoticed. ■ **2°:** Presents as "inguinal syndrome"—painful enlargement and inflammation of the inguinal nodes with fever, malaise, headache, and loss of appetite. ■ **3°:** Presents as "anogenital syndrome"—anal pruritus with discharge, proctocolitis, rectal stricture, rectovaginal fistula, and elephantiasis.	L-serotype *Chlamydia trachomatis*	Clinical.	Doxycycline 100 mg BID × 21 days.

Table 2.12-5.   **External Anogenital Lesions**

DISEASE/LESION	PRESENTATION	PATHOGEN	DIAGNOSIS	TREATMENT
Granuloma inguinale	Raised, firm red lesions.	*Calymmato-bacterium granulomatis*	Clinical, smears.	Doxycycline, TMP-SMX, or ciprofloxacin (for a minimum of 21 days).
Condylomata acuminata (genital warts)	Raised cauliflower-like lesions that are especially prevalent in immunocompromised patient populations.	HPV (primarily HPV 6 and HPV 11)	Usually clinical. Biopsy is definitive.	**Surgical:** Local excision, cryosurgery, laser removal. **Chemical:** TCA, podophyllin, 5-FU, podofilox. **Immunologic:** Imiquimod.
Molluscum contagiosum	Small, domed papules with an umbilicated, waxy core.	Poxviridae	Microscopic examination with Wright or Giemsa stain.	Desiccation, cryotherapy, curettage, imiquimod.

HISTORY/PE

- Determine the entire spectrum of vaginal symptoms, including change in discharge, malodor, pruritus, irritation, burning, swelling, dyspareunia, and dysuria.
- Normal secretions are as follows:
  - **Midcycle estrogen surge:** Clear, elastic, mucoid secretions.
  - **Luteal phase/pregnancy:** Thick and white; adhere to the vaginal wall.
- Conduct a thorough examination of the vulva, vaginal walls, and cervix.

DIAGNOSIS

- Samples from the speculum exam should be obtained for vaginal pH, amine ("whiff") test, wet mount (with saline), and 10% hydroxide (KOH) microscopy.
- In selected patients, vaginal cultures for *Trichomonas* or yeast can be helpful. A vaginal Gram stain for Nugent scoring of bacteria may be used to identify patients with bacterial vaginosis.
- To rule out cervicitis, DNA tests or cultures for *Neisseria gonorrhoeae* or *Chlamydia trachomatis* should be obtained in patients with a purulent discharge, numerous leukocytes on wet prep, cervical friability, and any symptoms of PID.

*Three out of four **Amsel's criteria** are required for the clinical diagnosis of bacterial vaginosis:*

- *Abnormal **whitish-gray discharge***
- *Vaginal **pH > 4.5***
- *Positive **amine ("whiff") test***
- ***Clue cells** comprise > 20% of epithelial cells on wet mount*

Cervicitis

- **Inflammation of the uterine cervix.** Because the female genital tract is contiguous from the vulva to the fallopian tubes, there is some overlap between vulvovaginitis and cervicitis. Etiologies are as follows:
  - **Infectious (most common):** *Chlamydia*, gonococcus, *Trichomonas*, HSV, HPV.
  - **Noninfectious:** Trauma, radiation exposure, malignancy.
- Hx/PE: Yellow-green mucopurulent discharge; ⊕ **cervical motion tenderness; absence of other signs of PID.**
- Dx/Tx: See the discussion of STDs.

Pelvic Inflammatory Disease (PID)

A polymicrobial infection of the **upper genital tract** associated with *Neisseria gonorrhoeae* (one-third of cases), *Chlamydia trachomatis* (one-third of cases),

TABLE 2.12-6. **Causes of Vaginitis**

	BACTERIAL VAGINOSIS	TRICHOMONAS	YEAST
Incidence	15–50% (most common).	5–50%.	15–30%.
Etiology	**Not an STI.** Reflects a shift in vaginal flora.	**An STI.** Protozoal flagellates affect the vagina, Skene's duct, and lower urinary tract as well as the lower GU tract in men.	Usually *Candida albicans*.
Risk factors	Pregnancy, > 1 sexual partner, female sexual partner, frequent douching.	Another STI. Risk factors include unprotected sex with multiple partners.	**DM, broad-spectrum antibiotic use, pregnancy, steroids,** HIV, OCP use, IUD use, young age at first intercourse, ↑ frequency of intercourse.
History	Odor, ↑ discharge.	↑ discharge, odor, pruritus, dysuria.	Pruritus, dysuria, burning, ↑ discharge.
Exam	Mild vulvar irritation.	"Strawberry petechiae" in the upper vagina/cervix (rare).	Erythematous, excoriated vulva/vagina.
Discharge	Homogenous, **grayish-white, fishy**/stale odor.	Profuse, malodorous, **yellow-green, frothy.**	Thick, white, curdy texture without odor.
Vaginal pH	> 4.5 (5.0–6.0).	> 4.5 (5.0–7.0).	Normal (~4.0).
Wet mount[a]	**"Clue cells"** (epithelial cells coated with bacteria; see Figure 2.12-5); shift in vaginal flora (↑ cocci, ↓ lactobacilli).	**Motile trichomonads** (flagellated organisms that are slightly larger than WBCs).	—
KOH prep	⊕ whiff test (fishy smell).	—	Hyphae (see Figure 2.12-5).
Treatment	PO metronidazole or PO clindamycin × 7 days. Vaginal metronidazole × 5 days or vaginal clindamycin × 7 days.	Single-dose PO metronidazole or tinidazole. Treat partners, avoid intercourse until partners have been treated, and test for other STDs.	**Uncomplicated:** Topical azole × 1–3 days or single-dose PO fluconazole. **Complicated** (≥ 4 episodes in one year, noncandidal, HIV, DM, immunocompromised, pregnancy): 7–14 days of topical antifungals or fluconazole × 2 doses, 72 hours apart. Treat azole-resistant cases with boric acid capsules QD x 2 weeks.

TABLE 2.12-6. **Causes of Vaginitis (continued)**

	BACTERIAL VAGINOSIS	TRICHOMONAS	YEAST
Complications	Chorioamnionitis/endometritis, infection, preterm delivery, miscarriage, PID, cellulitis when invasive procedures are done (e.g., biopsy, C-section, IUD placement, vaginal or abdominal hysterectomy).	Same as for bacterial vaginosis.	Oral azoles should be avoided in pregnancy.

ᵃ If there are many WBCs and no organism on saline smear, suspect *Chlamydia*.

and endogenous aerobes/anaerobes. The lifetime risk is 1–3%. Risk factors include non-Caucasian ethnicity, douching, smoking, and prior PID. A ↓ risk is associated with the use of OCPs or barrier methods. Occurs most often in young, nulliparous, sexually active women with multiple sex partners.

HISTORY/PE

- Presents with lower abdominal pain, **fever** and chills, menstrual disturbances, and a purulent cervical discharge.
- **Cervical motion (chandelier sign) and adnexal tenderness** are also seen.
- RUQ pain may indicate perihepatitis (Fitz-Hugh–Curtis syndrome).

DIAGNOSIS

- Diagnosis is complicated by the fact that many women have mild symptoms that are not readily recognized as PID.
- Labs show WBC > 10,000, ↑ ESR (> 15 mm/hr), and ↑ CRP.
- Cervical or vaginal discharge with WBCs on saline microscopy.
- Obtain an endocervical culture for *N. gonorrhoeae* and *C. trachomatis*.
- Order a β-hCG and ultrasound to rule out pregnancy and to evaluate the possibility of tubo-ovarian abscess.

The chandelier sign is defined as severe cervical motion tenderness that makes the patient "jump for the chandelier" on exam.

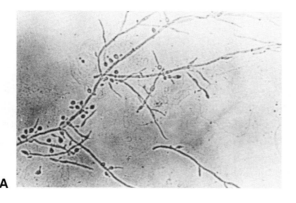
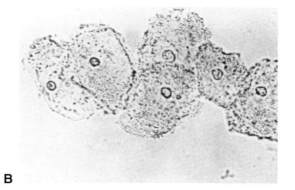

FIGURE 2.12-5. **Causes of vaginitis.**

(A) Candidal vaginitis. Branched and budding *Candida albicans* organisms are evident on KOH preparation of vaginal discharge. (B) *Gardnerella vaginalis*. Saline wet mount of vaginal fluid reveals granulations on vaginal epithelial cells ("clue cells") due to adherence of *G. vaginalis* organisms to the cell surface. (Reproduced, with permission, from DeCherney AH. *Current Obstetric & Gynecologic Diagnosis & Treatment*, 8th ed. Stamford, CT: Appleton & Lange, 1994, p. 692.)

TREATMENT

- **Antibiotic treatment should not be delayed** while awaiting culture results. All sexual partners should be examined and treated appropriately.
- **Outpatient antibiotic regimens** are as follows:
  - **Regimen A:** Cefoxitin with probenecid × 1 dose.
  - **Regimen B:** Ceftriaxone IM × 1 dose + doxycycline × 14 days.
  - **Regimen C:** Ofloxacin × 14 days + metronidazole × 14 days.
- **Admit the following for IV antibiotics:**
  - Patients in whom surgical emergencies such as appendicitis cannot be ruled out.
  - Those with tubo-ovarian abscess (admit for at least 24 hours before switching to outpatient).
  - Pregnant patients.
  - Patients who are unable to follow or tolerate an outpatient regimen.
  - Those who have failed to respond clinically to outpatient therapy.
  - Those with severe illness, nausea/vomiting, or high fever.
  - Immunodeficient patients (HIV-⊕ patients with low CD4 counts or those who are taking immunosuppressant drugs).
- **Inpatient antibiotic regimens:**
  - Cefoxitin or cefotetan + doxycycline × 14 days.
  - Clindamycin + gentamicin × 14 days.
- **Surgery:**
  - Tubo-ovarian abscess may require surgical excision (30% of cases) or transcutaneous/transvaginal aspiration. Unilateral salpingo-oophorectomy is acceptable for unilateral abscess.
  - Hysterectomy and BSO may be necessary for overwhelming infection or in cases of chronic disease with intractable pelvic pain.

COMPLICATIONS

- Some 25% of women with acute disease develop repeated episodes of infection, chronic pelvic pain, dyspareunia, **ectopic pregnancy,** or **infertility.**
- RUQ pain (Fitz-Hugh–Curtis syndrome) may indicate an associated perihepatitis (abnormal liver function, shoulder pain).
- The risk of infertility ↑ with repeated episodes of salpingitis and is estimated to approach 10% after the first episode, 25% after the second episode, and 50% after a third episode.

Toxic Shock Syndrome (TSS)

An acute illness caused by preformed *S. aureus* toxin (TSST-1) that can → scalded skin syndrome, bullous impetigo, necrotizing pneumonitis, and enterotoxin food poisoning. **More than 90% of patients are women of childbearing age;** often occurs within five days of the onset of a menstrual period in women who have used **tampons.** Nonmenstrual cases are nearly as common as menstrual cases; organisms from the nasopharynx, bones, vagina, rectum, and wounds have all been associated with the illness.

HISTORY/PE

- Presents with **abrupt onset of fever, vomiting,** and watery diarrhea.
- A **diffuse macular erythematous rash** is also seen.
- Nonpurulent conjunctivitis is common.
- **Desquamation, especially of the palms and soles,** generally occurs during recovery within 1–2 weeks of illness.

DIAGNOSIS

Blood cultures are ⊖ because symptoms result from preformed toxin and are not due to the invasive properties of the organism.

TREATMENT

- Rapid rehydration; removal of sources of toxin (e.g., removal of tampons, drainage of abscess).
- Antistaphylococcal drugs (nafcillin, oxacillin); management of renal or cardiac failure.

GYNECOLOGIC NEOPLASMS

The most common gynecologic cancers are endometrial, ovarian (carries the highest mortality), cervical, and vulvar. Table 2.12-7 outlines common findings associated with endometrial, cervical, vulvar, and ovarian cancers.

Uterine Leiomyoma (Fibroids)

The most common **benign** neoplasm of the female genital tract. The tumor is discrete, round, firm, and often multiple. It is composed of smooth muscle and connective tissue that is hormonally responsive; its size often ↑ in pregnancy and ↓ after menopause. Malignant transformation to **leiomyosarcoma is rare (0.1–0.5%).**

HISTORY/PE

- The majority of patients are asymptomatic.
- Symptomatic patients may present with the following:
    - **Bleeding:** Longer, heavier periods; anemia.
    - **Pressure:** Pelvic pressure and bloating; constipation and rectal pressure; urinary frequency or retention.
    - **Pain:** 2° dysmenorrhea, dyspareunia.
    - **Pelvic symptoms:** A firm, nontender, irregular enlarged ("lumpy-bumpy"), or cobblestone uterus may be seen.

DIAGNOSIS

- **CBC:** To look for anemia.
- **Ultrasound:** To look for **uterine myomas;** can also exclude ovarian masses.
- **MRI:** Can delineate intramural and submucous myomas.

TREATMENT

- **Pharmacologic:**
    - Medroxyprogesterone acetate or danazol to slow or stop bleeding.
    - GnRH analogs (leuprolide or nafarelin) to ↓ **the size of myomas, suppress further growth,** and ↓ **surrounding vascularity.**
- **Surgery:** Emergent surgery is indicated for torsion of a pedunculated myoma.
- **Women of childbearing years:** Myomectomy.
- **Women who have completed childbearing:** Total or subtotal abdominal or vaginal hysterectomy.
- Embolization (interventional radiology).

If a uterine mass continues to grow after menopause, pathologic evaluation is crucial to rule out malignancy.

TABLE 2.12-7. **Gynecologic Neoplasms**

	ENDOMETRIAL	CERVICAL	VULVAR	OVARIAN
Patients affected	Postmenopausal, 50–70 years of age.	Premenopausal, > 40 years of age.	Postmenopausal, > 50 years of age.	Postmenopausal, > 50 years of age.
History	Vaginal bleeding (80% of patients), pain (late finding).	Metrorrhagia, postcoital spotting, discharge (bloody or purulent, odorous, nonpruritic). May be asymptomatic.	Prolonged vulvar irritation; **pruritus;** history of genital warts.	Often asymptomatic, but may present with ↑ abdominal girth from ascites, GI and GU complaints, thrombophlebitis, and lower abdominal pain/pressure.
Exam	Palpable abdominal and pelvic masses.	Cervical ulceration; bladder/rectal dysfunction.	**Early:** Resembles chronic vulvar dermatitis. **Late:** Presents with a large, cauliflower-like or hard ulcerated area in the vulva.	**Early:** Pelvic exam may be normal or may present with a palpable adnexal mass and pedal edema. **Late:** Palpable mass, ascites.
Risk factors	**Excess estrogen:** Well-differentiated tumor with high survival rates.[a] Thin, multiparous African-American women have more aggressive tumors with a poorer prognosis.	HPV infection, venereal warts, early sexual activity, multiple sex partners, smoking, family history.	**HPV (types 16,18, 31),** infrequent medical exams, diabetes, obesity, hypertension, cardiovascular disease, immunosuppression.	Nulliparity, breast cancer, family history. OCP use is protective.
Screening tests	None (Pap smear is only 50% effective).	Annual Pap smear for sexually active women.		None (routine ultrasound and CA-125 are not cost-efficient).
Precursor lesion	Endometrial hyperplasia (treatment is progesterone).	Cervical intraepithelial neoplasia (CIN) is a common diagnosis; most often seen in women 25–40 years of age. Associated with HPV.	Vulvar intraepithelial neoplasia (VIN).	None.

TABLE 2.12-7.   **Gynecologic Neoplasms (continued)**

	ENDOMETRIAL	CERVICAL	VULVAR	OVARIAN
Diagnostic tests	**Endometrial/ endocervical biopsy;** Pap smear is not reliable. Vaginal ultrasound shows thickened endometrium → hypertrophy and neoplastic change.	⊕ **Pap smear;** punch +/– cone biopsy.	Punch biopsy. VIN I and II are associated with mild and moderate dysplasia with ↑ risk → advanced stages and carcinoma. VIN III = carcinoma in situ.	Ultrasound, abdominal CT, CA-125 for epithelial cancers; α-fetoprotein (AFP) and β-hCG for germ cell cancers.
Treatment	TAH/BSO with lymph node dissection; progesterone; radiotherapy. Treat advanced cases with chemotherapy.	**Early:** Chemoradiation; radical hysterectomy and lymph-adenectomy. **Advanced:** Irradiation/ chemotherapy (surgery would harm the bladder and rectum without being effective).	**Surgical:** ▪ **In situ:** Excise with wide margin. ▪ **Invasive:** (1) Radical vulvectomy and regional lymphadenectomy or (2) wide local excision of the 1° tumor with inguinal lymph node dissection. **Chemoradiation:** To ↓ tumor burden and for metastatic or recurrent disease.	TAH/BSO and peritoneal washing for cytology with or without pelvic and aortic node sampling; tumor debulking; chemotherapy.
Prevention	Progesterone to oppose estrogen; low-fat diet; weight control.	Safe sex (condoms) to ↓ the risk of HPV infection; smoking cessation; routine Pap smears.	Same as with cervical cancer.	OCPs; prophylactic BSO in patients with a strong family history.
Notes	Adenocarcinomas.	Some 5% are squamous cell carcinomas and 15% adenocarcinomas. **Uremia** is the most common cause of death in end-stage cervical cancer.	Approximately 87% are squamous cell carcinomas and 6% malignant melanomas; the remainder include basal cell carcinoma and Paget's disease.	Complications include ovarian rupture, torsion, hemorrhage, infections, and infarction. The most common cause of death is bowel obstruction.

[a] **Excess estrogen exposure** is associated with a history of unopposed estrogen use, late menopause, obesity, nulliparity, and tamoxifen use for breast cancer.

HIGH-YIELD FACTS

GYNECOLOGY

COMPLICATIONS

Infertility may be due to a myoma that distorts the uterine cavity and plays a role similar to that of an IUD.

Endometrial Cancer

Endometrial carcinoma is the most common gynecologic cancer in the United States. Table 2.11-8 compares the two types of endometrial cancer. Endometrial hyperplasia is the abnormal proliferation of glandular and stromal elements of the endometrium. When only architectural changes are present, the hyperplasia is categorized as either simple (glandular crowding absent) or complex (glandular crowding present). When cytologic atypia is present with architectural changes, the hyperplasia is categorized as either atypical simple or atypical complex. Each type of endometrial hyperplasia is associated with a different risk of progression to endometrial (type I) cancer:

- Simple hyperplasia: 1%.
- Complex hyperplasia: 3%.
- Atypical simple hyperplasia: 8%.
- Atypical complex hyperplasia: 29%.

TABLE 2.11-8. **Types of Endometrial Cancer**

	TYPE I: ENDOMETRIOID	TYPE II: SEROUS
Etiology	Related to unopposed estrogen stimulation (e.g., tamoxifen use, exogenous estrogen-only therapy).	Unrelated to estrogen; p53 mutation is present in 90% of cases.
Epidemiology	The most common female reproductive cancer in the United States (~35,000 cases/year); 80–85% of endometrial cancers.	Responsible for 15–20% of endometrial cancers.
Precursor lesion	Hyperplasia and atypical hyperplasia.	Endometrial intraepithelial carcinoma (EIC).
Mean age	55	67
Signs and symptoms	Abnormal vaginal bleeding, enlarged uterus.	N/A
Reproductive history	Nulliparity or low parity, infertility (chronic anovulation).	N/A
Metabolic syndrome (obesity, DM, hypertension)	Present	Absent
Tumor grade	Low	High
Myoinvasion	Superficial	Deep
Treatment	Age dependent for stage I—high-dose progestins for premenopausal women; TAH/BSO for peri- and postmenopausal women +/− radiation therapy.	TAH/BSO plus staging for all stages and ages (+ adjuvant chemotherapy for advanced stages).
Prognosis	Favorable	Poor

Ovarian Tumors

Most ovarian tumors are benign, but malignant tumors are the leading cause of death from reproductive tract cancer. Death most commonly results from **bowel obstruction.** The lifetime risk is 1.6%. Risk factors include the following:

- Age, low parity, ↓ fertility, delayed childbearing.
- A ⊕ family history. Patients with one affected first-degree relative have a 5% lifetime risk. With two or more affected first-degree relatives, the risk is 7%.
- The BRCA1 mutation carries a 45% lifetime risk of ovarian cancer. The BRCA2 mutation is associated with a 25% lifetime risk.
- **Lynch II syndrome,** or hereditary nonpolyposis colorectal cancer (HNPCC), is associated with an ↑ risk of colon, ovarian, endometrial, and breast cancer.
- **OCPs ↓ risk.**

HISTORY/PE

- Both benign and malignant ovarian neoplasms are generally asymptomatic.
- Mild, nonspecific GI symptoms or pelvic pressure/pain may be seen.
- Early disease is typically not detected on routine pelvic exam.
- Some 75% of woman present with **advanced malignant disease,** as evidenced by abdominal pain and bloating, a palpable abdominal mass, and ascites.
- Table 2.12-9 differentiates the benign and malignant characteristics of pelvic masses.

DIAGNOSIS

- **Tumor markers (see** Table 2.12-10): ↑ **CA-125** is associated with epithelial cell cancer (90% of ovarian cancers) but is used only as a marker for progression and recurrence.
    - **Premenopausal women:** ↑ CA-125 may point to benign disease such as endometriosis.
    - **Postmenopausal women:** ↑ CA-125 (> 35 units) indicates an ↑ likelihood that the ovarian tumor is malignant.
- **Transvaginal ultrasound:**
    - **Screen high-risk women.**
    - See Table 2.12-9 to differentiate benign and malignant ovarian/adnexal masses.

TREATMENT

Treatment of **ovarian masses** is as follows:

- **Premenarchal women:** Masses > 2 cm require exploratory laparotomy.
- **Premenopausal women:**
    - Observation for 4–6 weeks for asymptomatic, mobile, unilateral simple cystic masses < 8–10 cm. Most resolve spontaneously.
    - Surgical evaluation is warranted for masses > 8–10 cm as well as for those that are unchanged on repeat pelvic exam and ultrasound.
    - If malignancy is suspected, preoperative workup includes CXR, LFTs and TFTs, and basic hematology studies.
- **Postmenopausal women:**
    - Asymptomatic, unilateral simple cysts < 5 cm in diameter with a **normal CA-125** should be **closely followed with ultrasound.**
    - Palpable masses warrant surgical evaluation by exploratory laparotomy.

Any palpable ovarian or adnexal mass in a premenarchal or postmenopausal patient is suggestive of ovarian neoplasm.

TABLE 2.12-9. Benign vs. Malignant Pelvic Masses

FINDING	BENIGN	MALIGNANT
Exam: pelvic mass		
Mobility	Mobile	Fixed
Consistency	Cystic	Solid or firm
Location	Unilateral	Bilateral
Cul-de-sac	Smooth	Nodular
Transvaginal ultrasound:		
adnexal mass		
Size	< 8 cm	> 8 cm
Consistency	Cystic	Solid or cystic and solid
Septations	Unilocular	Multilocular
Location	Unilateral	Bilateral
Other	Calcifications	Ascites

Treatment of **ovarian cancer** is as follows:

- **Surgery:**
  - Surgical staging followed by TAH/BSO with omentectomy, peritoneal washings and biopsies, and pelvic and para-aortic lymphadenectomy.
  - Benign neoplasms warrant tumor removal or unilateral oophorectomy.
  - **Postoperative chemotherapy** is routine except for women with early-stage or low-grade ovarian cancer.
- Radiation therapy is effective for dysgerminomas.

PREVENTION

- Women with the BRCA1 gene mutation should be screened annually with ultrasound and CA-125 testing. Prophylactic oophorectomy is recommended by age 35 or whenever childbearing is completed.
- OCP use ↓ risk.

TABLE 2.12-10. Ovarian Tumor Markers

OVARIAN TUMOR	MARKER
Epithelial	CA-125
Endodermal sinus	AFP
Embryonal carcinoma	AFP, hCG
Choriocarcinoma	hCG
Dysgerminoma	LDH
Granulosa cell	Inhibin

Defined as the involuntary loss of urine due to either bladder or sphincteric dysfunction.

HISTORY/PE

- Table 2.12-11 outlines the types of incontinence along with their distinguishing features and treatment.
- Exclude fistula in cases of total incontinence. Look for neurologic abnormalities in cases of urge incontinence (spasticity, flaccidity, rectal sphincter tone) or distended bladder in overflow incontinence.

DIAGNOSIS

- UA and urine culture to exclude UTI.
- Voiding diary; possible urodynamic testing.
- Serum creatinine to exclude renal dysfunction.
- Cystogram to demonstrate fistula sites and descensus of the bladder neck.

> *Causes of urinary incontinence without specific urogenital pathology—*
>
> **DIAPPERS**
>
> **D**elirium/confusional state
> **I**nfection
> **A**trophic urethritis/vaginitis
> **P**harmaceutical
> **P**sychiatric causes (esp. depression)
> **E**xcessive urinary output (hyperglycemia, hypercalcemia, CHF)
> **R**estricted mobility
> **S**tool impaction

TABLE 2.12-11. Types of Incontinence

TYPE	HISTORY OF URINE LOSS	ETIOLOGY	TREATMENT
Total	Uncontrolled loss at all times and in all positions.	Sphincteric efficiency is lost (previous surgery, nerve damage, cancer infiltration). Abnormal connection between the urinary tract and the skin (fistula).	Surgery.
Stress	Activities that ↑ intra-abdominal pressure (coughing, sneezing, lifting); not common in the supine position.	Urethral sphincteric insufficiency due to laxity of pelvic floor musculature; common in multiparous women or after pelvic surgery.	Surgery centers on placing the bladder neck into the appropriate anatomical location. Medical management includes Kegel exercises and use of a pessary.
Urge[a]	Preceded by a strong, unexpected urge to void that is unrelated to position or activity.	Detrusor hyperreflexia or sphincter dysfunction due to inflammatory conditions or neurogenic disorders of the bladder.	Anticholinergic medications or TCAs, behavioral training (biofeedback).
Overflow[b]	Patients with chronic urinary retention.	Chronically distended bladder with ↑ intravesical pressure that just exceeds the outlet resistance, allowing a small amount of urine to dribble out.	Placement of urethral catheter in acute settings. Treat underlying diseases. Timed voiding.

[a]Etiologies include inhibited contractions, local irritation (cystitis, stone, tumor), and CNS causes.
[b]Etiologies include physical agents (tumor, stricture), neurologic factors (lesions), and medications.

HIGH-YIELD FACTS

GYNECOLOGY

Pediatrics

CHILD ABUSE

Includes neglect as well as physical, sexual, and emotional abuse. Suspect abuse if the history is discordant with physical findings or if there is a delay in obtaining appropriate medical care.

HISTORY/PE

- Abuse or neglect in infants may present as apnea, seizures, feeding intolerance, excessive irritability or somnolence, or failure to thrive (FTT).
- Neglect in older children may present as poor hygiene or behavioral abnormalities.
- Exam findings may include the following:
  - Injuries in atypical places (e.g., the face or thighs) or patterns (stocking-glove burns, cigarette burns, belt marks).
  - Spiral fractures of the humerus and femur (strongly suggest abuse in children < 3 years of age).
  - Epiphyseal/metaphyseal injuries in infants (can result from pulling or twisting of the limbs).
  - Posterior rib fractures.
  - Genital bleeding or discharge.

Consider abuse if the caretaker's story does not match the child's injury or developmental level.

DIAGNOSIS

- Rule out conditions that mimic abuse—e.g., bleeding disorders or mongolian spots (bruises), osteogenesis imperfecta (fractures), bullous impetigo (cigarette burns), and "coining" (an alternative treatment in certain cultures).
- A skeletal survey and bone scan can show fractures in various stages of healing.
- Test for gonorrhea, syphilis, chlamydia, and HIV if sexual abuse is suspected.
- Rule out shaken baby syndrome (SBS) by performing an ophthalmologic exam for retinal hemorrhages and noncontrast CT for subdural hematomas. Infants with SBS often do not exhibit external signs of abuse.
- Consider MRI to visualize white matter changes (diffuse axonal injury associated with violent shaking) and the extent of intra- and extracranial bleeds. MRI often requires the young patient to be intubated and sedated, while CT usually does not.

Spiral fractures suggest child abuse.

TREATMENT

- Document injuries.
- Notify child protective services (CPS) for evaluation and possible removal of the child from the home.
- Hospitalize if necessary to stabilize injuries or to protect the child.

CONGENITAL HEART DISEASE

Intrauterine risk factors for congenital heart disease include maternal alcohol and drug use, exogenous hormones (e.g., OCPs), lithium, and congenital infection. Disease is classified by the presence or absence of cyanosis:

- **Noncyanotic conditions** have left-to-right shunts in which oxygenated blood from the lungs is shunted back into the pulmonary circulation.
- **Cyanotic conditions** have right-to-left shunts in which deoxygenated blood is shunted into the systemic circulation.

> *Noncyanotic heart disease—*
>
> *The 3 D's*
>
> VS**D**
> AS**D**
> P**D**A

> *Cyanotic heart disease—*
>
> *The 5 T's and 1 P*
>
> **T**runcus arteriosus
> **T**ransposition of the great arteries
> **T**etralogy of Fallot
> **T**ricuspid atresia
> **T**otal anomalous pulmonary venous return
> **P**ulmonary atresia

Ventricular Septal Defect (VSD)

An opening in the ventricular septum allows blood to flow between ventricles. VSD is **the most common congenital heart defect.** It is more common in patients with Apert's syndrome (cranial deformities, fusion of the fingers and toes), Down syndrome, fetal alcohol syndrome, cri-du-chat syndrome, and trisomies 13 and 18.

HISTORY/PE

Symptoms depend on the degree of left-to-right shunting.

- Small defects are usually **asymptomatic** at birth, but exam reveals a harsh holosystolic murmur heard best at the lower left sternal border.
- Large defects can present with **frequent respiratory infections, dyspnea, FTT, and CHF;** if present, the holosystolic murmur is softer and more blowing but can be accompanied by a systolic thrill, crackles, ↑ S2, and a mid-diastolic apical murmur reflecting ↑ flow across the mitral valve.

DIAGNOSIS

Echocardiogram is diagnostic. ECG and CXR can demonstrate LVH with small defects and show both LVH and RVH with larger VSDs. CXR may show ↑ pulmonary vascular markings.

TREATMENT

- Most small VSDs close spontaneously; patients should be monitored via echocardiography.
- Surgical repair is indicated in symptomatic patients who fail medical management, children < 1 year of age with signs of pulmonary hypertension, and older children with large VSDs that have not reduced in size over time.
- Treat existing CHF with diuretics, inotropes, and ACEIs; treat respiratory infections as needed.
- **All VSD patients** should be given **antibiotic prophylaxis** prior to the use of dental, oropharyngeal, or GU instrumentation.

Atrial Septal Defect (ASD)

A condition in which an opening in the atrial septum allows blood to flow between the atria → left-to-right shunting. Associated with Holt-Oram syndrome (absent radii, ASD, first-degree heart block), fetal alcohol syndrome, and Down syndrome.

HISTORY/PE

- Ostium primum defects present in early childhood with findings of a murmur or fatigue with exertion. Ostium secundum defects tend to present in late childhood or early adulthood. Symptom onset and severity depend on the size of the defect.
- Symptoms of easy fatigability, frequent respiratory infections, and FTT can be observed, but patients are frequently asymptomatic.
- Exam reveals a right ventricular heave; a wide and fixed, split S2; and a systolic ejection murmur at the upper left sternal border (from ↑ flow across the pulmonary valve).

DIAGNOSIS

- Echocardiogram with color flow Doppler reveals blood flow between the atria (diagnostic), paradoxical ventricular wall motion, and a dilated right ventricle.
- ECG most commonly shows right axis deviation and RVH, although other patterns are possible depending on the type of defect. PR prolongation is common.
- CXR reveals cardiomegaly and ↑ pulmonary vascular markings.

TREATMENT

- Small defects may close spontaneously and do not require treatment.
- Antibiotic prophylaxis before dental procedures is required for ostium primum defects to prevent bacterial endocarditis.
- Surgical closure is indicated in infants with CHF and in patients with more than a 2:1 ratio of pulmonary to systemic blood flow. Early correction prevents complications such as arrhythmias, right ventricular dysfunction, and Eisenmenger's syndrome.

In Eisenmenger's syndrome, left-to-right shunt → pulmonary hypertension and shunt reversal.

Patent Ductus Arteriosus (PDA)

Failure of the ductus arteriosus to close in the first few days of life → a left-to-right shunt from the aorta to the pulmonary artery. Risk factors include maternal first-trimester rubella infection, prematurity, and female gender.

HISTORY/PE

- Typically asymptomatic; patients with large defects may present with FTT, recurrent lower respiratory tract infections, lower extremity clubbing, and CHF.
- Exam reveals a wide pulse pressure; a continuous "machinery murmur" at the second left intercostal space at the sternal border; a loud S2; and bounding peripheral pulses.

DIAGNOSIS

- A color flow Doppler demonstrating blood flow from the aorta into the pulmonary artery is diagnostic.
- With larger PDAs, echocardiography shows left atrial and left ventricular enlargement.
- ECG may show LVH, and CXR may show cardiomegaly.
- Small PDAs often have no signs of cardiomegaly.

Come **IN** and **CLOSE** the door—give **IN**domethacin to **CLOSE** a PDA.

TREATMENT

- Give indomethacin unless the PDA is needed for survival (e.g., transposition of the great vessels, tetralogy of Fallot, hypoplastic left heart) or if indomethacin is contraindicated (e.g., intraventricular hemorrhage).
- If indomethacin fails or if the child is > 6–8 months of age, surgical closure is required.

Coarctation of the Aorta

Constriction of a portion of the aorta → ↑ flow proximal to and ↓ flow distal to the coarctation, occurring just below the left subclavian artery in 98% of patients.

The condition is associated with Turner's syndrome, berry aneurysms, and male gender. **More than two-thirds of patients have a bicuspid aortic valve.**

HISTORY/PE

- Often presents in childhood with **asymptomatic hypertension.**
- Lower extremity claudication, syncope, epistaxis, and headache may be present.
- The classic physical exam finding is a systolic BP that is higher in the upper extremities; the difference in BP between the left and right arm can indicate the point of coarctation.
- Additional findings include weak femoral pulses, a short systolic murmur in the left axilla, and a forceful apical impulse.
- In infancy, critical coarctation requires a patent PDA for survival. Such infants may present in the first few weeks of life in a shocklike state when the PDA closes. Differential cyanosis may be seen with lower oxygen saturation in the left arm and lower extremities (postductal areas) as compared to the right arm (preductal area).

DIAGNOSIS

- Echocardiography and color flow Doppler are diagnostic.
- CXR in young children may demonstrate cardiomegaly and pulmonary congestion.
- In older children, the following compensatory changes may be seen: LVH on ECG; the **"3" sign on CXR** due to pre- and postdilatation of the coarctation segment with aortic wall indentation; and **"rib notching"** due to collateral circulation through the intercostal arteries.

TREATMENT

- If severe coarctation presents in infancy, the ductus arteriosus should be kept open with prostaglandin E_1 (PGE_1).
- Surgical correction or balloon angioplasty (controversial).
- Monitor for restenosis, aneurysm development, and aortic dissection.

Transposition of the Great Vessels

The most common cyanotic congenital heart lesion in the newborn. In this condition, the aorta is connected to the right ventricle and the pulmonary artery to the left ventricle, creating parallel pulmonary and systemic circulations. **Without a septal defect or a PDA, it is incompatible with life.** Risk factors include diabetic mothers and, rarely, **CATCH 22** (DiGeorge syndrome).

HISTORY/PE

- Critical illness and cyanosis typically occur immediately after birth. Reverse differential cyanosis may be present if left ventricular outflow tract obstruction (e.g., coarctation, aortic stenosis) is also present.
- Exam reveals tachypnea and progressive hypoxemia. Some patients have signs of CHF, and a single S2 is often present.

DIAGNOSIS

- Echocardiography.
- CXR may show a narrow heart base, absence of the main pulmonary artery segment ("egg-shaped silhouette"), and ↑ pulmonary vascular markings.

*Coarctation is a cause of 2°
hypertension in children.*

**DiGeorge
syndrome—**

CATCH 22

Cardiac abnormalities
Abnormal facies
Thymic aplasia
Cleft palate
Hypocalcemia
22q11 deletion

*Coarctation in infancy may
present with differential
cyanosis, while transposition
of the great arteries may
present with reverse
differential cyanosis.*

TREATMENT

- Start IV PGE₁ to maintain or open the PDA.
- Balloon atrial septostomy to create or enlarge an ASD if surgery is not feasible within the first few days of life or if the PDA cannot be maintained with prostaglandin.
- Surgical correction (arterial or atrial switch).

Tetralogy of Fallot

Consists of pulmonary stenosis, overriding aorta, RVH, and VSD. **The most common cyanotic congenital heart disease in children.** Early cyanosis results from right-to-left shunting across the VSD. As right-sided pressures ↓ in the weeks after birth, the shunt direction reverses and cyanosis may ↓. If the degree of pulmonary stenosis is severe, the right-sided pressures may remain high and cyanosis may worsen over time. Risk factors include maternal PKU and CATCH 22 syndrome.

HISTORY/PE

- Presents in infancy or early childhood with dyspnea and fatigability. Cyanosis is often not present at birth but develops over the first two years of life; the degree of cyanosis often reflects the degree of pulmonary stenosis.
- Infants are often asymptomatic until 4–6 months of age, when CHF may develop and may manifest as diaphoresis with feeding or tachypnea.
- Children often squat for relief (↑ systemic vascular resistance) during hypoxemic episodes ("tet spells").
- Hypoxemia may → FTT or mental status changes.
- Exam reveals a systolic ejection murmur at the left upper sternal border (right ventricular outflow obstruction), right ventricular heave, and a single S2.

DIAGNOSIS

- Echocardiography and catheterization.
- CXR shows a "boot-shaped" heart with ↓ pulmonary vascular markings. Remember that a VSD may result in ↑ pulmonary vascular markings
- ECG shows right-axis deviation and RVH.

TREATMENT

- Lesions with severe pulmonary stenosis or atresia require immediate PGE₁ to keep the PDA open and urgent surgical consultation.
- Treat hypercyanotic "tet spells" with O₂, propranolol, phenylephrine, knee-chest position, fluids, and morphine.
- Temporary palliation can be achieved through the creation of an artificial shunt (e.g., balloon atrial septostomy) before definitive surgical correction.

DEVELOPMENT

Developmental Milestones

Table 2.13-1 highlights major developmental milestones.

Failure to Thrive (FTT)

Defined as persistent weight below the fifth percentile for age or "falling off the growth curve" (i.e., crossing two major percentile lines on a growth chart). Risk factors include chronic illness, poverty, low maternal age, chaotic

---

Tetralogy of Fallot—PROVe

Pulmonary stenosis
RVH
Overriding aorta
VSD

*Transposition of the great vessels is the most common cyanotic heart disease of **newborns**. Tetralogy of Fallot is the most common cyanotic heart disease of **childhood**.*

Both transposition of the great vessels and tetralogy of Fallot are initially treated with PGE₁ and are definitively treated with surgical correction.

In infants presenting in a shocklike state within the first few weeks of life, look for:

1. *Sepsis*
2. *Inborn error of metabolism*
3. *Ductal-dependent congenital heart disease (as the ductus is closing)*

TABLE 2.13-1.   Developmental Milestones

AGE	GROSS MOTOR	FINE MOTOR	LANGUAGE	SOCIAL/COGNITIVE
2 months	Lifts head/chest when prone.	Tracks past midline.	Alerts to sound; coos.	Recognizes parent; social smile.
4–5 months	Rolls front to back, back to front (5 months).	Grasps rattle.	Orients to voice; begins to make consonant sounds, razzes.	Enjoys looking around; laughs.
6 months	Sits unassisted.	Transfers objects; raking grasp.	Babbles.	Stranger anxiety.
9–10 months	Crawls; pulls to stand.	Uses three-finger (immature) pincer grasp.	Says "mama/dada" (nonspecific).	Waves bye-bye; plays pat-a-cake.
12 months	Cruises (11 months); walks alone.	Uses two-finger (mature) pincer grasp.	Says "mama/dada" (specific).	Imitates actions.
15 months	Walks backward.	Uses cup.	Uses 4–6 words.	Temper tantrums.
18 months	Runs; kicks a ball.	Builds tower of 2–4 cubes.	Names common objects.	Copies parent in tasks (e.g., sweeping).
2 years	Walks up/down steps with help; jumps.	Builds tower of six cubes.	Uses two-word phrases.	Follows two-step commands; removes clothes.
3 years	Rides tricycle; climbs stairs with alternating feet (3–4 years).	Copies a circle; uses utensils.	Uses three-word sentences.	Brushes teeth with help; washes/dries hands.
4 years	Hops.	Copies a square.	Knows colors and some numbers.	Cooperative play; plays board games.
5 years	Skips; walks backward for long distances.	Ties shoelaces; knows left and right; prints letters.	Uses five-word sentences.	Domestic role playing; plays dress-up.

environments, genetic disease (e.g., CF), inborn errors of metabolism, endocrine disorders, and HIV. Classified as follows:

- **Organic:** When an underlying medical condition is present (GI dysfunction; infection; endocrine, cardiac, pulmonary, or neurologic disease).
- **Nonorganic (most cases):** When psychosocial factors are thought to be the cause (maternal depression, neglect).

HISTORY/PE

- Patients are of low weight for age and height and experience weight loss or minimal weight gain.

TABLE 2.13-2. Tanner Staging Criteria

	MALE	FEMALE
Tanner stage 1 (prepubertal)	Basal growth in height; no penis or testicular enlargement; no pubic hair.	Basal growth in height; breast papilla elevation, no pubic hair.
Tanner stage 2	Basal growth in height; minimal pubic hair; earliest ↑ in testicular enlargement.	Accelerated growth; development of breast buds and enlargement of areolae; minimal pubic hair on labia.
Tanner stage 3	Accelerated growth; moderate pubic hair over pubis; continued testicular enlargement; penis begins to lengthen; gynecomastia.	Peak growth rate; breasts and areolae enlarge; pubic hair develops across mons pubis; axillary hair growth.
Tanner stage 4	Peak growth rate; widened distribution of pubic hair; continued enlargement of penis (in length and circumference) and testicles; axillary hair growth and change in voice quality.	Growth rate ↓; areolae form 2° mound; pubic hair coarsens and widens in distribution.
Tanner stage 5	No further ↑ in height; adult pubic hair distribution; mature genital size; development of facial hair.	No further ↑ in height; adult breast contour with recession of 2° areola mound; adult pubic hair distribution.

- Take a careful diet history and observe caregiver-child interactions (particularly observation of feeding).

DIAGNOSIS/TREATMENT

- Diagnosis is based on a comparison of height, weight, and head circumference on a growth chart and subsequent comparison to population norms. For endocrine disorders, height is usually the most severely affected parameter.
- Look for signs of systemic disease. Tests included CBC, electrolytes, creatinine, albumin, and total protein. Consider a sweat chloride tests (for CF), UA and culture, stool culture/O&P, and assessment of bone age.
- Start a calorie count. Supplement nutrition if breast-feeding is inadequate.
- Hospitalize if there is evidence of neglect or severe malnourishment.

Hospitalize children if there is evidence of neglect or severe malnourishment.

Sexual Development

Begins in early adolescence, with breast buds appearing in girls between 8 and 13 years of age and testicular enlargement beginning in boys between 9 and 11 years of age. Table 2.13-2 outlines the Tanner staging criteria for sexual development.

GENETIC DISEASE

Tables 2.13-3 and 2.13-4 outline common genetic diseases and their associated abnormalities.

TABLE 2.13-3. **Genetic Diseases**

DISEASE	GENETIC ABNORMALITY	COMMON CHARACTERISTICS
Down syndrome	Trisomy 21 (most common) or translocation (higher risk of recurrence)	The most common chromosomal disorder and cause of mental retardation. Associated with advanced maternal age. Presents with mental retardation, a flat facial profile, prominent epicanthal folds, and simian crease. Associated with duodenal atresia, Hirschsprung's disease, and congenital heart disease (the most common malformation is atrioventricular canal, which includes an ASD and VSD with mitral and triscuspid valve abnormalities due to endocardial cushion defects). Associated with an ↑ risk of acute lymphocytic leukemia (ALL) and early-onset Alzheimer's. Patients are also at ↑ risk for atlantoaxial (C1–C2) instability.
Edwards' syndrome	Trisomy 18	Presents with severe mental retardation, rocker-bottom feet, low-set ears, micrognathia, clenched hands, and prominent occiput. Associated with congenital heart disease. May have horseshoe kidneys. Death usually occurs within one year of birth.
Patau's syndrome	Trisomy 13	Presents with severe mental retardation, microphthalmia, microcephaly, cleft lip/palate, abnormal forebrain structures (holoprosencephaly), "punched-out" scalp lesions, and polydactyly. Associated with congenital heart disease. Death usually occurs within one year of birth.
Klinefelter's syndrome (male)	45,XXY	Presence of inactivated X chromosome (Barr body). One of the most common causes of hypogonadism in males. Presents with testicular atrophy; a eunuchoid body shape; tall, long extremities; gynecomastia; and female hair distribution.
Turner's syndrome (female)	45,XO	The most common cause of 1° amenorrhea. No Barr body. Presents with short stature, ovarian dysgenesis, webbing of the neck, and coarctation of the aorta. May present with lymphedema of the hands and feet in the neonatal period. May have horseshoe kidney.
Double Y males	47,XYY	Observed with ↑ frequency among inmates of penal institutions. Phenotypically normal; patients are very tall with severe acne and antisocial behavior (seen in 1–2% of XYY males).
Phenylketonuria (PKU)	↓ phenylalanine hydroxylase or ↓ tetrahydrobiopterin cofactor	Screened for at birth; screening is valid only after the baby has had a protein meal (i.e., a normal breast or formula feed). Tyrosine becomes essential and phenylalanine builds up excess phenyl ketones. Presents with mental retardation, fair skin, eczema, and a musty or mousy urine odor. Blond-haired, blue-eyed infants. Associated with an ↑ risk of heart disease. Treat with ↓ phenylalanine and ↑ tyrosine in diet. A mother with PKU who wants to become pregnant must restrict her diet as above *before* conception.

TABLE 2.13-3.   Genetic Diseases (continued)

DISEASE	GENETIC ABNORMALITY	COMMON CHARACTERISTICS
Fragile X syndrome	An X-linked defect affecting the methylation and expression of FMR1 gene	The second most common cause of genetic mental retardation. Presents with macro-orchidism; a long face with a large jaw; large, everted ears; and autism. A triplet repeat disorder that may show genetic anticipation.

TABLE 2.13-4.   Lysosomal Storage Diseases

DISEASE	ETIOLOGY	MODE OF INHERITANCE
Fabry's disease	Caused by a deficiency of α-galactosidase A → accumulation of ceramide trihexoside in the heart, brain, and kidneys. Findings include renal failure and an ↑ risk of stroke and MI.	X-linked recessive.
Krabbe's disease	Absence of galactosylceramide and galactoside (due to galactosylceramidase deficiency) → accumulation of galactocerebroside in the brain. Optic atrophy, spasticity, early death.	Autosomal recessive.
Gaucher's disease	Caused by a deficiency of glucocerebrosidase → glucocerebroside accumulation in the brain, liver, spleen, and bone marrow (Gaucher's cells with characteristic "crinkled paper" enlarged cytoplasm). May present with hepatosplenomegaly, anemia, and thrombocytopenia. Type I, the more common form, is compatible with a normal life span and does not affect the brain.	Autosomal recessive.
Niemann-Pick disease	Deficiency of sphingomyelinase → buildup of sphingomyelin cholesterol in reticuloendothelial and parenchymal cells and tissues. Patients with type A die by the age of three.	Autosomal recessive. No man PICKs (Niemann-PICK) his nose with his sphinger.
Tay-Sachs disease	Absence of hexosaminidase → GM_2 ganglioside accumulation. May appear normal until 3–6 months of age, when weakness begins and development slows and regresses. Exaggerated startle response. Death occurs by the age of three. A cherry-red spot is visible on the macula. The carrier rate is 1 in 30 Jews of European descent (1 in 300 for others).	Tay-SaX lacks heXosaminidase.
Metachromatic leukodystrophy	Deficiency of arylsulfatase A → accumulation of sulfatide in the brain, kidney, liver, and peripheral nerves.	Autosomal recessive.
Hurler's syndrome	Deficiency of α-L-iduronidase → corneal clouding and mental retardation.	Autosomal recessive.
Hunter's syndrome	Deficiency of iduronate sulfatase. A mild form of Hurler's with no corneal clouding and mild mental retardation.	X-linked recessive. Hunters need to see (no corneal clouding) to aim for the X.

HIGH-YIELD FACTS

PEDIATRICS

Cystic Fibrosis (CF)

An autosomal-recessive disorder caused by mutations in the CFTR gene (chloride channel) on chromosome 7 and characterized by widespread exocrine gland dysfunction. CF is the most common severe genetic disease in the United States and is most common in Caucasians.

HISTORY/PE

- Fifty percent of cases present with FTT or respiratory compromise.
- Characterized by recurrent pulmonary infections (especially with *Pseudomonas* and *S. aureus*) with subsequent cyanosis, digital clubbing, cough, dyspnea, bronchiectasis, hemoptysis, chronic sinusitis, rhonchi, rales, hyperresonance to percussion, and nasal polyposis.
- Fifteen percent of infants present with meconium ileus. Patients usually have greasy stools and flatulence; other prominent GI symptoms include pancreatitis, rectal prolapse, esophageal varices, and biliary cirrhosis.
- GI symptoms are more prominent in infancy, while pulmonary manifestations predominate thereafter.
- Additional symptoms include type 2 DM, "salty taste," male infertility, and unexplained hyponatremia.
- Patients are at risk for fat-soluble vitamin deficiency (vitamins A, D, E, and K) due to malabsorption and may present with manifestations of these deficiencies.

DIAGNOSIS

Sweat chloride test > 60 mEq/L for those < 20 years of age and > 80 mEq/L in adults; genetic testing.

TREATMENT

- Pulmonary manifestations are managed with chest physical therapy, bronchodilators, corticosteroids, antibiotics, and DNase.
- Administer pancreatic enzymes and fat-soluble vitamins A, D, E, and K for malabsorption.
- Nutritional counseling and support are essential for health maintenance.
- Patients who have severe disease (but who can tolerate surgery) may be candidates for lung or pancreas transplants.

GASTROENTEROLOGY

Intussusception

A condition in which one portion of the bowel telescopes into an adjacent segment, usually proximal to the ileocecal valve (see Figure 2.13-1). The most common cause of bowel obstruction in the first two years of life (males > females); usually seen between three months and three years of age. The cause is often unknown. Risk factors include Meckel's diverticulum, intestinal lymphoma (> 6 years of age), Henoch-Schönlein purpura, parasites, polyps, adenovirus or rotavirus infection, celiac disease, and CF.

HISTORY/PE

- Presents with abrupt-onset, colicky abdominal pain in apparently healthy children, often accompanied by flexed knees and vomiting. The child may appear well in between episodes if intussusception is released.

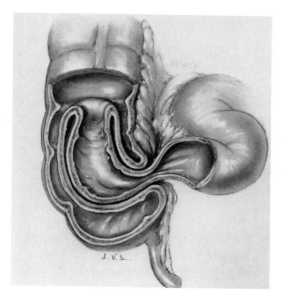

FIGURE 2.13-1.   Intussusception.

A segment of bowel telescopes into an adjacent segment, causing obstruction. (Reproduced, with permission, from Way LW. *Current Surgical Diagnosis & Treatment*, 10th ed. Stamford, CT: Appleton & Lange, 1994, p. 1222.)

- The classic triad is abdominal pain, vomiting, and blood per rectum (only one in three patients).
- Young infants may have pallor and sweating.
- Advanced signs include bloody mucus in stools (red "currant jelly" stool), lethargy, and fever. The condition may progress to shock as the blood flow to the affected segment is compromised.
- On exam, look for abdominal tenderness, ⊕ stool guaiac, and a palpable "sausage-shaped" RUQ abdominal mass.

Diagnosis/Treatment

- Correct any volume or electrolyte abnormalities and check CBC (for leukocytosis).
- Abdominal plain films (showing small bowel obstruction) and ultrasound may be helpful.
- Air-contrast barium enema is diagnostic and often curative. If the child is unstable or enema reduction is unsuccessful, perform surgical reduction and resection of gangrenous bowel.

Pyloric Stenosis

Hypertrophy of the pyloric sphincter → gastric outlet obstruction. More common in firstborn males; associated with tracheoesophageal fistula and with a maternal history of pyloric stenosis.

History/PE

- Nonbilious emesis typically begins around three weeks of age and progresses to projectile emesis after most to all feedings.

- Babies initially feed well but eventually suffer from malnutrition and dehydration.
- Exam may reveal a palpable olive-shaped, mobile, nontender epigastric mass and visible gastric peristaltic waves.

DIAGNOSIS

- Abdominal ultrasound showing a hypertrophic pylorus is diagnostic.
- Barium studies reveal a narrow pyloric channel ("string sign") or a pyloric beak.
- Check for hypochloremic, hypokalemic metabolic alkalosis due to persistent emesis.

TREATMENT

- Correct existing dehydration and acid-base/electrolyte abnormalities. NG tube placement may be necessary.
- Surgical correction with pyloromyotomy.

Meckel's Diverticulum

The most common congenital abnormality of the small intestine, affecting up to 2% of children. Most frequently occurs in children < 2 years of age.

HISTORY/PE

- Typically asymptomatic and often discovered incidentally.
- Classically presents with sudden, painless rectal bleeding.
- Abdominal pain typically signifies complications such as diverticulitis, volvulus, and intussusception.

> **Meckel's rule of 2's—**
>
> Most common in children under **2**
> **2** times as common in males
> Contains **2** types of tissue (pancreatic and gastric)
> **2** inches long
> Found within **2** feet of the ileocecal valve
> Occurs in **2%** of the population

DIAGNOSIS

A Meckel scintigraphy scan is diagnostic; plain films can be useful in diagnosing obstruction.

TREATMENT

- If there is active bleeding, treatment is excision of the diverticulum together with the adjacent intestinal segment.
- If asymptomatic but discovered intraoperatively, treatment is controversial but often involves excision.

Hirschsprung's Disease

Congenital lack of ganglion cells in the distal colon → uncoordinated peristalsis and ↓ motility. Associated with male gender, Down syndrome, Waardenburg's syndrome, and multiple endocrine neoplasia (MEN) type 2.

HISTORY/PE

- Neonates present with delayed passage of meconium, bilious vomiting, and FTT; children with less severe lesions may present later in life with chronic constipation.
- Physical exam may reveal abdominal distention and explosive discharge of stool following rectal exam.

- Plain films reveal proximally distended loops of bowel followed by the constricted, obstructed aganglionic segment.
- Anorectal manometry or rectal biopsy

TREATMENT

Surgical excision of the affected bowel segment is required to prevent megacolon.

Malrotation with Volvulus

Congenital malrotation of the midgut results in abnormal positioning of the small intestine (cecum in the right hypochondrium) and formation of fibrous bands (Ladd's bands). Bands predispose to obstruction and constriction of blood flow.

HISTORY/PE

- Often presents in the newborn period with bilious emesis, abdominal tenderness, and distention.
- Postsurgical adhesions can lead to obstruction and volvulus at any point in life.

DIAGNOSIS

- AXR may reveal the absence of intestinal gas but may also be normal.
- If the patient is stable, an upper GI is the study of choice. Ultrasound may be used, but sensitivity is determined by the experience of the ultrasonographer.

TREATMENT

- NG tube insertion to decompress the intestine.
- IV fluid hydration.
- Surgical repair (emergent when volvulus is present).

IMMUNOLOGY

Immunodeficiency Disorders

Congenital immunodeficiencies are rare and often present with chronic or recurrent infections (e.g., chronic thrush), unusual or opportunistic organisms, incomplete treatment response, or FTT. Categorization is based on the 1° immune system component that is abnormal (see Table 2.13-5):

- **B-cell deficiencies:** Most common (50%). Typically present **after six months of age** with recurrent sinopulmonary, GI, and urinary tract infections with encapsulated organisms (*H. influenzae, Streptococcus pneumoniae, Neisseria meningitidis*). Treated with IVIG (except for IgA deficiencies).
- **T-cell deficiencies:** Tend to present earlier (1–3 months) with **opportunistic and low-grade fungal, viral, and intracellular bacterial infections** (e.g., mycobacteria). 2° B-cell dysfunction may also be seen.
- **Phagocyte deficiencies:** Characterized by mucous membrane infections, abscesses, and poor wound healing. **Infections with catalase-⊕ organisms (e.g., *S. aureus*), fungi, and gram-⊖ enteric organisms are common.**

TABLE 2.13-5. **Pediatric Immunodeficiencies**

DISORDER	DESCRIPTION	INFECTION RISK/TYPE	DIAGNOSIS/TREATMENT
B cell			
X-linked agamma-globulinemia (**Bruton's**)	A **B-cell** deficiency in **boys** only.	Life-threatening; encapsulated *Pseudomonas, S. pneumoniae,* and *Haemophilus* infections.	Quantitative immunoglobulin levels. If low, confirm diagnosis with B- and T-cell subsets (absent B cells; T cells often high); absent tonsils and other lymphoid tissue may be a clue. Treat with prophylactic antibiotics and IVIG.
Common variable immunodeficiency	Immunoglobulin level drops in the **20s and 30s; usually a combined B- and T-cell defect.**	↑ pyogenic upper and lower respiratory infections; ↑ risk of lymphoma and autoimmune disease.	Quantitative Ig levels; confirm with B- and T-cell subsets; treat with IVIG.
IgA deficiency	Mild; the most common immunodeficiency.	Usually asymptomatic; patients may develop recurrent infections. Anaphylactic transfusion reaction due to anti-IgA antibodies is a common presentation.	Quantitative IgA levels; treat infections.
T cell			
Thymic aplasia (DiGeorge syndrome)	See mnemonic. Presents with tetany (2° to hypocalcemia) in the first days of life.	Variable risk of infection. ↑↑↑ infections with fungi and *Pneumocystis jiroveci* pneumonia (formerly *P. carinii*).	Absolute lymphocyte count; mitogen stimulation response; delayed hypersensitivity skin testing. Treat with bone marrow transplantation and IVIG for antibody deficiency; PCP prophylaxis. Thymus transplantation is an alternative.
Combined			
Ataxia-telangiectasia	**Oculocutaneous telangiectasias** and progressive **cerebellar ataxia.** Caused by a **DNA repair defect.**	↑ incidence of non-Hodgkin's lymphoma, leukemia, and gastric carcinoma.	No specific treatment; may require IVIG depending on the severity of the Ig deficiency.

TABLE 2.13-5. Pediatric Immunodeficiencies (continued)

DISORDER	DESCRIPTION	INFECTION RISK/TYPE	DIAGNOSIS/TREATMENT
Combined (continued)			
Severe combined immunodeficiency (SCID)	Severe lack of B and T cells.	Severe, frequent bacterial infections; chronic candidiasis; and opportunistic organisms.	Treat with bone marrow transplant or stem cell transplant and IVIG for antibody deficiency. **Needs PCP prophylaxis.**
Wiskott-Aldrich syndrome	An **X-linked** disorder with less severe B- and T-cell dysfunction. Patients have **eczema,** ↑ IgE/IgA, ↓ IgM, and **thrombocytopenia.** The classic presentation involves bleeding, eczema, and recurrent otitis media.	↑↑ risk of atopic disorders, lymphoma/leukemia, and infection from *S. pneumoniae*, *S. aureus*, and *H. influenzae* type b.	Treatment is supportive (IVIG and antibiotics). Patients rarely survive to adulthood. Patients with severe infections may be treated with a bone marrow transplant.
Phagocytic			
Chronic granulomatous disease (CGD)	An X-linked (2/3) or autosomal-recessive (1/3) disease with deficient superoxide production by PMNs and macrophages. Anemia, lymphadenopathy, and hypergamma-globulinemia may be present.	Chronic skin, pulmonary, GI, and urinary tract infections; osteomyelitis and hepatitis. Infecting organisms are catalase ⊕. ↑ risk of infection with *Aspergillus*. May have granulomas of the skin and GI/GU tracts.	Absolute neutrophil count with neutrophil assays. **The nitroblue tetrazolium test is diagnostic for CGD.** Treat with **daily TMP-SMX;** judicious use of antibiotics during infections. IFN-γ can ↓ the incidence of serious infection. Bone marrow transplantation and gene therapy are new therapies.
Leukocyte adhesion deficiency (LAD)	A defect in the chemotaxis of leukocytes.	Recurrent skin, mucosal, and pulmonary infections. May present as omphalitis in the newborn period with delayed separation of the umbilical cord.	No pus with minimal inflammation in wounds (due to a chemotaxis defect). High WBCs in blood. Bone marrow transplantation is curative.

HIGH-YIELD FACTS

PEDIATRICS

DISORDER	DESCRIPTION	INFECTION RISK/TYPE	DIAGNOSIS/TREATMENT
Phagocytic (continued) Chédiak-Higashi syndrome	An autosomal-recessive disorder → a defect in neutrophil chemotaxis. The syndrome includes oculocutaneous albinism, neuropathy, and neutropenia.	↑↑ incidence of overwhelming infections with *S. pyogenes*, *S. aureus,* and *Pseudomonas* spp.	Bone marrow transplant is the treatment of choice.
Complement C1 esterase deficiency (hereditary angioedema)	An autosomal-dominant disorder with recurrent episodes of angioedema lasting 2–72 hours and provoked by stress or trauma.	Can → life-threatening airway edema.	Total hemolytic complement (CH50) to assess the quantity and function of complement. Purified C1 esterase and FFP can be used prior to surgery.
Terminal complement deficiency (C5–C9)	Inability to form membrane attack complex (MAC).	Recurrent meningococcal or gonococcal infections. Rarely, lupus or glomerulonephritis.	Meningococcal vaccine and appropriate antibiotics.

- **Complement deficiencies:** Present in children with congenital asplenia or splenic dysfunction (sickle cell disease). Characterized by recurrent **bacterial** infections with **encapsulated organisms.**

Kawasaki Disease

Untreated Kawasaki disease can → coronary aneurysms.

A multisystemic acute vasculitis that primarily affects young children (80% are < 5 years of age), particularly those of Asian ancestry. Divided into acute, subacute, and chronic phases.

DIAGNOSIS

- **Acute phase:** Lasts 1–2 weeks and presents with the following symptoms (fever plus ≥ 4 of the criteria below are required for diagnosis):
    - Fever (usually > 40°C) for at least **five** days.
    - Bilateral, nonexudative, painless conjunctivitis.
    - Polymorphous rash (primarily truncal).
    - Cervical lymphadenopathy (often unilateral, with at least one node > 1.5 cm).
    - Diffuse mucous membrane erythema (e.g., "strawberry tongue").
    - Erythema of the palms and soles; indurative edema of the hands and feet; late desquamation of the fingertips (in subacute phase).
    - Other manifestations include sterile pyuria, gallbladder hydrops, hepatitis, and arthritis.

- **Subacute phase:** Begins after the abatement of fever and typically lasts for an additional 2–3 weeks. Subacute-phase manifestations are thrombocytosis and elevated ESR. Untreated children may begin to develop coronary artery aneurysms (40%); all patients should be assessed by echocardiography at diagnosis.
- **Chronic phase:** Begins when all clinical symptoms have disappeared, and lasts until ESR returns to baseline. **Untreated children are at risk of aneurysmal expansion and MI.**

TREATMENT

- High-dose aspirin (for inflammation and fever) and IVIG (to prevent aneurysms).
- Low-dose aspirin is then continued, usually for six weeks. Children who develop coronary aneurysms may require chronic anticoagulation with aspirin or other antiplatelet medications.
- Corticosteroids may be used in IVIG-refractory cases—**routine use is not recommended.**
- Consult a pediatric cardiologist to guide management.

> *Kawasaki disease symptoms—*
>
> ***"CRASH AND BURN"***
>
> **C**onjunctivitis
> **R**ash
> **A**denopathy
> **S**trawberry tongue
> **H**ands and feet (red, swollen, flaky skin)
> **B**urn (fever > 40°C for ≥ 5 days)

Juvenile Rheumatoid Arthritis (JRA)

An autoimmune disorder manifesting as arthritis with "morning stiffness" and gradual loss of motion that is present for at least six weeks in a patient < 16 years of age.

DIAGNOSIS

- **Pauciarticular (oligoarthritis):** Most common; ≤ 4 joints involved; usually ANA ⊕ and RF ⊖. Involves young females; **uveitis** is common and requires slit-lamp exam for evaluation; no systemic symptoms.
- **Polyarthritis:** Involves ≥ 5 joints. RF ⊕ is rare and indicates severe disease; younger children may be ANA ⊕ with milder disease. Systemic symptoms are rare.
- **Systemic-onset (Still's disease):** May present with recurrent high fever (usually > 39°C), hepatosplenomegaly, and rash; usually RF ⊖ and ANA ⊖.

TREATMENT

- NSAIDs.
- Steroids and immunosuppressive medications are second-line agents.
- Steroids are used if there is carditis.

INFECTIOUS DISEASE

Childhood Vaccinations

Table 2.13-6 summarizes recommended childhood immunizations. Contraindications and precautions are as follows:

- **Contraindications:**
  - Severe allergy to a vaccine component or a prior dose of vaccine.
  - Encephalopathy within seven days of prior pertussis vaccination.
  - Avoid live vaccines (oral polio vaccine, varicella, MMR) in immunocompromised and pregnant patients (exception: HIV patients may receive MMR and varicella).

TABLE 2.13-6. Immunization Schedule

Vaccine	Birth	2 Months	4 Months	6 Months	12–15 Months	15–18 Months	2 Years	4–6 Years	11–12 Years
HBV	X	X		X					
DTaP		X	X	X		X		X	
Hib		X	X	X	X				
IPV		X	X	X				X	
PPV		X	X	X	X				
MMR					X			X	
Varicella					X				
HAV							X		
Rotavirus		X	X						
Meningococcal									X
Influenza	Healthy children aged 6–23 months; other high-risk children annually.								

- Precautions:
  - Current moderate to severe illness (with or without fever).
  - Prior reactions to pertussis vaccine (fever > 40.5°C, shocklike state, persistent crying for > 3 hours within 48 hours of vaccination, or seizure within three days of vaccination).
  - A history of receiving IVIG in the past year.
- The following are **not** contraindications to vaccination:
  - Mild illness and/or low-grade fever.
  - Current antibiotic therapy.
  - Prematurity.

RSV is the most common cause of bronchiolitis.

Bronchiolitis

An acute inflammatory illness of the small airways that primarily affects infants and children < 2 years of age. **RSV is the most common cause.** Progression to respiratory failure is a potentially fatal complication. For severe RSV, risk factors include age < 6 months, male gender, prematurity, heart or lung disease, and immunodeficiency.

HISTORY/PE

- Presents with low-grade fever, rhinorrhea, cough, and apnea (in young infants).
- Exam reveals **tachypnea, wheezing,** crackles, prolonged expiration, and hyperresonance to percussion.

- CXR reveals hyperinflation of the lungs, interstitial infiltrates, and atelectasis.
- ELISA of nasal washings for RSV is highly sensitive and specific.

TREATMENT

- Treat mild disease with outpatient management using fluids and nebulizers if needed.
- Hospitalize in the setting of marked respiratory distress, O_2 saturation of < 92%, toxic appearance, dehydration/poor oral feeding, a history of prematurity (< 34 weeks), age < 3 months, underlying cardiopulmonary disease, or unreliable parents.
- Treat inpatients with contact isolation, hydration, and O_2. A trial of aerosolized albuterol may be attempted; continue albuterol therapy if effective.
- RSV prophylaxis with injectable poly- or monoclonal antibodies (RespiGam or Synagis) is recommended in winter for high-risk patients ≤ 2 years of age (e.g., those with a history of prematurity, chronic lung disease, or congenital heart disease).

Croup (Laryngotracheobronchitis)

An acute viral inflammatory disease of the larynx, primarily within the subglottic space. Pathogens include parainfluenza virus type 1 (most common), 2, and 3; RSV; influenza; and adenovirus. Bacterial superinfection may progress to tracheitis.

HISTORY/PE

Prodromal URI symptoms are typically followed by low-grade fever, mild dyspnea, inspiratory stridor that worsens with agitation, a hoarse voice, and a characteristic barking cough (usually at night).

DIAGNOSIS

- Clinical impression; often based on degree of stridor and respiratory distress.
- AP neck film may show the **classic "steeple sign" from subglottic narrowing** (see Figure 2.13-2), but the finding is **neither sensitive nor specific.**
- Table 2.13-7 differentiates croup from epiglottitis and tracheitis.

TREATMENT

- **Mild cases:** Outpatient management with cool mist therapy and fluids.
- **Moderate cases:** May require oral and IM corticosteroids and nebulized racemic epinephrine.
- **Severe cases** (e.g., respiratory distress at rest, inspiratory stridor): Hospitalize and give nebulized racemic epinephrine.

Epiglottitis

A serious and rapidly progressive infection of supraglottic structures (e.g., the epiglottis and aryepiglottic folds). Prior to immunization, *H. influenzae* type b was the 1° pathogen. Common causes now include *Streptococcus* spp., nontypable *H. influenzae*, and viral agents.

Epiglottitis can → life-threatening airway obstruction.

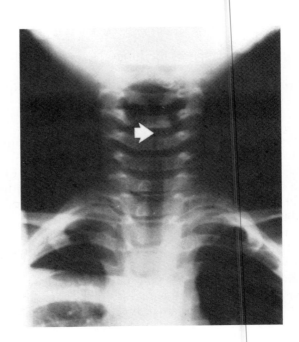

FIGURE 2.13-2. Croup.

The x-ray shows marked subglottic narrowing of the airway ("steeple sign"). (Reproduced, with permission, from Saunders CE. *Current Emergency Diagnosis & Treatment*, 4th ed. Stamford, CT: Appleton & Lange, 1992, p. 448.)

TABLE 2.13-7. Characteristics of Croup, Epiglottitis, and Tracheitis

	CROUP	EPIGLOTTITIS	TRACHEITIS
Age group affected	3 months to 3 years	3–7 years	3 months to 2 years
Incidence in children presenting with stridor	88%	8%	2%
Pathogen	Parainfluenza virus	*H. influenzae*	Often *S. aureus*
Onset	Prodrome (1–7 days)	Rapid (4–12 hours)	Prodrome (3 days) → acute decompensation (10 hours)
Fever severity	Low grade	High grade	Intermediate grade
Associated symptoms	Barking cough, hoarseness	Muffled voice, drooling	Variable respiratory distress
Position preference	None	Seated, neck extended	None
Response to racemic epinephrine	Stridor improves	None	None
CXR findings	"Steeple sign" on AP film	"Thumbprint sign'" on lateral film	Subglottic narrowing

HISTORY/PE

- Presents with acute-onset high fever (39–40°C), dysphagia, drooling, muffled voice, inspiratory retractions, cyanosis, and soft stridor.
- Patients sit with the neck hyperextended and the chin protruding ("sniffing dog" position) and lean forward in a "tripod" position to maximize air entry.
- Untreated infection can → life-threatening airway obstruction and respiratory arrest.

DIAGNOSIS

- Clinical impression. The differential diagnosis must include diffuse and localized causes of airway obstruction (see Tables 2.13-7 and 2.13-8).
- **The airway must be secured before definitive diagnosis.** In light of potential laryngospasm and airway compromise, **do not examine the throat unless an anesthesiologist or otolaryngologist is present.**
- Definitive diagnosis is made via direct fiberoptic visualization of a cherry-red, swollen epiglottis and arytenoids.
- Lateral x-ray shows a swollen epiglottis obliterating the valleculae ("thumbprint sign"; see Figure 2.13-3).

TREATMENT

- This disease is a true emergency. Keep the patient (and parents) calm, call anesthesia, and transfer the patient to the OR.
- Treat with endotracheal intubation or tracheostomy and IV antibiotics (ceftriaxone or cefuroxime).

TABLE 2.13-8. Comparison of Retropharyngeal Abscess and Peritonsillar Abscess

	RETROPHARYNGEAL ABSCESS	PERITONSILLAR ABSCESS
Age group affected	Six months to six years.	Usually > 10 years of age.
History/PE	Muffled "hot potato" voice; trismus; drooling; cervical lymphadenopathy. Usually unilateral; may see mass in the posterior pharyngeal wall on visual inspection.	Muffled "hot potato" voice; trismus; drooling; displacement of the affected tonsil medially and laterally.
Pathogen	Group A streptococcus (most common); *S. aureus*; *Bacteroides*.	Group A streptococcus (most common); *S. aureus*; *S. pneumoniae*; anaerobes.
Preferred position	Supine with the neck extended (sitting up or flexing the neck worsens symptoms).	None.
Diagnosis	On lateral neck x-ray, the soft tissue plane should be ≤ 50% of the width of the corresponding vertebral body. Contrast CT of the neck helps differentiate abscess from cellulitis.	Usually clinical.
Treatment	Aspiration or incision and drainage of abscess; antibiotics.	Incision and drainage +/– tonsillectomy; antibiotics.

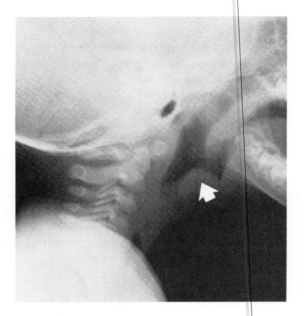

FIGURE 2.13-3. **Epiglottitis.**

The classic swollen epiglottis ("thumbprint sign"; arrow) and obstructed airway are seen on lateral neck x-ray. (Reproduced, with permission, from Saunders CE. *Current Emergency Diagnosis & Treatment*, 4th ed. Stamford, CT: Appleton & Lange, 1992, p. 447.)

Meningitis

Bacterial meningitis occurs most often in children under three years of age; common organisms include S. *pneumoniae,* N. *meningitidis,* and *E. coli.* Enteroviruses are the most common agents of viral meningitis and occur in children of all ages. Risk factors include sinofacial infections, trauma, and sepsis.

HISTORY/PE

- Bacterial meningitis classically presents with the triad of **headache, high fever, and nuchal rigidity.**
- Viral meningitis is typically preceded by a prodromal illness that includes fever, sore throat, and fatigue.
- Kernig's sign (pain on knee extension when the hip is flexed) and Brudzinski's sign (pain with passive neck flexion) are nonspecific signs of meningeal irritation. Additional physical exam findings may include signs of ↑ ICP (papilledema, cranial nerve palsies) or petechial rash (N. *meningitidis*).

DIAGNOSIS

- Head CT to rule out ↑ ICP (risk of brain stem herniation)
- Perform an LP; send cell count with differential, glucose and protein levels, Gram stain, and culture.

TREATMENT

- Empiric antibiotic therapy regimens (ceftriaxone, vancomycin, ampicillin) should be administered until bacterial meningitis can be excluded.
- Neonates should receive ampicillin and cefotaxime or gentamicin.
- Older children should receive ceftriaxone and vancomycin.

Pertussis

A bacterial infection caused by *Bordetella pertussis* (whooping cough), a gram-negative bacillus.

HISTORY/PE

- Has three stages: catarrhal (mild URI symptoms); paroxysmal (paroxysms of cough with inspiratory whoop and post-tussive emesis); and convalescent (symptoms wane).
- Patients most often present in the paroxysmal stage but are most contagious in the catarrhal stage.
- The classic presentation is an infant < 6 months of age with post-tussive emesis and apnea. Common sources of infection are adolescents and young adults.

DIAGNOSIS

- Labs show an elevated WBC with lymphocytosis (often ≥ 70%)
- Culture is the gold standard.

TREATMENT

- Hospitalize infants < 6 months of age.
- Give erythromycin × 14 days to patients and close contacts (including day care contacts).
- Patients should not return to school or day care until five days of antibiotics have been administered or until three weeks have elapsed if no therapy has been initiated.

Viral Exanthems

Table 2.13-9 outlines the clinical presentation of common viral exanthems.

NEONATOLOGY

Apgar Scoring

A rapid scoring system that helps evaluate the need for neonatal resuscitation. Each of five parameters (see the mnemonic **APGAR**) is assigned a score of 0–2 at one and five minutes after birth.

- Scores of 8–10 typically reflect good cardiopulmonary adaptation.
- Scores of 4–7 indicate the possible need for resuscitation. Infants should be observed, stimulated, and possibly given ventilatory support.
- Scores of 0–3 indicate the need for immediate resuscitation.

Apgar scoring—

APGAR:

Appearance (color)
Pulse (heart rate)
Grimace (reflex irritability)
Activity (muscle tone)
Respiratory effort

TABLE 2.13-9. **Viral Exanthems**

DISEASE	CAUSE	CHARACTERISTICS	COMPLICATIONS
Erythema infectiosum (fifth disease)	Parvovirus B19	**Prodrome:** None; fever is often absent or low grade. **Rash: "Slapped-cheek"** erythematous rash. An erythematous, pruritic, maculopapular rash starts on the arms and spreads to the trunk and legs. **Worsens with fever and sun exposure.**	Arthritis, hemolytic anemia, encephalopathy. Congenital infection is associated with fetal hydrops and death. Aplastic crisis may be precipitated in children with ↑ RBC turnover (e.g., sickle cell anemia, hereditary spherocytosis) or in those with ↓ RBC production (e.g., severe iron deficiency anemia).
Measles	Paramyxovirus	**Prodrome:** Low-grade fever with cough, coryza, and conjunctivitis (the "**3 C's**"); Koplik's spots (small irregular red spots with central gray specks) appear on the buccal mucosa after 1–2 days. **Rash:** An erythematous maculopapular rash spreads from the head toward the feet.	**Common:** Otitis media, pneumonia, laryngotracheitis. **Rare:** Subacute sclerosing panencephalitis.
Rubella	Rubella virus	**Prodrome:** Asymptomatic or tender, generalized lymphadenopathy. **Rash:** Presents with an erythematous, tender maculopapular rash that also starts on the face and spreads distally. In contrast to measles, children with rubella often have only a low-grade fever and do not appear as ill. Polyarthritis may be seen in adolescents.	Encephalitis, thrombocytopenia (rare complication of postnatal infection). Congenital infection is associated with congenital anomalies.
Roseola infantum	HHV-6	**Prodrome:** Acute onset of high fever (> 40°C); no other symptoms for 3–4 days. **Rash: A maculopapular rash appears as fever breaks** (begins on the trunk and quickly spreads to the face and extremities) and often lasts < 24 hours.	**Febrile seizures** may occur as a result of rapid fever onset.
Varicella	Varicella-zoster virus (VZV)	**Prodrome:** Mild fever, anorexia, and malaise precede the rash by 24 hours. **Rash:** Generalized, pruritic, "teardrop" vesicular periphery; lesions are often at different stages of healing. Infectious from 24 hours before eruption until lesions crust over.	Progressive varicella with meningoencephalitis and hepatitis occurs in immunocompromised children. Congenital infection is associated with congenital anomalies.

TABLE 2.13-9. Viral Exanthems (continued)

DISEASE	CAUSE	CHARACTERISTICS	COMPLICATIONS
Varicella zoster	VZV	**Prodrome:** Reactivation of varicella infection; starts as pain along an affected sensory nerve. **Rash:** Pruritic "teardrop" vesicular rash in a dermatomal distribution. Uncommon unless the patient is immunocompromised.	Encephalopathy, aseptic meningitis, pneumonitis, thrombotic thrombocytopenic purpura, Guillain-Barré syndrome, cellulitis, arthritis.
Hand-foot-and-mouth disease	Coxsackie A	**Prodrome:** Fever, anorexia, oral pain. **Rash:** Oral ulcers; maculopapular vesicular rash on the hands and feet and sometimes on the buttocks.	None (self-limited).

Congenital Malformations

Table 2.13-10 describes selected congenital malformations.

Neonatal Jaundice

Elevated serum bilirubin concentration (> 5 mg/dL) due to ↑ hemolysis or ↓ excretion. Subtypes are as follows:

- **Conjugated (direct) hyperbilirubinemia:** Always pathologic.
- **Unconjugated (indirect) hyperbilirubinemia:** May be physiologic or pathologic. See Table 2.13-11 for differentiating characteristics.
- **Kernicterus:** A complication of unconjugated hyperbilirubinemia that results from irreversible bilirubin deposition in the basal ganglia, pons, and cerebellum. It typically occurs at levels of > 25–30 mg/dL and can be fatal. Risk factors include prematurity, asphyxia, and sepsis.

Direct hyperbilirubinemia is always pathologic.

HISTORY/PE

- The differential includes the following:
    - **Conjugated:** Extrahepatic cholestasis (biliary atresia, choledochal cysts), intrahepatic cholestasis (neonatal hepatitis, inborn errors of metabolism, TPN cholestasis), ToRCHeS infections (see the Infectious Disease section).
    - **Unconjugated:** Physiologic jaundice, hemolysis, breast milk jaundice, ↑ enterohepatic circulation (e.g., GI obstruction), disorders of bilirubin metabolism, sepsis.
- The history should focus on diet (breast milk or formula), intrauterine drug exposure, and family history (hemoglobinopathies, enzyme deficiencies, or RBC defects).
- Physical exam may reveal signs of hepatic or GI dysfunction (abdominal distention, delayed passage of meconium, light-colored stools, dark urine), infection, or hemoglobinopathies (cephalohematomas, bruising, pallor, petechiae, and hepatomegaly).
- **Kernicterus** presents with lethargy, poor feeding, a high-pitched cry, hypertonicity, and seizures; jaundice may follow a cephalopedal progression as bilirubin concentrations ↑.

TABLE 2.13-10. **Selected Congenital Malformations**

MALFORMATION	PRESENTATION/DIAGNOSIS/TREATMENT
Tracheoesophageal fistula	Tract between the trachea and esophagus. Associated with defects such as esophageal atresia and **VACTERL** (**V**ertebral, **A**nal, **C**ardiac, **T**racheal, **E**sophageal, **R**enal, **L**imb) anomalies. **Presentation:** Polyhydramnios in utero, ↑ oral secretions, inability to feed, gagging, respiratory distress. **Diagnosis:** CXR showing an NG tube coiled in the esophagus identifies esophageal atresia. The presence of air in the GI tract is suggestive; confirm with bronchoscopy. **Treatment:** Surgical repair.
Congenital diaphragmatic hernia	GI tract segments protrude through the diaphragm into the thorax; 90% are posterior left (Bochdalek). **Presentation:** Respiratory distress (from pulmonary hypoplasia and pulmonary hypertension); sunken abdomen; bowel sounds over the left hemithorax. **Diagnosis:** Ultrasound in utero; confirmed by postnatal CXR. **Treatment:** High-frequency ventilation or extracorporeal membrane oxygenation to manage pulmonary hypertension; surgical repair.
Gastroschisis	Herniation of the intestine only through the abdominal wall next to the umbilicus (usually on the right) with no sac. **Presentation:** Polyhydramnios in utero; often premature; associated with GI stenoses or atresia. **Treatment:** A surgical emergency! Single-stage closure is possible in only 10% of cases.
Omphalocele	Herniation of abdominal viscera through the abdominal wall at the umbilicus into a sac covered by peritoneum and amniotic membrane. **Presentation/diagnosis:** Polyhydramnios in utero; often premature; associated with other GI and cardiac defects. Seen in Beckwith-Wiedemann syndrome and trisomies. **Treatment:** C-section can prevent sac rupture; if the sac is intact, postpone surgical correction until the patient is fully resuscitated. Keep the sac covered/stable with petroleum and gauze. Intermittent NG suction to prevent abdominal distention.
Duodenal atresia	Complete or partial failure of the duodenal lumen to recanalize during gestational weeks 8–10. **Presentation:** Polyhydramnios in utero; bilious emesis within hours after first feeding; associated with Down syndrome and other cardiac/GI anomalies (e.g., annular pancreas, malrotation, imperforate anus). **Diagnosis:** Abdominal radiographs show the **"double-bubble"** sign (air bubbles in the stomach and duodenum) proximal to the site of the atresia. **Treatment:** Surgical repair.

DIAGNOSIS

- CBC with peripheral blood smear; blood typing of mother and infant (for ABO or Rh incompatibility); Coombs' test and bilirubin levels.
- Ultrasound and/or HIDA scan can confirm suspected cholestatic disease.
- For direct hyperbilirubinemia, check LFTs, bile acids, blood cultures, sweat test, and tests for aminoacidopathies and α_1-antitrypsin deficiency.
- A jaundiced neonate who is febrile, hypotensive, and/or tachypneic needs a full sepsis workup and ICU monitoring.

TABLE 2.3.11. Physiologic vs. Pathologic Jaundice

PHYSIOLOGIC JAUNDICE	PATHOLOGIC JAUNDICE
Not present until 72 hours after birth.	Present in the first 24 hours of life.
Bilirubin ↑ < 5 mg/dL/day.	Bilirubin ↑ > 0.5 mg/dL/hour.
Bilirubin peaks at < 14–15 mg/dL.	Bilirubin ↑ to > 15 mg/dL.
Direct bilirubin is < 10% of total.	Direct bilirubin is > 10% of total.
Resolves by one week in term infants and two weeks in preterm infants.	Persists beyond one week in term infants and two weeks in preterm infants.

TREATMENT

- Treat underlying causes (e.g., infection).
- Treat unconjugated hyperbilirubinemia with **phototherapy** (for mild elevations) or **exchange transfusion** (for severe elevations). Start phototherapy earlier (10–15 mg/dL) for preterm infants. Phototherapy with conjugated hyperbilirubinemia can → skin bronzing.

Respiratory Distress Syndrome (RDS)

The most common cause of respiratory failure in preterm infants (affects > 70% of infants born at 28–30 weeks' gestation). Surfactant deficiency → poor lung compliance and atelectasis. Risk factors include maternal DM, male gender, and the second born of twins.

HISTORY/PE

Presents in the first 48–72 hours of life with a respiratory rate > 60/min, progressive hypoxemia, cyanosis, nasal flaring, intercostal retractions, and expiratory grunting.

DIAGNOSIS

- Check ABGs, CBC, and blood cultures to rule out infection.
- Diagnosis is based mainly on characteristic CXR findings:
  - **RDS:** "Ground-glass" appearance and **air bronchograms** on CXR.
  - **Transient tachypnea of the newborn:** Retained amniotic fluid → prominent perihilar streaking in interlobular fissures.
  - **Meconium aspiration:** Coarse, irregular infiltrates; hyperexpansion and pneumothoraces.
  - **Congenital pneumonia:** Nonspecific patchy infiltrates; neutropenia, tracheal aspirate, and Gram stain suggest the diagnosis.

TREATMENT

- Continuous positive airway pressure (CPAP) or intubation and mechanical ventilation.
- Artificial surfactant administration ↓ mortality.

RDS is the most common cause of respiratory failure in preterm infants.

- Pretreat mothers at risk for preterm delivery with corticosteroids; monitor fetal lung maturity via lecithin-sphingomyelin ratio and phosphatidylglycerol.

COMPLICATIONS

Persistent PDA and bronchopulmonary dysplasia. Retinopathy of prematurity, intraventricular hemorrhage, and necrotizing enterocolitis are complications of treatment.

Cerebral Palsy

A range of nonhereditary disorders of movement and posture; the most common movement disorder in children. In most cases the cause in unknown, but it often results from perinatal neurologic insult. Risk factors include low birth weight, intrauterine exposure to maternal infection, prematurity, perinatal asphyxia, trauma, brain malformation, and neonatal cerebral hemorrhage. Categories include the following:

- **Pyramidal (spastic):** Spastic paresis of any or all limbs. Accounts for 75% of cases. Mental retardation is present in up to 90% of cases.
- **Extrapyramidal (dyskinetic):** A result of damage to extrapyramidal tracts. Subtypes are ataxic (difficulty coordinating purposeful movements), choreoathetoid, and dystonic (uncontrollable jerking, writhing, or posturing). Abnormal movements worsen with stress and disappear during sleep.

HISTORY/PE

- May be associated with seizure disorders, behavioral disorders, hearing or vision impairment, learning disabilities, and speech deficits.
- Affected limbs may show hyperreflexia, pathologic reflexes (e.g., Babinski), ↑ tone/contractures, weakness, and/or underdevelopment.
- Toe walking and scissor gait are common. Hip dislocations and scoliosis may be seen.

DIAGNOSIS

Clinical impression. Ultrasound or CT may be useful in infants to identify intracranial hemorrhage or structural malformations. MRI is diagnostic in older children. EEG may be useful in patients with seizures.

TREATMENT

- Special education, physical therapy, braces, and surgical release of contractures may help.
- Treat spasticity with diazepam, dantrolene, or baclofen. Baclofen pumps and posterior rhizotomy may alleviate severe contractures.

Febrile Seizures

Usually occur in children between six months and five years of age who have no evidence of intracranial infection or other cause. Risk factors include a rapid ↑ in temperature and a history of febrile seizures in a close relative. Febrile seizures recur in 30% of patients.

HISTORY/PE

- Seizures usually occur during the onset of fever and may be the first sign of an underlying illness (e.g., otitis media, roseola).
- Classified as simple or complex:
    - **Simple:** A short-duration (< 15-minute), generalized seizure with one seizure in a 24-hour period. High fever (> 39°C) and fever onset within hours of the seizure are typical.
    - **Complex:** A long-duration (> 15-minute) or focal seizure, or multiple seizures in a 24-hour period. Low-grade fever for several days before seizure onset may be present.

DIAGNOSIS

- Focus on finding a source of infection. LP is indicated if there are clinical signs of CNS infection (e.g., altered consciousness, meningismus, tense/bulging anterior fontanelle) after ruling out ↑ ICP.
- No lab studies are needed if presentation is consistent with febrile seizures in children > 18 months of age.
- For atypical presentations, obtain electrolytes, serum glucose, blood cultures, UA, and CBC with differential.
- The utility of EEG and MRI in evaluating complex febrile seizures is controversial. Children presenting with complex seizures may be at ↑ risk of developing seizure disorders.

Perform LP if CNS infection is suspected in a patient with a febrile seizure.

TREATMENT

- Use antipyretic therapy (avoid aspirin in light of the risk of Reye's syndrome) and treat any underlying illness. Note that antipyretic therapy does not ↓ the occurrence of febrile seizures.
- For complex seizures, perform a thorough neurologic evaluation. Chronic anticonvulsant therapy (e.g., diazepam or phenobarbital) may be necessary.

ONCOLOGY

Leukemia

A hematopoietic malignancy of lymphocytic or myeloblastic origin. The most common childhood malignancy; 97% of cases are acute leukemias (ALL > AML). ALL is most common in male Caucasian children between two and five years of age; AML is seen most frequently in male African-American children throughout childhood. Associated with trisomy 21, Fanconi's anemia, prior radiation, severe combined immunodeficiency, and congenital bone marrow failure states.

ALL is the most common childhood malignancy.

HISTORY/PE

- Symptoms are abrupt in onset.
- Symptoms are initially nonspecific (anorexia, fatigue) and are followed by bone pain, fever (from neutropenia), anemia, ecchymoses, petechiae, and/or hepatosplenomegaly.
- CNS metastases may be associated with headache, vomiting, and papilledema.
- AML can present with a chloroma, a greenish soft-tissue tumor on the skin or spinal cord.

DIAGNOSIS

■ CBC, coagulation studies, and peripheral blood smear (high numbers of blast cells).
■ Obtain a bone marrow aspirate for immunophenotyping and genetic analysis, which can help confirm the diagnosis.
■ CXR to rule out a mediastinal mass.

TREATMENT

Chemotherapy based; tumor lysis syndrome (hyperkalemia, hyperuricemia) is common prior to and during the initiation of treatment.

Watch for tumor lysis syndrome at the onset of any chemotherapy regimen.

Neuroblastoma

An embryonal tumor of neural crest origin. More than half of patients are < 2 years of age, and 70% of patients have distant metastases at presentation. Associated with neurofibromatosis, Hirschsprung's disease, and the N-myc oncogene.

HISTORY/PE

■ Lesion sites are most commonly abdominal, thoracic, and cervical (in descending order).
■ Symptoms may vary with location and may include a **nontender** abdominal mass (may cross the midline), Horner's syndrome, hypertension, or cord compression (from a paraspinal tumor).
■ Patients may have anemia, FTT, and fever.
■ Site-specific metastases may → bone marrow suppression, proptosis, hepatomegaly, subcutaneous nodules, and opsoclonus/myoclonus.

DIAGNOSIS

■ CT scan; fine-needle aspirate of tumor.
■ Elevated 24-hour urinary catecholamines (VMA and HVA).
■ Bone marrow aspirate; BUN/creatinine.

TREATMENT

Local excision plus postsurgical chemotherapy and/or radiation.

Wilms' Tumor

A renal tumor of embryonal origin that is most commonly seen in children 2–5 years of age. Associated with Beckwith-Wiedemann syndrome (hemihypertrophy, macroglossia, visceromegaly), neurofibromatosis, and WAGR syndrome (**W**ilms', **A**niridia, **G**enitourinary abnormalities, mental **R**etardation).

Wilms' tumor is associated with aniridia and hemihypertrophy.

HISTORY/PE

■ Presents as an **asymptomatic, nontender,** smooth abdominal mass.
■ Abdominal pain, fever, hypertension, and microscopic or gross hematuria are seen.

DIAGNOSIS

■ CBC, BUN, creatinine, and UA.

- Abdominal ultrasound.
- CT scans of the chest and abdomen are used to detect metastases.

TREATMENT

Local resection with postsurgical chemotherapy and radiation depending on stage and histology.

Ewing's Sarcoma

A sarcoma of neuroectodermal origin. Arises in bone; most commonly seen in **Caucasian male adolescents.** Associated with a chromosome 11:22 translocation.

HISTORY/PE

- Symptoms include local pain and swelling.
- Tumors commonly target the **midshaft** of long bones—the femur, pelvis, fibula, and humerus (in descending order).
- **Systemic manifestations** (fever, anorexia, fatigue) are common in children with metastases.

DIAGNOSIS

- Labs reveal leukocytosis and elevated ESR.
- A lytic bone lesion ("onion skin" appearance if the tumor penetrates through the cortex) or a soft tissue can be seen on x-ray.

TREATMENT

Local excision plus chemotherapy and radiation.

Osteosarcoma

A tumor arising from osteoblasts of mesenchymal origin. Most commonly seen in **male adolescents.**

HISTORY/PE

- Presents with local pain and swelling; physical exam can show a palpable mass and ↓ range of motion.
- **Systemic symptoms** are **rare.**
- The most common tumor sites are the **metaphyses of long bones**—the distal femur, proximal tibia, and proximal humerus. Metastases to the lung occur in 20% of patients.

DIAGNOSIS

- Obtain CBC, BUN, creatinine, UA, and LDH (an elevated LDH has poor prognostic significance).
- Elevated serum alkaline phosphatase.
- **"Sunburst" lytic bone lesions** are seen on CT and/or MRI.
- Obtain a chest CT to rule out pulmonary metastases.

TREATMENT

Local resection plus postsurgical chemotherapy to treat micrometastases.

Psychiatry

Generalized Anxiety Disorder

- Uncontrollable, excessive anxiety or worry about activities or events in life → significant impairment or distress.
- The male-to-female ratio is 1:2; clinical onset is usually in the early 20s.
- Hx/PE: Presents with anxiety on most days (**six or more months**) and with **three or more somatic symptoms** (restlessness, fatigue, difficulty concentrating, irritability, muscle tension, disturbed sleep).
- Tx:
    - Lifestyle changes, psychotherapy, medication. SSRIs, venlafaxine, and buspirone are most often used (see Table 2.14-1). Benzodiazepines may be used for immediate symptom relief.
    - Taper benzodiazepines as soon as long-term treatment (e.g., with SSRIs), is initiated given the high risk of tolerance and dependence.
    - Patient education is essential.

Obsessive-Compulsive Disorder (OCD)

- Characterized by obsessions and/or compulsions that → significant distress and dysfunction in social or personal areas.
- Typically presents in late adolescence or early adulthood; prevalence is equal in males and females. Often a chronic condition that is difficult to treat.
- Hx/PE:
    - **Obsessions: Persistent, unwanted, and intrusive ideas, thoughts, impulses, or images** that → marked anxiety or distress (e.g., fear of contamination, fear of harm to oneself or to loved ones) and occur despite the patient's attempts to prevent them.
    - **Compulsions: Repeated mental acts or behaviors** that neutralize anxiety from obsessions (e.g., hand washing, elaborate rituals for ordinary tasks, counting, excessive checking).

Many OCD patients initially present to a nonpsychiatrist— e.g., seeing a dermatologist with a skin complaint 2° to overwashing hands.

TABLE 2.14-1. Anxiolytic Medications

Drug Class	Indications	Side Effects
SSRIs (fluoxetine, sertraline, paroxetine, citalopram, escitalopram)	First-line treatment for generalized anxiety disorder, OCD, and PTSD.	Nausea, GI upset, somnolence, sexual dysfunction, agitation.
Buspirone	Generalized anxiety disorder, OCD, PTSD.	Seizures with chronic use. No tolerance, dependence, or withdrawal.
β-blockers	Performance anxiety, PTSD.	Bradycardia, hypotension.
Benzodiazepines	Anxiety, insomnia, alcohol withdrawal, muscle spasm.	↓ sleep duration; risk of abuse, tolerance, and dependence.
Flumazenil	Antidote to benzodiazepine intoxication.	Resedation; nausea, dizziness, vomiting, and pain at the injection site.

- Patients **recognize these behaviors as excessive and irrational products of their own minds** (vs. obsessive-compulsive personality disorder, or OCPD; see Table 2.14-2). Patients wish they could get rid of the obsessions and/or compulsions.
- **Tx:** Pharmacotherapy (clomipramine or SSRIs; see Table 2.14-1) and cognitive-behavioral therapy (CBT) using exposure and desensitization relaxation techniques. Patient education is imperative.

Panic Disorder

- Characterized by recurrent, unexpected panic attacks.
- Two to three times more common in females than in males. **Agoraphobia** is present in 30–50% of cases. Average age of onset is 25, but may occur at any age.
- Hx/PE:
    - **Panic attacks:** Discrete **periods of intense fear or discomfort** in which at least four of the following symptoms develop abruptly and peak within 10 minutes: chest pain, **palpitations, diaphoresis,** nausea, tachypnea, trembling, dizziness, **fear of dying** or "going crazy," depersonalization, or hot flashes.
    - Patients present with **one or more months** of concern about having additional attacks or significant behavior change as a result of the attacks—e.g., avoiding situations that may precipitate attacks.
    - **Elucidate if a patient has panic disorder with or without agoraphobia.**
- Tx:
    - CBT, pharmacotherapy (e.g., SSRIs, TCAs).
    - Benzodiazepines (e.g., clonazepam) may be used for immediate relief, but avoid long-term use because of the potential for addiction and tolerance (see Table 2.14-1).
    - Taper benzodiazepine as soon as long-term treatment (e.g., SSRIs) is initiated.

Agoraphobia:
- *Defined as fear of being alone in public places.*
- *May be diagnosed alone or as panic disorder with agoraphobia.*

Phobias (Social and Specific)

- Defined as follows:
    - **Social phobia:** Characterized by marked fear provoked by **social or performance situations** in which embarrassment may occur. It may be specific (e.g., public speaking, urinating in public) or general (e.g., social interaction) and often begins in adolescence.
    - **Specific phobia:** Anxiety is provoked by exposure to a **feared object or situation** (e.g., animals, heights, airplanes). Most cases begin in childhood.

TABLE 2.14-2. OCD vs. OCPD

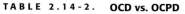

OCD	OCPD
Characterized by obsessions and/or compulsions.	Patients are excessively conscientious and inflexible.
Patients **recognize** the obsessions/compulsions and want to be rid of them (ego-dystonic).	Patients **do not recognize** their behavior as problematic (ego-syntonic).

- **Hx/PE:** Excessive or unreasonable fear and/or avoidance of an object or situation that is persistent and → significant distress or impairment in function. A related history of traumatic events or panic attacks may be present. Patients recognize that their fear is excessive.
- **Tx:**
    - **Specific phobias:** **CBT** involving desensitization through incremental exposure to the feared object or situation and relaxation techniques. Other options include supportive, family, and insight-oriented psychotherapy.
    - **Social phobias:** CBT, SSRIs, low-dose benzodiazepines, or β-blockers (for performance anxiety) may be used (see Table 2.14-1).

Post-traumatic Stress Disorder (PTSD)

- Follows exposure to an extreme, life-threatening traumatic event (e.g., assault, combat, witnessing a violent crime) that evoked intense fear, helplessness, or horror.
- **Hx/PE:**
    - Characterized by **reexperiencing of the event** (e.g., nightmares), **avoidance** of stimuli associated with the trauma, **numbed responsiveness** (e.g., detachment, anhedonia), and ↑ **arousal** (e.g., hypervigilance, exaggerated startle) → significant distress or impairment in functioning.
    - Symptoms must persist for **> 1 month.**
    - Survivor guilt, irritability, poor concentration, amnesia, personality change, sleep disturbance, substance abuse, depression, and suicidality may be present.
- **Tx:**
    - SSRIs are first line; buspirone, TCAs, and MAOIs may be helpful (see Table 2.14-1).
    - Short-term agents **targeting anxiety** include β-blockers, benzodiazepines, and α_2-agonists (e.g., clonidine).
    - **Psychotherapy** and **support groups** are useful.

COGNITIVE DISORDERS

Affect memory, orientation, judgment, and attention.

Dementia

An impairment in **cognitive** functioning with **global deficits. Level of consciousness is stable.** Prevalence is highest in those > 85 years of age. The course is persistent and progressive. The most common causes are **Alzheimer's disease** (50%) and **multi-infarct dementia** (25%). Other causes are outlined in the mnemonic **DEMENTIAS.**

HISTORY/PE

Diagnostic criteria include **memory impairment and one or more** of the following:

- **Aphasia:** Language impairment.
- **Apraxia:** Inability to perform motor activities.
- **Agnosia:** Inability to recognize previously known objects.
- **Impaired executive function (problems with planning, organizing,** and **abstracting)** in the presence of a **clear sensorium.**

Causes of dementia—

DEMENTIAS

Degenerative diseases (Parkinson's, Huntington's)
Endocrine (thyroid, parathyroid, pituitary, adrenal)
Metabolic (alcohol, electrolytes, vitamin B$_{12}$ deficiency, glucose, hepatic, renal, Wilson's disease)
Exogenous (heavy metals, carbon monoxide, drugs)
Neoplasia
Trauma (subdural hematoma)
Infection (meningitis, encephalitis, endocarditis, syphilis, HIV, prion diseases, Lyme disease)
Affective disorders (pseudodementia)
Stroke/**S**tructure (vascular dementia, ischemia, vasculitis, normal pressure hydrocephalus)

- Personality, mood, and behavior changes are common (e.g., wandering and aggression).

DIAGNOSIS

- A careful history and physical is critical. Serial mini-mental status exams should be performed.
- Rule out treatable causes of dementia; obtain CBC, RPR, CMP, TFTs, HIV, B_{12}/folate, ESR, UA, and a head CT or MRI.
- Table 2.14-3 outlines key characteristics distinguishing dementia from delirium.

TREATMENT

- Provide **environmental cues** and a rigid structure for the patient's daily life.
- **Cholinesterase inhibitors** are used to treat. Low-dose **antipsychotics** may be used for agitation. **Avoid benzodiazepines,** which may worsen disinhibition and confusion.
- Family, caregiver, and patient education and support are imperative.

Delirium

An acute **disturbance of consciousness** with **altered cognition** that develops over a short period of time (usually hours to days). Children, the elderly, and hospitalized patients (e.g., **ICU psychosis**) are particularly susceptible. Major causes are outlined in the mnemonic **I WATCH DEATH.** Symptoms are potentially reversible if the underlying cause can be treated.

HISTORY/PE

- Presents with acute onset of **waxing and waning consciousness** with lucid intervals and **perceptual disturbances** (hallucinations, illusions, delusions).
- Patients may be combative, anxious, paranoid, or stuporous.
- Also characterized by a ↓ attention span and short-term memory; a reversed sleep-wake cycle; and ↑ symptoms at night (sundowning).

> **The 4 A's of dementia:**
>
> **A**mnesia
> **A**praxia
> **A**phasia
> **A**gnosia

> **Major causes of delirium—**
>
> **I WATCH DEATH**
>
> **I**nfection
> **W**ithdrawal
> **A**cute metabolic/ substance **A**buse
> **T**rauma
> **C**NS pathology
> **H**ypoxia
> **D**eficiencies
> **E**ndocrine
> **A**cute vascular/MI
> **T**oxins/drugs
> **H**eavy metals

It is common for delirium to be superimposed on dementia.

TABLE 2.14-3. **Delirium vs. Dementia**

	DELIRIUM	DEMENTIA
Level of attention	Impaired (fluctuating).	Usually alert.
Onset	Acute.	Gradual.
Course	Fluctuating from hour to hour.	Progressive deterioration.
Consciousness	Clouded.	Intact.
Hallucinations	Present (often visual or tactile).	Occur in approximately 30% of patients in highly advanced disease.
Prognosis	Reversible.	Largely irreversible, but up to 15% of cases are due to treatable causes and are reversible.

DIAGNOSIS

- Check vitals, pulse oximetry, and glucose; perform physical and neurologic exams.
- Note recent medications (insulin, anticholinergics, steroids, narcotics, or benzodiazepines), substance use, prior episodes, medical problems, signs of organ failure (kidney, liver), and infection (**occult UTI is common in the elderly**; check UA).
- Order lab and radiologic studies to identify a possible underlying cause.

TREATMENT

- **Treat underlying causes** (delirium is often reversible).
- Normalize fluids and electrolytes.
- **Optimize the sensory environment.**
- Use low-dose **antipsychotics** (e.g., haloperidol) for agitation and psychotic symptoms.
- Conservative use of **physical restraints** may be necessary to prevent harm to the patient or others.

MOOD DISORDERS

Also known as **affective disorders.**

Major Depressive Disorder

A mood disorder characterized by one or more major depressive episodes (MDEs). The **male-to-female ratio is 1:2**; lifetime prevalence ranges from 15% to 25%. Onset is usually in the mid-20s; in the elderly, prevalence ↑ with age. **Chronic illness and stress** ↑ risk. Up to 15% of patients die by suicide.

HISTORY/PE

Diagnosis requires **depressed mood or anhedonia (loss of interest/pleasure) and five or more signs/symptoms** from the **SIG E CAPS** mnemonic present **for a two-week period.** Table 2.14-4 outlines the differential diagnosis of conditions that may be mistaken for depression. Selected depression subtypes include the following:

- **Psychotic features:** Typically **mood-congruent** delusions/hallucinations.
- **Postpartum:** Occurs within one month postpartum; has a 10% incidence and a high risk of recurrence. Psychotic symptoms are common.
- **Atypical:** Characterized by weight gain, hypersomnia, and rejection sensitivity.
- **Seasonal:** Depressive episodes tend to occur during a particular season, most commonly winter. Responds well to light therapy +/− antidepressants.
- **Double depression:** MDE in a patient with dysthymia. Has a poorer prognosis than MDE alone.

TREATMENT

- **Pharmacotherapy:** Effective in 50–70% of patients. Allow 2–6 weeks to take effect; treat for ≥ 6 months (see Table 2.14-5).
- **Electroconvulsive therapy (ECT):**
  - Safe, highly effective, often lifesaving therapy that is reserved for refractory depression or psychotic depression, or if a rapid improvement in mood is needed.

Symptoms of a depressive episode—

SIG E CAPS

Sleep (hypersomnia or insomnia)
Interest (loss of interest or pleasure in activities)
Guilt (feelings of worthlessness or inappropriate guilt)
Energy (↓) or fatigue
Concentration (↓)
Appetite (↑ or ↓) or weight (↑ or ↓)
Psychomotor agitation or retardation
Suicidal ideation

MDEs can be present in major depressive disorder or in bipolar disorder types I and II.

Cheese and red wine can precipitate a hypertensive crisis when consumed while a patient is on an MAOI.

TCA toxicity—

Tri-C's:

Convulsions
Coma
Cardiac arrhythmias

TABLE 2.14-4. Differential Diagnosis of Major Depression

DISEASE	DISTINGUISHING FEATURES
Mood disorder due to a medical condition	Hypothyroidism, Parkinson's disease, CNS neoplasm, other neoplasm (e.g., pancreatic cancer), stroke (especially ACA stroke), dementias, parathyroid disorders.
Substance-induced mood disorder	Illicit drugs, alcohol, antihypertensives, corticosteroids, OCPs.
Adjustment disorder with depressed mood	A constellation of symptoms resembling an MDE occurring within three months of an identifiable stressor.
Normal bereavement	Occurs after the loss of a loved one. No severe impairment/suicidality; usually resolves in one year, but varies with cultural norms. May → major depressive disorder requiring treatment.
Dysthymia	Milder, chronic depression with depressed mood present most of the time for at least two years; often treatment resistant.

TABLE 2.14-5. Indications and Side Effects of Common Antidepressants

DRUG	INDICATIONS	SIDE EFFECTS
SSRIs Fluoxetine Sertraline Paroxetine Citalopram Fluvoxamine	Depression and anxiety.	Sexual side effects, GI distress, agitation, insomnia, tremor, diarrhea. **Serotonin syndrome** (fever, myoclonus, mental status changes, cardiovascular collapse) can occur if SSRIs are used with MAOIs.
Atypicals Bupropion Venlafaxine Mirtazapine Nefazodone Trazodone	Depression, anxiety, and chronic pain.	**Bupropion:** ↓ seizure threshold; minimal sexual side effects. **Contraindicated in bulimics.** **Venlafaxine:** Diastolic hypertension. **Mirtazapine:** Weight gain, sedation. **Nefazodone:** Sedation, headache, dry mouth. **Trazodone:** Highly sedating; priapism.
TCAs Nortriptyline Desipramine Amitriptyline Imipramine	Depression, anxiety disorder, chronic pain, migraine headaches, enuresis (imipramine).	**Lethal** with overdose owing to cardiac conduction arrhythmias. Monitor for 3–4 days in the ICU following an OD. **Anticholinergic** effects (dry mouth, constipation, urinary retention, sedation).
MAOIs Phenelzine Tranylcypromine	Depression, especially atypical.	Hypertensive crisis if taken with high-**tyramine** foods (cheese, red wine). Sexual side effects, orthostatic hypotension, weight gain.

Mixed states and mania are psychiatric emergencies 2° to impaired judgment and great risk of harm to self and others.

To diagnose a mixed affective episode, manic and depressive symptoms must be prominent most of the time for one week or more.
Irritability *is usually a prominent feature.*

> **Symptoms of mania—**
>
> **DIG FAST**
>
> **D**istractibility
> **I**nsomnia (↓ need for sleep)
> **G**randiosity (↑ self-esteem)/more **G**oal directed
> **F**light of ideas (or racing thoughts)
> **A**ctivities/psychomotor **A**gitation
> **S**exual indiscretions/ other pleasurable activities
> **T**alkativeness/pressured speech

Chronic lithium use can → hypothyroidism and nephrotoxicity. Lamotrigine can → a life-threatening skin rash.

- May also be used for mania and psychosis; usually requires 6–12 treatments.
- Adverse effects include postictal confusion, arrhythmias, headache, and **anterograde amnesia.**
- Contraindications include recent MI/stroke, intracranial mass, and high anesthetic risk (a relative contraindication).
- **Psychotherapy: Psychotherapy combined with antidepressants is more effective than either treatment alone.**
- **Phototherapy:** Effective for patients whose depression has a seasonal pattern.

Bipolar Disorders

Prevalence is approximately 1%, and the male-to-female ratio is 1:1. A family history of bipolar illness significantly ↑ risk. Average age of onset is 20, and the frequency of mood episodes tends to ↑ with age. Up to 10–15% of those affected die by suicide. Subtypes are as follows:

- **Bipolar I: At least one manic or mixed episode** (usually requiring hospitalization).
- **Bipolar II: At least one MDE and one hypomanic episode** (less intense than mania). Patients do not meet the criteria for full manic or mixed episodes.
- **Rapid cycling:** Four or more episodes (MDE, manic, mixed, or hypomanic) in one year.
- **Cyclothymic:** Chronic and less severe, with alternating periods of hypomania and moderate depression for > 2 years.

HISTORY/PE

- The mnemonic **DIG FAST** outlines the clinical presentation of mania.
- Patients may report excessive engagement in pleasurable activities (e.g., excessive spending or sexual activity), reckless behaviors, and/or psychotic features.
- **Antidepressant use may trigger manic episodes.**

DIAGNOSIS

- A manic episode is **one week or more** of **persistently elevated, expansive, or irritable mood** plus **three DIG FAST symptoms. Psychotic symptoms** are common in mania.
- Symptoms are not due to a substance or medical condition and → significant impairment socially, occupationally, or familially.
- Hypomania is similar but does not involve marked functional impairment or psychotic symptoms and does not require hospitalization.

TREATMENT

- **Mania:** Antipsychotics (see Table 2.14-6) and mood stabilizers (see Table 2.14-7). Benzodiazepines may be useful in refractory agitation.
- **Bipolar depression:** Mood stabilizers +/− antidepressants. **Start mood stabilizers first** (see Table 2.14-7) to avoid inducing mania. ECT may be used to treat refractory cases.

PERSONALITY DISORDERS

Personality can be defined as an individual's set of emotional and behavioral traits, which are generally stable and predictable. Personality disorders are de-

TABLE 2.14-6. Antipsychotic Medications

Drug Class	Indications	Side Effects
Typical antipsychotics Haloperidol Droperidol Fluphenazine Thioridazine Chlorpromazine	Psychotic disorders, acute agitation, acute mania, Tourette's syndrome.	**Extrapyramidal symptoms** (EPS): **See Table 2.14-8.** **Hyperprolactinemia.** **Anticholinergic effects:** Dry mouth, urinary retention, constipation. Seizures, hypotension, sedation, and QTc prolongation. **Thioridazine:** Irreversible retinal pigmentation. **Neuroleptic malignant syndrome:** Fever, muscle rigidity, autonomic instability, clouded consciousness. **Stop medication;** provide supportive care in the **ICU;** administer **dantrolene** or **bromocriptine (see Table 2.14-8).**
Atypical antipsychotics Clozapine Risperidone Quetiapine Olanzapine Ziprasidone Aripiprazole	Currently first-line treatment for schizophrenia given fewer EPS and anticholinergic effects. Clozapine is reserved for severe treatment resistance and severe tardive dyskinesia.	Weight gain, type 2 DM, somnolence, sedation, and QTc prolongation. **Clozapine: Agranulocytosis** requiring weekly CBC monitoring.

fined when one's traits become chronically rigid and maladaptive, and affect most aspects of one's life (see the mnemonic **MEDIC**). Onset occurs by early adulthood. These are defined under Axis II. Specific disorders are outlined in Table 2.14-9.

TABLE 2.14-7. Mood Stabilizers

Drug Class	Indications	Side Effects
Lithium	Mood stabilizer. Used for acute mania (in combination with antipsychotics); prophylaxis in bipolar disorders; and augmentation in depression treatment.	Thirst, polyuria, diabetes insipidus, tremor, weight gain, hypothyroidism, nausea, diarrhea, seizures, teratogenicity (if used in the first trimester), acne, vomiting. Narrow threapeutic window. **Lithium toxicity:** ataxia, dysarthria, and delirium.
Carbamazepine	Second-line mood stabilizer; anticonvulsant.	Nausea, skin rash, leukopenia, AV block. Rarely, aplastic anemia (monitor CBC biweekly). Stevens-Johnson syndrome.
Valproic acid	Bipolar disorder; anticonvulsant.	GI (nausea, vomiting), tremor, sedation, alopecia, weight gain. Rarely, pancreatitis, thrombocytopenia, fatal hepatotoxicity, and agranulocytosis.
Lamotrigine	Second-line mood stabilizer; anticonvulsant.	Blurred vision, GI distress, Stevens-Johnson syndrome.

TABLE 2.14-8. Extrapyramidal Symptoms and Treatment

EPS	DESCRIPTION	TREATMENT
Acute dystonia	Involuntary muscle contraction or spasm (e.g., torticollis, oculogyric crisis).	Anticholinergics (benztropine or diphenhydramine); to prevent, administer these medications prophylactically.
Akathisia	Subjective/objective restlessness, which is perceived as being distressing.	↓ neuroleptic and try β-blockers (propranolol). Benzodiazepines or anticholinergics may help.
Dyskinesia	Pseudoparkinsonism (e.g., shuffling gait, cogwheel rigidity).	Give an anticholinergic (benztropine) or a dopamine agonist (amantadine). ↓ dose of neuroleptic or discontinue (if tolerated).
Tardive dyskinesia	Stereotypic oral-facial movements. Likely from dopamine receptor sensitization. Often irreversible (50%).	Discontinue or ↓ the dose of neuroleptic; attempt treatment with more appropriate drugs; and consider changing neuroleptic (e.g., to clozapine or risperidone). **Giving anticholinergics or decreasing neuroleptics may initially worsen tardive dyskinesia.**

Characteristics of personality disorders—

MEDIC

Maladaptive
Enduring
Deviates from cultural norms
Inflexible
Causes impairment in social or occupational functioning

DIAGNOSIS

- Ask about attitudes, mood variability, activities, and reaction to stress.
- Patients have chronic problems dealing with responsibilities, roles, and stressors. They may also deny their behavior, have difficulty understanding the cause of their problems, have difficulty changing their behavior patterns, and frequently refuse psychiatric care.

TREATMENT

- **Psychotherapy** is the mainstay of therapy.
- **Pharmacotherapy** is reserved for cases with comorbid mood, anxiety, or psychotic disorders.

PSYCHOTIC DISORDERS

Evolution of EPS:

4 hours: Acute dystonia
4 days: Akinesia
4 weeks: Akathisia
4 months: Tardive dyskinesia

Schizophrenia

Characterized by hallucinations, delusions, disordered thoughts, behavioral disturbances, and disrupted social functioning with a clear sensorium. Prevalence is approximately 1%; the male-to-female ratio is 1:1. **Peak onset is earlier in males (ages 18–25) than in females (ages 25–35)**; has an ↑ incidence in those born in winter or early spring. Schizophrenia in first-degree relatives also ↑ risk. Etiologic theories focus on neurotransmitter abnormalities such as dopamine dysregulation (frontal hypoactivity; limbic hyperactivity; efficacy of dopamine antagonists) and brain abnormalities on CT and MRI (enlarged ventricles and ↓ cortical volume). **Ten percent of those affected commit suicide.** Subtypes are as follows:

- **Paranoid:** Delusions (often of persecution of the patient) and/or hallucinations are present. Cognitive function is usually preserved. Associated with the best overall prognosis.

TABLE 2.14-9.   Signs and Symptoms of Personality Disorders

Cluster	Disorders	Characteristics	Clinical Dilemma/Strategy
Cluster A: **"weird"**	Paranoid	Distrustful, suspicious; interpret others' motives as malevolent.	Patients are suspicious and distrustful of doctors and rarely seek medical attention.
	Schizoid	Isolated, detached "loners." Restricted emotional expression.	Be clear, honest, noncontrolling, and nondefensive. Avoid humor. Maintain emotional distance.
	Schizotypal	Odd behavior, perceptions, and appearance. Magical thinking; ideas of reference.	
Cluster B: **"wild"**	Borderline	Unstable mood, relationships, and self-image; feelings of emptiness. Impulsive. History of suicidal ideation or self-harm.	Patients change the rules and demand attention. Patients are manipulative and demanding, and will split staff members.
	Histrionic	Excessively emotional and attention seeking. Sexually provocative; theatrical.	Be firm: Stick to treatment plan. Be fair: Do not be punitive or derogatory.
	Narcissistic	Grandiose, need admiration, have sense of entitlement. Lack empathy.	Be consistent: Do not change rules.
	Antisocial	Violate rights of others, social norms, and laws. Impulsive; lack remorse. Begins in childhood as conduct disorder.	
Cluster C: **"worried and wimpy"**	Obsessive-compulsive	Preoccupied with perfectionism, order, and control at the expense of efficiency. Inflexible morals, values.	Patients are controlling and may sabotage their treatment. Words may be inconsistent with actions.
	Avoidant	Socially inhibited; rejection sensitive. Fear being disliked or ridiculed.	Avoid power struggles. Give clear recommendations, but do not push patients into decisions.
	Dependent	Submissive, clingy; need to be taken care of. Difficulty making decisions. Feel helpless.	

- **Disorganized:** Speech and behavior patterns are highly disordered and disinhibited with flat affect. The thought disorder is pronounced, and the patient has poor contact with reality. Carries the worst prognosis.
- **Catatonic:** A rare form characterized by psychomotor disturbance with two or more of the following: excessive motor activity, immobility, extreme negativism, mutism, waxy flexibility, echolalia, or echopraxia.

HISTORY/PE

- Two or more of the following are present continuously for **six or more months** with **social or occupational dysfunction:**
    - ⊕ **symptoms:** Hallucinations (most often auditory), delusions, disorganized speech, bizarre behavior, and thought disorder.
    - ⊖ **symptoms:** Flat affect, ↓ emotional reactivity, poverty of speech, lack of purposeful actions, and anhedonia.
- The differential includes the following:
    - **Schizophreniform disorder:** Symptoms of schizophrenia with a duration of < 6 months.

- **Schizoaffective disorder:** Combines the symptoms of schizophrenia with a major affective disorder (major depressive disorder or bipolar disorder).

TREATMENT

- **Antipsychotics** (see Table 2.14-6); **long-term follow-up.**
- Supportive psychotherapy, training in social skills, vocational rehabilitation, and illness education may help.
- ⊖ symptoms may be more difficult to treat.

CHILDHOOD AND ADOLESCENT DISORDERS

Attention-Deficit Hyperactivity Disorder (ADHD)

A persistent pattern of excessive inattention and/or hyperactivity/impulsivity. More common in males; typically presents between ages 3 and 13. Often shows a familial pattern.

HISTORY/PE

Children must exhibit ADHD symptoms in two or more settings (e.g., home and school).

Diagnosis requires **six or more symptoms** from each category listed below for **six or more months** in **at least two settings** → significant social and academic impairment. Some symptoms must be present in patients **before age seven.**

- **Inattention: Poor attention span** in schoolwork/play; poor attention to detail or careless mistakes; does not listen when spoken to; has **difficulty following instructions or finishing tasks;** loses items needed to complete tasks; forgetful and **easily distracted.**
- **Hyperactivity/impulsivity: Fidgets;** leaves seat in classroom; runs around inappropriately; cannot play quietly; talks excessively; **does not wait turn; interrupts others.**

TREATMENT

- Initial treatment may be nonpharmacologic (e.g., behavior modification). Sugar and food additives are **not** considered etiologic factors.
- Pharmacologic treatment includes the following:
    - **Psychostimulants: Methylphenidate,** dextroamphetamine. Adverse effects include insomnia, irritability, ↓ appetite, tic exacerbation, and ↓ growth velocity (normalizes when medication is stopped).
    - **Antidepressants** (e.g., SSRIs, nortriptyline, bupropion) and α₂-agonists (e.g., **clonidine**).

Autism Spectrum Disorders

More common in males. May be associated with **tuberous sclerosis and fragile X syndrome.** Symptom severity and IQ vary widely.

HISTORY/PE

- Characterized by abnormal or **impaired social interaction and communication** together with **restricted activities and interests,** evident **before age three.**
- Patients fail to develop normal social behaviors (e.g., social smile, eye contact) and lack interest in relationships.

- The development of spoken language is delayed or absent.
- Children show **stereotyped speech and behavior** (e.g., hand flapping) and restricted interests (e.g., preoccupation with parts of objects).
- Other pervasive developmental disorders include the following:
    - **Asperger's syndrome:** An autism-like disorder of social impairment and repetitive activities, behaviors, and interests **without marked language or cognitive delays.**
    - **Rett's disorder:** A genetic neurodegenerative disorder of females with progressive impairment (e.g., language, head growth, coordination) **after five months of normal development.**
    - **Childhood disintegrative disorder:** Severe developmental **regression** after > 2 years of normal development (e.g., language, motor skills, social skills, bladder/bowel control, play).

TREATMENT

- Intensive special education, **behavioral management,** and symptom-targeted medications (e.g., neuroleptics for aggression; SSRIs for stereotyped behavior).
- Family support and counseling are crucial.

Disruptive Behavioral Disorders

- Includes conduct disorder and oppositional defiant disorder.
- More common among males and in patients with a history of abuse.
- Hx/PE:
    - **Conduct disorder:**
        - A repetitive, persistent pattern of **violating the basic rights of others** or age-appropriate **societal norms or rules** for **one year or more.** Behaviors may be **aggressive** (e.g., rape, robbery, animal cruelty) or **nonaggressive** (e.g., stealing, lying, deliberately annoying people).
        - May progress to antisocial personality disorder in adulthood.
    - **Oppositional defiant disorder:**
        - A pattern of **negativistic, defiant, disobedient, and hostile behavior** toward authority figures (e.g., losing temper, arguing) for six or more months.
        - **May progress to conduct disorder.**
- **Tx:** Individual and family therapy.

*C*onduct disorder is seen in
*C*hildren.

*A*ntisocial personality disorder
is seen in *A*dults.

Learning Disabilities

- Occur more frequently in males and in those of low SES; often exhibit a familial pattern.
- Hx/PE:
    - **Academic functioning is substantially lower than expected for age, intelligence, and education** as measured by standardized test achievement in reading, mathematics, or written expression.
    - Learning problems significantly interfere with schooling and daily activities.
    - Always rule out physical disorders (e.g., deafness) and social factors (e.g., non–English speakers).
- **Tx:** Interventions include **remedial classes** or **individualized learning strategies.**

Mental Retardation

- Associated with male gender, chromosomal abnormalities, congenital infections, teratogens, inborn errors of metabolism, and alcohol/illicit substances during pregnancy.
- Hx/PE:
    - Patients have significantly subaverage intellectual functioning (**an IQ of < 70**) with **deficits in adaptive functioning** (e.g., hygiene, social skills); onset is before the age of 18.
    - Levels of severity are **mild** (IQ 50–70; **85% of cases),** moderate (IQ 35–49), severe (IQ 20–34), and profound (IQ < 20).
- Tx:
    - 1° prevention consists of educating the general public about possible causes of mental retardation and providing optimal prenatal screening and health care to mothers and their children.
    - Treatment measures include family counseling and support; speech and language therapy; occupational/physical therapy; behavioral intervention; educational assistance; and social skills training.

Coprolalia: Repetition of obscene words.

Tourette's Syndrome

- More common in males; shows a genetic predisposition. **Associated with ADHD, learning disorders,** and **OCD.**
- Hx/PE:
    - Begins prior to age 18.
    - Characterized by **multiple motor** (e.g., blinking, grimacing) and **vocal** (e.g., grunting, coprolalia) **tics** occurring many times per day, recurrently, for > 1 year with social or occupational impairment.
- Tx: Treatments include **dopamine receptor antagonists** (haloperidol, pimozide) or clonidine. Behavioral therapy may be of benefit, and counseling can aid in social adjustment and coping. Stimulants can worsen or precipitate tics.

More than 15% of the U.S. adult population has a serious substance use problem.

MISCELLANEOUS DISORDERS

Substance Abuse/Dependence

Both substance abuse and substance dependence are maladaptive patterns of substance abuse that → clinically significant impairment. Substance abuse is distinguished from substance dependence as follows:

- **Substance abuse:** Requires one or more of the following in one year:
    - **Failure to fulfill responsibilities** at work, school, or home.
    - Use in **physically hazardous** situations (e.g., driving while intoxicated).
    - **Legal problems** during the time of substance use.
    - Continued substance use despite recurrent social or interpersonal problems 2° to the effects of such use (e.g., frequent arguments with spouse over the substance use).
- **Substance dependence:** Requires three or more of the following in one year:
    - **Tolerance** and using progressively larger amounts to obtain the same desired effect.
    - **Withdrawal** symptoms when not taking the substance.
    - Failed **attempts to cut down use or abstain** from the substance.
    - Significant time spent obtaining the substance (e.g., visiting many doctors to obtain a prescription for pain pills).

Features of substance dependence—

WITHDraw IT

Three or more of seven within a 12-month period:
Withdrawal
Interest or **I**mportant activities given up or reduced
Tolerance
Harm (physical and psychosocial) with continued use
Desire to cut down/control
Intended time/amount exceeded
Time spent obtaining/using the substance is ↑

- Isolation from life activities.
- Taking greater amounts of the substance than intended.
- Continued substance abuse despite recurrent physical or psychological problems 2° to the effect of the substance use.

DIAGNOSIS/TREATMENT

- Substance use is often denied or underreported, so seek out collateral information from family and friends.
- Check urine and blood toxicology screens, LFTs, and serum EtOH level.
- The management of intoxication for selected drugs is described in Table 2.14-10.

A diagnosis of substance dependence trumps a diagnosis of substance abuse.

Alcoholism

- Occurs more often in **men** (4:1) and in those 21–34 years of age, although the incidence in women is rising. Also associated with a ⊕ family history.
- Hx/PE: See Table 2.14-10 for the symptoms of intoxication and withdrawal. Look for palmar erythema or telangiectasias as well as for other signs and symptoms of end-organ complications.
- Dx: Screen with the **CAGE** questionnaire. Monitor vital signs for evidence of withdrawal. Lab tests may reveal ↑ LFTs, LDH, and MCV.
- Tx:
  - Rule out medical complications; correct electrolyte abnormalities.
  - Start a **benzodiazepine taper** for withdrawal symptoms.
  - Give **multivitamins and folic acid; administer thiamine** before glucose (which depletes thiamine) to prevent Wernicke's encephalopathy.
  - Give anticonvulsants to patients with a seizure history.
  - Group therapy, disulfiram, or naltrexone can aid patients with dependence.
  - Long-term rehabilitative therapy (e.g., Alcoholic Anonymous).
- Cx: **GI bleeding, pancreatitis, liver disease,** DTs, alcoholic hallucinosis, peripheral neuropathy, Wernicke's encephalopathy, Korsakoff's psychosis, fetal alcohol syndrome, cardiomyopathy, anemia, aspiration pneumonia, ↑ risk of sustaining trauma (e.g., subdural hematoma).

> **CAGE** *questionnaire:*
>
> 1. Have you ever felt the need to **C**ut down on your drinking?
> 2. Have you ever felt **A**nnoyed by criticism of your drinking?
> 3. Have you ever felt **G**uilty about drinking?
> 4. Have you ever had to take a morning **E**ye opener?
>
> More than one "yes" answer makes alcoholism likely.

Anorexia Nervosa

- Risk factors include female gender, low self-esteem, and high SES. Also associated with OCD, major depressive disorder, anxiety, and careers such as modeling, gymnastics, ballet, and running.
- Hx/PE: Diagnosed as follows (see also Table 2.14-11):
  - Body weight is **< 85% of that expected.**
  - Patients present with **refusal to maintain normal body weight,** an intense **fear of weight gain,** a distorted body image (**patients perceive themselves as fat**), and **amenorrhea.**
  - Patients **restrict** (e.g., fasting, excessive exercise) or **binge and purge** (through vomiting, laxatives, and diuretics).
  - Signs and symptoms include **lanugo,** dry skin, bradycardia, lethargy, hypotension, cold intolerance, and hypothermia (as low as 35°C).
- Dx: Measure height and weight; check **CBC, electrolytes,** endocrine levels, and **ECG.** Perform a **psychiatric evaluation** to screen patients for comorbid conditions.

Bulimic patients tend to be more disturbed by their behavior than anorexics and are more easily engaged in therapy.

Anorexic patients deny health risks associated with their behavior, making them resistant to treatment.

TABLE 2.14-10. **Signs and Symptoms of Substance Abuse**

Drug	Intoxication	Withdrawal
Alcohol	Disinhibition, emotional lability, slurred speech, ataxia, aggression, blackouts, hallucinations, memory impairment, impaired judgment, coma.	Tremor, tachycardia, hypertension, malaise, nausea, seizures, DTs, agitation.
Opioids	Euphoria → apathy, CNS depression, constipation, **pupillary constriction,** and respiratory depression (life-threatening in overdose). Naloxone/naltrexone will block opioid receptors and reverse effects (beware of antagonist clearing before opioids, particularly with long-acting opioids such as methadone).	Dysphoria, insomnia, anorexia, myalgias, fever, lacrimation, diaphoresis, dilated pupils, rhinorrhea, piloerection, nausea, vomiting, stomach cramps, diarrhea, yawning.
Amphetamines	Psychomotor agitation, impaired judgment, hypertension, **pupillary dilation,** tachycardia, fever, diaphoresis, anxiety, angina, euphoria, prolonged wakefulness/attention, arrhythmias, delusions, seizures, hallucinations. Can give haloperidol for severe agitation and symptom-targeted medications (e.g., antiemetics, NSAIDs).	Postuse "crash" with anxiety, lethargy, headache, stomach cramps, hunger, fatigue, depression/dysphoria, sleep disturbance, nightmares.
Cocaine	Psychomotor agitation, euphoria, impaired judgment, tachycardia, **pupillary dilation,** hypertension, paranoia, hallucinations, sudden death. Treat with haloperidol for severe agitation along with symptom-specific medications (e.g., to control hypertension).	Postuse "crash" with hypersomnolence, depression, malaise, severe craving, angina, suicidality, ↑ appetite, nightmares.
Phencyclidine hydrochloride (PCP)	**Assaultiveness,** belligerence, psychosis, violence, impulsiveness, psychomotor agitation, fever, tachycardia, **vertical/horizontal nystagmus,** hypertension, impaired judgment, ataxia, seizures, delirium. Give benzodiazepines or haloperidol for severe symptoms; otherwise reassure.	Recurrence of intoxication symptoms due to reabsorption in the GI tract; sudden onset of severe, random violence.
LSD	Marked anxiety or depression, delusions, visual hallucinations, flashbacks, pupillary dilation, impaired judgment, diaphoresis, tachycardia, hypertension, heightened senses (e.g., colors become more intense). Supportive counseling; traditional antipsychotics for psychotic symptoms; benzodiazepines for anxiety.	
Marijuana	Euphoria, slowed sense of time, imparied judgment, social withdrawal, ↑ appetite, dry mouth, conjunctival injection, hallucinations, anxiety, paranoia, amotivational syndrome.	

TABLE 2.14-10. Signs and Symptoms of Substance Abuse (continued)

DRUG	INTOXICATION	WITHDRAWAL
Barbiturates	Low safety margin; respiratory depression.	Anxiety, seizures, delirium, life-threatening cardiovascular collapse.
Benzodiazepines	Interactions with alcohol, amnesia, ataxia, somnolence, mild respiratory depression.	Rebound anxiety, seizures, tremor, insomnia, hypertension, tachycardia, **death.**
Caffeine	Restlessness, insomnia, diuresis, muscle twitching, arrhythmias, tachycardia, flushed face, psychomotor agitation.	Headache, lethargy, depression, weight gain, irritability, craving.
Nicotine	Restlessness, insomnia, anxiety, arrhythmias.	Irritability, headache, anxiety, weight gain, craving, bradycardia, difficulty concentrating, insomnia.

- Tx:
    - Initially, monitor caloric intake to restore nutritional state and to stabilize weight; then focus on **weight gain.**
    - Hospitalize if necessary to restore nutritional status, rehydrate, and correct electrolyte imbalances.
    - Once the patient is medically stable, initiate individual, family, and group **psychotherapy.** Treat comorbid depression and anxiety.
- Cx: Mitral valve prolapse, arrhythmias, hypotension, bradycardia, **amenorrhea** (missing three consecutive cycles), nephrolithiasis, osteoporosis, multiple stress fractures, pancytopenia, thyroid abnormalities (see Table 2.14-12). Mortality from **suicide** or medical complications is > 10%.

There are two types of anorexia nervosa:

- *Restricting type*
- *Binging/purge-eating type*

Bulimia Nervosa

- More common among women; associated with low self-esteem, mood disorders, and OCD.

TABLE 2.14-11. Anorexia vs. Bulimia

	ANOREXIA NERVOSA	BULIMIA NERVOSA
Body image	Disturbed body image; use extensive measures to avoid weight gain (e.g., purging, excess exercise).	Same.
Binge eating	May occur.	Same.
Weight	Patients are underweight (≥ 15% below expected weight).	Patients are of normal weight or are overweight.
Attitude toward illness	Patients are typically not distressed by their illness and may thus be resistant to treatment.	Patients are typically distressed about their symptoms and are thus easier to treat.

TABLE 2.14-12. **Common Medical Complications of Eating Disorders**

Constitutional	Cardiac	GI	GU	Other
Cachexia	Arrhythmias	Dental erosions and decay	Amenorrhea	**Dermatologic:** Lanugo
Hypothermia	Sudden death		Nephrolithiasis	**Hematologic:** Leukopenia
Fatigue	Hypotension	Abdominal pain		**Neurologic:** Seizures
Electrolyte abnormalities	Bradycardia	Delayed gastric emptying		**Musculoskeletal:** Osteoporosis, stress fractures
	Prolonged QT interval			

Bupropion should be avoided in the treatment of patients with eating disorders, as it is associated with a ↓ in seizure threshold.

- **Hx/PE:** Diagnostic criteria are as follows (see also Table 2.14-11):
  - **Patients have normal weight or are overweight.** For at least two times a week for three or more months, patients have episodes of **binge eating** and **compensatory behaviors** that include **purging** or **fasting.**
  - Patients are usually **ashamed** and conceal their behaviors.
  - **Signs** include **dental enamel erosion, enlarged parotid glands,** and **scars on the dorsal hand surfaces** (from inducing vomiting). Patients usually have normal body weight.
- **Tx: Psychotherapy** focuses on behavior modification and body image. **Antidepressants** may be effective for both depressed and nondepressed patients.
- **Cx:** See Table 2.14-12.

Sexual Disorders

SEXUAL CHANGES WITH AGING

- **Interest** in sexual activity **usually does not ↓ with aging.**
- Men usually require ↑ stimulation of the genitalia for longer periods of time to reach orgasm; intensity of orgasm ↓, and the length of the refractory period before the next orgasm ↑.
- In women, estrogen levels ↓ after menopause → vaginal dryness and thinning, which may → discomfort during coitus. May be treated with HRT, estrogen vaginal suppositories, or other vaginal creams.

PARAPHILIAS

- Preoccupation or engagement in unusual sexual fantasies, urges, or behaviors for > 6 months with clinically significant impairment in one's life. Includes criminal sex offenders (e.g., pedophilia); see Table 2.14-13. Found almost exclusively in men, and usually begins before or during puberty.
- Sexual excitement is derived from unique exposures to certain situations, individuals, or objects.
- **Tx:** Treatment includes insight-oriented psychotherapy and behavioral therapy. Antiandrogens (e.g., Depo-Provera) have been used for hypersexual paraphilic activity.

GENDER IDENTITY DISORDERS

- **Strong, persistent cross-gender identification** and **discomfort with one's assigned sex or gender role of the assigned sex** in the absence of intersexual disorders. Patients may have a history of dressing like the opposite sex, taking sex hormones, or pursuing surgeries to reassign their sex.

TABLE 2.14-13.   **Features of Common Paraphilias**

DISORDER	CLINICAL MANIFESTATIONS
Exhibitionism	Sexual arousal from exposing one's genitals to a stranger.
Pedophilia	Urges or behaviors involving sexual activities with children.
Voyeurism	Observing unsuspecting persons unclothed or involved in sex.
Fetishism	Use of nonliving objects (often clothing) for sexual arousal.
Transvestic fetishism	Cross-dressing for sexual arousal.
Frotteurism	Touching or rubbing one's genitalia against a nonconsenting person (common in subways).
Sexual sadism	Sexual arousal from inflicting suffering on sexual partner.
Sexual masochism	Sexual arousal from being hurt, humiliated, bound, or threatened.

- More common in males than in females. Associated with depression, anxiety, substance abuse, and personality disorders, which may be addressed and treated.
- Tx: Treatment is complex and includes educating the patient about culturally acceptable behavior patterns. Other options include sex-reassignment surgery or hormonal treatment (e.g., estrogen for males, testosterone for females). Supportive psychotherapy is helpful.

SEXUAL DYSFUNCTION

- Problems in sexual **arousal, desire, or orgasm; or pain** with sexual intercourse.
- Prevalence is 30%; one-third of cases are attributable to biological factors and another third to psychological factors.
- Tx: Treatment depends on the particular condition.

Sleep Disorders

Up to one-third of all American adults suffer from some type of sleep disorder during their lives. The term *dyssomnia* describes any condition that → a disturbance in the normal rhythm or pattern of sleep. Insomnia is the most common example. **Risk factors** include female gender, the presence of mental and medical disorders, substance abuse, and advanced age.

1° INSOMNIA

- **Affects up to 30% of the general population;** causes sleep disturbance that is not attributable to physical or mental conditions. It is often exacerbated by anxiety, and patients may become preoccupied with getting enough sleep.

- **Dx**: Patients present with a history of **nonrestorative sleep** or **difficulty initiating or maintaining sleep** that is present at least three times a week for one month.
- **Tx**:
  - First-line therapy includes the initiation of **good sleep hygiene** measures, which include the following:
    - Establishment of a regular sleep schedule
    - Limit caffeine intake
    - Avoidance of daytime naps
    - Warm baths in the evening
    - Use of the bedroom for sleep and sexual activity only
    - Exercising early in the day
    - Relaxation techniques
    - Avoidance of large meals near bedtime
  - Pharmacotherapy is considered second-line therapy and should be **initiated with care for short periods of time** (< 2 weeks). Pharmacologic agents include diphenhydramine (Benadryl), zolpidem (Ambien), zaleplon (Sonata), and trazodone (Desyrel).

1° HYPERSOMNIA

- **Dx**: Diagnosed when a patient complains of **excessive daytime sleepiness or nighttime sleep** that occurs for > 1 month. The excessive somnolence cannot be attributable to medical or mental illness, medications, poor sleep hygiene, insufficient sleep, or narcolepsy.
- **Tx**:
  - First-line therapy includes **stimulant drugs** such as amphetamines.
  - Antidepressants such as SSRIs may be useful in some patients.

NARCOLEPSY

- May affect up to 0.16% of the population. Onset typically occurs by young adulthood, generally before the age of 30. Some forms of narcolepsy may have a genetic component.
- **Dx**:
  - Manifestations include **excessive daytime somnolence** and ↓ **REM sleep latency** on a daily basis for at least three months. **Sleep attacks** are the classic symptom; patients cannot avoid falling asleep.
  - The characteristic excessive sleepiness may be associated with the following:
    - **Cataplexy**: Sudden loss of muscle tone → collapse.
    - **Hypnagogic hallucinations**: Occur as the patient is falling asleep.
    - **Hypnopompic hallucinations**: Occur as the patient awakens.
    - **Sleep paralysis**: Brief paralysis upon awakening.
- **Tx**: Treat with a regimen of **scheduled daily naps** plus **stimulant drugs** such as amphetamines; give SSRIs for cataplexy.

SLEEP APNEA

- Occurs 2° to **disturbances in breathing** during sleep that → **excessive daytime somnolence** and **sleep disruption**. Etiologies can be either central or peripheral.
  - **Central sleep apnea (CSA)**: A condition in which both airflow and respiratory effort cease. CSA is linked to **morning headaches**, mood changes, and repeated awakenings during the night.

- **Obstructive sleep apnea (OSA):** A condition in which airflow ceases as a result of obstruction along the respiratory passages. OSA is strongly associated with **snoring.** Risk factors include **male gender, obesity,** prior upper airway surgeries, a deviated nasal septum, a large uvula or tongue, and retrognathia (recession of the mandible).
  - In both forms, arousal → cessation of the apneic event.
- Associated with **sudden death in infants and elderly,** headaches, depression, ↑ systolic blood pressure, and **pulmonary hypertension.**
- **Dx:** Sleep studies **(polysomnography)** document the number of arousals, obstructions, and episodes of ↓ O₂ saturation; distinguish OSA from CSA, and identify possible movement disorders, seizures, or other sleep disorders.
- **Tx:**
  - **OSA:** Nasal continuous positive airway pressure (CPAP). Weight loss if obese. In children, most cases are due to tonsillar/adenoidal hypertrophy, which is corrected surgically.
  - **CSA:** Mechanical ventilation (e.g., BPAP) with a backup rate for severe cases.

CIRCADIAN RHYTHM SLEEP DISORDER

- A spectrum of disorders characterized by a **misalignment between desired and actual sleep** periods. Subtypes include jet-lag type, shift-work type, delayed sleep-phase type, and unspecified.
- **Tx:**
  - Jet-lag type usually **resolves** within 2–7 days **without specific treatment.**
  - Shift-work type may respond to **light therapy.**
  - Oral melatonin may be useful if given 5 1/2 hours prior to the desired bedtime.

Somatoform and Factitious Disorders

Patients often present with **medically unexplained somatic symptoms,** generally with varying etiologies.

- **Somatoform disorders:** Patients have **no conscious control over symptoms.** The five main categories are outlined in Table 2.14-14.
- **Factitious disorders:** Patients fabricate symptoms or cause self-injury to assume the sick role (1° gain). More common in men; Munchausen's syndrome is an example that is common among **health care workers.**
- **Malingering:** Patients **intentionally cause** or feign symptoms for **2° gain** of **financial benefit** or **housing.**

Sexual and Physical Abuse

- Most frequently affects women < 35 years of age who fill the following criteria:
  - Are experiencing marital discord and are substance abusers or have a partner who is a substance abuser; or
  - Are pregnant, are of low SES, or have obtained a restraining order.
- Victims of childhood abuse are more likely to become adult victims of abuse.
- **Hx/PE:**
  - Patients typically have **multiple somatic complaints, frequent ER** visits, and **unexplained injuries** with **delayed medical treatment.** They may also **avoid eye contact** or act afraid or hostile.

Sexual abusers are usually male and are often known to the victim (and are often family members).

TABLE 2.14-14. **Somatoform Disorders**

Somatization disorder	Multiple, chronic somatic symptoms from different organ systems with multiple GI, sexual, neurologic, and pain complaints. Frequent clinical contacts and/or surgeries; significant functional impairment. The male-to-female ratio is 1:20. Onset is usually before age of 30. Schedule regular appointments with the identified 1° caregiver who maintains communication with consultants and specialists; psychotherapy.
Conversion disorder	Symptoms or deficits of voluntary motor or sensory function (e.g., blindness, seizure, paralysis) incompatible with medical processes. Close temporal relationship to stress or intense emotion. More common in young females and in lower socioeconomic and less educated groups. Usually resolves spontaneously, but psychotherapy may help.
Hypochondriasis	Preoccupation with or fear of having a serious disease despite medical reassurance → significant distress/impairment. Often involves a history of prior physical disease. Men and women are equally affected. Onset is in adulthood. Manage with group therapy and schedule regular appointments with the patient's 1° caregiver.
Body dysmorphic disorder	Preoccupation with imagined physical defect or abnormality → significant distress/impairment. Patients often present to dermatologists or plastic surgeons. Has a slight female predominance. May be associated with depression, and SSRIs may be of benefit.
Pain disorder	Intensity or profile of pain symptoms is inconsistent with physiologic processes. Close temporal relationship with psychological factors. More common in females. Peak onset is at 40–50 years of age. May be associated with depression. Treatment includes rehabilitation (e.g., physical therapy), psychotherapy, and behavioral therapy. Analgesia is usually not helpful. TCAs and venlafaxine may be therapeutic.

- Children may exhibit precocious sexual behavior, **genital or anal trauma, STDs**, UTIs, and psychiatric problems.
- Other clues include a partner who answers questions for the patient or refuses to leave the exam room.
- **Tx:** Perform a screening assessment of the patient's safety domestically and in their close personal relationships. Provide **medical care,** emotional **support, and counseling;** educate the patient about **support services** and refer appropriately. **Documentation** is crucial.

Suicidality

- Accounts for 30,000 deaths per year in the United States; the eighth overall cause of death in the United States. One suicide occurs every 20 minutes.
- Risk factors include male gender, age greater than 45 years, psychiatric disorders (major depression, presence of psychotic symptoms), a history of an admission to a psychiatric institution, previous suicide attempt, a history of violent behavior, ethanol or substance abuse, recent severe stressors, and a family suicide history (see the mnemonic **SAD PERSONS**). Women are more likely to attempt suicide, whereas men are more likely to succeed by virtue of their ↑ use of more lethal methods.
- **Dx:**
  - Perform a comprehensive psychiatric evaluation.
  - Ask about family history, previous attempts, ambivalence toward death, and hopelessness.

Risk factors for suicide—

SAD PERSONS

Sex (male)
Age (older)
Depression
Previous attempt
Ethanol/substance abuse
Rational thought
Sickness (chronic illness)
Organized plan/access to weapons
No spouse
Social support lacking

- Ask directly about suicidal ideation, intent, and plan, and look for available means.
- **Tx:** A patient who endorses suicidality requires emergent inpatient hospitalization even against his will. Suicide risk may ↑ after antidepressant therapy is initiated because a patient's energy to act on suicidal thoughts can return before the depressed mood lifts.

Suicide is the third leading cause of death (after homicide and accidents) among 15- to 24-year-olds in the United States.

HIGH-YIELD FACTS

PSYCHIATRY

Pulmonary

Figure 2.15-1 contrasts obstructive with restrictive lung disease. The etiologies of restrictive lung disease are shown in the mnemonic **PAINT**.

Interstitial Lung Disease

A heterogeneous group of disorders characterized by **inflammation** and/or **fibrosis** of the **interalveolar septum**. In advanced disease, there are cystic spaces in the lung periphery ("honeycombing"). Causes include idiopathic interstitial pneumonias, collagen vascular disease, granulomatous disorders, drugs, hypersensitivity disorders, pneumoconiosis, and eosinophilic pulmonary syndromes.

HISTORY/PE

Presents with **shallow, rapid breathing**; dyspnea with exercise; and a nonproductive **cough.** Patients may have cyanosis, inspiratory squeaks, fine or "Velcro" crackles, finger clubbing, or right heart failure.

DIAGNOSIS

- **CXR:** Reticular, nodular, or ground-glass pattern; honeycomb pattern (severe disease).

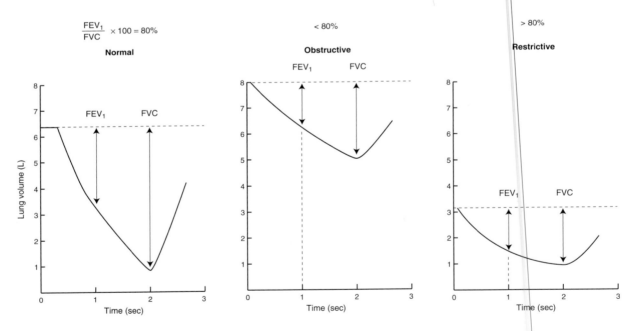

FIGURE 2.15-1. **Obstructive vs. restrictive lung disease.**

Note: Obstructive lung volumes > normal ($\uparrow$ TLC, $\uparrow$ FRC, $\uparrow$ RV); restrictive lung volumes < normal. In both obstructive and restrictive disease, FEV_1 and FVC are reduced, but in obstructive disease, FEV_1 is more dramatically reduced, resulting in a $\downarrow$ FEV_1/FVC ratio.

- $\downarrow$ TLC, $\downarrow$ FVC, $\downarrow$ DL$_{CO}$, normal FEV$_1$/FVC. Serum markers of connective tissue diseases should be obtained if clinically indicated.

TREATMENT

Supportive. Avoid exposure to causative agents. Some inflammatory diseases respond to **corticosteroids** or other anti-inflammatory/immunosuppressive agents.

Systemic Sarcoidosis

A multisystem disease of unknown etiology characterized by **noncaseating granulomas.** Most commonly found in **African-American females** and northern European Caucasians; most often arises in the third or fourth decade of life.

HISTORY/PE

Commonly presents with **fever, cough, malaise,** weight loss, dyspnea, and **arthritis.** The lungs, liver, eyes, skin (erythema nodosum, violaceous skin plaques), nervous system, heart, and kidney may be affected. Symptoms may be **GRUELING** (see mnemonic).

DIAGNOSIS

- **CXR:** Radiographic findings are used to determine the stage of the disease and include the following:
    - Bilateral hilar lymphadenopathy alone (stage I).
    - Hilar adenopathy + pulmonary infiltrates (stage II).
    - Pulmonary infiltrates alone (stage III).
- **Biopsy: Lymph node biopsy** or transbronchial/video-assisted thoracoscopic **lung biopsy** reveals **noncaseating granulomas.**
- **PFTs:** $\downarrow$ lung volumes (restrictive pattern) and $\downarrow$ diffusion capacity.
- **Other findings:** $\uparrow$ **serum ACE levels** (neither sensitive nor specific), **hypercalcemia,** hypercalciuria, $\uparrow$ alkaline phosphatase (with liver involvement), lymphopenia, cranial nerve defects, arrhythmias.

TREATMENT

Systemic **corticosteroids** are indicated for constitutional symptoms, hypercalcemia, or extrathoracic organ involvement.

Hypersensitivity Pneumonitis

- Risk factors include environmental exposure to antigens → alveolar thickening and granulomas. Types and etiologies are listed in Table 2.15-1.
- Hx/PE:
    - **Acute:** Presents with dyspnea, fever, malaise, shivering, and cough starting 4–6 hours after exposure.
    - **Chronic:** Patients present with progressive dyspnea; exam reveals fine bilateral rales.
- **Dx:** CXR is normal or shows miliary nodular infiltrate (acute); fibrosis is seen in the upper lobes (chronic).
- **Tx:** Avoid ongoing exposure to inciting agents; give steroids to $\downarrow$ inflammation.

Interventions associated with interstitial lung disease include busulfan, nitrofurantoin, amiodarone, bleomycin, radiation, and long-term high O$_2$ concentration (e.g., ventilators).

Features of sarcoid—

GRUELING

Granulomas
a**R**thritis
Uveitis
Erythema nodosum
Lymphadenopathy
Interstitial fibrosis
Negative TB test
Gammaglobulinemia

TABLE 2.15-1. Antigens of Hypersensitivity Pneumonitis

DISORDER	ANTIGEN
Farmer's lung	Spores of actinomycetes from moldy hay.
Bird fancier's lung	Antigens from feathers, excreta, serum.
Mushroom worker's lung	Spores of actinomycetes from compost.
Malt worker's lung	Spores of *Aspergillus clavatus* in grain.
Grain handler's lung	Grain weevil dust.
Bagassosis	Spores of actinomycetes from sugarcane.
Air conditioner lung	Spores of actinomycetes from air conditioners.

Pneumoconiosis

- Risk factors include prolonged occupational exposure and inhalation of small inorganic dust particles.
- **Hx/PE/Dx:** Table 2.15-2 outlines the findings and diagnostic criteria associated with common pneumoconioses.
- **Tx:** Supportive therapy and supplemental O_2.

Usual Interstitial Pneumonia (Idiopathic Pulmonary Fibrosis)

Usual interstitial pneumonia is one of the most common forms of interstitial pneumonia.

- The most common form of **idiopathic interstitial pneumonia.** Has an unrelenting progression, with death usually occurring within 5–10 years.
- **Hx/PE:**
  - Presents with **exertional dyspnea** and a nonproductive **cough.**
  - Exam may reveal inspiratory crackles and/or clubbing.
- **Dx:**
  - **High-resolution CT:** Patchy opacities at the lung bases, often with honeycombing.
  - **PFTs:** Restrictive pattern.
  - **Surgical biopsy** (usually required to confirm the diagnosis): Interstitial inflammation, fibrosis, and honeycombing.
- **Tx:** Options include steroids, cytotoxic agents (azathioprine, cyclophosphamide), antifibrotic agents (have not been shown to improve survival), and lung transplant.

Eosinophilic Pulmonary Syndromes

- A diverse group of disorders characterized by eosinophilic **pulmonary infiltrates** and **peripheral blood eosinophilia.** Includes **allergic bronchopulmonary aspergillosis, Löffler's syndrome,** and **acute eosinophilic pneumonia.**
- **Hx/PE:** Presents with dyspnea, cough, and/or fever.
- **Dx:** CBC reveals peripheral eosinophilia; CXR shows pulmonary infiltrates.

TABLE 2.1 5-2.   Pneumoconioses

	HISTORY	DIAGNOSIS	COMPLICATIONS
Asbestosis	Work involving manufacture of tile or brake linings, insulation, construction, demolition, or shipbuilding. Presents 15–20 years after initial exposure.	**CXR:** Linear opacities at lung bases and interstitial fibrosis; calcified pleural plaques are indicative of benign pleural disease.	↑ risk of mesothelioma (rare) and lung cancer; risk of lung cancer higher in smokers.
Coal mine disease	Work in underground coal mines.	**CXR:** Small nodular opacities (< 1 cm) in upper lung zones. **Spirometry:** Consistent with restrictive disease.	Progressive massive fibrosis.
Silicosis	Work in mines or quarries or with glass, pottery, or silica.	**CXR:** Small (< 1-cm) nodular opacities in upper lung zones. **Eggshell calcifications. Spirometry:** Consistent with restrictive disease.	↑ risk of TB; need annual TB skin test. Progressive massive fibrosis.
Berylliosis	Work in high-technology fields such as aerospace, nuclear, and electronics plants; ceramics industries; foundries; plating facilities; dental material sites; and dye manufacturing.	**CXR:** Diffuse infiltrates; hilar adenopathy.	Requires chronic steroid treatments.

- **Tx:** Removal of the extrinsic cause or treatment of underlying infection if identified. Corticosteroid treatment may be used if no cause is identified.

OBSTRUCTIVE LUNG DISEASE

The causes of obstructive lung disease are described in the mnemonic **ABCT.**

Asthma

Reversible airway obstruction 2° to bronchial **hyperreactivity**, airway **inflammation, mucous plugging,** and **smooth muscle hypertrophy.**

HISTORY/PE

- Presents with **cough,** dyspnea, **episodic wheezing,** and/or chest tightness. Symptoms often worsen at night or early in the morning.
- Male gender and older age are additional historical risk factors.
- Exam reveals tachypnea, tachycardia, ↓ breath sounds, **wheezing, prolonged expiratory duration** (↓ I/E ratio), ↓ O_2 saturation (late sign), hyperresonance, **accessory muscle use,** and possible pulsus paradoxus.

> *Causes of obstructive pulmonary disease—*
>
> **ABCT**
>
> **A**sthma
> **B**ronchiectasis
> **C**ystic fibrosis
> **T**racheal or bronchial obstruction

Asthma triggers include allergens, URIs, cold air, exercise, drugs, and stress.

HIGH-YIELD FACTS

PULMONARY

Beware—all that wheezes is
not asthma!

Asthma should be suspected
in children with multiple
episodes of croup and URIs
associated with dyspnea.

Meds for asthma
exacerbations—

ASTHMA

Albuterol
Steroids
Theophylline
Humidified O_2
Magnesium
Anticholinergics

DIAGNOSIS

- **ABGs: Mild hypoxia** and **respiratory alkalosis.** Normalizing PCO_2 in an acute exacerbation warrants close observation, as it may indicate fatigue and impending respiratory failure.
- **Spirometry/PFTs: Peak flow is diminished** acutely; $\downarrow$ FEV_1/FVC; $\uparrow$ residual volume and TLC.
- **CBC:** Possible eosinophilia.
- **CXR:** Hyperinflation.
- **Methacholine challenge:** Tests for bronchial hyperresponsiveness; useful when PFTs are normal.

TREATMENT

In general, avoid allergens or any potential exacerbating factor. Management is as follows (see also Tables 2.15-3 and 2.15-4):

- **Acute:** O_2, **bronchodilating agents** (short-acting inhaled β_2-agonists are first-line therapy), ipratropium (never use alone), systemic **steroids.** Intubation is appropriate for severe cases.
- **Chronic:** Measure lung function (FEV_1, peak flow, ABGs) to guide management. Administer long-acting inhaled **bronchodilators** and/or inhaled steroids, systemic **steroids,** cromolyn, or **theophylline. Montelukast** and other leukotriene antagonists are oral adjuncts to inhalant therapy.

Bronchiectasis

A disease caused by cycles of infection and inflammation in the bronchi/bronchioles that $\rightarrow$ permanent fibrosis, remodeling, and **dilation of bronchi.**

TABLE 2.15-3. Common Asthma Medications and Their Mechanisms

Nonspecific β-agonists	**Isoproterenol:** Relaxes bronchial smooth muscle (β_2). Tachycardia (β_1) is an adverse effect.
β_2-agonists	**Albuterol:** Relaxes bronchial smooth muscle (β_2). Use during acute exacerbations. **Salmeterol:** Long-acting agent for prophylaxis.
Methylxanthines	**Theophylline:** Likely causes bronchodilation by inhibiting phosphodiesterase, thereby decreasing cAMP hydrolysis. Usage is limited because of its narrow therapeutic index (cardiotoxicity, neurotoxicity).
Muscarinic antagonists	**Ipratropium:** Competitive block of muscarinic receptors, preventing bronchoconstriction.
Cromolyn	Prevents release of mediators from mast cells. Useful for exercise-induced bronchospasm. Effective only for the prophylaxis of asthma; not effective during an acute asthmatic attack. Toxicity is rare.
Corticosteroids	**Beclomethasone, prednisone:** Inhibit the synthesis of virtually all cytokines; inactivate NF-κB, the transcription factor that induces the production of TNF-α, among other inflammatory agents. **Inhaled** corticosteroids are the first-line treatment for long-term control of asthma.
Antileukotrienes	**Zileuton:** A 5-lipoxygenase pathway inhibitor. Blocks conversion of arachidonic acid to leukotrienes. **Zafirlukast:** Blocks leukotriene receptors.

TABLE 2.15-4. Medications for Chronic Treatment of Asthma

Type	Symptoms (Day/Night)	FEV$_1$	Medications
Severe persistent	Continual Frequent	≤ 60%	High-dose inhaled corticosteroids + long-acting inhaled β$_2$-agonists. Possible PO steroids. PRN short-acting bronchodilator.
Moderate persistent	Daily > 1 night/week	60–80%	Low- to medium-dose inhaled corticosteroids + long-acting inhaled β$_2$-agonists. PRN short-acting bronchodilator.
Mild persistent	> 2/week but < 1/day > 2 nights/month	≥ 80%	Low-dose inhaled corticosteroids. PRN short-acting bronchodilator.
Mild intermittent	≤ 2 days/week ≤ 2 nights/month	≥ 80%	No daily medications. PRN short-acting bronchodilator.

HISTORY/PE

- Presents with chronic **cough** with frequent bouts of yellow or green **sputum** production, dyspnea, and possible hemoptysis and halitosis.
- Associated with a history of pulmonary infections (e.g., *Pseudomonas*, *Haemophilus*, TB), hypersensitivity (allergic bronchopulmonary aspergillosis), CF, immunodeficiency, localized airway obstruction (foreign body, tumor), aspiration, autoimmune disease (e.g., rheumatoid arthritis, SLE), or IBD.
- Exam reveals rales, wheezes, rhonchi, purulent mucus, and occasional hemoptysis.

DIAGNOSIS

- CXR: ↑ bronchovascular markings; **tram lines** (parallel lines outlining dilated bronchi as a result of peribronchial inflammation and fibrosis); areas of **honeycombing.**
- **High-resolution CT: Dilated airways** and ballooned cysts at the end of the bronchus (mostly lower lobes). Spirometry shows a ↓ FEV$_1$/FVC ratio.

TREATMENT

- Antibiotics for bacterial infections; consider inhaled corticosteroids.
- Maintain bronchopulmonary hygiene (cough control, postural drainage, chest physiotherapy).
- Consider lobectomy or lung transplantation for severe disease.

Chronic Obstructive Pulmonary Disease (COPD)

Characterized by ↓ lung function with airflow obstruction. Generally due to chronic bronchitis or emphysema, which are distinguished as follows:

- **Chronic bronchitis:** Productive cough for > 3 months per year for two consecutive years.
- **Emphysema:** Terminal airway destruction and dilation that may be due to **smoking** (centrilobular) or to **α$_1$-antitrypsin deficiency** (panlobular).

> *Differential diagnosis—*
>
> **BRONCHIECTASIS**
>
> **B**ronchial cyst
> **R**epeated gastric acid aspiration
> **O**r due to foreign bodies
> **N**ecrotizing pneumonia
> **C**hemical corrosive substances
> **H**ypogammaglobulinemia
> **I**mmotile cilia syndrome
> **E**osinophilia (pulmonary)
> **C**ystic fibrosis
> **T**uberculosis (1°) or *Mycobacterium avium-intracellulare*
> **A**topic bronchial asthma
> **S**treptococcal pneumonia
> **I**n Young's syndrome
> **S**taphylococcal pneumonia

Administer O_2 to COPD
patients with chronic
hypercapnia with care, as
high concentrations of O_2 may
suppress their hypoxic
respiratory drive.

Treatment for COPD—

COPD

Corticosteroids
Oxygen
Prevention (cigarette
smoking cessation,
pneumococcal and
influenza vaccines)
Dilators (β_2-agonists,
anticholinergics)

HISTORY/PE

- Symptoms are minimal or nonspecific until the disease is advanced.
- The clinical spectrum includes the following:
  - **Emphysema ("pink puffer"): Dyspnea, pursed lips,** minimal cough, ↓ breath sounds, late hypercarbia/hypoxia; patients often have a thin, wasted appearance. Pure emphysematous patients tend to have fewer reactive airways between exacerbations.
  - **Chronic bronchitis ("blue bloater"): Productive cough;** cyanosis with mild dyspnea. Patients are often overweight with peripheral edema, rhonchi, and early hypercarbia/hypoxia. Look for barrel chest, use of accessory chest muscles, JVD, end-expiratory **wheezing,** or muffled breath sounds.

DIAGNOSIS

- **CXR:** ↓ lung markings with flat diaphragms, **hyperinflated lungs,** and a thin-appearing heart and mediastinum. Parenchymal **bullae** or subpleural **blebs** (pathognomonic of emphysema) are also seen (see Figure 2.15-2).
- **PFTs:** ↓ FEV_1/FVC, normal or ↓ FVC, normal or ↑ TLC (emphysema, asthma), ↓ DL_{CO} (in emphysema).
- **ABGs: Hypoxemia** with **acute** or **chronic respiratory acidosis** (↑ Pco_2).
- **Blood cultures:** Obtain if the patient is febrile.
- **Gram stain and sputum culture:** Obtain in the setting of fever or productive cough.

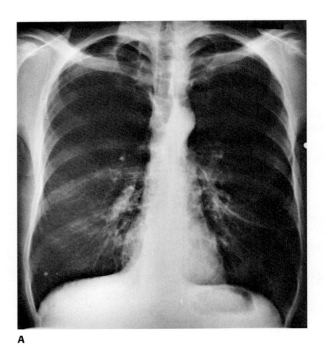

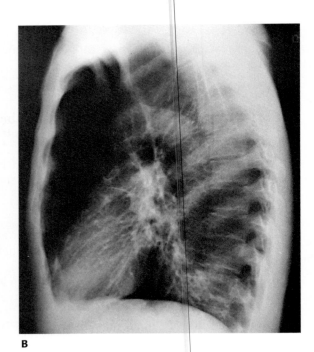

A

B

FIGURE 2.15-2. **Chronic obstructive pulmonary disease.**

Note the hyperinflated and hyperlucent lungs, flat diaphragms, increased AP diameter, narrow mediastinum, and large upper bullae on (A) AP and (B) lateral CXRs. (Reproduced, with permission, from Stobo J et al. *The Principles and Practice of Medicine,* 23rd ed. Stamford, CT: Appleton & Lange, 1997, p. 135.)

TREATMENT

- **Acute exacerbations:** O_2, inhaled **β-agonists** (albuterol) and **anticholinergics** (ipratropium, tiotropium), IV +/– inhaled **steroids, antibiotics.** Severe cases may benefit from noninvasive ventilation. Consider intubation in the setting of severe hypoxemia or hypercapnia, impending respiratory fatigue, or changes in mental status.
- **Chronic: Smoking cessation,** supplemental O_2 (if resting PaO_2 is ≤ 55 mmHg or SaO_2 is ≤ 89%), inhaled **β-agonists,** anticholinergics (tiotropium), systemic or inhaled steroids. Give **pneumococcal** and **flu vaccines.**

Supplemental oxygen is the only therapy proven to improve survival in patients with COPD.

ACUTE RESPIRATORY FAILURE

Hypoxemia

- Causes include right-to-left shunt, hypoventilation, low inspired O_2 content (important only at altitudes), **ventilation-perfusion (V/Q) mismatch,** and **diffusion impairment.**
- **Hx/PE:** Findings depend on the etiology. ↓ **HbO₂ saturation,** cyanosis, tachypnea, shortness of breath, pleuritic chest pain, and altered mental status may be seen.
- **Dx:**
  - **Pulse oximetry:** Demonstrates ↓ HbO_2 saturation.
  - **CXR:** To rule out ARDS, atelectasis, or an infiltrative process (e.g., pneumonia) and to look for signs of pulmonary embolism.

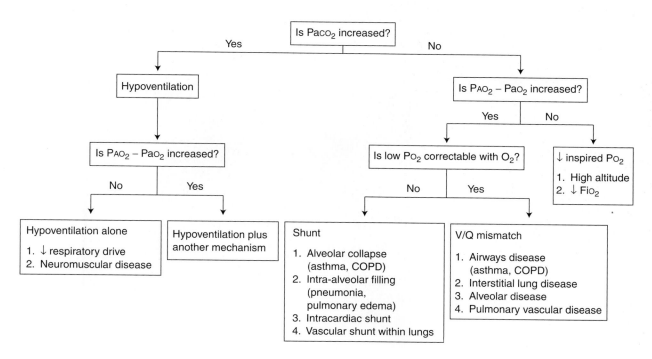

FIGURE 2.15-3. **Determination of the mechanism of hypoxia.**

(Reproduced, with permission, from Kasper DL et al (eds). *Harrison's Principles of Internal Medicine,* 16th ed. New York: McGraw-Hill, 2005.)

- **ABGs:** To evaluate PaO_2 and to calculate the **alveolar-arterial (A-a) oxygen gradient** ($[(P_{atm} - 47) \times FiO_2] - [(PaCO_2/0.8) - PaO_2]$). An ↑ A-a gradient suggests a V/Q mismatch or a diffusion impairment. Figure 2.15-3 summarizes the approach toward hypoxemic patients.
- **Tx:**
  - Based on the underlying etiology.
  - Administer O_2 before initiating evaluation.
  - **If the patient is on a ventilator,** ↑ O_2 saturation by ↑ FiO_2, ↑ **positive end-expiratory pressure (PEEP),** or ↑ the I/E ratio.
  - **Hypercapnic patients:** ↑ minute ventilation.

Acute Respiratory Distress Syndrome (ARDS)

Acute respiratory failure with refractory **hypoxemia,** ↓ **lung compliance,** and noncardiogenic **pulmonary edema.** The pathogenesis is thought to be endothelial injury. Common triggers include sepsis, pneumonia, aspiration, multiple blood transfusions, inhaled/ingested toxins, and trauma. Overall mortality is 30–40%.

HISTORY/PE

Presents with **acute-onset** (12–48 hours) tachypnea, dyspnea, and tachycardia, +/− fever, cyanosis, labored breathing, diffuse high-pitched rales, and hypoxemia in the setting of one of the systemic inflammatory causes or exposure. Additional findings are as follows:

- **Phase 1 (acute injury):** Normal physical exam; possible respiratory alkalosis.
- **Phase 2 (6–48 hours):** Hyperventilation, hypocapnia, widening A-a oxygen gradient.
- **Phase 3:** Acute respiratory failure, tachypnea, dyspnea, ↓ lung compliance, scattered rales, diffuse chest infiltrates on CXR (see Figure 2.15-4).

> **ARDS diagnosis:**
>
> **A**cute onset
> **R**atio (PaO_2/FiO_2) ≤ 200
> **D**iffuse infiltration
> **S**wan-Ganz wedge
>   pressure < 18 mmHg

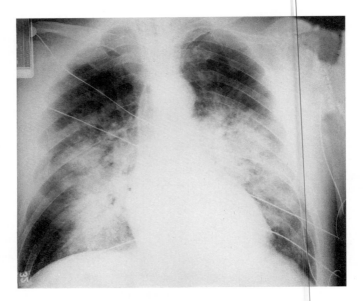

FIGURE 2.15-4. **AP CXR showing a diffuse alveolar filling pattern due to ARDS.**

(Reproduced, with permission, from Kasper DL et al (eds). *Harrison's Principles of Internal Medicine,* 16th ed. New York: McGraw-Hill, 2005, p. 1497.)

- **Phase 4:** Severe hypoxemia unresponsive to therapy; ↑ intrapulmonary shunting; metabolic and respiratory acidosis.

DIAGNOSIS

The criteria for ARDS diagnosis (according to the American-European Consensus Conference definition) are as follows:

- Acute onset of respiratory distress.
- **PaO_2/FiO_2 ratio ≤ 200 mmHg.**
- Bilateral pulmonary infiltrates on CXR.
- **No evidence of cardiac origin** (capillary wedge pressure < 18 mmHg or no clinical evidence for elevated left atrial pressure).

TREATMENT

There is no standard successful treatment. **Treat the underlying disease and maintain adequate perfusion and O_2 delivery to the organs.** Minimize injury induced by mechanical ventilation by ventilating with **low tidal volumes.** Use PEEP to recruit collapsed alveoli and titrate PEEP and FiO_2 to achieve adequate oxygenation. Goal oxygenation is PaO_2 > 60 mmHg or SaO_2 > 90% on FiO_2 ≤ 0.6.

PULMONARY VASCULAR DISEASE

Pulmonary Hypertension/Cor Pulmonale

- Pulmonary hypertension is defined as a mean pulmonary arterial pressure of > 25 mmHg. It is classified as 1° (if the etiology is unknown) or 2°. 1° pulmonary hypertension most often occurs in young or middle-aged women. The main causes of 2° pulmonary hypertension include the following:
    - Increased pulmonary venous pressure from left-sided **heart failure** or mitral valve disease.
    - Increased pulmonary blood flow 2° to **congenital heart disease** with left-to-right shunt.
    - **Hypoxic vasoconstriction** 2° to chronic lung disease (e.g., COPD).
    - **Thromboembolic** disease.
    - Remodeling of pulmonary vessels 2° to structural lung disease.
- **Hx/PE:**
    - Presents with dyspnea on exertion, fatigue, lethargy, syncope with exertion, chest pain, and symptoms of right-sided CHF (edema, abdominal distention).
    - Inquire about a history of COPD, interstitial lung disease, heart disease, sickle cell anemia, emphysema, and pulmonary emboli.
    - Exam reveals a loud, palpable S2 (often split), a systolic ejection murmur, an S4, or a parasternal heave.
- **Dx:** CXR shows enlargement of central pulmonary arteries; ECG demonstrates RVH. Echocardiogram and right heart catheterization may show signs of right ventricular overload and may aid in the diagnosis of the underlying cause.
- **Tx:** Supplemental O_2, anticoagulation, vasodilators, and diuretics if symptoms of right-sided CHF are present. Treat underlying causes of 2° pulmonary hypertension.

Pulmonary Thromboembolism

Occlusion of the pulmonary vasculature by a blood clot. Ninety-five percent of emboli originate from DVTs in the deep leg veins. Often → pulmonary in-

The main disorder of the pulmonary vasculature is pulmonary hypertension, which is defined as a mean P_{PA} > 25 mmHg (normal = 15 mmHg). Causes include left heart failure, mitral valve disease, and ↑ resistance in the pulmonary veins, including hypoxic vasoconstriction.

farction, right heart failure, and hypoxemia. **Virchow's triad** consists of the following:

- **Stasis:** Immobility, CHF, obesity, surgery, ↑ central venous pressure.
- **Endothelial injury:** Trauma, surgery, recent fracture, previous DVT.
- **Hypercoagulable states:** Pregnancy/postpartum, OCP use, coagulation disorders (e.g., protein C/protein S deficiency, factor V Leiden), malignancy, severe burns.

> **VIRchow's triad for venous thrombosis:**
>
> **V**ascular trauma
> **I**ncreased coagulability
> **R**educed blood flow (stasis)

HISTORY/PE

- Presents with sudden-onset dyspnea, **pleuritic chest pain, low-grade fever,** cough, and hemoptysis (rarely).
- **Pulmonary embolism:**
    - Hypoxia and hypocarbia with resulting respiratory alkalosis.
    - Presents with tachypnea, tachycardia, and fever.
    - Exam reveals a loud P2 and prominent jugular a waves with right heart failure.
- **Venous thrombosis:** Unilateral swelling; Homans' sign (calf pain on forced dorsiflexion); cords on the calf.

DIAGNOSIS

Dyspnea, tachycardia, and a normal CXR in a hospitalized and/or bedridden patient should raise suspicion of pulmonary embolism.

- **ABGs: Respiratory alkalosis** (due to hyperventilation) with $P_{O_2} < 80$ mmHg.
- **CXR:** Usually normal, but may show atelectasis, pleural effusion, **Hampton's hump** (a wedge-shaped infarct), or **Westermark's sign** (oligemia in the embolized lung zone).
- **ECG:** Not diagnostic; most commonly reveals **sinus tachycardia.** The classic triad of **S1Q3T3**—acute right heart strain with an S wave in lead I, a Q wave in lead III, and an inverted T wave in lead III—is uncommon.
- **V/Q scan:** May reveal segmental areas of mismatch. Results are reported with a designated probability of pulmonary embolism (low, indeterminate, or high) and are interpreted on the basis of clinical suspicion.
- **Helical (spiral) CT with IV contrast:** Sensitive for pulmonary embolism in the proximal pulmonary arteries, but less so in the distal segmental arteries.
- **Angiogram:** The gold standard, but more invasive and rarely done (see Figure 2.15-5).
- **D-dimer:** Sensitive but not specific in patients at risk for DVT or pulmonary embolism.
- **Venous ultrasound of the lower extremity:** Can detect a clot that may have given off the pulmonary embolism. Serial ultrasounds have a high diagnostic specificity.

TREATMENT

- **Heparin:** Bolus and then weight-based continuous infusion or low-molecular-weight heparin (LMWH) SQ.
- **Warfarin:** For long-term anticoagulation, usually given for six months unless the underlying predisposing factor persists (then given indefinitely). Follow INR (goal = 2–3).
- **IVC filter:** Indicated for patients with documented DVT in a lower extremity if anticoagulation is contraindicated or if patients experience recurrent emboli while anticoagulated.
- **Thrombolysis:** Indicated only in cases of massive DVT or pulmonary embolism causing right heart failure and hemodynamic instability (contraindicated in patients with recent surgery or bleeding).

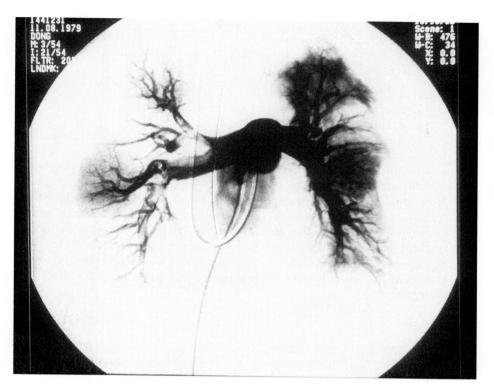

FIGURE 2.15-5. Pulmonary embolus.

A large filling defect in the pulmonary artery is evident on pulmonary angiogram.

- **DVT prophylaxis:** Treat bedridden medical patients and surgical patients; use **SQ heparin,** LMWH, intermittent pneumatic compression of the lower extremities (less effective), and **early ambulation (most effective).**

NEOPLASMS OF THE LUNGS

Lung Nodules

- **Hx/PE:** Often asymptomatic, or patients may present with chronic cough, dyspnea, and shortness of breath. Always inquire about smoking and exposure history.
- **Dx:**
  - **Serial CXRs:** Determine the location, progression, and extent of the nodule.
  - **Chest CT:** Determine the nature, extent, and infiltrating nature of the nodule.
  - **Characteristics favoring carcinoma:** Age > 45–50; smoking history; history of malignancy; new or larger lesions; absence of calcification or irregular calcification; size > 2 cm; irregular margins.
  - **Characteristics favoring a benign lesion:** Age < 35; no change from old films; central/uniform/laminated/popcorn calcification; size < 2 cm; smooth margins.
- **Tx:** Surgical resection is indicated for nodules at high risk for malignancy. Low-risk nodules can be followed with CXR or CT every three months for one year and then every six months for another year. An invasive diagnostic procedure is indicated if the size of the nodule ↑.

Lung Cancer

The leading cause of cancer death in the United States. Risk factors include tobacco smoke (except for bronchoalveolar carcinoma) and radon or asbestos exposure. Types are as follows:

Main locations for lung cancer metastasis—

BLAB

Bone
Liver
Adrenals
Brain

- **Small cell lung cancer (SCLC):**
    - Highly correlated with **cigarette exposure.**
    - **Central location.**
    - **Neuroendocrine origin;** associated with paraneoplastic syndromes (see Table 2.15-5).
    - Commonly presents with metastases (intrathoracic and extrathoracic sites such as brain, liver, and bone).
- **Non–small cell lung cancer (NSCLC): Less propensity to metastasize.**
- **Adenocarcinoma:** The most common lung cancer; **peripheral** location. Includes **bronchoalveolar carcinoma,** which is associated with multiple nodules, interstitial infiltration, and prolific sputum production.
- **Squamous cell carcinoma:** Central location; 98% are seen in smokers.
- **Large cell/neuroendocrine carcinomas:** Least common; associated with a poor prognosis.

HISTORY/PE

- Presents with cough, hemoptysis, dyspnea, wheezing, postobstructive pneumonia, chest pain, weight loss, and possible abnormalities on respiratory exam (crackles, atelectasis).

T A B L E   2 . 1 5 - 5 .   Paraneoplastic Syndromes of Lung Cancer

CLASSIFICATION	SYNDROME	HISTOLOGIC TYPE
Endocrine/metabolic	Cushing's syndrome (ACTH)	Small cell
	SIADH → hyponatremia	Small cell
	Hypercalcemia (PTHrP)	Squamous cell
	Gynecomastia	Large cell
Skeletal	Hypertrophic pulmonary osteoarthropathy	Non–small cell
	Digital clubbing	Non–small cell
Neuromuscular	Peripheral neuropathy	Small cell
	Subacute cerebellar degeneration	Small cell
	Myasthenia (Eaton-Lambert syndrome)	Small cell
	Dermatomyositis	All
Cardiovascular	Thrombophlebitis	Adenocarcinoma
	Nonbacterial verrucous endocarditis	Adenocarcinoma
Hematologic	Anemia	All
	DIC	All
	Eosinophilia	All
	Thrombocytosis	All
	Hypercoagulability	Adenocarcinoma
Cutaneous	Acanthosis nigricans	All
	Erythema gyratum repens	All

- Other findings include **Horner's syndrome** (miosis, ptosis, anhidrosis) in patients with Pancoast's tumor at the apex of the lung; **superior vena cava syndrome** (obstruction of the SVC with supraclavicular venous engorgement); **hoarseness** (due to recurrent laryngeal nerve involvement); and many **paraneoplastic syndromes** (see Table 2.15-5).

DIAGNOSIS

- CXR or **chest CT.**
- Fine-needle aspiration (CT guided) for peripheral lesions and **bronchoscopy** (biopsy or brushing) for central lesions.
- Thoracoscopic biopsy may be performed, with conversion to open thoracotomy if the lesion is found to be malignant.

TREATMENT

- **SCLC: Unresectable.** Often responds to radiation and chemotherapy initially but always recurs; lower median survival rate than NSCLC. Usually metastasized at the time of diagnosis.
- **NSCLC: Surgical resection** in early stages (IA, IB, IIA, IIB, and possibly IIIA). The extent of resection is based on lesion size; the presence of metastases; and the patient's age, general health, and lung function. Supplement surgery with radiation or chemotherapy (depending on the stage). Palliation (radiation and/or chemotherapy) for symptomatic but unresectable disease.

Chemotherapy is the mainstay of treatment for small cell lung cancer.

PLEURAL DISEASE

Pleural Effusion

Abnormal **accumulation of fluid in the pleural space.** Classified as follows:

- **Transudate:** Due to ↑ pulmonary capillary wedge pressure (PCWP) or ↓ oncotic pressure.
- **Exudate:** Due to ↑ pleural vascular permeability.

Table 2.15-6 lists the possible causes of both transudates and exudates.

HISTORY/PE

Presents with **dyspnea,** pleuritic chest pain, and/or cough. Exam reveals **dullness to percussion** and ↓ **breath sounds** over the effusion. A pleural friction rub may be present.

TABLE 2.15-6.   Causes of Pleural Effusions

TRANSUDATES	EXUDATES
CHF	Pneumonia (parapneumonic effusion)
Cirrhosis	TB
Nephrotic syndrome	Malignancy
	Pulmonary embolism
	Collagen vascular disease (rheumatoid arthritis, SLE)
	Pancreatitis
	Trauma

DIAGNOSIS

- CXR shows costophrenic angle blunting.
- **Thoracentesis** is indicated for new effusions > 1 cm in decubitus view.
- The effusion is an exudate if it meets the following criteria:
  - The ratio of pleural to serum protein is > 0.5 **or**
  - The ratio of pleural to serum LDH is > 0.6 **or**
  - Pleural fluid LDH is more than two-thirds the upper normal limit of serum LDH
- A parapneumonic effusion is classified as complicated in the setting of a ⊕ Gram stain or culture **or** a pH < 7.2 **or** a glucose level of < 60. The presence of **pus** indicates an **empyema**.

TREATMENT

Treatment is directed toward the underlying condition causing the effusion. Complicated parapneumonic effusions and empyemas require **chest tube drainage** in addition to **antibiotic therapy**.

Complicated parapneumonic effusions necessitate chest tube drainage.

Presentation of pneumothorax:

P-THORAX

Pleuritic pain
Tracheal deviation
Hyperresonance
Onset sudden
Reduced breath sounds (and dyspnea)
Absent fremitus
X-ray shows collapse

Pneumothorax

A collection of air in the pleural space that can → pulmonary collapse. Subtypes are as follows:

- **1° spontaneous pneumothorax:** Due to rupture of subpleural apical blebs (usually found in **tall, thin young males**).
- **2° pneumothorax:** Due to COPD, TB, trauma, *Pneumocystis carinii* pneumonia (PCP), and iatrogenic factors (thoracentesis, subclavian line placement, positive-pressure mechanical ventilation, bronchoscopy).
- **Tension pneumothorax:** A pulmonary or chest wall defect acts as a **one-way valve,** drawing air into the pleural space during inspiration but trapping air during expiration. Etiologies include penetrating trauma, infection, and positive-pressure mechanical ventilation. Shock and death result unless the condition is immediately recognized and treated.

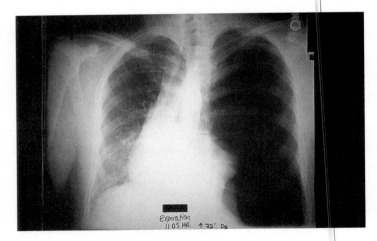

FIGURE 2.15-6.   Tension pneumothorax.

Note the hyperlucent lung field, hyperexpanded lower diaphragm, collapsed lung, tracheal deviation, mediastinal shift, and compression of the opposite lung on AP CXR.

HISTORY/PE

- Presents with acute onset of **unilateral pleuritic chest pain** and **dyspnea**.
- Exam reveals tachypnea, **diminished or absent breath sounds, hyperresonance**, and ↓ **tactile fremitus.**
- Suspect tension pneumothorax in the presence of respiratory distress, falling O_2 saturation, hypotension, distended neck veins, and **tracheal deviation.**

DIAGNOSIS

CXR shows the presence of a visceral pleural line and/or **lung retraction** from the chest wall (best seen in end-expiratory films; see Figure 2.15-6).

TREATMENT

- Small pneumothoraces may resorb spontaneously. Supplemental O_2 therapy is helpful.
- Large, symptomatic pneumothoraces require chest tube placement.
- Tension pneumothorax requires immediate needle decompression (second intercostal space at the midclavicular line) followed by a chest tube.

Renal/Genitourinary

In hypernatremia, patients may not drink enough free water to replace insensible losses.

Hypernatremia causes—

the 6 D's:

Diuretics
Dehydration
Diabetes insipidus
Docs (iatrogenic)
Diarrhea
Disease (e.g., kidney, sickle cell)

Hypernatremia

Serum sodium > 145 mEq/L. Usually due to water loss rather than sodium gain.

HISTORY/PE

- Presents with **thirst** (due to hypertonicity) as well as with oliguria or polyuria (depending on the etiology).
- **Neurologic symptoms** include mental status changes, weakness, focal neurologic deficits, and seizures.
- Exam reveals **"doughy" skin** and signs of volume depletion.

DIAGNOSIS

- Assess volume status by conducting a clinical exam and measuring urine volume and osmolality.
    - **Hypertonic Na⁺ gain:** Due to hypertonic saline/tube feeds or ↑ aldosterone.
    - **Pure water loss:** Due to central or nephrogenic **diabetes insipidus (DI)**; characterized by large volumes of dilute urine. Don't neglect dermal and respiratory-insensible losses.
    - **Hypotonic fluid loss:** Due to ↓ intake, diuretics, intrinsic renal disease, GI losses (**diarrhea**), burns, and osmotic diuresis (mannitol).
- A minimal volume (approximately 500 mL/day) of maximally concentrated urine (> 800 mOsm/kg) suggests adequate renal response without adequate free-water replacement.

TREATMENT

- Treat the underlying causes and replace free-water deficit with hypotonic saline, D5W, or oral water, depending on volume status.
- Correction of chronic hypernatremia (> 36–48 hours) should be accomplished **gradually over 48–72 hours** to prevent neurologic damage 2° to cerebral swelling.

Hyponatremia

Serum sodium < 136 mEq/L.

HISTORY/PE

- May be asymptomatic or may present with **confusion, lethargy,** muscle cramps, hyporeflexia, and nausea.
- Can progress to seizures, coma, or brain stem herniation.

DIAGNOSIS

Hyponatremia can be categorized according to serum and urine osmolality as well as by volume status (i.e., by clinical exam). Osmolality is classified as follows:

- **High (> 295 mEq/L):** Hyperglycemia, hypertonic infusion (e.g., mannitol).
- **Normal (280–295 mEq/L):** Hypertriglyceridemia, paraproteinemia (pseudohyponatremia).

- **Low (< 280 mEq/L):** Applies to the majority of cases. Hypotonic etiologies are listed in Table 2.16-1.

TREATMENT

- Specific treatments are outlined in Table 2.16-1.
- Chronic hyponatremia (> 72 hours' duration) should be corrected slowly (no more than 0.5–1.0 mEq/L/hr) in order to prevent central pontine myelinolysis (quadriplegia and pseudobulbar palsy).

Hyperkalemia

Serum potassium > 5 mEq/L. Etiologies are as follows:

- **Spurious:** Hemolysis of blood samples, fist clenching during blood draws, extreme leukocytosis or thrombocytosis, rhabdomyolysis.
- **↓ excretion:** Renal insufficiency, drugs (e.g., spironolactone, triamterene, ACEIs, trimethoprim, NSAIDs), mineralocorticoid deficiency/type IV renal tubular acidosis (RTA).
- **Cellular shifts:** Tissue injury, insulin deficiency, acidosis, drugs (e.g., succinylcholine, digitalis, arginine, β-blockers).
- **Iatrogenic.**

HISTORY/PE

May be asymptomatic or may present with nausea, vomiting, **intestinal colic, areflexia, weakness,** flaccid paralysis, and paresthesias.

DIAGNOSIS

- Confirm hyperkalemia with a **repeat blood draw.** In the setting of extreme leukocytosis or thrombocytosis, check plasma potassium.
- ECG findings include **tall, peaked T waves;** PR prolongation; wide QRS; and loss of P waves (see Figure 2.16-1). Can progress to **sine waves,** ventricular fibrillation, and cardiac arrest.

TREATMENT

- Values of > 6.5 mEq/L or ECG changes (especially PR prolongation or wide QRS) require emergent treatment.
- The mnemonic **C BIG K** summarizes the treatment of hyperkalemia.
  - First give **calcium gluconate** for cardiac cell membrane stabilization.
  - Give **bicarbonate and/or insulin and glucose** to temporarily shift potassium into cells.

> **Treatment of hyperkalemia—**
>
> **C BIG K**
>
> **C**alcium
> **B**icarbonate
> **I**nsulin
> **G**lucose
> **K**ayexalate

TABLE 2.16-1. **Evaluation and Treatment of Hypotonic Hyponatremia**

VOLUME STATUS	ETIOLOGIES	TREATMENT
Hypervolemic	Renal failure, nephrotic syndrome, cirrhosis, CHF.	Water restriction.
Euvolemic	SIADH, hypothyroidism, renal failure, drugs, psychogenic polydipsia, adrenal insufficiency.	Water restriction.
Hypovolemic	Diuretics, vomiting, diarrhea, third spacing, dehydration.	Replete volume with normal saline.

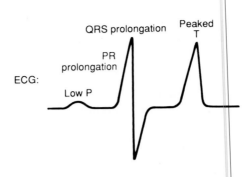

FIGURE 2.16-1. Hyperkalemia on ECG.

Electrocardiographic manifestations include peaked T waves, PR prolongation, and a widened QRS complex. (Reproduced, with permission, from Cogan MG. *Fluid and Electrolytes*, 1st ed. Stamford, CT: Appleton & Lange, 1991, p. 170.)

- β-agonists promote cellular reuptake of potassium.
- **Kayexalate** and loop diuretics (e.g., furosemide) to remove potassium from the body.
- Dialysis is appropriate for patients with renal failure or for severe, refractory cases.

Hypokalemia

Hypokalemia is usually due to renal or GI losses.

Serum potassium < 3.6 mEq/L. Etiologies are as follows:

- **Transcellular shifts:** Insulin, β_2-agonists, alkalosis, familial hypokalemic periodic paralysis.
- **GI losses:** Diarrhea, chronic laxative abuse, vomiting, NG suction.
- **Renal losses:** Diuretics (e.g., loop or thiazide), 1° mineralocorticoid excess or 2° hyperaldosteronism, ↓ circulating volume, Bartter's syndrome, drugs (e.g., gentamicin, amphotericin), DKA, hypomagnesemia, type I RTA (defective distal H^+ secretion).

HISTORY/PE

Presents with fatigue, **muscle weakness or cramps, ileus,** hyporeflexia, paresthesias, rhabdomyolysis, and ascending paralysis.

DIAGNOSIS

- Twenty-four-hour or spot urine potassium may distinguish renal from GI losses.
- ECG may show **T-wave flattening, U waves** (an additional wave after the T wave), and ST-segment depression → AV block and subsequent cardiac arrest.
- Consider RTA in the setting of metabolic acidosis.

TREATMENT

- Treat the underlying disorder.
- Oral and/or IV **potassium repletion.**
- Replace magnesium, as this deficiency complicates potassium repletion.
- Monitor ECG and plasma potassium levels frequently during replacement.

Hypercalcemia

Serum calcium > 10.2 mg/dL. The most common causes are **hyperparathyroidism and malignancy** (e.g., breast cancer, squamous cell carcinoma, multiple myeloma). Other causes are summarized in the mnemonic **CHIMPANZEES.**

HISTORY/PE

May present with **bones** (fractures), **stones** (kidney stones), abdominal **groans** (anorexia, constipation), and **psychiatric overtones** (weakness, fatigue, altered mental status).

DIAGNOSIS

Order a total/ionized calcium, albumin, phosphate, PTH, parathyroid hormone–related peptide (PTHrP), vitamin D, and ECG (may show a **short QT interval**).

TREATMENT

- **IV hydration** followed by **furosemide** to ↑ calcium excretion.
- Calcitonin, bisphosphonates (e.g., pamidronate), glucocorticoids, and dialysis are used for severe or refractory cases. **Avoid thiazide diuretics,** which ↑ tubular reabsorption of calcium.

Hypocalcemia

Serum calcium < 8.5 mg/dL. Etiologies include hypoparathyroidism (postsurgical, idiopathic), malnutrition, hypomagnesemia, acute pancreatitis, vitamin D deficiency, and pseudohypoparathyroidism.

HISTORY/PE

- Presents with **abdominal muscle cramps,** dyspnea, **tetany, perioral and acral paresthesias,** and convulsions.
- Facial spasm elicited from tapping of the facial nerve (**Chvostek's sign**) and carpal spasm after arterial occlusion by a BP cuff (**Trousseau's sign**) are classic findings that are most commonly seen in severe hypocalcemia.

DIAGNOSIS

- Order an ionized Ca^{2+}, Mg^+, PTH, albumin, and possibly calcitonin. If the patient is post-thyroidectomy, review the operative note to determine the number of parathyroid glands removed.
- ECG may show a **prolonged QT interval.**

TREATMENT

- Treat the underlying disorder.
- Magnesium repletion.
- Administer oral **calcium supplements;** give IV calcium for severe symptoms.

Hypomagnesemia

Serum magnesium < 1.5 mEq/L. Etiologies are as follows:

- ↓ **intake:** Malnutrition, malabsorption, short bowel syndrome, TPN.

Loops (furosemide) Lose calcium.

Serum calcium may be falsely low in hypoalbuminemia.

The classic case of hypocalcemia is a patient who develops cramps and tetany following thyroidectomy.

- ↑ **loss:** Diuretics, diarrhea, vomiting, hypercalcemia, drugs (amphotericin), alcoholism.
- **Miscellaneous: DKA,** pancreatitis.

HISTORY/PE

- Symptoms are generally related to concurrent hypocalcemia and hypokalemia; they include anorexia, nausea, vomiting, muscle cramps, and weakness.
- In severe cases, symptoms may also include hyperactive reflexes, paresthesias, irritability, confusion, lethargy, seizures, and arrhythmias.

DIAGNOSIS

- Labs may show concurrent hypocalcemia and hypokalemia.
- ECG may reveal prolonged PR and QT intervals.

TREATMENT

- IV and oral supplements.
- Hypokalemia and hypocalcemia will not correct without magnesium correction.

ACID-BASE DISORDERS

See Figure 2.16-2 for a diagnostic algorithm for acid-base disorders.

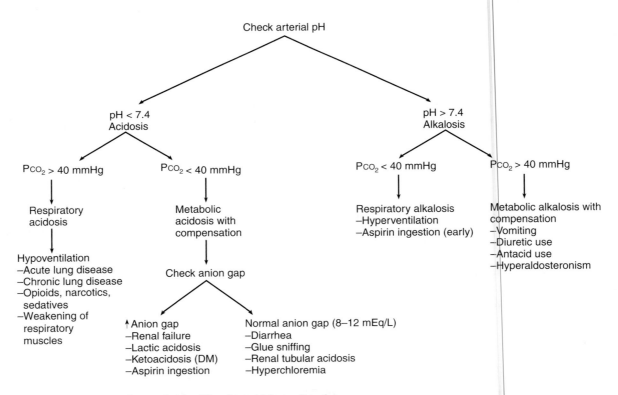

FIGURE 2.16-2. **Diagnostic algorithm for acid-base disorders.**

TABLE 2.16-2. Types of RTA

	TYPE I (DISTAL)	TYPE II (PROXIMAL)	TYPE IV (DISTAL)
Defect	H^+ secretion.	HCO_3^- reabsorption.	Aldosterone deficiency or resistance $\rightarrow$ defects in Na^+ reabsorption and H^+ and K^+ excretion.
Serum K^+	High or low.	Low.	High.
Urinary pH	> 5.3.	5.3 initially; < 5.3 once serum is acidic.	< 5.3.
Etiologies (most common)	Hereditary, amphotericin, cirrhosis, autoimmune disorders, sickle cell disease, lithium.	Hereditary, carbonic anhydrase inhibitors, Fanconi's syndrome, multiple myeloma.	Hyporeninemic hypoaldosteronism; chronic kidney disease from DM, hypertension, and HIV.
Treatment	Potassium citrate.	Potassium citrate.	Furosemide, fludrocortisone, and low-potassium diet in patients with aldosterone deficiency.
Complications	Nephrolithiasis.	Rickets, osteomalacia.	Hyperkalemia.

RENAL TUBULAR ACIDOSIS (RTA)

A net ↓ in either tubular H^+ secretion or HCO_3^- reabsorption that → a **non–anion gap metabolic acidosis**. There are three main types of RTA; **type IV (distal)** is the **most common form** (see Table 2.16-2).

ACUTE RENAL FAILURE (ARF)

An abrupt ↓ in renal function → the retention of creatinine and BUN. ↓ urine output (i.e., oliguria, defined as < 500 cc/day) is not required for ARF. ARF is categorized as follows (see also Table 2.16-3):

TABLE 2.16-3. Causes of Acute Renal Failure

PRERENAL	RENAL (INTRINSIC)	POSTRENAL
Hypovolemia (hemorrhage, dehydration, burns)	Acute tubular necrosis (ATN)	Prostatic disease
Cardiogenic shock	Acute/allergic interstitial nephritis	Nephrolithiasis
Sepsis	Glomerulonephritis	Pelvic tumors
Anaphylaxis	Thromboembolism	Recent pelvic surgery
Drugs		Retroperitoneal fibrosis
Renal artery stenosis		
Cirrhosis with ascites (hepatorenal syndrome)		

- **Prerenal:** ↓ renal perfusion.
- **Intrinsic:** Injury within the nephron unit.
- **Postrenal:** Urinary outflow obstruction. Generally, both kidneys must be obstructed before one can see a significant ↑ in BUN and creatinine.

HISTORY/PE

- Symptoms of **uremia** include malaise, fatigue, confusion, oliguria, anorexia, and nausea.
- Exam may show a **pericardial rub, asterixis, hypertension,** ↓ urine output, and an ↑ respiratory rate (compensation of metabolic acidosis or from pulmonary edema 2° to volume overload).
- Category-specific symptoms are as follows:
    - **Prerenal:** Thirst, orthostatic hypotension, tachycardia, ↓ skin turgor, dry mucous membranes, reduced axillary sweating, stigmata of comorbid conditions.
        - **Intrinsic:** Associated with a history of drug exposure (aminoglycosides, NSAIDs) or exposure to contrast media or toxins (e.g., myoglobin, myeloma protein).
        - **Acute interstitial nephritis:** Fever, arthralgias, and a pruritic, erythematous rash. Methicillin is the classic association.
        - **Atheroemboli:** Subcutaneous nodules, livedo reticularis, digital ischemia.
        - **Glomerulonephritis:** Oliguria, edema, hypertension.
    - **Postrenal:** Prostatic disease, suprapubic pain, distended bladder and flank pain.

DIAGNOSIS

- Check serum electrolytes. Examine the urine for RBCs, WBCs, casts (see Table 2.16-4), and **urine eosinophils.**
- An $Fe_{Na} < 1\%$, a $U_{Na} < 20$, a urine specific gravity > 1.020, or a BUN/creatinine ratio > 20 suggests a prerenal etiology.
- A urinary catheter and renal ultrasound can help rule out obstruction. Ultrasound can also identify kidneys that are ↓ in size, as occurs with chronic renal failure.
- In patients with oliguria, the Fe_{Na} can help identify prerenal failure and distinguish it from intrinsic renal disease.
- Obtain a renal biopsy only when the cause of intrinsic renal disease is unclear.

Patients with ARF may have a normal urine volume.

Renal ischemia, toxins, hemoglobinuria, or myoglobinuria may → ATN.

An $Fe_{Na} < 1\%$ indicates that the kidneys are trying to conserve sodium, suggesting a prerenal etiology.

TABLE 2.16-4. Findings on Microscopic Urine Examination in Acute Renal Failure

URINE SEDIMENT	ETIOLOGY	CLASSIFICATION
Hyaline casts	Normal finding, but an ↑ amount suggests volume depletion	Prerenal
Red cell casts, dysmorphic red cells	Glomerulonephritis	Intrinsic
White cells, eosinophils	Allergic interstitial nephritis, atheroembolic disease	Intrinsic
Granular casts, renal tubular cells, "muddy-brown cast"	ATN	Intrinsic
White cells, white cell casts	Pyelonephritis	Postrenal

TREATMENT

- Balance fluids and electrolytes.
- In acute or allergic interstitial nephritis, adjust or discontinue offending medications.
- Dialyze if indicated (see the mnemonic **AEIOU**) using hemodialysis. Peritoneal dialysis should be considered only for long-term dialysis patients.

COMPLICATIONS

- Chronic renal failure may result, requiring dialysis to prevent the buildup of **K$^+$, H$^+$, and toxic metabolites.**
- Patients who are dialysis dependent are at ↑ risk for a number of disorders, including CAD.

DIURETICS

Table 2.16-5 summarizes the actions and side effects of commonly used diuretics.

> **Indications for urgent dialysis—**
>
> **AEIOU**
>
> **A**cidosis
> **E**lectrolyte abnormalities (hyperkalemia)
> **I**ngestions (salicylates, theophylline, methanol, barbiturates, lithium, ethylene glycol)
> **O**verload (fluid)
> **U**remic symptoms (pericarditis, encephalopathy, bleeding, nausea, pruritus, myoclonus)

TABLE 2.16-5. Mechanism of Action and Side Effects of Diuretics

TYPE	DRUGS	SITE OF ACTION	MECHANISM OF ACTION	SIDE EFFECTS
Carbonic anhydrase inhibitors	Acetazolamide	Proximal convoluted tubule.	Inhibits carbonic anhydrase, ↑ H$^+$ reabsorption, blocks Na$^+$/H$^+$ exchange.	Hyperchloremic metabolic acidosis, sulfa allergy.
Osmotic agents	Mannitol, urea	Entire tubule.	↑ tubular fluid osmolarity.	Pulmonary edema due to CHF and anuria.
Loop agents	Furosemide, ethacrynic acid, bumetanide, torsemide	Ascending loop of Henle.	Inhibits Na$^+$/K$^+$/2 Cl$^-$ transporter.	Water loss, metabolic alkalosis, ↓ K$^+$, ↓ **Ca^{2+}**, **ototoxicity,** sulfa allergy (e.g., except ethacrynic acid, hyperuricemia).
Thiazide agents	Hydrochlorothiazide, chlorothiazide	Distal convoluted tubule.	Inhibits Na$^+$/Cl$^-$ transporter.	Water loss, metabolic alkalosis, ↓ **Na$^+$**, ↓ K$^+$, ↑ glucose, ↑ **Ca^{2+}**, ↑ uric acid, sulfa allergy, pancreatitis.
K$^+$-sparing agents	Spironolactone, triamterene, amiloride	Cortical collecting tubule.	Aldosterone receptor antagonist (spironolactone), block sodium channel (triamterene, amiloride).	Metabolic acidosis, ↑ K$^+$, antiandrogenic effects, including gynecomastia (spironolactone).

GLOMERULAR DISEASE

Nephritic Syndrome

A disorder of glomerular inflammation, also called glomerulonephritis. Proteinuria may be present but is usually < 1.5 g/day. Causes are summarized in Table 2.16-6.

Think nephritic syndrome if the patient has hematuria, hypertension, and oliguria.

HISTORY/PE

The classic findings are oliguria, macroscopic/microscopic hematuria (smoky-brown urine), hypertension, and **edema.**

DIAGNOSIS

- UA shows hematuria and possibly mild proteinuria.
- Patients have a ↓ GFR with elevated BUN and creatinine. Complement, ANA, ANCA, and anti-GBM antibody levels should be measured to determine the underlying etiology.
- Renal biopsy may be useful for histologic evaluation.

TREATMENT

- Treat hypertension, fluid overload, and uremia with salt and water restriction, diuretics, and, if necessary, dialysis.
- **Corticosteroids** are useful in reducing glomerular inflammation in some cases.

Nephrotic Syndrome

Proteinuria, hypoalbuminemia, edema, hyperlipidemia, and hyperlipiduria are due to the initial ↑ permeability of the glomerulus to protein.

Defined as **proteinuria (≥ 3.5 g/day), generalized edema, hypoalbuminemia,** and **hyperlipidemia.** Approximately one-third of all cases are the result of systemic diseases such as DM, SLE, or amyloidosis. Causes are summarized in Table 2.16-7.

HISTORY/PE

- Presents with **generalized edema** and **foamy urine.** In severe cases, dyspnea and ascites may develop.
- Patients have ↑ susceptibility to infection as well as a predisposition to hypercoagulable states with an ↑ risk for venous thrombosis and pulmonary embolism.

DIAGNOSIS

- UA shows **proteinuria** (≥ 3.5 g/day) and lipiduria.
- Blood chemistry shows ↓ **albumin** (< 3 g/dL) and hyperlipidemia.
- Evaluation should include workup for 2° causes.
- Renal biopsy is used to definitively diagnose the underlying etiology.

TREATMENT

- Treat with **protein and salt restriction,** diuretic therapy, and antihyperlipidemics.
- **ACEIs** ↓ proteinuria and diminish the progression of renal disease in patients with diabetic nephropathy.
- Vaccinate with 23-polyvalent pneumococcus vaccine (PPV23), as patients are at ↑ risk of *Streptococcus pneumoniae* infection.

TABLE 2.16-6. Causes of Nephritic Syndrome

	DESCRIPTION	HISTORY/PE	LABS/HISTOLOGY	TREATMENT/PROGNOSIS
Immune complex				
Postinfectious glomerulo-nephritis	Often associated with a recent group A β-hemolytic **streptococcal infection** (within two weeks).	Oliguria, edema, hypertension, smoky-brown urine.	Low serum C3, ↑ **ASO titer, lumpy-bumpy immuno-fluorescence.**	Supportive. Almost all children and most adults have a complete recovery.
IgA nephropathy (Berger's disease)	**Most common type;** associated with upper respiratory or GI infections. Commonly seen in young men; may be seen in Henoch-Schönlein purpura.	Episodic gross hematuria or persistent microscopic hematuria.	Normal C3.	Glucocorticoids for select patients; ACEIs in patients with proteinuria. Some 20% of cases progress to end-stage renal disease (ESRD).
Pauci-immune				
Wegener's granulomatosis	Granulomatous inflammation of the respiratory tract and kidney with necrotizing vasculitis.	Fever, weight loss, hematuria, hearing disturbances, respiratory and sinus symptoms. Cavitary pulmonary lesions bleed and → **hemoptysis.**	Presence of **c-ANCA** (cell-mediated immune response). Renal biopsy shows segmental necrotizing glomerulonephritis with few immunoglobulin deposits on immuno-fluorescence.	High-dose corticosteroids and cytotoxic agents. Patients tend to have frequent relapses.
Anti-GBM disease				
Goodpasture's syndrome	Glomerulonephritis with pulmonary hemorrhage; peak incidence in men in their mid-20s.	**Hemoptysis,** dyspnea, possible respiratory failure.	**Linear anti-GBM deposits** on immuno-fluorescence; iron deficiency anemia; hemosiderin-filled macrophages in sputum; pulmonary infiltrates on CXR.	Plasma exchange therapy; pulsed steroids. May progress to ESRD.
Alport's syndrome	Hereditary glomerulonephritis; presents in boys 5–20 years of age.	Asymptomatic hematuria associated with **nerve deafness** and eye disorders.	GBM splitting on electron microscopy.	Progresses to renal failure. Anti-GBM nephritis may recur after transplant.

TABLE 2.16-7.   Causes of Nephrotic Syndrome

	DESCRIPTION	HISTORY/PE	LABS/HISTOLOGY	TREATMENT/PROGNOSIS
Minimal change disease	The most common cause of nephritic syndrome in children. Idiopathic etiology; 2° causes include NSAIDs and hematologic malignancies.	Tendency toward infections and thrombotic events.	Light microscopy appears **normal;** electron microscopy shows **fusion of epithelial foot processes** with lipid-laden renal cortices.	Steroids; excellent prognosis.
Focal segmental glomerular sclerosis	Idiopathic, IV drug use, HIV infection, obesity.	The typical patient is a young black male with uncontrolled hypertension.	Microscopic hematuria; biopsy shows sclerosis in capillary tufts.	Prednisone, cytotoxic therapy.
Membranous nephropathy	**The most common nephropathy in Caucasian adults.** 2° causes includes solid tumor malignancies (especially in patients > 60 years of age) and immune complex disease.	Associated with HBV, syphilis, malaria, and gold.	**"Spike-and-dome"** appearance due to granular deposits of IgG and C3 at the basement membrane.	Prednisone and cytotoxic therapy for severe disease.
Diabetic nephropathy	Two characteristic forms: diffuse hyalinization and nodular glomerulosclerosis **(Kimmelstiel-Wilson lesions).**	Generally have long-standing, poorly controlled DM with evidence of retinopathy or neuropathy.	Thickened GBM; ↑ **mesangial matrix.**	Tight control of blood sugar; ACEIs for type 1 DM and ARBs for type 2 DM.
Lupus nephritis	Classified as WHO types I–VI. Both nephrotic and nephritic. The severity of renal disease often determines overall prognosis.	Proteinuria or RBCs on UA may be found during evaluation of SLE patients.	Mesangial proliferation; subendothelial immune complex deposition.	Prednisone and cytotoxic therapy may ↓ disease progression.
Renal amyloidosis	1° (plasma cell dyscrasia) and 2° (infectious or inflammatory) are the most common.	Patients may have multiple myeloma or a chronic inflammatory disease (e.g., rheumatoid arthritis, TB).	Fat pad biopsy; seen with **Congo red stain; apple-green** birefringence under polarized light.	Prednisone and melphalan. Bone marrow transplant may be used for multiple myeloma.

TABLE 2.16-7. Causes of Nephrotic Syndrome (continued)

	DESCRIPTION	HISTORY/PE	LABS/HISTOLOGY	TREATMENT/PROGNOSIS
Membranoproliferative nephropathy	Can also be nephritic syndrome. Type I is associated with HCV, cryoglobulinemia, lupus, and subacute bacterial endocarditis.	Slow progression to renal failure.	"Tram-track," double-layered basement membrane. Type I has subendothelial deposits and mesangial deposits; all three types have low serum C3; type II by way of C3 nephritic factor.	Corticosteroids and cytotoxic agents may help.

DIABETES INSIPIDUS (DI)

Failure to concentrate urine as a result of central or nephrogenic ADH dysfunction. Subtypes are as follows:

- **Central DI:** The posterior pituitary fails to secrete ADH. Causes include **tumor,** ischemia (Sheehan's syndrome), traumatic cerebral injury, infection, and autoimmune disorders.
- **Nephrogenic DI:** The kidneys fail to respond to circulating ADH. Causes include renal diseases and drugs (e.g., **lithium,** demeclocycline).

For unknown reasons, patients with DI prefer ice-cold beverages.

HISTORY/PE

- Presents with **polydipsia, polyuria,** and **persistent thirst** with dilute urine.
- Patients may present with hypernatremia and dehydration, but if given unlimited access to water, they are typically normonatremic.

DIAGNOSIS

- During a **water deprivation test,** patients excrete a high volume of dilute urine.
- Desmopressin acetate (DDAVP), a synthetic analog of ADH, can be used to distinguish central from nephrogenic DI.
    - **Central DI:** DDAVP challenge will ↓ **urine output and** ↑ **urine osmolarity.**
    - **Nephrogenic DI:** DDAVP challenge will not significantly ↓ urine output.
- MRI may show a pituitary or hypothalamic mass in central DI.

TREATMENT

- Treat the underlying cause.
    - **Central DI:** Administer DDAVP intranasally.
    - **Nephrogenic DI:** Salt restriction and water intake are the 1° treatment. Thiazide diuretics are used to promote mild volume depletion and to stimulate proximal reabsorption of salt and water.

A common cause of euvolemic hyponatremia that results from **stimulated ADH release independent of serum osmolality.**

HISTORY/PE

Associated with **CNS disease** (e.g., head injury, tumor), **pulmonary disease** (e.g., sarcoid, pneumonia), ectopic tumor production/paraneoplastic syndrome (e.g., small cell carcinoma), drugs (e.g., antipsychotics, antidepressants), or surgery.

DIAGNOSIS

Fluid restriction is the cornerstone of SIADH treatment.

- Diagnose on the basis of a urine osmolality > 50–100 mOsm/kg with concurrent serum hyposmolarity in the absence of a physiologic reason for ↑ ADH (e.g., CHF, cirrhosis, hypovolemia).
- **Urinary sodium ≥ 20 mEq/L** demonstrates that the patient is not hypovolemic.

TREATMENT

- **Restrict fluid** and address the underlying cause.
- If hyponatremia is severe (< 110 mEq/L) or the patient is significantly symptomatic (e.g., comatose, seizing), cautiously give hypertonic saline.
- **Demeclocycline** can help normalize serum sodium by antagonizing the action of ADH in the collecting duct.
- Chronic correction depends on treatment of the underlying disorder.

Renal calculi. Stones are most commonly calcium oxalate but may also be calcium phosphate, struvite, uric acid, or cystine (see Table 2.16-8). Risk factors include a ⊕ family history, **low fluid intake,** gout, postcolectomy/postileostomy, specific enzyme disorders, RTA (due to alkaline urinary pH), and hyperparathyroidism. Most common in older males.

HISTORY/PE

- Presents with **acute onset of severe, colicky flank pain** that may **radiate to the testes or vulva** and is associated with nausea and vomiting.
- Patients are unable to get comfortable and shift position frequently (as opposed to those with peritonitis, who lie still).

DIAGNOSIS

- UA may show gross or **microscopic hematuria** (15% do not have hematuria) and an **altered urine pH.**
- Obtain an AXR in patients with known radiopaque stones and possibly a **renal ultrasound** to look for obstruction (ultrasound is also preferred for pregnant patients, in whom radiation should be avoided).
- **Noncontrast abdominal CT scans** may diagnose stones and other causes of flank pain.
- An **IVP** can be used to confirm the diagnosis if there is a lack of contrast filling below the stone.

TABLE 2.16-8. **Types of Nephrolithiasis**

TYPE	FREQUENCY	ETIOLOGY AND CHARACTERISTICS	TREATMENT
Calcium oxalate/ calcium phosphate	83%	The most common causes are **idiopathic hypercalciuria,** elevated urine uric acid 2° to diet, and 1° hyperparathyroidism. Alkaline urine. Radiopaque.	Hydration, thiazide diuretic.
Struvite (Mg-NH$_4$-PO$_4$)	9%	"Triple phosphate stones." Associated with urease-producing organisms (e.g., *Proteus*). Form staghorn calculi. Alkaline urine. Radiopaque.	Hydration; treat UTI if present.
Uric acid	7%	Associated with gout and high purine turnover states. Acidic urine (pH < 5.5). **Radiolucent.**	Hydration; alkalinize urine with citrate, which is converted to HCO$_3^-$ in the liver; dietary purine restriction and allopurinol.
Cystine	1%	Due to a defect in renal transport of certain amino acids (COLA—cystine, ornithine, lysine, and arginine). **Hexagonal crystals.** Radiopaque.	Hydration, alkalinize urine, penicillamine.

TREATMENT

- **Hydration and analgesia** are the initial treatment.
- Kidney stones < 5 mm in diameter can pass through the urethra; stones < 3 cm in diameter can be treated with **extracorporeal shock-wave lithotripsy (ESWL)** or percutaneous nephrolithotomy.
- Preventive measures include hydration; additional prophylaxis is dependent on stone composition.

POLYCYSTIC KIDNEY DISEASE (PCKD)

Characterized by the presence of renal cysts as well as by cysts in the spleen, liver, and pancreas. The two major forms are as follows:

- **Autosomal dominant:**
  - Most common.
  - Usually asymptomatic until patients are > 30 years of age.
  - One-half of autosomal-dominant PCKD patients will have ESRD requiring dialysis by age 60.
  - Associated with an ↑ risk of cerebral aneurysm, especially in patients with a ⊕ family history.
- **Autosomal recessive:** Less common but more severe. Presents in infants and young children with renal failure, liver fibrosis, and portal hypertension; may lead to death in the first few years of life.

HISTORY/PE

- **Pain and hematuria** are the most common presenting symptoms. Sharp, localized pain may result from cyst rupture, infection, or passage of renal calculi.

- Additional findings include **hypertension, hepatic cysts, cerebral berry aneurysms,** diverticulosis, and mitral valve prolapse.
- Patients may have large, palpable kidneys on abdominal exam.

DIAGNOSIS

Based on ultrasound or CT scan. Multiple bilateral cysts will be present throughout the renal parenchyma, and renal enlargement will be visualized.

TREATMENT

- **Prevent complications and ↓ the rate of progression to ESRD.** Early management of UTIs is critical to prevent renal cyst infection. BP control is necessary to ↓ hypotension-induced renal damage.
- Dialysis and renal transplantation are used to manage patients with ESRD.

HYDRONEPHROSIS

Dilation of renal calyces resulting from ↑ pressure in the distal urinary tract → kidney/ureter damage. Usually occurs 2° to ureteral obstruction. In pediatric patients, the obstruction is often at the ureteropelvic junction. In adults, it may be due to BPH, tumors, aortic aneurysms, or renal calculi.

HISTORY/PE

May be asymptomatic, or may present with flank/back pain, ↓ urine output, abdominal pain, and UTIs.

DIAGNOSIS

- Ultrasound or IVP to detect dilation of the renal calyces and/or ureter.
- ↑ BUN and creatinine provide evidence of 2° renal failure.

TREATMENT

- Surgically correct any anatomic obstruction; use laser or sound wave lithotripsy if calculi are causing obstruction.
- Ureteral stent placement across the obstructed area of the urinary tract and/or percutaneous nephrostomy tube placement to relieve pressure may be appropriate if the urinary outflow tract is not sufficiently cleared of obstruction.

URETERAL REFLUX

Retrograde projection of urine from the bladder to the ureters and kidneys. Often caused by insufficient tunneling of ureters into submucosal bladder tissue → ineffective restriction of retrograde urine flow during bladder contraction. Classified as follows:

- **Mild reflux (grades I–II):** No ureteral or renal pelvic dilation. Often resolves spontaneously.
- **Moderate to severe reflux (grade III–V):** Ureteral dilation with associated calyceal blunting in severe cases

HISTORY/PE

Patients present with recurrent UTIs.

DIAGNOSIS

Obtain a **voiding cystourethrogram** to detect abnormalities at ureteral insertion sites and to classify the grade of reflux. All children < 7 years of age presenting with their first UTI should undergo a voiding cystourethrogram to screen for reflux.

TREATMENT

Treat infections aggressively. Treat mild reflux with daily prophylactic antibiotics until reflux resolves at puberty. Ureteral implantation may be considered in severe reflux. Inadequate treatment can → progressive renal scarring and ESRD.

CRYPTORCHIDISM

Failure of the testes to fully descend into the scrotum. **Prematurity is a risk factor.**

HISTORY/PE

Bilateral cryptorchidism is associated with oligospermia and infertility.

DIAGNOSIS

The testes **cannot be manipulated into the scrotal sac** with gentle pressure (vs. retracted testes) and may be palpated anywhere along the inguinal canal or in the abdomen.

TREATMENT

- **Orchiopexy** after age one (in all but 1% of males, the testes will descend by that age) but before age five (to preserve fertility).
- If discovered later, treat with orchiectomy to avoid the risk of testicular cancer.

EPIDIDYMITIS

Inflammation of the epididymis associated with testicular enlargement and tenderness. Often results from **STIs, prostatitis, and/or urinary reflux.** Must be differentiated from **testicular torsion,** a surgical emergency.

HISTORY/PE

Presents with epididymal tenderness, tender/enlarged testicle(s), fever, scrotal thickening and erythema, and pyuria. Pain often ↓ with scrotal elevation as opposed to torsion.

DIAGNOSIS

UA reveals pyuria; urine culture or culture of urethral discharge (if present) reveals *Neisseria gonorrhoeae, E. coli,* or *Chlamydia.*

TREATMENT

Treat the underlying infection, generally with **tetracycline, fluoroquinolones,** or other antibiotics appropriate to specific culture and sensitivities. Treat pain/discomfort with NSAIDs and scrotal support.

ERECTILE DYSFUNCTION (ED)

Found in 10–25% of middle-aged and elderly men; has a significant impact on the well-being of affected individuals. Pathophysiologically classified as failure to initiate (e.g., psychological, endocrinologic, neurologic), failure to fill (e.g., arteriogenic), or failure to store (e.g., veno-occlusive dysfunction). Risk factors include **DM, atherosclerosis, medications** (e.g., β-blockers, SSRIs), hypertension, heart disease, surgery or radiation for prostate cancer, and spinal cord injury.

HISTORY/PE

- Because patients rarely volunteer this complaint, physicians should make a specific inquiry.
- Ask about risk factors, **medication use,** recent life changes, and psychological stressors.
- The distinction between psychological and organic ED is based on the presence of **nocturnal or early-morning erections** (if present, it is nonorganic) and on **situation dependence** (i.e., occurring with only one partner).
- Evaluate for **neurologic dysfunction** (e.g., anal tone, lower extremity sensation) and for **hypogonadism** (e.g., small testes, loss of 2° sexual characteristics).

DIAGNOSIS

- **Testosterone** and **gonadotropin levels** may be abnormal.
- Check prolactin levels, as elevated **prolactin** can → ↓ androgen activity.

TREATMENT

- Patients with psychological ED may benefit from psychotherapy or sex therapy involving discussion and exercises with the appropriate partner.
- Oral **sildenafil (Viagra), vardenafil (Levitra), and tadalafil (Cialis)** are phosphodiesterase-5 (PDE5) inhibitors that → prolonged action of cGMP-mediated smooth muscle relaxation and ↑ blood flow in the corpora cavernosa. PDE5 inhibitors are effective for a broad range of etiologies but are contraindicated in patients taking nitroglycerin.
- **Testosterone** is a useful therapy for patients with hypogonadism of testicular or pituitary origin; it is discouraged for patients with normal testosterone levels.
- Vacuum pumps, intracavernosal injections, and surgical implantation of semirigid or inflatable penile prostheses are alternatives for patients who fail PDE5 therapy.

BENIGN PROSTATIC HYPERPLASIA (BPH)

BPH most commonly occurs in the central (periurethral) zone of the prostate and may not be detected on DRE.

Enlargement of the prostate that is a normal part of the aging process and is seen in **> 80% of men by age 80.** Most commonly presents in men **> 50 years of age.**

HISTORY/PE

- In BPH, the enlarged prostate may → obstructive and irritative symptoms.
  - **Obstructive:** Hesitancy, weak stream, intermittent stream, incomplete emptying, urinary retention, bladder fullness.

446

- **Irritative:** Nocturia, daytime frequency, urge incontinence, opening hematuria.
- On DRE, the prostate is uniformly enlarged with a rubbery texture. If the prostate is hard or has irregular lesions, cancer should be suspected.

DIAGNOSIS

- Potentially dangerous causes of urinary symptoms must be ruled out before BPH is diagnosed.
- Conduct a **DRE** to screen for masses; if findings are suspicious, evaluate for prostate cancer.
- Obtain a **UA and urine culture** to rule out infection and hematuria.
- Measure **creatinine levels** to rule out obstructive uropathy and renal insufficiency.
- PSA testing and cystoscopy are not recommended for longitudinal BPH monitoring.

TREATMENT

- **Reassurance** for mild symptoms.
- **Medical therapy** with α-blockers (terazosin) and 5α-reductase inhibitors (finasteride) to reduce mild to moderate symptoms.
- Transurethral resection of the prostate (TURP) or open prostatectomy for patients with moderate to severe symptoms.

PROSTATE CANCER

The **most common cancer in men** and the **second leading cause of cancer death** in men (after lung cancer). Risk factors include advanced age and a ⊕ family history.

HISTORY/PE

- Usually **asymptomatic**, but may present with obstructive urinary symptoms (e.g., **urinary retention**, a ↓ in the force of the urine stream) as well as with lymphedema due to obstructing metastases, constitutional symptoms, and **back pain due to bone metastases.**
- DRE may reveal a **palpable nodule** or an area of induration. Early carcinoma is usually not detectable on exam.
- A tender prostate suggests prostatitis.

DIAGNOSIS

- Suggested by clinical findings and/or a markedly ↑ **PSA** (> 4 ng/mL).
- Definitive diagnosis is made with **ultrasound-guided transrectal biopsy.**
- Tumors are graded by the **Gleason histologic system,** which sums the scores (from 1 to 5) of the two most dysplastic samples (10 is the highest grade).
- Look for metastases with CXR and **bone scan.**

TREATMENT

- Treatment is controversial, as many cases of prostate cancer are slow to progress. Treatment choice is based on the aggressiveness of the tumor and the patient's mortality risk.
- **Watchful waiting** may be the best approach for elderly patients with low-grade tumors.

The major side effect of α-blockers is orthostatic hypotension.

An annual DRE after the age of 50 is the recommended screening method for prostate cancer.

Leading causes of cancer death in men:

1. Lung cancer
2. Prostate cancer
3. Colorectal cancer
4. Pancreatic cancer
5. Leukemia

Elevated PSA may be due to BPH, prostatitis, UTI, prostatic trauma, or carcinoma.

- **Radical prostatectomy** and **radiation therapy** (e.g., brachytherapy or external beam) are associated with an ↑ risk of incontinence and/or impotence.
- **PSA,** while controversial as a screening test, is used to follow patients post-treatment to evaluate for disease recurrence.
- Treat metastatic disease with **androgen ablation** (e.g., GnRH agonists, orchiectomy, flutamide) and chemotherapy.

PREVENTION

- All males > 50 years of age should have an **annual DRE.** Screening should begin earlier in African-American males and in those with a first-degree relative with prostate cancer.
- Screening with PSA is common, but its utility remains controversial.

BLADDER CANCER

> **Differential for hematuria—**
>
> **S2I3T3**
>
> **S**trictures
> **S**tones
> **I**nfection
> **I**nflammation
> **I**nfarction
> **T**umor
> **T**rauma
> **T**B

The second most common urologic cancer and **the most frequent malignant tumor of the urinary tract;** usually a **transitional cell carcinoma.** Most prevalent in men during the sixth and seventh decades. Risk factors include smoking, diets rich in meat and fat, schistosomiasis, chronic treatment with cyclophosphamide, and exposure to aniline dye (a benzene derivative).

HISTORY/PE

- **Gross hematuria** is the most common presenting symptom.
- Other urinary symptoms, such as frequency, urgency, and dysuria, may also be seen, but most patients are asymptomatic in the early stages of disease.

DIAGNOSIS

- **Cystoscopy with biopsy is diagnostic.**
- UA often shows hematuria (macro- or microscopic); cytology may show dysplastic cells.
- IVP can examine the upper urinary tract as well as defects in bladder filling.
- MRI, CT, and bone scan are important tools with which to define invasion and metastases.

TREATMENT

Treatment depends on the extent of spread beyond the bladder mucosa.

- **Carcinoma in situ:** Intravesicular chemotherapy.
- **Superficial cancers:** Complete transurethral resection or intravesicular chemotherapy with mitomycin-C or BCG (the vaccine for TB).
- **Large, high-grade recurrent lesions:** Intravesicular chemotherapy.
- **Invasive cancers without metastases:** Radical cystectomy or radiotherapy for patients who are deemed poor candidates for radical cystectomy as well as for those with unresectable local disease.
- **Invasive cancers with distant metastases:** Chemotherapy alone.

RENAL CELL CARCINOMA

An adenocarcinoma from tubular epithelial cells (~ 80–90% of all malignant tumors of the kidney). Tumors can spread along the renal vein to the IVC and can metastasize to lung and bone. Risk factors include male **gender, smoking, obesity, acquired cystic kidney disease in ESRD,** and von Hippel–Lindau disease.

HISTORY/PE

- Presents with the triad of **hematuria, flank pain,** and a **palpable flank mass.**
- Many patients have **fever** or other constitutional symptoms. Varicocele is seen in men.
- **Anemia is common at presentation, but polycythemia** due to ↑ erythropoietin production may be seen in 5–10% of patients.

DIAGNOSIS

Ultrasound and/or CT to characterize the renal mass (usually complex cysts or solid tumor).

TREATMENT

- **Surgical resection** may be curative in localized disease.
- Response rates from chemotherapy are only 15–30%.

The classic triad of renal cell carcinoma is hematuria, flank pain, and a palpable flank mass.

TESTICULAR CANCER

A heterogeneous group of neoplasms. Some 95% of testicular tumors derive from **germ cells,** and **virtually all are malignant. Cryptorchidism** is associated with an ↑ risk of neoplasia in both testes. **Klinefelter's syndrome** is also a risk factor. Testicular cancer is the most common malignancy in men 25–34 years of age.

HISTORY/PE

- Patients most often present with **painless enlargement of the testes.**
- Most testicular cancers occur between the ages of 15 and 30, but seminomas have a peak incidence between 40 and 50 years of age.

DIAGNOSIS

- **Testicular** ultrasound.
- CXR and abdominal/pelvic CT to evaluate for metastasis.
- **Tumor markers** are useful for diagnosis and in monitoring treatment response.
    - β-hCG is always elevated in choriocarcinoma and is elevated in 10% of seminomas.
    - α-fetoprotein (AFP) is often elevated in nonseminomatous germ cell tumors, particularly endodermal sinus (yolk sac) tumors.

β-hCG = choriocarcinoma.

AFP = endodermal sinus tumor.

TREATMENT

- Radical orchiectomy.
- Seminomas are **exquisitely radiosensitive** and also respond to chemotherapy.
- Platinum-based chemotherapy is used for nonseminomatous germ cell tumors.

Selected Topics in Emergency Medicine

Acute management of a trauma patient can be remembered with the mnemonic **ABCDE. Airway patency and adequacy of ventilation take precedence over other treatment.**

1° Survey

- **Airway:**
  - Start with supplemental O_2 by nasal cannula or face mask for conscious patients. Use a chin-lift or jaw-thrust maneuver to reposition the tongue in an unconscious patient. An oropharyngeal or nasopharyngeal airway may facilitate bag-mask ventilation.
  - Perform intubation in patients with apnea, ↓ mental status, impending airway compromise (e.g., significant maxillofacial trauma or inhalation injury in fires), severe closed-head injuries, failed bag-mask ventilation, or a Glasgow Coma Scale score of < 8.
  - Perform a surgical airway (cricothyroidotomy) in patients who cannot be intubated or in whom there is significant maxillofacial trauma.
  - Maintain cervical spine stabilization/immobilization in trauma patients until the spine is appropriately cleared through exam and radiographic studies. However, **never allow this concern to delay airway management.**
- **Breathing:** Thorough cardiac and pulmonary exams will identify the five thoracic causes of immediate death: **tension pneumothorax, cardiac tamponade, open pneumothorax, massive hemothorax,** and **airway obstruction.**
- **Circulation:**
  - Place a 16-gauge IV in each antecubital fossa.
  - Isotonic fluids (LR or NS) are repleted in a **3:1 ratio (fluid to blood loss).** Start with a fluid bolus of 1–2 L in adults; then recheck vitals and continue repletion as indicated.
  - For severe intravascular depletion, transfuse with packed RBCs.
- **Disability/Exposure:**
  - Disability (CNS dysfunction) is assessed and quantified with the Glasgow Coma Scale.
  - Exposure requires that the patient is completely disrobed and assessed for injury and temperature status.

2° Survey

- Once the patient is stable, perform a full examination.
- Order a trauma radiology series (AP chest, AP pelvis, and AP/lateral/odontoid C-spine views that adequately visualize the T1 vertebra).
- Place a Foley catheter after urethral injury has been ruled out. Place NG tube.
- Order pertinent labs based on the mechanism of injury, suspicion of intoxication or OD, and past medical history.

Evaluation and treatment depend on the location and extent of the injury.

1° survey of a trauma patient—

ABCDE

Airway
Breathing
Circulation
Disability
Exposure

Immediately evaluate trauma patients for tension pneumothorax, cardiac tamponade, open pneumothorax, massive hemothorax, and airway obstruction.

Neck

- Intubate early.
- Treatment varies according to zone and whether the platysma has been violated (see Figure 2.17-1).
    - **Zone 1:** Aortography.
    - **Zone 2:** Mandatory exploration is no longer required if the platysma has been violated. Perform two-dimensional Doppler studies and selective exploration.
    - **Zone 3:** Aortography and triple endoscopy.

Chest

- Unstable patients with penetrating thoracic injuries require immediate **intubation** and bilateral **chest tubes.** Thoracotomy may be necessary if the patient remains unstable despite resuscitative efforts.
- Leave any impaled objects in place until the patient is taken to the OR, as such objects may tamponade further blood loss.
- Beware of pneumothorax, tension pneumothorax, hemothorax, cardiac tamponade, aortic disruption, diaphragmatic tear, and esophageal injury.
- If a previously stable chest trauma patient suddenly dies, suspect **air embolism.**
- New diastolic murmur after chest trauma suggests aortic dissection.

Abdomen

- The absence of pain does not rule out an abdominal injury.
- Gunshot wounds require immediate exploratory laparotomy.
- Stab wounds in a hemodynamically unstable patient or in a patient with peritoneal signs or evisceration require immediate exploratory laparotomy.
- Stab wounds in a hemodynamically stable patient warrant a CT scan or focused abdominal sonography for trauma (FAST scan).

Leave any impaled objects in place until the patient is taken to the OR.

ED thoracotomy is indicated only if there is loss of vital signs en route to or after arrival in the ED.

Suspect air embolism when a previously stable chest trauma patient suddenly dies.

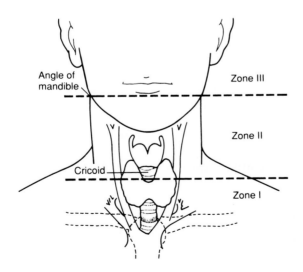

FIGURE 2.17-1. Zones of the neck.

(Reproduced, with permission, from Way LW [ed]. *Current Surgical Diagnosis & Treatment,* 10th ed. Stamford, CT: Appleton & Lange, 1994, p. 223.)

HIGH-YIELD FACTS

EMERGENCY MEDICINE

Musculoskeletal

- If there is no neurovascular injury on exam, debride and repair. If vascular injury is suspected, do an arteriogram first.
- **Early wound irrigation** and **tissue debridement,** not antibiotic therapy, are the most important steps in the treatment of contaminated wounds. However, do administer antibiotics and tetanus prophylaxis.

BLUNT AND DECELERATION TRAUMA

Chest

AORTIC DISRUPTION

Aortic disruption is often associated with first and second rib, scapular, and sternal fractures.

A **rapid deceleration injury** that is most commonly seen after high-speed motor vehicle accidents, ejection from vehicles, and falls from heights. Since complete aortic rupture is rapidly fatal (85% die at the scene), trauma patients with an aortic disruption injury usually have a contained hematoma within the adventitia. Laceration is most common just proximal to the ligamentum arteriosum. **Always suspect aortic disruption if there are scapular, sternal, or first and second rib fractures.**

DIAGNOSIS

- **Immediate CXR:** Reveals a **widened mediastinum** (> 8 cm), **loss of aortic knob, pleural cap,** deviation of the trachea and esophagus to the right, and depression of the left main stem bronchus.
- CT evaluation and/or transesophageal echocardiography (TEE) prior to surgery.
- **Aortography is the gold standard for evaluation.**

TREATMENT

Basic trauma management (ABCs); emergent surgery for defect repair.

FLAIL CHEST

- Three or more adjacent ribs fractured at two points causing paradoxical inward movement of the flail segment with inspiration.
- **Hx/PE:** Present with crepitus and abnormal chest wall movement. Abnormal chest wall movement may not be appreciated if the patient is splinting because of pain.
- **Dx:** CXR, O_2 saturation, and blood gases.
- **Tx:** O_2, narcotic analgesia.
- **Cx: Respiratory compromise** due to underlying pulmonary contusion.

Abdomen/Pelvis

- The **spleen** and **liver** are the **most commonly injured organs following blunt abdominal trauma.** Symptoms are consistent with signs of blood loss and include hypotension, tachycardia, and peritonitis. Suspect spleen or liver injury when lower rib fractures are present.
- Pancreatic rupture should be suspected after a direct epigastric blow (handlebar injury).

- **Diaphragmatic rupture** may occur with blunt or penetrating trauma. Difficult to diagnose and often missed. **Kehr's sign** may be ⊕. X-ray may demonstrate abdominal viscera in the thorax.
- The **kidneys** are the **most commonly injured GU organ in trauma**, with injuries including renal contusion, laceration, fracture, and pedicle injury.
- In hemodynamically stable patients, abdominal blunt trauma can be diagnosed with FAST scan, CT scan, and serial abdominal exams.
- In hemodynamically unstable patients, abdominal blunt trauma should be treated with immediate exploratory laparotomy to look for signs of perforation or evisceration.

Kehr's sign: referred left shoulder pain due to diaphragmatic irritation.

PELVIC FRACTURES

Most commonly occur after traumas such as motor vehicle accidents. Require immediate attention by the orthopedist owing to their life-threatening potential.

DIAGNOSIS

- May present with an unstable pelvis upon compression.
- Pelvic x-rays may confirm the fracture; in a stable patient, a CT scan of the pelvis will better define the extent of injury.
- If hypotension and shock are present, an exsanguinating hemorrhage is likely. In the field, MAST (military antishock trousers; rarely used today) can be used to maintain adequate BP and organ perfusion.

TREATMENT

- Consider embolization of bleeding vessels, emergent external pelvic fixation, or, in a hemodynamically stable patient, internal fixation. Give blood early. Hemorrhage → death in 50% of patients.
- Pelvic injuries can be associated with urethral injury.
  - Make note of **blood at the urethral meatus; a high-riding, "ballotable" prostate;** or **lack of a prostate.**
  - If present, a **retrograde urethrogram** must be performed to rule out injury before a Foley catheter is placed.
- Never explore a pelvic or retroperitoneal hematoma. Follow with serial hemoglobin and hematocrit.

CARDIAC LIFE SUPPORT BASICS

Table 2.17-1 summarizes the basic management of cardiac arrhythmias in an acute setting.

ACUTE ABDOMEN

Acute-onset abdominal pain has many potential etiologies and may require immediate medical or surgical intervention. Sharp, focal pain generally implies a parietal (peritoneal) etiology; dull, diffuse pain is commonly of visceral (organ) origin. Figure 2.17-2 identifies the common causes of acute abdomen.

HISTORY/PE

- Obtain a complete history, including the elements indicated in the mnemonic **OPQRST.**

Possible causes of PEA—

the 5 H's and 5 T's

Hypovolemia
Hypoxia
Hydrogen ion: Acidosis
Hyper/**H**ypo: K+, other metabolic
Hypothermia
Tablets: Drug OD, ingestion
Tamponade: Cardiac
Tension pneumothorax
Thrombosis: Coronary
Thrombosis: Pulmonary embolism

Aspects of a pain history—

OPQRST

Onset
Precipitating factors
Quality
Radiation
Symptoms
Temporal course/**T**reatment modalities

TABLE 2.17-1. Management of Cardiac Arrhythmias[a]

ARRHYTHMIA	TREATMENT
Asystole	Epinephrine and atropine.
Ventricular fibrillation or ventricular tachycardia	Desynchronized shock with 360 J → 360-J shock → epinephrine → 360-J shock → amiodarone **or** lidocaine → 360-J shock → epinephrine. Vasopressin may be given in place of the first or second dose of epinephrine. If stable, give amiodarone.
Pulseless electrical activity (PEA)	Epinephrine and atropine; simultaneously search for underlying cause (see the **5 H's and 5 T's** mnemonic). Give atropine for bradycardic PEA.
Supraventricular tachycardia (SVT)	If unstable, perform electrical cardioversion. If stable, control rate with maneuvers (Valsalva maneuver, carotid sinus massage, or cold stimulus). If resistant to maneuvers, consider adenosine.
Atrial fibrillation/flutter	If unstable, shock starting at 100 J. If stable, control rate with diltiazem or β-blockers, convert rhythm (if < 48 hours, convert electrically or chemically; if > 48 hours, anticoagulate or perform TEE prior to conversion), and anticoagulate. Do not give nodal blockers if there is evidence of Wolff-Parkinson-White syndrome (δ waves) on prior ECG.
Bradycardia	If symptomatic, give atropine and consider dopamine, epinephrine, or glucagon. If Mobitz II or third-degree heart block is present, place a transvenous pacemaker.

[a]In all cases, disruptions of CPR should be minimized. After a shock or administration of a drug, five cycles of CPR should be given before checking for a pulse or rhythm.

If the patient remembers the exact moment of pain onset, think perforation.

Pneumonia can present as right or left upper quadrant abdominal pain.

- Obtain a full gynecologic history for females (including last menstrual period, pregnancy, and any STD symptoms).
- **Perforation** → sudden onset of diffuse, severe pain.
- **Obstruction** → acute onset of severe, radiating, colicky pain.
- **Inflammation** → gradual onset (over 10–12 hours) of constant, ill-defined pain.
- **Associated symptoms** include the following:
  - Anorexia, nausea, vomiting, changes in bowel habits, hematochezia, and melena suggest GI etiologies.
  - Fever and cough suggest pneumonia.
  - Hematuria and costovertebral angle tenderness suggest a GU etiology.
  - If associated with meals, consider mesenteric ischemia, PUD, biliary disease, pancreatitis, or bowel pathology.
  - A family history of abdominal pain may indicate familial Mediterranean fever or acute intermittent porphyria.

DIAGNOSIS

- If peritoneal signs, shock, or impending shock is present, emergent exploratory laparotomy is necessary.

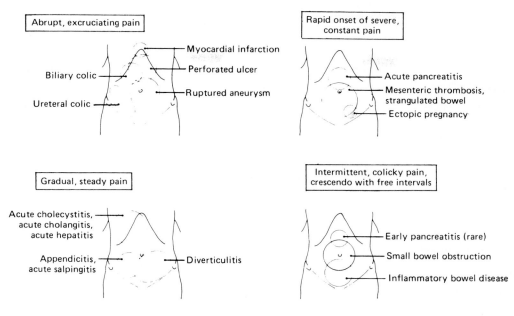

FIGURE 2.17-2. Acute abdomen.

The location and character of pain are helpful in the differential diagnosis of the acute abdomen. (Reproduced, with permission, from Way LW [ed]. *Current Surgical Diagnosis & Treatment*, 10th ed. Stamford, CT: Appleton & Lange, 1994, p. 444.)

- If the patient is stable, a complete physical exam—including a **rectal exam** and, in women, a **pelvic exam**—is mandatory.
- Obtain electrolytes, LFTs, amylase, lipase, **urine or serum β-hCG**, UA, and a CBC with differential.
- Consider a CXR, KUB, CT, and/or rectal contrast studies. **Avoid PO contrast studies if a complete bowel obstruction is suspected.** In women, ultrasound can be used to evaluate for ectopic pregnancy and ovarian torsion.

All female patients with an acute abdomen require a pelvic exam and a pregnancy test to rule out PID, ectopic pregnancy, and ovarian torsion.

TREATMENT

- Hemodynamically unstable patients must have an **emergent exploratory laparotomy.**
- In stable patients, expectant management may include NPO status, NG tube placement, IV fluids, placement of a Foley catheter (to monitor urine output and fluid status), and vital sign monitoring with serial abdominal exams and serial labs.
- Type and cross all unstable patients.

ACUTE APPENDICITIS

The inciting event is obstruction of the appendiceal lumen with subsequent inflammation and infection. Rising intraluminal pressure → vascular compromise of the appendix, ischemia, necrosis, and possible perforation. Etiologies include hypertrophied lymphoid tissue (55–65%), fecalith (35%), foreign body, tumor (e.g., carcinoid tumor), and parasites. Incidence peaks in the early teens, and the male-to-female ratio is 2:1.

McBurney's point is located two-thirds of the distance from the anterior superior iliac spine to the umbilicus.

457

"Hamburger sign": If a patient wants to eat, consider a diagnosis other than appendicitis. Anorexia is 80% specific for appendicitis.

Psoas sign: *Passive extension of the hip → RLQ pain.*

Obturator sign: *Passive internal rotation of the flexed hip → RLQ pain.*

Rovsing's sign: *Deep palpation of the LLQ → RLQ pain.*

Use the "rule of 9's" to estimate %BSA in adults:

Head and each arm = 9%
Back and chest each = 18%
Each leg = 18%
Perineum = 1%

HISTORY/PE

- Dull periumbilical pain lasting 1–12 hours → sharp RLQ pain at McBurney's point.
- Also presents with nausea, vomiting, anorexia ("hamburger sign"), and low-grade fever.
- Psoas, obturator, and Rovsing's signs are insensitive tests that may be ⊕.
- **Perforated appendix:** Partial pain relief is possible, but peritoneal signs (e.g., rebound, guarding, hypotension, ↑ WBC count, fever) will ultimately develop.
- Children, the elderly, pregnant women, and those with retrocecal appendices may have atypical presentations → misdiagnosis and ↑ mortality.

DIAGNOSIS

- Clinical impression.
- Look for fever, mild leukocytosis (11,000–15,000 cells/μL) with left shift, and UA with a few RBCs and/or WBCs.
- If the clinical diagnosis is unequivocal, no imaging studies are necessary. Otherwise, studies include the following:
    - **KUB:** Fecalith or loss of psoas shadow.
    - **Ultrasound:** Enlarged, noncompressible appendix.
    - **CT scan with contrast (95–98% sensitive):** Periappendiceal streaking.

TREATMENT

- The patient should be NPO and should receive IV hydration and antibiotics with anaerobic and gram-⊖ coverage.
- Immediate open or laparoscopic appendectomy is the definitive treatment. If appendicitis is not found, complete exploration of the abdomen is performed.
- **Perforation:** Administer antibiotics until the patient is afebrile with a normalized WBC count; the wound should be closed by delayed 1° closure.
- **Abscess:** Treat with broad-spectrum antibiotics and percutaneous drainage; an elective appendectomy should be performed 6–8 weeks later.

BURNS

The **second leading cause of death in children.** Categorized by depth of tissue destruction.

- **First degree:** Only the epidermis is involved. The area is painful and erythematous, but blisters are not present, and capillary refill is intact.
- **Second degree:** The epidermis and partial thickness of the dermis are involved. The area is painful, and blisters are present.
- **Third degree:** The epidermis, the full thickness of the dermis, and potentially deeper tissues are involved. The area is painless, white, and charred.

HISTORY/PE

- Patients may present with obvious skin wounds, but significant deep destruction may not be visible, especially with electrical burns.
- Perform a thorough airway and lung exam to assess for inhalation injury.

DIAGNOSIS

- Assess the ABCs. If airway compromise is impending, intubate.
- Be vigilant for shock, inhalation injury, and carbon monoxide poisoning.
- Evaluate the percentage of body surface area (%BSA) involved.

- Supportive measures; tetanus, stress ulcer prophylaxis, and IV narcotic analgesia.
- For second- and third-degree burns, fluid repletion using the **Parkland formula** is critical; adjust repletion on the basis of additional insensible losses to maintain at least 1 cc/kg/hr of urine output.
- Topical silver sulfadiazine and mafenide may be used prophylactically; however, there is no proven benefit associated with the use of PO/IV antibiotics or steroids.

COMPLICATIONS

- Shock and superinfection, with the latter most likely due to *Pseudomonas*.
- Criteria for transfer to a burn center include the following:
  - Full-thickness burn > 5% of BSA.
  - Partial-thickness burn > 10% BSA.
  - Any full- or partial-thickness burn over critical areas (face, hands, feet, genitals, perineum, major joints).
  - Circumferential burns; chemical, electrical, or lightning injury; inhalation injury.
  - Any special psychosocial or rehabilitative care needs.

> **Parkland formula:** Fluids for the first 24 hours = 4 × patient's weight in kg × %BSA. Give 50% of fluids over the first eight hours and the remaining 50% over the following 16 hours.

POSTOPERATIVE FEVER

- Occurs in 40% of all postoperative patients. Remember the mnemonic "Wind, Water, Walking, Wounds, and Wonder drugs."
- ↓ the risk of postoperative fever with incentive spirometry, pre- and postoperative antibiotics when indicated, short-term Foley catheter use, early ambulation, and DVT prophylaxis (e.g., anticoagulation, compression stockings).
- Fevers before postoperative day 3 are unlikely to be infectious unless *Clostridium* or β-hemolytic streptococci are involved.

> **The 5 W's of post-operative fever:**
> **W**ind: Atelectasis, pneumonia
> **W**ater: UTI
> **W**alking: DVT
> **W**ounds: Wound infection, abscess
> **W**onder drugs: Drug reaction

SHOCK

Defined as **inadequate oxygenation to maintain vital organ function.** The multiple etiologies are differentiated by their cardiovascular effects and treatment options (see Table 2.17-2).

TOXICOLOGY

Carbon Monoxide Poisoning

A **hypoxemic poisoning syndrome** seen in patients who have been exposed to automobile exhaust, smoke inhalation, barbecues, or old appliances in poorly ventilated locations.

HISTORY/PE

- Hypoxemia, **cherry-red skin** (rare), confusion, **headaches.** Coma or seizures occur in severe cases.
- Chronic low-level exposure may cause **flulike symptoms** with generalized myalgias, nausea, and headaches. Ask about symptoms in others living in the same house.
- **Suspect smoke inhalation** in the presence of **singed nose hairs, facial burns, hoarseness, wheezing,** or **carbonaceous sputum.**

TABLE 2.17-2. Types of Shock

Type of Shock	Major Causes	Cardiac Output	PCWP[a]	PVR[b]	Treatment
Hypovolemic	Trauma, blood loss, inadequate fluid repletion, third spacing, burns.	↓	↓	↑	Replete with isotonic solution (e.g., LR or NS) and blood in a 3:1 (fluid-to-blood) ratio.
Cardiogenic	Tension pneumothorax, CHF, cardiac tamponade, arrhythmia, structural heart disease (severe mitral regurgitation, VSD), MI (> 40% of LV function).	↓	↑	↑	Identify the cause and treat if possible. Give pressors such as dopamine and, if necessary, dobutamine or norepinephrine.
Septic	Bacteremia, especially gram-⊖ organisms.	↑	↓	↓	Administer fluid and antibiotics. Consider a Swan-Ganz catheter. Give dopamine or norepinephrine. Obtain cultures prior to administration of antibiotics if possible.
Anaphylactic	Bee stings, medication, food allergies.	↑	↓	↓	Give diphenhydramine. If severe, administer 1:1000 epinephrine.

[a] PCWP = pulmonary capillary wedge pressure.
[b] PVR = peripheral vascular resistance.

DIAGNOSIS

- Check an ABG and serum carboxyhemoglobin level (normal is < 5% in nonsmokers and < 10% in smokers).
- Perform laryngoscopy or bronchoscopy if smoke inhalation is suspected.
- Check an ECG in the elderly and in patients with a history of cardiac disease.

TREATMENT

- Treat with 100% O_2 until asymptomatic.
- Use **hyperbaric O_2** for pregnant patients, nonresponders, those with neurologic symptoms, or those with severely ↑ carboxyhemoglobin to facilitate displacement of carbon monoxide from hemoglobin.
- Patients with **smoke inhalation** may require early intubation, since upper airway edema can rapidly → complete obstruction.

Common Drug Interactions/Reactions

Table 2.17-3 outlines drug interactions and reactions that are commonly encountered in a clinical setting.

TABLE 2.17-3. Drug Interactions and Reactions

INTERACTION/REACTION	DRUGS
Induction of P-450 enzymes	Barbiturates, phenytoin, carbamazepine, rifampin, quinidine, griseofulvin.
Inhibition of P-450 enzymes	Cimetidine, ketoconazole, INH, grapefruit, erythromycin, sulfonamides.
Metabolism by P-450 enzymes	Benzodiazepines, amide anesthetics, metoprolol, propranolol, nifedipine, phenytoin, quinidine, theophylline, warfarin, barbiturates.
↑ risk of digoxin toxicity	Quinidine, cimetidine, amiodarone, calcium channel blockers.
Competition for albumin-binding sites	Warfarin, ASA, phenytoin.
Blood dyscrasias	Ibuprofen, quinidine, methyldopa, chemotherapeutic agents.
Hemolysis in G6PD-deficient patients	Sulfonamides, INH, ASA, ibuprofen, nitrofurantoin, primaquine, pyrimethamine, chloramphenicol.
Gynecomastia	**S**pironolactone, **E**strogens, **D**igitalis, **C**imetidine, chronic **A**lcohol use, **K**etoconazole: "**S**ome **E**xcellent **D**rugs **C**reate **A**wesome **K**nockers."
Stevens-Johnson syndrome	Ethosuximide, sulfonamides.
Photosensitivity	Tetracycline, amiodarone, sulfonamides.
Drug-induced SLE	Procainamide, hydralazine, INH, penicillamine, chlorpromazine, methyldopa, quinidine.

Drug Overdose

Table 2.17-4 summarizes antidotes and treatments for substances commonly encountered in overdoses and intoxications.

Major Drug Side Effects

Table 2.17-5 outlines the major side effects of select drugs.

Management of Drug Withdrawal

Table 2.17-6 summarizes common drug withdrawal symptoms and treatment.

TABLE 2.17-4. **Specific Antidotes**

Toxin	Antidote/Treatment
Acetaminophen	*N*-acetylcysteine.
Acid/alkali ingestion	Upper endoscopy to evaluate for stricture.
Anticholinesterases, organophosphates	Atropine, pralidoxime.
Antimuscarinic/anticholinergic agents	Physostigmine.
Arsenic, mercury, gold	Succimer, dimercaprol.
β-blockers	Glucagon.
Barbiturates (phenobarbital)	Urine alkalinization, dialysis, activated charcoal.
Benzodiazepines	Flumazenil.
Black widow bite	Calcium gluconate, methocarbamol.
Carbon monoxide	100% O_2, hyperbaric O_2.
Copper, arsenic, lead, gold	Penicillamine.
Cyanide	Amyl nitrate, sodium nitrate, sodium thiosulfate.
Digitalis	Stop digitalis, normalize K^+, lidocaine (for torsades), anti-digitalis Fab.
Heparin	Protamine sulfate.
Iron salts	Deferoxamine.
Isoniazid (INH)	Pyridoxine.
Lead	Succimer, CaEDTA, dimercaprol.
Methanol, ethylene glycol (antifreeze)	EtOH, fomepizole, dialysis, calcium gluconate for ethylene glycol.
Methemoglobin	Methylene blue.
Opioids	Naloxone.
Phencyclidine hydrochloride (PCP)	NG suction.
Salicylates	Urine alkalinization, dialysis, activated charcoal.
TCAs	Sodium bicarbonate for QRS prolongation; diazepam or lorazepam for seizures; cardiac monitor for arrhythmias.
Theophylline	Activated charcoal. Consider repeat doses.
tPA, streptokinase	Aminocaproic acid.
Warfarin	Vitamin K, FFP.

TABLE 2.17-5. **Drug Side Effects**

DRUG	SIDE EFFECTS
ACEIs	**Cough,** rash, proteinuria, angioedema, taste changes, teratogenic effects.
Amantadine	Ataxia, **livedo reticularis.**
Aminoglycosides	Ototoxicity, nephrotoxicity (acute tubular necrosis).
Amiodarone	Pulmonary fibrosis, peripheral deposition → bluish discoloration, arrhythmias, hypo-/hyperthyroidism, corneal deposition.
Amphotericin	Fever/chills, nephrotoxicity, bone marrow suppression, anemia.
Antipsychotics	Sedation, acute dystonic reaction, akathisia, parkinsonism, tardive dyskinesia, **neuroleptic malignant syndrome.**
Azoles (e.g., fluconazole)	Inhibition of P-450 enzymes.
AZT	Thrombocytopenia, megaloblastic anemia.
β-blockers	Asthma exacerbation, masking of hypoglycemia, impotence, bradycardia, AV block, CHF.
Benzodiazepines	Sedation, dependence, respiratory depression.
Bile acid resins	GI upset, malabsorption of vitamins and medications.
Calcium channel blockers	Peripheral edema, constipation, cardiac depression.
Carbamazepine	Induction of P-450 enzymes, **agranulocytosis,** aplastic anemia, liver toxicity.
Chloramphenicol	**Gray baby syndrome,** aplastic anemia.
Cisplatin	Nephrotoxicity, acoustic nerve damage.
Clonidine	Dry mouth; **severe rebound headache and hypertension.**
Clozapine	Agranulocytosis.
Corticosteroids	Mania (acute), immunosuppression, bone mineral loss, thinning of skin, easy bruising, myopathy (chronic), cataracts.
Cyclophosphamide	Myelosuppression, **hemorrhagic cystitis.**
Digoxin	GI disturbance, **yellow visual changes, arrhythmias** (e.g., junctional tachycardia or SVT).
Doxorubicin	**Cardiotoxicity (cardiomyopathy).**
Ethyl alcohol	Renal dysfunction.
Fluoroquinolones	Cartilage damage in children; Achilles tendon rupture in adults.
Furosemide	Ototoxicity, hypokalemia, nephritis, gout.

HIGH-YIELD FACTS

EMERGENCY MEDICINE

TABLE 2.17-5. **Drug Side Effects (continued)**

DRUG	SIDE EFFECTS
Gemfibrozil	Myositis, reversible ↑ in LFTs.
Halothane	Hepatotoxicity, **malignant hyperthermia.**
HCTZ	Hypokalemia, hyponatremia, hyperuricemia, hyperglycemia, hypercalcemia.
HMG-CoA reductase inhibitors	Myositis, reversible ↑ in LFTs.
Hydralazine	Drug-induced SLE.
Hydroxychloroquine	Retinopathy.
INH	Peripheral neuropathy **(prevent with pyridoxine/vitamin B₆),** hepatotoxicity, inhibition of P-450 enzymes, seizures with overdose, hemolysis in G6PD deficiency.
MAOIs	**Hypertensive tyramine reaction, serotonin syndrome** (with meperidine).
Methanol	Blindness.
Methotrexate	Hepatic fibrosis, pneumonitis, anemia.
Methyldopa	⊕ Coombs' test, drug-induced SLE.
Metronidazole	Disulfiram reaction, vestibular dysfunction, **metallic taste.**
Niacin	**Cutaneous flushing.**
Nitroglycerin	Hypotension, tachycardia, headache, tolerance.
Penicillamine	Drug-induced SLE.
Penicillin/β-lactams	Hypersensitivity reactions.
Phenytoin	Nystagmus, diplopia, ataxia, **gingival hyperplasia,** hirsutism, teratogenic effects.
Prazosin	First-dose hypotension.
Procainamide	Drug-induced SLE.
Propylthiouracil	Agranulocytosis, aplastic anemia.
Quinidine	Cinchonism (headache, tinnitus), thrombocytopenia, arrhythmias (e.g., **torsades de pointes**).
Reserpine	Depression.
Rifampin	Induction of P-450 enzymes; **orange-red body secretions.**
Salicylates	Fever; hyperventilation with **respiratory alkalosis and metabolic acidosis;** dehydration, diaphoresis, hemorrhagic gastritis.

TABLE 2.17-5. Drug Side Effects (continued)

DRUG	SIDE EFFECTS
SSRIs	Anxiety, **sexual dysfunction,** serotonin syndrome if taken with MAOIs.
Succinylcholine	**Malignant hyperthermia,** hyperkalemia.
TCAs	Sedation, coma, anticholinergic effects, seizures and arrhythmias.
Tetracyclines	Tooth discoloration, photosensitivity, Fanconi's syndrome, GI distress.
Trimethoprim	Megaloblastic anemia, leukopenia, granulocytopenia.
Valproic acid	Teratogenicity → neural tube defects, rare fatal hepatotoxicity.
Vancomycin	Nephrotoxicity, ototoxicity, **"red man syndrome"** (histamine release; not an allergy).
Vinblastine	Severe myelosuppression.
Vincristine	Peripheral neuropathy, paralytic ileus.

TABLE 2.17-6. Symptoms and Treatment of Drug Withdrawal

DRUG	WITHDRAWAL SYMPTOMS	TREATMENT
Alcohol	Tremor (6–12 hours). Tachycardia, hypertension, agitation, seizures (within 48 hours). Hallucinations, **DTs**—severe autonomic instability → tachycardia, hypertension, delirium, and possibly death (within 2–7 days). Mortality is 15–20%.	**Benzodiazepines;** haloperidol for hallucinations; **thiamine,** folate, and multivitamin replacement (do not affect withdrawal, but most alcoholics are deficient).
Barbiturates	Anxiety, seizures, delirium, tremor; cardiac and respiratory depression.	**Benzodiazepines.**
Benzodiazepines	Rebound anxiety, seizures, tremor, insomnia.	**Benzodiazepines.** Monitor for DTs.
Cocaine/amphetamines	Depression, hyperphagia, hypersomnolence.	Supportive treatment. Avoid pure β-blockers (may → unopposed α activity, causing hypertension).
Opioids	Anxiety, insomnia, flulike symptoms, piloerection, fever, rhinorrhea, lacrimation, yawning, nausea, stomach cramps, diarrhea, mydriasis.	Clonidine and/or buprenorphine for moderate symptoms; methadone for severe symptoms. Naltrexone for patients who are drug free for 7–10 days.

HIGH-YIELD FACTS

EMERGENCY MEDICINE

Table 2.17-7 summarizes the signs and symptoms of key vitamin deficiencies.

TABLE 2.17-7. **Vitamin Functions and Deficiencies**

VITAMIN	SIGNS/SYMPTOMS OF DEFICIENCY
Vitamin A	Night blindness, dry skin.
Vitamin B$_1$ (thiamine)	Beriberi (polyneuritis, dilated cardiomyopathy, high-output CHF, edema), Wernicke-Korsakoff syndrome.
Vitamin B$_2$ (riboflavin)	Angular stomatitis, cheilosis, corneal vascularization.
Vitamin B$_3$ (niacin)	Pellagra (diarrhea, dermatitis, dementia).
Vitamin B$_5$ (pantothenate)	Dermatitis, enteritis, alopecia, adrenal insufficiency.
Vitamin B$_6$ (pyridoxine)	Convulsions, hyperirritability; required during administration of INH.
Vitamin B$_{12}$ (cobalamin)	Macrocytic, megaloblastic anemia; neurologic symptoms (e.g., optic neuropathy, subacute combined degeneration, paresthesias); glossitis.
Vitamin C	Scurvy (e.g., swollen gums, bruising, anemia, poor wound healing).
Vitamin D	Rickets in children (bending bones), osteomalacia in adults (soft bones), hypocalcemic tetany.
Vitamin E	↑ fragility of RBCs.
Vitamin K	Neonatal hemorrhage; ↑ PT and aPTT, normal BT.
Biotin	Dermatitis, enteritis. Can be caused by ingestion of **raw eggs** or antibiotic use.
Folic acid	The **most common vitamin deficiency in the United States.** Sprue; macrocytic, megaloblastic anemia without neurologic symptoms.
Magnesium	Weakness, muscle cramps, exacerbation of hypocalcemic tetany, CNS hyperirritability → tremors, choreoathetoid movement.
Selenium	Keshan disease (cardiomyopathy).

Rapid Review

Classic ECG finding in atrial flutter.	"Sawtooth" P waves
Definition of unstable angina.	Angina is new, is worsening, or occurs at rest
Antihypertensive for a diabetic patient with proteinuria.	ACEI
Beck's triad for cardiac tamponade.	Hypotension, distant heart sounds, and JVD
Drugs that slow AV node transmission.	β-blockers, digoxin, calcium channel blockers
Hypercholesterolemia treatment that → flushing and pruritus.	Niacin
Treatment for atrial fibrillation.	Anticoagulation, rate control, cardioversion
Treatment for ventricular fibrillation.	Immediate cardioversion
Autoimmune complication occurring 2–4 weeks post-MI.	Dressler's syndrome: fever, pericarditis, ↑ ESR
IV drug use with JVD and holosystolic murmur at the left sternal border. Treatment?	Treat existing heart failure and replace the tricuspid valve
Diagnostic test for hypertrophic cardiomyopathy.	Echocardiogram (showing thickened left ventricular wall and outflow obstruction)
A fall in systolic BP of > 10 mmHg with inspiration.	Pulsus paradoxus (seen in cardiac tamponade)
Classic ECG findings in pericarditis.	Low-voltage, diffuse ST-segment elevation
Definition of hypertension.	BP > 140/90 on three separate occasions two weeks apart
Eight surgically correctable causes of hypertension.	Renal artery stenosis, coarctation of the aorta, pheochromocytoma, Conn's syndrome, Cushing's syndrome, unilateral renal parenchymal disease, hyperthyroidism, hyperparathyroidism
Evaluation of a pulsatile abdominal mass and bruit.	Abdominal ultrasound and CT
Indications for surgical repair of abdominal aortic aneurysm.	> 5.5 cm, rapidly enlarging, symptomatic, or ruptured
Treatment for acute coronary syndrome.	Morphine, O_2, sublingual nitroglycerin, ASA, IV β-blockers, heparin
What is the metabolic syndrome?	Abdominal obesity, high triglycerides, low HDL, hypertension, insulin resistance, prothrombotic or proinflammatory states

Appropriate diagnostic test? ■ A 50-year-old male with angina can exercise to 85% of maximum predicted heart rate. ■ A 65-year-old woman with left bundle branch block and severe osteoarthritis has unstable angina.	Exercise stress treadmill with ECG Pharmacologic stress test (e.g., dobutamine echo)
Target LDL in a patient with diabetes.	< 70
Signs of active ischemia during stress testing.	Angina, ST-segment changes on ECG, or ↓ BP
ECG findings suggesting MI.	ST-segment elevation (depression means ischemia), flattened T waves, and Q waves
A young patient has angina at rest with ST-segment elevation. Cardiac enzymes are normal.	Prinzmetal's angina
Common symptoms associated with silent MIs.	CHF, shock, and altered mental status
The diagnostic test for pulmonary embolism.	V/Q scan
An agent that reverses the effects of heparin.	Protamine
The coagulation parameter affected by warfarin.	PT
A young patient with a family history of sudden death collapses and dies while exercising.	Hypertrophic cardiomyopathy
Endocarditis prophylaxis regimens.	Oral surgery—amoxicillin; GI or GU procedures—ampicillin and gentamicin before and amoxicillin after
The 6 P's of ischemia due to peripheral vascular disease.	Pain, pallor, pulselessness, paralysis, paresthesia, poikilothermia
Virchow's triad.	Stasis, hypercoagulability, endothelial damage
The most common cause of hypertension in young women.	OCPs
The most common cause of hypertension in young men.	Excessive EtOH

DERMATOLOGY

"Stuck-on" appearance.	Seborrheic keratosis
Red plaques with silvery-white scales and sharp margins.	Psoriasis
The most common type of skin cancer; the lesion is a pearly-colored papule with a translucent surface and telangiectasias.	Basal cell carcinoma
Honey-crusted lesions.	Impetigo

A febrile patient with a history of diabetes presents with a red, swollen, painful lower extremity.	Cellulitis
$\oplus$ Nikolsky's sign.	Pemphigus vulgaris
$\ominus$ Nikolsky's sign.	Bullous pemphigoid
A 55-year-old obese patient presents with dirty, velvety patches on the back of the neck.	Acanthosis nigricans. Check fasting blood sugar to rule out diabetes
Dermatomal distribution.	Varicella zoster
Flat-topped papules.	Lichen planus
Iris-like target lesions.	Erythema multiforme
A lesion characteristically occurring in a linear pattern in areas where skin comes into contact with clothing or jewelry.	Contact dermatitis
Presents with a herald patch, Christmas-tree pattern.	Pityriasis rosea
A 16-year-old presents with an annular patch of alopecia with broken-off, stubby hairs.	Alopecia areata (autoimmune process)
Pinkish, scaling, flat lesions on the chest and back. KOH prep has a "spaghetti-and-meatballs" appearance.	Pityriasis versicolor
Four characteristics of a nevus suggestive of melanoma.	Asymmetry, border irregularity, color variation, large diameter
Premalignant lesion from sun exposure that can → squamous cell carcinoma.	Actinic keratosis
"Dewdrop on a rose petal."	Lesions of 1° varicella
"Cradle cap."	Seborrheic dermatitis. Treat with antifungals
Associated with *Propionibacterium acnes* and changes in androgen levels.	Acne vulgaris
A painful, recurrent vesicular eruption of mucocutaneous surfaces.	Herpes simplex
Inflammation and epithelial thinning of the anogenital area, predominantly in postmenopausal women.	Lichen sclerosus
Exophytic nodules on the skin with varying degrees of scaling or ulceration; the second most common type of skin cancer.	Squamous cell carcinoma

The most common cause of hypothyroidism.	Hashimoto's thyroiditis
Lab findings in Hashimoto's thyroiditis.	High TSH, low T_4, antimicrosomal antibodies
Exophthalmos, pretibial myxedema, and ↓ TSH.	Graves' disease
The most common cause of Cushing's syndrome.	Iatrogenic steroid administration. The second most common cause is Cushing's disease
A patient presents with signs of hypocalcemia, high phosphorus, and low PTH.	Hypoparathyroidism
"Stones, bones, groans, psychiatric overtones."	Signs and symptoms of hypercalcemia
A patient complains of headache, weakness, and polyuria; exam reveals hypertension and tetany. Labs reveals hypernatremia, hypokalemia, and metabolic alkalosis.	1° hyperaldosteronism (due to Conn's syndrome or bilateral adrenal hyperplasia)
A patient presents with tachycardia, wild swings in BP, headache, diaphoresis, altered mental status, and a sense of panic.	Pheochromocytoma
Should α- or β-antagonists be used first in treating pheochromocytoma?	α-antagonists (phentolamine and phenoxybenzamine)
A patient with a history of lithium use presents with copious amounts of dilute urine.	Nephrogenic diabetes insipidus (DI)
Treatment of central DI.	Administration of DDAVP ↓ serum osmolality and free water restriction
A postoperative patient with significant pain presents with hyponatremia and normal volume status.	SIADH due to stress
An antidiabetic agent associated with lactic acidosis.	Metformin
A patient presents with weakness, nausea, vomiting, weight loss, and new skin pigmentation. Labs show hyponatremia and hyperkalemia. Treatment?	1° adrenal insufficiency (Addison's disease). Treat with replacement glucocorticoids, mineralocorticoids, and IV fluids
Goal hemoglobin A_{1c} for a patient with DM.	< 7.0
Treatment of DKA.	Fluids, insulin, and aggressive replacement of electrolytes (e.g., K^+)
Why are β-blockers contraindicated in diabetics?	They can mask symptoms of hypoglycemia

Bias introduced into a study when a clinician is aware of the patient's treatment type.	Observational bias
Bias introduced when screening detects a disease earlier and thus lengthens the time from diagnosis to death.	Lead-time bias
If you want to know if race affects infant mortality rate but most of the variation in infant mortality is predicted by socioeconomic status, then socioeconomic status is a _____.	Confounding variable
The number of true positives divided by the number of patients with the disease is _____.	Sensitivity
Sensitive tests have few false negatives and are used to rule _____ a disease.	Out
PPD reactivity is used as a screening test because most people with TB (except those who are anergic) will have a $\oplus$ PPD. Highly sensitive or specific?	Highly sensitive for TB
Chronic diseases such as SLE—higher prevalence or incidence?	Higher prevalence
Epidemics such as influenza—higher prevalence or incidence?	Higher incidence
Cross-sectional survey—incidence or prevalence?	Prevalence
Cohort study—incidence or prevalence?	Incidence and prevalence
Case-control study—incidence or prevalence?	Neither
Describe a test that consistently gives identical results, but the results are wrong.	High reliability, low validity
Difference between a cohort and a case-control study.	Cohort studies can be used to calculate relative risk (RR), incidence, and/or odds ratio (OR). Case-control studies can be used to calculate an OR
Attributable risk?	The incidence rate (IR) of a disease in exposed – the IR of a disease in unexposed
Relative risk?	The IR of a disease in a population exposed to a particular factor ÷ the IR of those not exposed
Odds ratio?	The likelihood of a disease among individuals exposed to a risk factor compared to those who have not been exposed

Number needed to treat?	1 ÷ (rate in untreated group − rate in treated group)
In which patients do you initiate colorectal cancer screening early?	Patients with IBD; those with familial adenomatous polyposis (FAP)/hereditary nonpolyposis colorectal cancer (HNPCC); and those who have first-degree relatives with adenomatous polyps (< 60 years of age) or colorectal cancer
The most common cancer in men and the most common cause of death from cancer in men.	Prostate cancer is the most common cancer in men, but lung cancer causes more deaths
The percentage of cases within one SD of the mean? Two SDs? Three SDs?	68%, 95.5%, 99.7%
Birth rate?	Number of live births per 1000 population
Fertility rate?	Number of live births per 1000 women 15–44 years of age
Mortality rate?	Number of deaths per 1000 population
Neonatal mortality?	Number of deaths from birth to 28 days per 1000 live births
Postnatal mortality?	Number of deaths from 28 days to one year per 1000 live births
Infant mortality?	Number of deaths from birth to one year of age per 1000 live births (neonatal + postnatal mortality)
Fetal mortality?	Number of deaths from 20 weeks' gestation to birth per 1000 total births
Perinatal mortality?	Number of deaths from 20 weeks' gestation to one month of life per 1000 total births
Maternal mortality?	Number of deaths during pregnancy to 90 days postpartum per 100,000 live births

ETHICS

True or false: Once patients sign a statement giving consent, they must continue treatment.	False. Patients may change their minds at any time. Exceptions to the requirement of informed consent include emergency situations and patients without decision-making capacity
A 15-year-old pregnant girl requires hospitalization for preeclampsia. Should her parents be informed?	No. Parental consent is not necessary for the medical treatment of pregnant minors
A doctor refers a patient for an MRI at a facility he/she owns.	Conflict of interest

Involuntary psychiatric hospitalization can be undertaken for which three reasons?	The patient is a danger to self, a danger to others, or gravely disabled (unable to provide for basic needs)
True or false: Withdrawing life-sustaining care is ethically distinct from withholding sustaining care.	False. Withdrawing and withholding life are the same from an ethical standpoint
When can a physician refuse to continue treating a patient on the grounds of futility?	When there is no rationale for treatment, maximal intervention is failing, a given intervention has already failed, and treatment will not achieve the goals of care
An eight-year-old child is in a serious accident. She requires emergent transfusion, but her parents are not present.	Treat immediately. Consent is implied in emergency situations
Conditions in which confidentiality must be overridden.	Real threat of harm to third parties; suicidal intentions; certain contagious diseases; elder and child abuse
Involuntary commitment or isolation for medical treatment may be undertaken for what reason?	When treatment noncompliance represents a serious danger to public health (e.g., active TB)
A 10-year-old child presents in status epilepticus, but her parents refuse treatment on religious grounds.	Treat because the disease represents an immediate threat to the child's life. Then seek a court order
A son asks that his mother not be told about her recently discovered cancer.	A patient's family cannot require that a doctor withhold information from the patient

GASTROINTESTINAL

Patient presents with sudden onset of severe, diffuse abdominal pain. Exam reveals peritoneal signs and AXR reveals free air under the diaphragm. Management?	Emergent laparotomy to repair perforated viscus, likely stomach
The most likely cause of acute lower GI bleed in patients > 40 years old.	Diverticulosis
Diagnostic modality used when ultrasound is equivocal for cholecystitis.	HIDA scan
Sentinel loop on AXR.	Acute pancreatitis
Risk factors for cholelithiasis.	Fat, female, fertile, forty, flatulent
Inspiratory arrest during palpation of the RUQ.	Murphy's sign, seen in acute cholecystitis

Identify key organisms causing diarrhea:	
■ Most common organism	*Campylobacter*
■ Recent antibiotic use	*Clostridium difficile*
■ Camping	*Giardia*
■ Traveler's diarrhea	ETEC
■ Church picnics/mayonnaise	*S. aureus*
■ Uncooked hamburgers	*E. coli* O157:H7
■ Fried rice	***Bacillus cereus***
■ Poultry/eggs	*Salmonella*
■ Raw seafood	*Vibrio*, HAV
■ AIDS	*Isospora, Cryptosporidium, Mycobacterium avium* complex (MAC)
■ Pseudoappendicitis	*Yersinia*
A 25-year-old Jewish male presents with pain and watery diarrhea after meals. Exam shows fistulas between the bowel and skin and nodular lesions on his tibias.	Crohn's disease
Inflammatory disease of the colon with ↑ risk of colon cancer.	Ulcerative colitis
Extraintestinal manifestations of IBD.	Uveitis, ankylosing spondylitis, pyoderma gangrenosum, erythema nodosum, 1° sclerosing cholangitis
Medical treatment for IBD.	5-aminosalicylic acid agents and steroids during acute exacerbations
Difference between Mallory-Weiss and Boerhaave tears.	Mallory-Weiss—superficial tear in the esophageal mucosa; Boerhaave—full-thickness esophageal rupture
Charcot's triad.	RUQ pain, jaundice, and fever/chills in the setting of ascending cholangitis
Reynolds' pentad.	Charcot's triad plus shock and mental status changes, with suppurative ascending cholangitis
Medical treatment for hepatic encephalopathy.	↓ protein intake, lactulose, neomycin
First step in the management of a patient with acute GI bleed.	Establish the ABCs
A four-year-old child presents with oliguria, petechiae, and jaundice following an illness with bloody diarrhea. Most likely diagnosis and cause?	Hemolytic-uremic syndrome (HUS) due to *E. coli* O157:H7
Post-HBV exposure treatment.	HBV immunoglobulin
Classic causes of drug-induced hepatitis.	TB medications (INH, rifampin, pyrazinamide), acetaminophen, and tetracycline

A 40-year-old obese female with elevated alkaline phosphatase, elevated bilirubin, pruritus, dark urine, and clay-colored stools.	Biliary tract obstruction
Hernia with highest risk of incarceration—indirect, direct, or femoral?	Femoral hernia
A 50-year-old man with a history of alcohol abuse presents with boring epigastric pain that radiates to the back and is relieved by sitting forward. Management?	Confirm the diagnosis of acute pancreatitis with elevated amylase and lipase. Make the patient NPO and give IV fluids, O_2, analgesia, and "tincture of time"

HEMATOLOGY/ONCOLOGY

Four causes of microcytic anemia.	**TICS**—**T**halassemia, **I**ron deficiency, anemia of **C**hronic disease, and **S**ideroblastic anemia
An elderly male with hypochromic, microcytic anemia is asymptomatic. Diagnostic tests?	Fecal occult blood test and sigmoidoscopy; suspect colorectal cancer
Precipitants of hemolytic crisis in patients with G6PD deficiency.	Sulfonamides, antimalarial drugs, fava beans
The most common inherited cause of hypercoagulability.	Factor V Leiden mutation
The most common inherited hemolytic anemia.	Hereditary spherocytosis
Diagnostic test for hereditary spherocytosis.	Osmotic fragility test
Pure RBC aplasia.	Diamond-Blackfan anemia
Anemia associated with absent radii and thumbs, diffuse hyperpigmentation, café-au-lait spots, microcephaly, and pancytopenia.	Fanconi's anemia
Medications and viruses that → aplastic anemia.	Chloramphenicol, sulfonamides, radiation, HIV, chemotherapeutic agents, hepatitis, parvovirus B19, EBV
How to distinguish polycythemia vera from 2° polycythemia.	Both have ↑ hematocrit and RBC mass, but polycythemia vera should have normal O_2 saturation and low erythropoietin levels
Thrombotic thrombocytopenic purpura (TTP) pentad?	**Pentad of TTP—"FAT RN"**: **F**ever, **A**nemia, **T**hrombocytopenia, **R**enal dysfunction, **N**eurologic abnormalities
HUS triad?	Anemia, thrombocytopenia, and acute renal failure
Treatment for TTP.	Emergent large-volume plasmapheresis, corticosteroids, antiplatelet drugs

HIGH-YIELD FACTS

RAPID REVIEW

Treatment for idiopathic thrombocytopenic purpura (ITP) in children.	Usually resolves spontaneously; may require IVIG and/or corticosteroids
Which of the following are ↑ in DIC: fibrin split products, D-dimer, fibrinogen, platelets, and hematocrit.	Fibrin split products and D-dimer are elevated; platelets, fibrinogen, and hematocrit are ↓.
An eight-year-old boy presents with hemarthrosis and ↑ PTT with normal PT and bleeding time. Diagnosis? Treatment?	Hemophilia A or B; consider desmopressin (for hemophilia A) or factor VIII or IX supplements
A 14-year-old girl presents with prolonged bleeding after dental surgery and with menses, normal PT, normal or ↑ PTT, and ↑ bleeding time. Diagnosis? Treatment?	von Willebrand's disease; treat with desmopressin, FFP, or cryoprecipitate
A 60-year-old African-American male presents with bone pain. Workup for multiple myeloma might reveal?	Monoclonal gammopathy, Bence Jones proteinuria, "punched-out" lesions on x-ray of the skull and long bones
Reed-Sternberg cells.	Hodgkin's lymphoma
A 10-year-old boy presents with fever, weight loss, and night sweats. Examination shows anterior mediastinal mass. Suspected diagnosis?	Non-Hodgkin's lymphoma
Microcytic anemia with ↓ serum iron, ↓ total iron-binding capacity (TIBC), and normal or ↑ ferritin.	Anemia of chronic disease
Microcytic anemia with ↓ serum iron, ↓ ferritin, and ↑ TIBC.	Iron deficiency anemia
An 80-year-old man presents with fatigue, lymphadenopathy, splenomegaly, and isolated lymphocytosis. Suspected diagnosis?	Chronic lymphocytic leukemia (CLL)
A late, life-threatening complication of chronic myelogenous leukemia (CML).	Blast crisis (fever, bone pain, splenomegaly, pancytopenia)
Auer rods on blood smear.	Acute myelogenous leukemia (AML)
AML subtype associated with DIC.	M3
Electrolyte changes in tumor lysis syndrome.	↓ Ca^{2+}, ↑ K^+, ↑ phosphate, ↑ uric acid
Treatment for AML M3.	Retinoic acid
A 50-year-old male presents with early satiety, splenomegaly, and bleeding. Cytogenetics show t(9,22). Diagnosis?	CML
Heinz bodies?	Intracellular inclusions seen in thalassemia, G6PD deficiency, and postsplenectomy
An autosomal-recessive disorder with a defect in the GPIIbIIIa platelet receptor and ↓ platelet aggregation.	Glanzmann's thrombasthenia

Virus associated with aplastic anemia in patients with sickle cell anemia.	Parvovirus B19
A 25-year-old African-American male with sickle cell anemia has sudden onset of bone pain. Management of pain crisis?	O_2, analgesia, hydration, and, if severe, transfusion
A significant cause of morbidity in thalassemia patients. Treatment?	Iron overload; use deferoxamine

INFECTIOUS DISEASE

The three most common causes of fever of unknown origin (FUO).	Infection, cancer, and autoimmune disease
Four signs and symptoms of streptococcal pharyngitis.	Fever, pharyngeal erythema, tonsillar exudate, lack of cough
A nonsuppurative complication of streptococcal infection that is not altered by treatment of 1° infection.	Postinfectious glomerulonephritis
Asplenic patients are particularly susceptible to these organisms.	Encapsulated organisms—pneumococcus, meningococcus, *Haemophilus influenzae, Klebsiella*
The number of bacteria on a clean-catch specimen to diagnose a UTI.	10^5 bacteria/mL
Which healthy population is susceptible to UTIs?	Pregnant women. Treat this group aggressively because of potential complications
A patient from California or Arizona presents with fever, malaise, cough, and night sweats. Diagnosis? Treatment?	Coccidioidomycosis. Amphotericin B
Nonpainful chancre.	1° syphilis
A "blueberry muffin" rash is characteristic of what congenital infection?	Rubella
Meningitis in neonates. Causes? Treatment?	Group B strep, *E. coli, Listeria.* Treat with gentamicin and ampicillin
Meningitis in infants. Causes? Treatment?	Pneumococcus, meningococcus, *H. influenzae.* Treat with cefotaxime and vancomycin
What should always be done prior to LP?	Check for ↑ ICP; look for papilledema
CSF findings: ■ Low glucose, PMN predominance ■ Normal glucose, lymphocytic predominance ■ Numerous RBCs in serial CSF samples ■ ↑ gamma globulins	 Bacterial meningitis Aseptic (viral) meningitis Subarachnoid hemorrhage (SAH) MS

Initially presents with a pruritic papule with regional lymphadenopathy and evolves into a black eschar after 7–10 days. Treatment?	Cutaneous anthrax. Treat with penicillin G or ciprofloxacin
Findings in 3° syphilis.	Tabes dorsalis, general paresis, gummas, Argyll Robertson pupil, aortitis, aortic root aneurysms
Characteristics of 2° Lyme disease.	Arthralgias, migratory polyarthropathies, Bell's palsy, myocarditis
Cold agglutinins.	*Mycoplasma*
A 24-year-old male presents with soft white plaques on his tongue and the back of his throat. Diagnosis? Workup? Treatment?	Candidal thrush. Workup should include an HIV test. Treat with nystatin oral suspension
Begin *Pneumocystis carinii* pneumonia (PCP) prophylaxis in an HIV-positive patient at what CD4 count? *Mycobacterium avium-intracellulare* (MAI) prophylaxis?	≤ 200 for PCP (with TMP-SMX); $\leq 50-100$ for MAI (with clarithromycin/azithromycin)
Risk factors for pyelonephritis.	Pregnancy, vesicoureteral reflux, anatomic anomalies, indwelling catheters, kidney stones
Neutropenic nadir postchemotherapy.	7–10 days
Erythema migrans.	Lesion of 1° Lyme disease
Classic physical findings for endocarditis.	Fever, heart murmur, Osler's nodes, splinter hemorrhages, Janeway lesions, Roth's spots
Aplastic crisis in sickle cell disease.	Parvovirus B19
Ring-enhancing brain lesion on CT with seizures	*Taenia solium* (cysticercosis)
Name the organism:	
▪ Branching rods in oral infection.	*Actinomyces israelii*
▪ Painful chancroid.	*Haemophilus ducreyi*
▪ Dog or cat bite.	*Pasteurella multocida*
▪ Gardener.	*Sporothrix schenckii*
▪ Pregnant women with pets.	*Toxoplasma gondii*
▪ Meningitis in adults.	*Neisseria meningitidis*
▪ Meningitis in elderly.	*Streptococcus pneumoniae*
▪ Alcoholic with pneumonia.	*Klebsiella*
▪ "Currant jelly" sputum.	*Klebsiella*
▪ Infection in burn victims.	*Pseudomonas*
▪ Osteomyelitis from foot wound puncture.	*Pseudomonas*
▪ Osteomyelitis in a sickle cell patient.	*Salmonella*

A 55-year-old man who is a smoker and a heavy drinker presents with a new cough and flulike symptoms. Gram stain shows no organisms; silver stain of sputum shows gram-negative rods. What is the diagnosis?	*Legionella* pneumonia
A middle-aged man presents with acute-onset monoarticular joint pain and bilateral Bell's palsy. What is the likely diagnosis, and how did he get it? Treatment?	Lyme disease, *Ixodes* tick, doxycycline
A patient develops endocarditis three weeks after receiving a prosthetic heart valve. What organism is suspected?	*S. aureus* or *S. epidermidis.*

MUSCULOSKELETAL

A patient presents with pain on passive movement, pallor, poikilothermia, paresthesias, paralysis, and pulselessness. Treatment?	All-compartment fasciotomy for suspected compartment syndrome
Back pain that is exacerbated by standing and walking and relieved with sitting and hyperflexion of the hips.	Spinal stenosis
Joints in the hand affected in rheumatoid arthritis.	MCP and PIP joints; DIP joints are spared
Joint pain and stiffness that worsen over the course of the day and are relieved by rest.	Osteoarthritis
Genetic disorder associated with multiple fractures and commonly mistaken for child abuse.	Osteogenesis imperfecta
Hip and back pain along with stiffness that improves with activity over the course of the day and worsens at rest. Diagnostic test?	Suspect ankylosing spondylitis. Check HLA-B27
Arthritis, conjunctivitis, and urethritis in young men. Associated organisms?	Reactive (Reiter's) arthritis. Associated with *Campylobacter*, *Shigella, Salmonella, Chlamydia,* and *Ureaplasma*
A 55-year-old man has sudden, excruciating first MTP joint pain after a night of drinking red wine. Diagnosis, workup, and chronic treatment?	Gout. Needle-shaped, negatively birefringent crystals are seen on joint fluid aspirate. Chronic treatment with allopurinol or probenecid
Rhomboid-shaped, positively birefringent crystals on joint fluid aspirate.	Pseudogout
An elderly female presents with pain and stiffness of the shoulders and hips; she cannot lift her arms above her head. Labs show anemia and ↑ ESR.	Polymyalgia rheumatica
An active 13-year-old boy has anterior knee pain. Diagnosis?	Osgood-Schlatter disease

Bone is fractured in fall on outstretched hand.	Distal radius (Colles' fracture)
Complication of scaphoid fracture.	Avascular necrosis
Signs suggesting radial nerve damage with humeral fracture.	Wrist drop, loss of thumb abduction
A young child presents with proximal muscle weakness, waddling gait, and pronounced calf muscles.	Duchenne muscular dystrophy
A first-born female who was born in breech position is found to have asymmetric skin folds on her newborn exam. Diagnosis? Treatment?	Developmental dysplasia of the hip. If severe, consider a Pavlik harness to maintain abduction
An 11-year-old obese, African-American boy presents with sudden onset of limp. Diagnosis? Workup?	Slipped capital femoral epiphyses. AP and frog-leg lateral view
The most common 1° malignant tumor of bone.	Multiple myeloma

NEUROLOGY

Unilateral, severe periorbital headache with tearing and conjunctival erythema.	Cluster headache
Prophylactic treatment for migraine.	β-blockers, Ca^{2+} channel blockers, TCAs
The most common pituitary tumor. Treatment?	Prolactinoma. Dopamine agonists (e.g., bromocriptine)
A 55-year-old patient presents with acute "broken speech." What type of aphasia? What lobe and vascular distribution?	Broca's aphasia. Frontal lobe, left MCA distribution
The most common cause of SAH.	Trauma; the second most common is berry aneurysm
A crescent-shaped hyperdensity on CT that does not cross the midline.	Subdural hematoma—bridging veins torn
A history significant for initial altered mental status with an intervening lucid interval. Diagnosis? Most likely etiology? Treatment?	Epidural hematoma. Middle meningeal artery. Neurosurgical evacuation
CSF findings with SAH.	Elevated ICP, RBCs, xanthochromia
Albuminocytologic dissociation.	Guillain-Barré (↑ protein in CSF with only a modest ↑ in cell count)
Cold water is flushed into a patient's ear, and the fast phase of the nystagmus is toward the opposite side. Normal or pathological?	Normal
The most common 1° sources of metastases to the brain.	Lung, breast, skin (melanoma), kidney, GI tract

May be seen in children who are accused of inattention in class and confused with ADHD.	Absence seizures
The most frequent presentation of intracranial neoplasm.	Headache
The most common cause of seizures in children (2–10 years).	Infection, febrile seizures, trauma, idiopathic
The most common cause of seizures in young adults (18–35 years).	Trauma, alcohol withdrawal, brain tumor
First-line medication for status epilepticus.	IV benzodiazepine
Confusion, confabulation, ophthalmoplegia, ataxia.	Wernicke's encephalopathy due to a deficiency of thiamine
What % lesion is an indication for carotid endarterectomy?	Seventy percent if the stenosis is symptomatic
The most common causes of dementia.	Alzheimer's and multi-infarct
Combined UMN and LMN disorder.	ALS
Rigidity and stiffness with resting tremor and masked facies.	Parkinson's disease
The mainstay of Parkinson's therapy.	Levodopa/carbidopa
Treatment for Guillain-Barré syndrome.	IVIG or plasmapheresis
Rigidity and stiffness that progress to choreiform movements, accompanied by moodiness and altered behavior.	Huntington's disease
A six-year-old girl presents with a port-wine stain in the V2 distribution as well as with mental retardation, seizures, and leptomeningeal angioma.	Sturge-Weber syndrome. Treat symptomatically. Possible focal cerebral resection of affected lobe
Café-au-lait spots on skin.	Neurofibromatosis 1
Hyperphagia, hypersexuality, hyperorality, and hyperdocility.	Klüver-Bucy syndrome (amygdala)
Administer to a symptomatic patient to diagnose myasthenia gravis.	Edrophonium

OBSTETRICS

1° causes of third-trimester bleeding.	Placental abruption and placenta previa
Classic ultrasound and gross appearance of complete hydatidiform mole.	Snowstorm on ultrasound. "Cluster-of-grapes" appearance on gross examination
Chromosomal pattern of a complete mole.	46,XX

Molar pregnancy containing fetal tissue.	Partial mole
Symptoms of placental abruption.	Continuous, painful vaginal bleeding
Symptoms of placenta previa.	Self-limited, painless vaginal bleeding
When should a vaginal exam be performed with suspected placenta previa?	Never
Antibiotics with teratogenic effects.	Tetracycline, fluoroquinolones, aminoglycosides, sulfonamides
Shortest AP diameter of the pelvis.	Obstetric conjugate: between the sacral promontory and the midpoint of the symphysis pubis
Medication given to accelerate fetal lung maturity.	Betamethasone or dexamethasone × 48 hours
The most common cause of postpartum hemorrhage.	Uterine atony
Treatment for postpartum hemorrhage.	Uterine massage; if that fails, give oxytocin
Typical antibiotics for group B streptococcus (GBS) prophylaxis.	IV penicillin or ampicillin
A patient fails to lactate after an emergency C-section with marked blood loss.	Sheehan's syndrome (postpartum pituitary necrosis)
Uterine bleeding at 18 weeks' gestation; no products expelled; membranes ruptured; cervical os open.	Inevitable abortion
Uterine bleeding at 18 weeks' gestation; no products expelled; cervical os closed.	Threatened abortion

GYNECOLOGY

The first test to perform when a woman presents with amenorrhea.	β-hCG; the most common cause of amenorrhea is pregnancy
Term for heavy bleeding during and between menstrual periods.	Menometrorrhagia
Cause of amenorrhea with normal prolactin, no response to estrogen-progesterone challenge, and a history of D&C.	Asherman's syndrome
Therapy for polycystic ovarian syndrome.	Weight loss and OCPs
Medication used to induce ovulation.	Clomiphene citrate
Diagnostic step required in a postmenopausal woman who presents with vaginal bleeding.	Endometrial biopsy

Indications for medical treatment of ectopic pregnancy.	Stable, unruptured ectopic pregnancy of < 3.5 cm at < 6 weeks' gestation
Medical options for endometriosis.	OCPs, danazol, GnRH agonists
Laparoscopic findings in endometriosis.	"Chocolate cysts," powder burns
The most common location for an ectopic pregnancy.	Ampulla of the oviduct
How to diagnose and follow a leiomyoma.	Ultrasound
Natural history of a leiomyoma.	Regresses after menopause
A patient has ↑ vaginal discharge and petechial patches in the upper vagina and cervix.	*Trichomonas* vaginitis
Treatment for bacterial vaginosis.	Oral or topical metronidazole
The most common cause of bloody nipple discharge.	Intraductal papilloma
Contraceptive methods that protect against PID.	OCP and barrier contraception
Unopposed estrogen is contraindicated in which cancers?	Endometrial or estrogen receptor–⊕ breast cancer
A patient presents with recent PID with RUQ pain.	Consider Fitz-Hugh–Curtis syndrome
Breast malignancy presenting as itching, burning, and erosion of the nipple.	Paget's disease
Annual screening for women with a strong family history of ovarian cancer.	CA-125 and transvaginal ultrasound
A 50-year-old woman leaks urine when laughing or coughing. Nonsurgical options?	Kegel exercises, estrogen, pessaries for stress incontinence
A 30-year-old woman has unpredictable urine loss. Examination is normal. Medical options?	Anticholinergics (oxybutynin) or β-adrenergics (metaproterenol) for urge incontinence.
Lab values suggestive of menopause.	↑ serum FSH
The most common cause of female infertility.	Endometriosis
Two consecutive findings of atypical squamous cells of undetermined significance (ASCUS) on Pap smear. Follow-up evaluation?	Colposcopy and endocervical curettage
Breast cancer type that ↑ the future risk of invasive carcinoma in both breasts.	Lobular carcinoma in situ

Nontender abdominal mass associated with elevated VMA and HVA.	Neuroblastoma
The most common type of tracheoesophageal fistula (TEF). Diagnosis?	Esophageal atresia with distal TEF (85%). Unable to pass NG tube
Not contraindications to vaccination.	Mild illness and/or low-grade fever, current antibiotic therapy, and prematurity
Tests to rule out shaken baby syndrome.	Ophthalmologic exam, CT, and MRI
A neonate has meconium ileus.	CF or Hirschsprung's disease
Bilious emesis within hours after the first feeding.	Duodenal atresia
A two-month-old presents with nonbilious projectile emesis. What are the appropriate steps in management?	Correct metabolic abnormalities. Then correct pyloric stenosis with pyloromyotomy
The most common 1° immunodeficiency.	Selective IgA deficiency
An infant has a high fever and onset of rash as fever breaks. What is he at risk for?	Febrile seizures (roseola infantum)
What is the immunodeficiency? ■ A boy has chronic respiratory infections. Nitroblue tetrazolium test is ⊕. ■ A child has eczema, thrombocytopenia, and high levels of IgA. ■ A four-month-old boy has life-threatening *Pseudomonas* infection.	Chronic granulomatous disease Wiskott-Aldrich syndrome Bruton's X-linked agammaglobulinemia
Acute-phase treatment for Kawasaki disease.	High-dose aspirin for inflammation and fever; IVIG to prevent coronary artery aneurysms
Treatment for mild and severe unconjugated hyperbilirubinemia.	Phototherapy (mild) or exchange transfusion (severe)
Sudden onset of mental status changes, emesis, and liver dysfunction after taking aspirin.	Reye's syndrome
A child has loss of red light reflex. Diagnosis?	Suspect retinoblastoma
Vaccinations at a six-month well-child visit.	HBV, DTaP, Hib, IPV, PCV
Tanner stage 3 in a six-year-old female.	Precocious puberty
Infection of small airways with epidemics in winter and spring.	RSV bronchiolitis
Cause of neonatal RDS.	Surfactant deficiency

A condition associated with red "currant-jelly" stools.	Intussusception
A congenital heart disease that cause 2° hypertension.	Coarctation of the aorta
First-line treatment for otitis media.	Amoxicillin × 10 days
The most common pathogen causing croup.	Parainfluenza virus type 1
A homeless child is small for his age and has peeling skin and a swollen belly.	Kwashiorkor (protein malnutrition)
Defect in an X-linked syndrome with mental retardation, gout, self-mutilation, and choreoathetosis.	Lesch-Nyhan syndrome (purine salvage problem with HGPRTase deficiency)
A newborn female has continuous "machinery murmur."	Patent ductus arteriosus (PDA)

PSYCHIATRY

First-line pharmacotherapy for depression.	SSRIs
Antidepressants associated with hypertensive crisis.	MAOIs
Galactorrhea, impotence, menstrual dysfunction, and ↓ libido.	Patient on dopamine antagonist
A 17-year-old female has left arm paralysis after her boyfriend dies in a car crash. No medical cause is found.	Conversion disorder
Name the defense mechanism: ■ A mother who is angry at her husband yells at her child. ■ A pedophile enters a monastery. ■ A woman calmly describes a grisly murder. ■ A hospitalized 10-year-old begins to wet his bed.	Displacement Reaction formation Isolation Regression
Life-threatening muscle rigidity, fever, and rhabdomyolysis.	Neuroleptic malignant syndrome
Amenorrhea, bradycardia, and abnormal body image in a young female.	Anorexia
A 35-year-old male has recurrent episodes of palpitations, diaphoresis, and fear of going crazy.	Panic disorder
The most serious side effect of clozapine.	Agranulocytosis
A 21-year-old male has three months of social withdrawal, worsening grades, flattened affect, and concrete thinking.	Schizophreniform disorder (diagnosis of schizophrenia requires ≥ 6 months of symptoms)
Key side effects of atypical antipsychotics.	Weight gain, type 2 DM, QT prolongation

A young weight lifter receives IV haloperidol and complains that his eyes are deviated sideways. Diagnosis? Treatment?	Acute dystonia (oculogyric crisis). Treat with benztropine or diphenhydramine
Medication to avoid in patients with a history of alcohol withdrawal seizures.	Neuroleptics
A 13-year-old male has a history of theft, vandalism, and violence toward family pets.	Conduct disorder
A five-month-old girl has ↓ head growth, truncal dyscoordination, and ↓ social interaction.	Rett's disorder
A patient hasn't slept for days, lost $20,000 gambling, is agitated, and has pressured speech. Diagnosis? Treatment?	Acute mania. Start a mood stabilizer (e.g., lithium)
After a minor fender bender, a man wears a neck brace and requests permanent disability.	Malingering
A nurse presents with severe hypoglycemia; blood analysis reveals no elevation in C peptide.	Factitious disorder (Munchausen syndrome)
A patient continues to use cocaine after being in jail, losing his job, and not paying child support.	Substance abuse
A violent patient has vertical and horizontal nystagmus.	Phencyclidine hydrochloride (PCP) intoxication
A woman who was abused as a child frequently feels outside of or detached from her body.	Depersonalization disorder
A man has repeated, intense urges to rub his body against unsuspecting passengers on a bus.	Frotteurism (a paraphilia)
A schizophrenic patient takes haloperidol for one year and develops uncontrollable tongue movements. Diagnosis? Treatment?	Tardive dyskinesia. ↓ or discontinue haloperidol and consider another antipsychotic (e.g., risperidone, clozapine)
A man unexpectedly flies across the country, takes a new name, and has no memory of his prior life.	Dissociative fugue

PULMONARY

Risk factors for DVT.	Stasis, endothelial injury, and hypercoagulability (Virchow's triad)
Criteria for exudative effusion.	Pleural/serum protein > 0.5; pleural/serum LDH > 0.6
Causes of exudative effusion.	Think of leaky capillaries. Malignancy, TB, bacterial or viral infection, pulmonary embolism with infarct, and pancreatitis

Causes of transudative effusion.	Think of intact capillaries. CHF, liver or kidney disease, and protein-losing enteropathy
Normalizing P_{CO_2} in a patient having an asthma exacerbation may indicate?	Fatigue and impending respiratory failure
Dyspnea, lateral hilar lymphodenopathy on CXR, noncaseating granulomas, increased ACE, and hypercalcemia.	Sarcoidosis
PFT showing ↓ FEV_1/FVC.	Obstructive pulmonary disease (e.g., asthma)
PFT showing ↑ FEV_1/FVC.	Restrictive pulmonary disease
Honeycomb pattern on CXR. Diagnosis? Treatment?	Diffuse interstitial pulmonary fibrosis. Supportive care. Steroids may help
Treatment for SVC syndrome.	Radiation
Treatment for mild, persistent asthma.	Inhaled β-agonists and inhaled corticosteroids
Acid-base disorder in pulmonary embolism.	Hypoxia and hypocarbia (respiratory alkalosis)
Non–small cell lung cancer (NSCLC) associated with hypercalcemia.	Squamous cell carcinoma
Lung cancer associated with SIADH.	Small cell lung cancer (SCLC)
Lung cancer highly related to cigarette exposure.	SCLC
A tall white male presents with acute shortness of breath. Diagnosis? Treatment?	Spontaneous pneumothorax. Spontaneous regression. Supplemental O_2 may be helpful
Treatment of tension pneumothorax.	Immediate needle thoracostomy
Characteristics favoring carcinoma in an isolated pulmonary nodule.	Age > 45–50 years; lesions new or larger in comparison to old films; absence of calcification or irregular calcification; size > 2 cm; irregular margins
Hypoxemia and pulmonary edema with normal pulmonary capillary wedge pressure.	ARDS
↑ risk of what infection with silicosis?	*Mycobacterium tuberculosis*
Causes of hypoxemia.	Right-to-left shunt, hypoventilation, low inspired O_2 tension, diffusion defect, V/Q mismatch
Classic CXR findings for pulmonary edema.	Cardiomegaly, prominent pulmonary vessels, Kerley B lines, "bat's-wing" appearance of hilar shadows, and perivascular and peribronchial cuffing

Renal tubular acidosis (RTA) associated with abnormal H$^+$ secretion and nephrolithiasis.	Type I (distal) RTA
RTA associated with abnormal HCO_3^- and rickets.	Type II (proximal) RTA
RTA associated with aldosterone defect.	Type IV (distal) RTA
"Doughy skin."	Hypernatremia
Differential of hypervolemic hyponatremia.	Cirrhosis, CHF, nephritic syndrome
Chvostek's and Trousseau's signs.	Hypocalcemia
The most common causes of hypercalcemia.	Malignancy and hyperparathyroidism
T-wave flattening and U waves.	Hypokalemia
Peaked T waves and widened QRS.	Hyperkalemia
First-line treatment for moderate hypercalcemia.	IV hydration and loop diuretics (furosemide)
Type of ARF in a patient with $Fe_{Na} < 1\%$.	Prerenal
A 49-year-old male presents with acute-onset flank pain and hematuria.	Nephrolithiasis
The most common type of nephrolithiasis.	Calcium oxalate
A 20-year-old man presents with a palpable flank mass and hematuria. Ultrasound shows bilateral enlarged kidneys with cysts. Associated brain anomaly?	Cerebral berry aneurysms (autosomal-dominant PCKD)
Hematuria, hypertension, and oliguria.	Nephritic syndrome
Proteinuria, hypoalbuminemia, hyperlipidemia, hyperlipiduria, edema.	Nephrotic syndrome
The most common form of nephritic syndrome.	Membranous glomerulonephritis
The most common form of glomerulonephritis.	IgA nephropathy (Berger's disease)
Glomerulonephritis with deafness.	Alport's syndrome
Glomerulonephritis with hemoptysis.	Wegener's granulomatosis and Goodpasture's syndrome
Presence of red cell casts in urine sediment.	Glomerulonephritis/nephritic syndrome
Eosinophils in urine sediment.	Allergic interstitial nephritis
Waxy casts in urine sediment and Maltese crosses (seen with lipiduria).	Nephrotic syndrome

Drowsiness, asterixis, nausea, and a pericardial friction rub.	Uremic syndrome seen in patients with renal failure
A 55-year-old man is diagnosed with prostate cancer. Treatment options?	Wait, surgical resection, radiation and/or androgen suppression
Low urine specific gravity in the presence of high serum osmolality.	DI
Treatment of SIADH?	Fluid restriction, demeclocycline
Hematuria, flank pain, and palpable flank mass.	Renal cell carcinoma (RCC)
Testicular cancer associated with β-hCG, AFP.	Choriocarcinoma
The most common type of testicular cancer.	Seminoma—a type of germ cell tumor
The most common histology of bladder cancer.	Transitional cell carcinoma
Complication of overly rapid correction of hyponatremia.	Central pontine myelinolysis
Salicylate ingestion → in what type of acid-base disorder?	Anion gap acidosis and 1° respiratory alkalosis due to central respiratory stimulation
Acid-base disturbance commonly seen in pregnant women.	Respiratory alkalosis
Three systemic diseases → nephrotic syndrome.	DM, SLE, and amyloidosis
Elevated erythropoietin level, elevated hematocrit, and normal O_2 saturation suggest?	RCC or other erythropoietin-producing tumor; evaluate with CT scan
A 55-year-old man presents with irritative and obstructive urinary symptoms. Treatment options?	Likely BPH. Options include no treatment, terazosin, finasteride, or surgical intervention (TURP)

SELECTED TOPICS IN EMERGENCY MEDICINE

Class of drugs that may cause syndrome of muscle rigidity, hyperthermia, autonomic instability, and extrapyramidal symptoms.	Antipsychotics (neuroleptic malignant syndrome)
Side effects of corticosteroids.	Acute mania, immunosuppression, thin skin, osteoporosis, easy bruising, myopathies
Treatment for DTs.	Benzodiazepines
Treatment for acetaminophen overdose.	N-acetylcysteine
Treatment for opioid overdose.	Naloxone
Treatment for benzodiazepine overdose.	Flumazenil
Treatment for neuroleptic malignant syndrome.	Dantrolene or bromocriptine

Treatment for malignant hypertension.	Nitroprusside
Treatment of AF.	Rate control, rhythm conversion, and anticoagulation
Treatment of supraventricular tachycardia (SVT).	If stable, rate control with carotid massage or other vagal stimulation; if unsuccessful, consider adenosine.
Causes of drug-induced SLE.	INH, penicillamine, hydralazine, procainamide, chlorpromazine, methyldopa, quinidine
Macrocytic, megaloblastic anemia with neurologic symptoms.	B_{12} deficiency
Macrocytic, megaloblastic anemia without neurologic symptoms.	Folate deficiency
A burn patient presents with cherry-red flushed skin and coma. Sao_2 is normal, but carboxyhemoglobin is elevated. Treatment?	Treat CO poisoning with 100% O_2 or with hyperbaric O_2 if severe poisoning or pregnant
Blood in the urethral meatus or high-riding prostate.	Bladder rupture or urethral injury
Test to rule out urethral injury.	Retrograde cystourethrogram
Radiographic evidence of aortic disruption or dissection.	Widened mediastinum (> 8 cm), loss of aortic knob, pleural cap, tracheal deviation to the right, depression of left main stem bronchus
Radiographic indications for surgery in patients with acute abdomen.	Free air under the diaphragm, extravasation of contrast, severe bowel distention, space-occupying lesion (CT), mesenteric occlusion (angiography)
The most common organism in burn-related infections.	*Pseudomonas*
Method of calculating fluid repletion in burn patients.	Parkland formula
Acceptable urine output in a trauma patient.	50 cc/hour
Acceptable urine output in a stable patient.	30 cc/hour
Cannon "a" waves.	Third-degree heart block
Signs of neurogenic shock.	Hypotension and bradycardia
Signs of ↑ ICP (Cushing's triad).	Hypertension, bradycardia, and abnormal respirations
↓ CO, ↓ pulmonary capillary wedge pressure (PCWP), ↑ peripheral vascular resistance (PVR).	Hypovolemic shock
↓ CO, ↑ PCWP, ↑ PVR.	Cardiogenic shock
↑ CO, ↓ PCWP, ↓ PVR.	Septic or anaphylactic shock

Treatment of septic shock.	Fluids and antibiotics
Treatment of cardiogenic shock.	Identify cause; pressors (e.g., dopamine)
Treatment of hypovolemic shock.	Identify cause; fluid and blood repletion
Treatment of anaphylactic shock.	Diphenhydramine or epinephrine 1:1000
Supportive treatment for ARDS.	Continuous positive airway pressure
Signs of air embolism.	A patient with chest trauma who was previously stable suddenly dies
Trauma series.	AP chest, AP/lateral C-spine, AP pelvis

Top-Rated Review Resources

This section is a database of recommended clinical science review books, sample examination books, and commercial review courses marketed to medical students studying for the USMLE Step 2. For each book, we list the **Title** of the book, the **First Author** (or editor), the **Current Publisher,** the **Copyright Year,** the **Edition,** the **Number of Pages,** the **ISBN Code,** the **Approximate List Price,** the **Format** of the book, and the **Number of Test Questions.** Most entries also include Summary Comments that describe their style and utility for studying. Finally, each book receives a **Rating.** The books are sorted into a comprehensive section as well as into sections corresponding to the seven clinical disciplines (internal medicine, neurology, OB/GYN, pediatrics, psychiatry, and surgery). Within each section, books are arranged first by Rating, then by Author, and finally by Title.

For this sixth edition of *First Aid for the USMLE Step 2 CK,* the database of review books has been completely revised, with in-depth summary comments on more than 100 books and software. A letter rating scale with six different grades reflects the detailed student evaluations. Each book receives a rating as follows:

A+	Excellent for boards review.
A	
A–	Very good for boards review; choose among the group.

B+	
B	Good, but use only after exhausting better sources.
B–	

The **Rating** is meant to reflect the overall usefulness of the book in preparing for the USMLE Step 2 examination. This is based on a number of factors, including:

- The cost of the book
- The readability of the text
- The appropriateness and accuracy of the book
- The quality and number of sample questions
- The quality of written answers to sample questions
- The quality and appropriateness of the illustrations (e.g., graphs, diagrams, photographs)
- The length of the text (longer is not necessarily better)
- The quality and number of other books available in the same discipline
- The importance of the discipline on the USMLE Step 2 examination

Please note that **the rating does not reflect the quality of the book for purposes other than reviewing for the USMLE Step 2 examination.** Many books with low ratings are well written and informative but are not ideal for boards preparation. We have also avoided listing or commenting on the wide variety of general textbooks available in the clinical sciences.

Evaluations are based on the cumulative results of formal and informal surveys of hundreds of medical students from medical schools across the country. The summary comments and overall ratings represent a consensus opinion, but there may have been a large range of opinions or limited student feedback on any particular book.

Please note that the data listed are subject to change because:

- Publishers' prices change frequently.
- Individual bookstores often charge an additional markup.
- New editions come out frequently, and the quality of updating varies.
- The same book may be reissued through another publisher.

We actively encourage medical students and faculty to submit their opinions and ratings of these clinical science review books so that we may update our database (see "How to Contribute," p. xv). In addition, we ask that publishers and authors submit review copies of clinical science review books, including new editions and books not included in our database, for evaluation. We also solicit reviews of new books or suggestions for alternate modes of study that may be useful in preparing for the examination, such as flash cards, computer-based tutorials, commercial review courses, and Internet Web sites.

DISCLAIMER/CONFLICT OF INTEREST STATEMENT

No material in this book, including the ratings, reflects the opinion or influence of the publisher. All errors and omissions will gladly be corrected if brought to the attention of the authors through the publisher. Please note that the *Underground Clinical Vignettes* series are publications by the authors of this book.

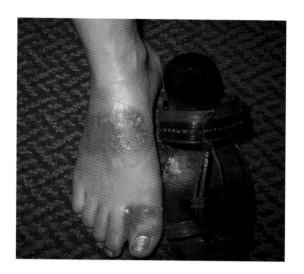

Contact dermatitis. Erythematous papules, vesicles, and serous weeping localized to areas of contact with the offending agent are characteristic. (Reproduced, with permission, from Hurwitz RM, *Pathology of the Skin: Atlas of Clinical–Pathological Correlation*, 1st ed. Stamford, CT: Appleton & Lange, 1991.)

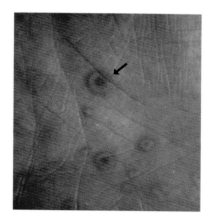

Erythema multiforme. The classic target lesion has a dull red center, pale zone, and darker outer ring (arrow). This acute self-limited reaction may occur with infection, antibiotic use, exposure to radiation or chemicals, or malignancy. (Reproduced, with permission, from Bondi EE, *Dermatology: Diagnosis and Therapy*, 1st ed., Stamford, CT: Appleton & Lange, 1991: 392.)

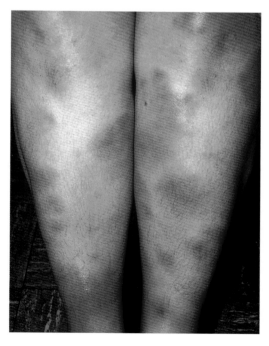

Erythema nodosum. The erythematous plaques and nodules are commonly located on pretibial areas. Lesions are painful and indurated and heal spontaneously without ulceration. (Reproduced, with permission, from Hurwitz RM, *Pathology of the Skin: Atlas of Clinical–Pathological Correlation*, 1st ed., Stamford, CT: Appleton & Lange, 1991: 132.)

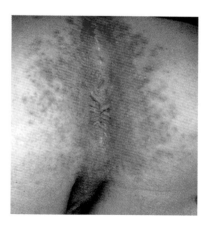

Candidial intertrigo. Erythematous areas surrounded by satellite pustules are restricted to warm, moist intertriginous areas. (Reproduced, with permission, from Bondi EE, *Dermatology: Diagnosis and Therapy*, 1st ed., Stamford, CT: Appleton & Lange, 1991: 390.)

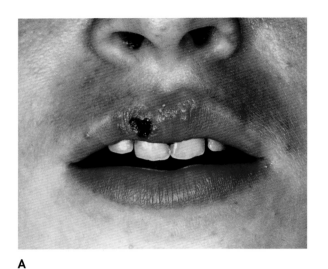

A

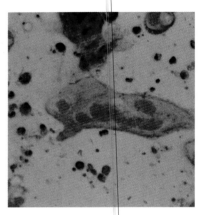

B

Herpes simplex. (A) Primary infection. Grouped vesicles on an erythematous base on the patient's lips and oral mucosa may progress to pustules before resolving. (B) Tzanck smear. The multinucleated giant cells from vesicular fluid provide a presumptive diagnosis of HSV infection. However, the Tzanck smear cannot distinguish between HSV and VZV infection. (Reproduced, with permission, from Hurwitz RM, *Pathology of the Skin: Atlas of Clinical–Pathological Correlation*, 1st ed., Stamford, CT: Appleton & Lange, 1991: 145; and Bondi EE, *Dermatology: Diagnosis and Therapy*, 1st ed., Stamford, CT: Appleton & Lange, 1991: 396.)

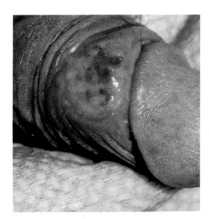

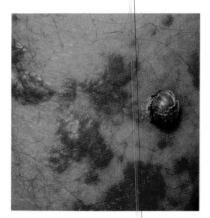

Primary syphilis. The chancre, which appears at the site of infection, is an ulcerated papule with a smooth, clean base; raised, indurated borders; and scant discharge. (Reproduced, with permission, from Bondi EE, *Dermatology: Diagnosis and Therapy*, 1st ed., Stamford, CT: Appleton & Lange, 1991: 394.)

Kaposi's sarcoma. Manifests as red to purple nodules and surrounding pink to red macules. The latter appear most often in immunosuppressed patients. (Reproduced, with permission, from Bondi EE, *Dermatology: Diagnosis and Therapy*, 1st ed., Stamford, CT: Appleton & Lange, 1991: 393.)

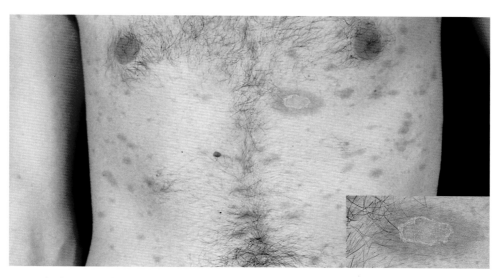

Pityriasis rosea. Pink plaques with an oval configuration are seen that follow the lines of cleavage. Inset: Herald patch. The collarette of scale is more obvious on this magnification. (Reproduced, with permission, from Wolff K, Johnson RA, Suurmond D. *Fitzpatrick's Color Atlas and Synopsis of Clinical Dermatology,* 5th ed. New York: McGraw-Hill, 2005:119.)

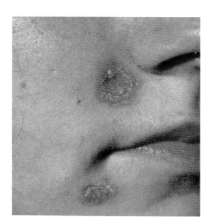

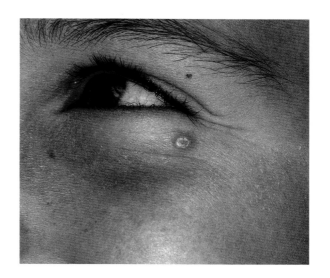

Impetigo. Dried pustules with superficial golden-brown crust are most commonly found around the nose and mouth. (Reproduced, with permission, from Bondi EE, *Dermatology: Diagnosis and Therapy,* 1st ed., Stamford, CT: Appleton & Lange, 1991: 390.)

Molluscum contagiosum. The dome-shaped, fleshy, umbilicated papule on the child's eyelid is characteristic. (Reproduced, with permission, from Hurwitz RM, *Pathology of the Skin: Atlas of Clinical–Pathological Correlation,* 1st ed., Stamford, CT: Appleton & Lange, 1991: 149.)

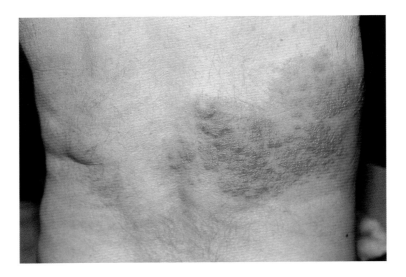

Herpes zoster. The unilateral dermatomal distribution of the grouped vesicles on an erythematous base is characteristic. (Reproduced, with permission, from Wolff K, Johnson RA, Suurmond D. *Fitzpatrick's Color Atlas & Synopsis of Clinical Dermatology,* 5th ed. New York, McGraw-Hill, 2005: 823.)

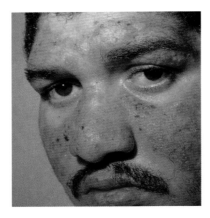

Malar rash of systemic lupus erythematosus. The malar rash is a red to purple continuous plaque extending across the bridge of the nose and to both cheeks. (Reproduced, with permission, from Bondi EE, *Dermatology: Diagnosis and Therapy,* 1st ed., Stamford, CT: Appleton & Lange, 1991: 395.)

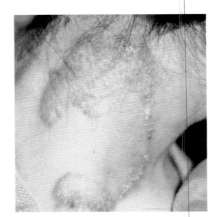

Tinea corporis. Ring-shaped, erythematous, scaling macules with central clearing are characteristic. (Reproduced, with permission, from Bondi EE, *Dermatology: Diagnosis and Therapy,* 1st ed., Stamford, CT: Appleton & Lange, 1991: 389.)

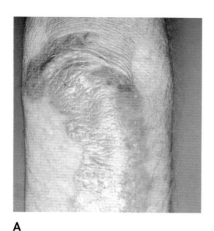

A

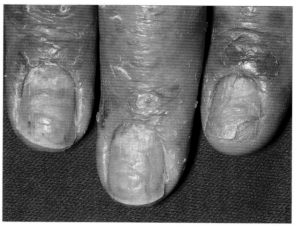

B

Psoriasis. (A) Skin changes. The classic sharply demarcated dark red plaques with silvery scales are commonly located on extensor surfaces (e.g., elbows, knees). (B) Nail changes. Note the pitting, onycholysis, and oil spots. (Reproduced, with permission, from Bondi EE, *Dermatology: Diagnosis and Therapy,* 1st ed., Stamford, CT: Appleton & Lange, 1991: 389; and Hurwitz RM, *Pathology of the Skin: Atlas of Clinical–Pathological Correlation,* 1st ed., Stamford, CT: Appleton & Lange, 1991.)

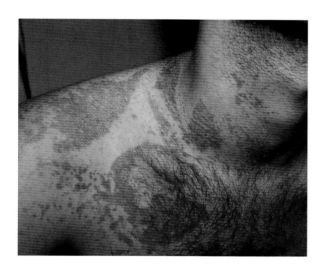

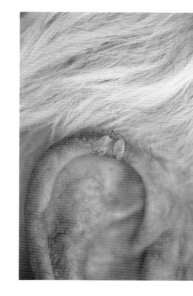

Tinea versicolor. These pinkish scaling macules commonly appear on the chest and back. Lesions may also be lightly pigmented or hypopigmented depending on the patient's skin color and sun exposure. (Courtesy of the Department of Dermatology, Wilford Hall USAF Medical Center and Brooke Army Medical Center, San Antonio, Texas.)

Actinic keratosis. The discrete patch has an erythematous base and rough white scaling. Actinic keratosis is a premalignant lesion that may progress to squamous cell carcinoma. It is most commonly found in sun-exposed areas. (Reproduced, with permission, from Hurwitz RM, *Pathology of the Skin: Atlas of Clinical–Pathological Correlation,* 1st ed., Stamford, CT: Appleton & Lange, 1991: 354.)

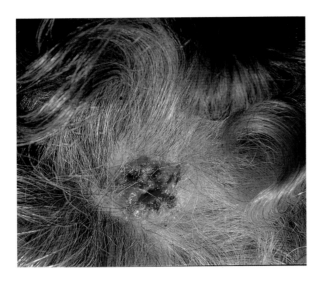

Squamous cell carcinoma. Note the crusting and ulceration of this erythematous plaque. Most lesions are exophytic nodules with erosion or ulceration. (Reproduced, with permission, from Hurwitz RM, *Pathology of the Skin: Atlas of Clinical–Pathological Correlation,* 1st ed., Stamford, CT: Appleton & Lange, 1991: 360.)

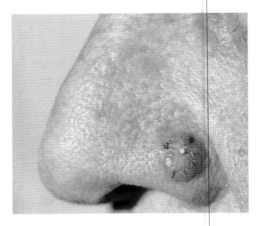

Nodular basal cell carcinoma. A smooth, pearly nodule with telangiectasias. (Reproduced, with permission, from Wolff K, Johnson RA, Suurmond D. *Fitzpatrick's Color Atlas and Synopsis of Clinical Dermatology,* 5th ed. New York: McGraw-Hill, 2005:283.)

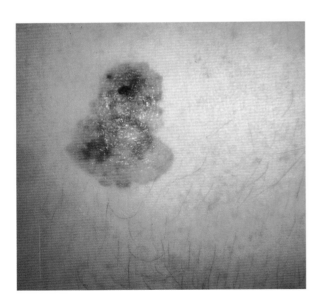

Melanoma. Note the **a**symmetry, **b**order irregularity, **c**olor variation, and large **d**iameter of this plaque. (Reproduced, with permission, from Hurwitz RM, *Pathology of the Skin: Atlas of Clinical–Pathological Correlation,* 1st ed., Stamford, CT: Appleton & Lange, 1991: 432.)

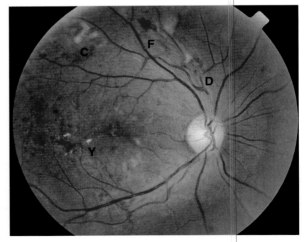

Nonproliferative diabetic retinopathy. Flame hemorrhages (F), dot-blot hemorrhages (D), cotton-wool spots (C), and yellow exudate (Y) result from small vessel damage and occlusion.

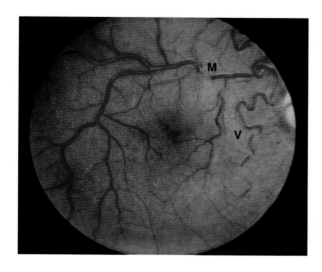

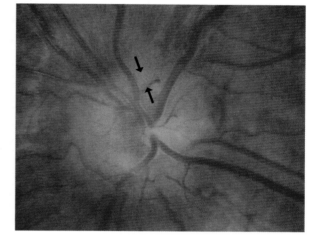

Hypertensive retinopathy. Note the tortuous retinal veins (V) and venous microaneurysms (M). Other findings include hemorrhages, retinal infarcts, detachment of the retina, and disk edema.

Papilledema. Look for blurred disk margins due to edema of the optic disk (arrows).

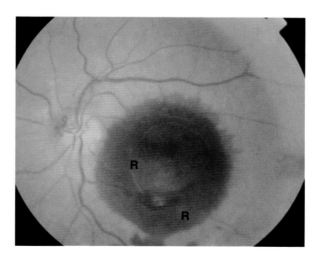

Subretinal hemorrhage. Note the preretinal blood and overlying retinal vessels (R). Subretinal hemorrhages may be seen in any condition with abnormal vessel proliferation (e.g., diabetes, hypertension) or in trauma.

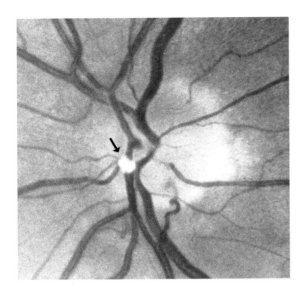

Cholesterol emboli. Cholesterol emboli (Hollenhorst plaque; arrow) usually arise in atherosclerotic carotid arteries and often lodge at the bifurcation of retinal arteries. (Reproduced, with permission, from Vaughan D, *General Ophthalmology,* 14th ed., Stamford, CT: Appleton & Lange, 1995: 299.)

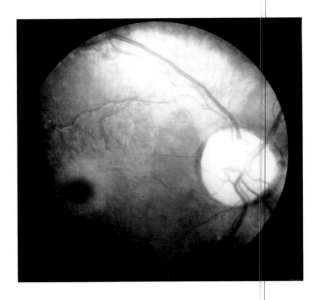

Tay–Sachs. Cherry-red spot. The red spot in the macula may be seen in Tay–Sachs disease, Niemann–Pick disease, central retinal artery occlusion, and methanol toxicity. (Reproduced, with permission, from Vaughan D, *General Ophthalmology,* 14th ed., Stamford, CT: Appleton & Lange, 1995: 293.)

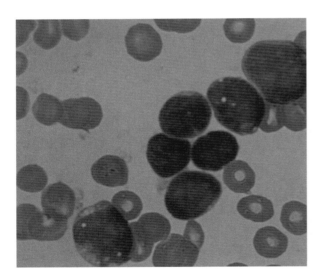

Acute lymphoblastic leukemia. Peripheral blood smear reveals numerous large, uniform lymphoblasts, which are large cells with a high nuclear-to-cytoplasmic ratio. Some lymphoblasts have visible clefts in their nuclei. (Courtesy of Dr. Peter McPhedran, Yale Department of Hematology.)

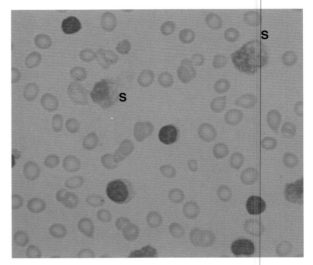

Chronic lymphocytic leukemia. The numerous, small, mature lymphocytes and smudge cells (S; fragile malignant lymphocytes are disrupted during blood smear preparation) are characteristic. (Courtesy of Dr. Peter McPhedran, Yale Department of Hematology.)

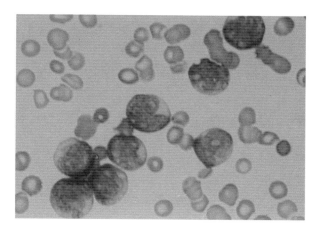

Acute myelocytic leukemia. Large, uniform myeloblasts with round or kidney-shaped nuclei and prominent nucleoli are characteristic. (Courtesy of Dr. Peter McPhedran, Yale Department of Hematology.)

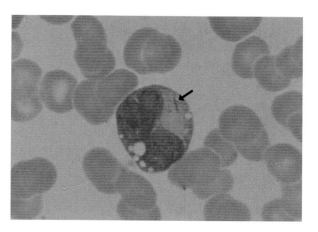

Auer rod in acute myelocytic leukemia. The red rod-shaped structure (arrow) in the cytoplasm of the myeloblast is pathognomonic. (Courtesy of Dr. Peter McPhedran, Yale Department of Hematology.)

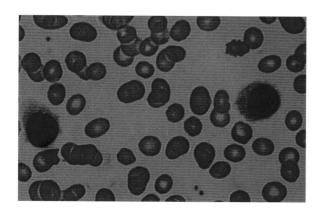

Hairy cell leukemia. Note the hairlike cytoplasmic projections from neoplastic lymphocytes. Villous lymphoma can also look like this. (Courtesy of Dr. Peter McPhedran, Yale Department of Hematology.)

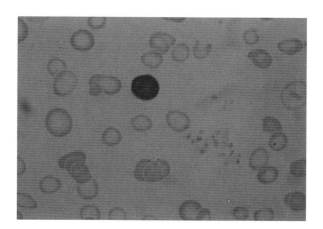

Iron deficiency anemia. Note the microcytic, hypochromic red blood cells ("doughnut cells") with enlarged areas of central pallor. (Courtesy of Dr. Peter McPhedran, Yale Department of Hematology.)

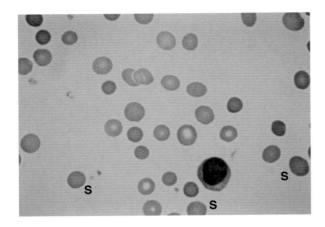

Spherocytes. These RBCs (S) lack areas of central pallor. Spherocytes are seen in autoimmune hemolysis and hereditary spherocytosis. (Courtesy of Dr. Peter McPhedran, Yale Department of Hematology.)

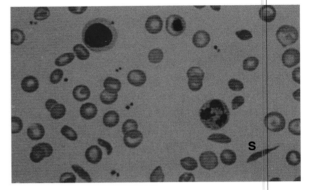

Sickle cells. Sickle-shaped RBCs (S) are almost always seen on the blood smear, regardless of whether the patient is having a sickle cell crisis or not. Anisocytosis, poikilocytosis, target cells, and nucleated RBCs can also be seen. (Courtesy of Dr. Peter McPhedran, Yale Department of Hematology.)

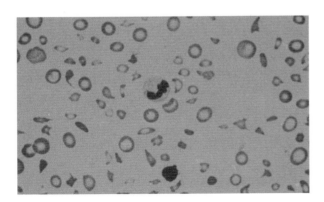

Schistocytes. These fragmented red blood cells may be seen in microangiopathic hemolytic anemia and mechanical hemolysis. (Courtesy of Dr. Peter McPhedran, Yale Department of Hematology.)

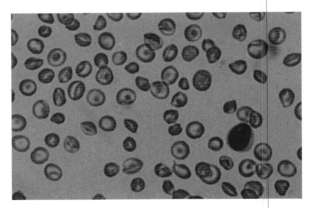

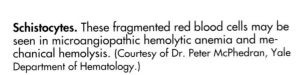

Target cells. The dense zone of hemoglobin in the RBC center is characteristic. Target cells are seen in hemoglobin C or S disease, thalassemia, severe liver disease, and severe iron deficiency anemia as well as postsplenectomy. (Courtesy of Dr. Peter McPhedran, Yale Department of Hematology.)

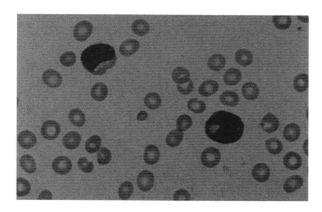

Mononucleosis. These atypical lymphocytes, with abundant blue cytoplasm, no granules, and variably shaped nuclei, are classically seen in EBV and CMV infections. (Courtesy of Dr. Peter McPhedran, Yale Department of Hematology.)

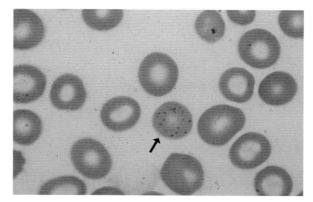

Basophilic stippling. The basophilic granules (arrow) within the red blood cells are a nonspecific finding that may suggest megaloblastic anemia, lead poisoning, or reticulocytes. (Reproduced, with permission, from Lichtman MA, Williams Hematology, 7th ed., New York: McGraw-Hill, 2006, Plate IV-3.)

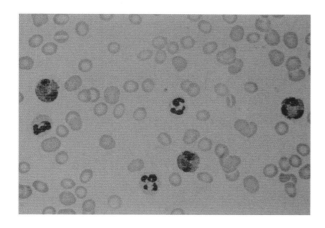

Eosinophilia. Eosinophils have red-staining cytoplasmic granules. Eosinophilia may be seen in atopic diseases, parasitic infections, collagen vascular diseases, medications, malignancies such as Hodgkin's disease, and endocrinopathies like adrenal insufficiency. (Courtesy of Dr. Peter McPhedran, Yale Department of Hematology.)

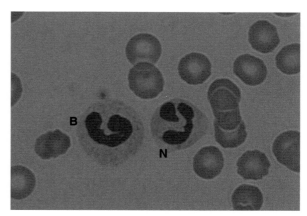

Neutrophil (N) and band (B). The more immature band form has a stretched, nonlobulated nucleus rather than a segmented nucleus. Bands are nonspecific markers of stress. (Courtesy of Dr. Peter McPhedran, Yale Department of Hematology.)

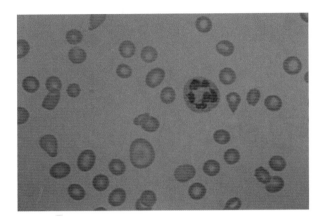

Hypersegmentation. The nucleus of this hypersegmented neutrophil has six lobes (six or more nuclear lobes are required). This is a characteristic finding of megaloblastic anemia. (Courtesy of Dr. Peter McPhedran, Yale Department of Hematology.)

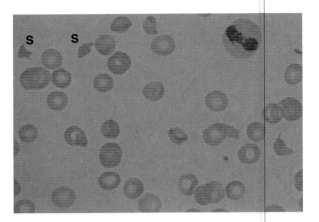

Thrombotic thrombocytopenic purpura (TTP). Note the schistocytes (S) and paucity of platelets. TTP is characterized by microangiopathic hemolytic anemia, thrombocytopenia, fever, neurologic abnormalities, and renal failure. (Courtesy of Dr. Peter McPhedran, Yale Department of Hematology.)

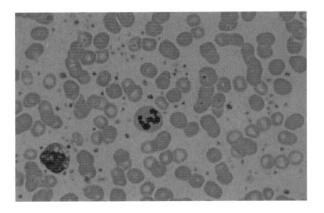

Thrombocytosis. Numerous platelets are seen in myeloproliferative disorders, severe iron deficiency anemia, inflammation, and postsplenectomy states. (Courtesy of Dr. Peter McPhedran, Yale Department of Hematology.)

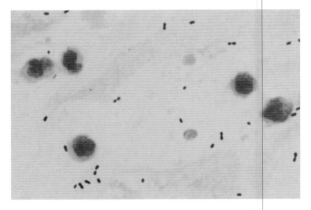

Streptococcus pneumoniae. This is a sputum sample from a patient with pneumonia. Note the characteristic lancet-shaped gram-positive diplococci.

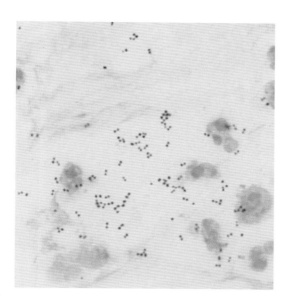

Staphylococcus aureus. These clusters of gram-positive cocci were isolated from the sputum of a patient with pneumonia.

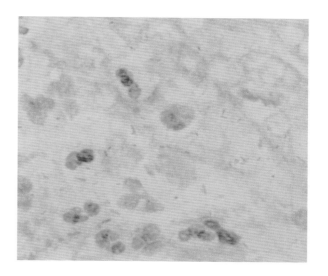

Pseudomonas aeruginosa. This sputum sample from a patient with pneumonia revealed gram-negative rods. The large number of neutrophils and relative paucity of epithelial cells indicate that this sample is not contaminated with oropharyngeal flora.

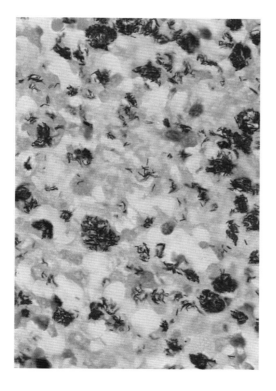

Tuberculosis (AFB smear). Note the red color of the tubercle bacilli an acid-fast staining of a sputum sample ("red snappers"). (Reproduced, with permission, from Milikowski C, *Color Atlas of Basic Histopathology*, 1st ed., Stamford, CT: Appleton & Lange, 1997: 193.)

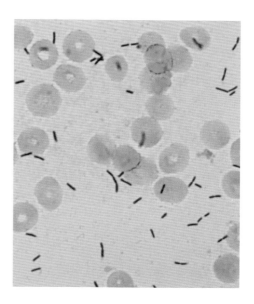

Listeria. These numerous rod-shaped bacilli were isolated from the blood of a patient with *Listeria* meningitis.

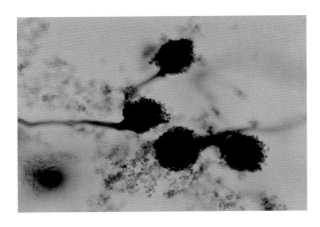

Aspergillosis. Note the characteristic appearance of *Aspergillus* spores in radiating columns.

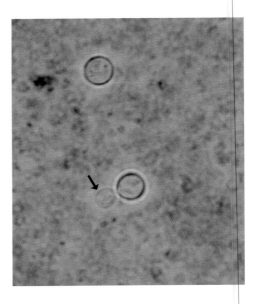

Cryptococcus. Note the budding yeast (arrow) and wide capsule of cryptococcus isolated from CSF.

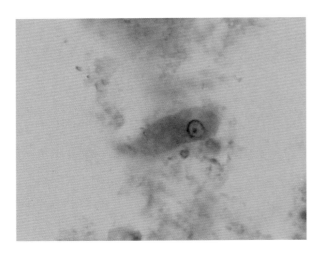

Entamoeba. *Entamoeba* cysts have large nuclei. This is a sample from diarrheal stool.

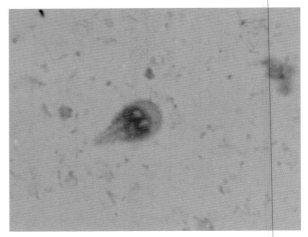

***Giardia* trophozoite in stool.** The trophozoite exhibits a classic pear shape with two nuclei imparting an owl's-eye appearance.

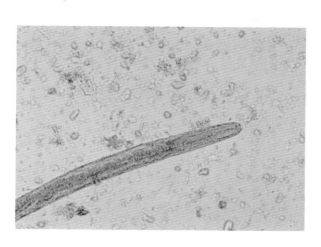

Strongyloides. These filarial larvae were found in the stool of a patient with watery diarrhea.

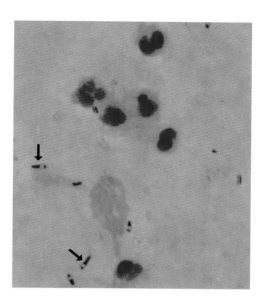

***Clostridium* wound infection.** The lucency at the end of each gram-positive bacillus is the terminal spore (arrow). This sample was isolated from an infected wound site.

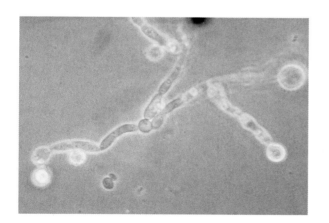

KOH mount of *Candida albicans.* (Reproduced, with permission, from Wolff K, Johnson RA, Suurmond D. *Fitzpatrick's Color Atlas & Synopsis of Clinical Dermatology,* 5th ed. New York: McGraw-Hill, 2005: 717.)

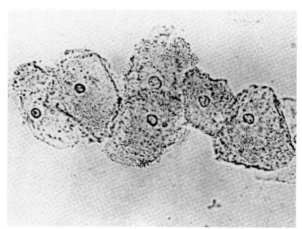

Gardnerella vaginalis. Saline wet mount of vaginal fluid reveals granulations on vaginal epithelial cells ("clue cells") due to adherence of *G. vaginalis* organisms to the cell surface. (Reproduced, with permission, from DeCherney A, *Current Obstetrics and Gynecology Diagnosis and Treatment,* 8th ed., Stamford, CT: Appleton and Lange, 1994: 692.)

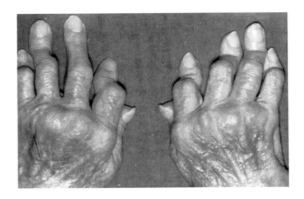

Rheumatoid arthritis. The swan-neck deformities of the digits and severe involvement of the proximal interphalangeal joints are characteristic. (Reproduced, with permission, from Chandrasoma P, *Concise Pathology,* 3rd ed., Stamford, CT: Appleton & Lange, 1998: 978.)

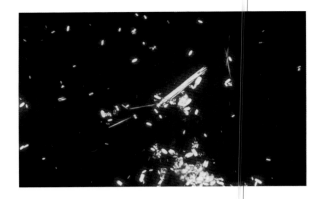

Gout. Negatively birefringent crystals. (Reproduced, with permission, from Milikowshi C, *Color Atlas of Basic Histopathology,* 1st ed., Stamford, CT: Appleton & Lange, 1997: 546.)

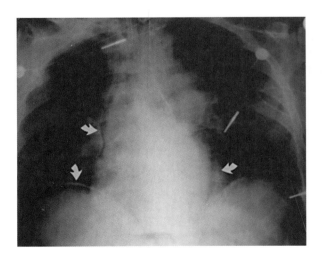

Pneumomediastinum. The lucency outlining the left heart border on chest x-ray suggests air in the mediastinum. (Reproduced, with permission, from Goldfrank LR, *Toxic Emergencies,* 6th ed., Stamford, CT: Appleton & Lange, 1998: 285.)

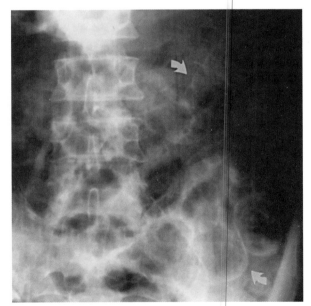

Pneumoperitoneum. The lucency outlining small bowel on abdominal x-ray indicated the abnormal presence of air. (Reproduced, with permission, from Goldfrank LR, *Toxic Emergencies,* 6th ed., Stamford, CT: Appleton & Lange, 1998: 285.)

A

Boards & Wards
AYALA

$36.95   Review

Lippincott Williams & Wilkins, 2007, 3rd ed., 363 pages,
ISBN 1405105097

Concise book in outline format, packed with key information across
the various fields of medicine. **Pros:** Very high yield. Nice use of tables and charts. Good for quick study and last-minute review. Can be
used during clinical rotations as well as in preparation for Step 2.
Cons: Small print. Not tremendously detailed, but covers many topics. Requires more in-depth books for further explanation. **Summary:**
Good, comprehensive review, although it lacks some detail.

A

USMLE Step 2 Mock Exam
BROCHERT

$29.95   Test/750 q

Elsevier, 2004, 2nd ed., 348 pages, ISBN 1560536101

Consists of 750 vignette-style questions in 15 test blocks. **Pros:** Questions are case based and offer a good approximation of real boards
questions. Questions cover high-yield topics, and explanations are
terse but adequate. Many questions also include images and associated laboratory findings. **Cons:** Explanations may not be adequate for
those who require an in-depth review of certain topics. **Summary:** Excellent vignette-type questions in mock exam format.

A⁻

USMLE Step 2 Secrets
BROCHERT

$34.95   Review

Elsevier, 2004, 2nd ed., 296 pages, ISBN 156053608X

Typical Secrets-series format, with questions and answers organized by
specialty. **Pros:** Concise review of many high-yield topics. Good use of
clinical images, including patient photos, blood smears, and radiographs. Gives clinical pearls that help differentiate and diagnose
common clinical presentations. **Cons:** No clinical vignettes; simply
lists questions that might be posed on the wards. Does not follow Step
2 format. Expensive. Content overlaps with that of other books by
Brochert. **Summary:** Overall, good content for self-quizzing and
study, but does not substitute for a formal review or practice tests.
Portable book that stresses relevant topics in a quick, easy format.

REVIEW RESOURCES

COMPREHENSIVE

A⁻

First Aid Cases for the USMLE Step 2

LE

McGraw-Hill, 2006, 272 pages, ISBN 0071464115

Review of high-yield clinical vignettes for Step 2. **Pros:** Cases provide detailed answers to high-yield topics and are arranged in an easy-to-follow format. Emphasizes the most likely diagnosis, the next step, and initial management answers. **Cons:** Some topics are either not covered or given only brief treatment. **Summary:** Good review with emphasis on vignette-style case presentation and boards-relevant answers, but not sufficient as a stand-alone text for review.

$34.95   Review

B⁺

Underground Clinical Vignettes: Nine-Volume Set

BHUSHAN

Lippincott Williams & Wilkins, 2005, 3rd ed., 942 pages, ISBN 140510418X

Nine-volume set containing clinical case scenarios of the various specialties, including OB/GYN, neurology, internal medicine, surgery, emergency medicine, psychiatry, and pediatrics, along with an extensive color atlas supplement. **Pros:** Well organized by focus points: pathogenesis, epidemiology, management, complications, and associated diseases. Recently revised and updated. **Cons:** Not comprehensive; use as a supplement to review. **Summary:** Organized and easy-to-read clinical vignettes. Excellent as a supplement to studying, but not sufficient by itself. More economical to purchase the nine-volume set than individual volumes.

$143.95   Review

B⁺

Lange Q&A: USMLE Step 2

CHAN

McGraw-Hill, 2005, 5th ed., 384 pages, ISBN 0071447709

Review questions organized by specialty along with two comprehensive practice exams. **Pros:** Overall question content is good, with broad coverage of high-yield topics. Well illustrated. **Cons:** Vignettes are brief, with short explanations. Some questions are too detailed and do not reflect the level of actual Step 2 questions. **Summary:** Good overall review questions on high-yield topics make it well suited to focused specialty review. Good buy for the number of questions.

$39.95   Test/1060 q

B⁺

Lange Practice Tests: USMLE Step 2

GOLDBERG

McGraw-Hill, 2005, 3rd ed., 288 pages, ISBN 0071446168

Comprehensive test questions. **Pros:** Great source of high-yield questions covering all topics. Many questions include clinically relevant radiographs and photographs of pathology. Adequate explanations. **Cons:** Some questions are not vignette style and do not reflect boards format. **Summary:** Good compilation of test questions that focus on high-yield material, but some questions still do not reflect boards style. Good source of supplemental questions.

$39.95   Test/900 q

NMS Review for USMLE Step 2 CK

Iʙsᴇɴ

Lippincott Williams & Wilkins, 2006, 3rd ed., 654 pages,
ISBN 0781765226

$44.95   Test/900 q

Comprehensive review book in question-and-answer format. **Pros:**
Clear, concise, and broad coverage of high-yield topics, presented in a
format similar to that of the actual Step 2 exam. Complete explanations. **Cons:** Questions are more detailed than needed for the boards.
Lacks illustrations or images. **Summary:** Good source of Step 2–style
questions with appropriate format and content, but questions may focus on details not emphasized on the actual exam.

Step-Up to USMLE Step 2

ᴠᴀɴ Kʟᴇᴜɴᴇɴ

Lippincott Williams & Wilkins, 2006, 1st ed., 294 pages,
ISBN 0781757924

$39.95   Review

Step 2 test review typical of the Step-Up series format, organized by systems. **Pros:** Comprehensive yet concise boards review resource with
many tables organizing the information and quick facts isolated in the
page margins. **Cons:** Not very detailed, but covers most boards exam
topics and serves as a good source of study organization. **Summary:**
Good, comprehensive review for Step 2 with many quick-study features.

Crush the Boards Step 2

Bʀᴏᴄʜᴇʀᴛ

Elsevier, 2002, 2nd ed., 200 pages, ISBN 1560535423

$32.95   Review

Comprehensive review of many high-yield topics, organized by specialty. **Pros:** Good emphasis on key points. Conversational style is easy
to read. Good use of charts and diagrams. Covers surgical topics in
more depth than similar books. **Cons:** Not comprehensive. No practice questions or vignettes. Not enough detail to be used alone for
Step 2 preparation. **Summary:** Solid review of key points and frequently tested topics. Should probably be supplemented with other
review material and practice tests.

Medical Boards Step 2 Made Ridiculously Simple

Cᴀʀʟ

MedMaster, 2003, 3rd ed., 353 pages, ISBN 0940780526

$29.95   Review

General review of topics for the Step 2 exam. Outline format with tables and brief discussions. **Pros:** Quick review. Useful in areas that
might otherwise be overlooked—e.g., ophthalmology, dermatology,
and ENT. Helpful for last-minute review. **Cons:** The table format of
the book does not provide substantive details but aids in the memorization of lists. **Summary:** Highlights most high-yield topics, but
should not be used alone for review.

REVIEW RESOURCES

COMPREHENSIVE

B

Lange Outline Review: USMLE Step 2

GOLDBERG

$39.95   Review

McGraw-Hill, 2006, 5th ed., 568 pages, ISBN 0071451927

Comprehensive boards review book with chapters organized by clinical disciplines. **Pros:** Comprehensive review source with extensive coverage of clinical topics with an organized, in-depth review of each. **Cons:** Covers some low-yield topics. Includes relatively few images, figures, or tables. **Summary:** Solid, single-source, comprehensive review for Step 2.

B

Cracking the Boards

MARIANI

$29.95   Review

Princeton Review, 2000, 2nd ed., 544 pages, ISBN 0375761640

Clinical vignette review organized by specialty with more than 400 vignette-style questions. **Pros:** Well organized, with a uniform format throughout the book and numerous charts. Appropriate emphasis on treatment. Questions reflect the style of the Step 2 exam and present classic clinical cases. **Cons:** Few images. **Summary:** Useful review that follows the emphasis of Step 2 on clinical vignettes.

B−

Rx: Prescription for the Boards USMLE Step 2

FEIBUSCH

$34.95   Review

Lippincott Williams & Wilkins, 2002, 3rd ed., 512 pages, ISBN 0781734002

Text review based on the widely used USMLE content outline. **Pros:** Covers high-yield core and specialty topics. Well-designed format. **Cons:** Not enough detail for each topic. Provides a framework for studying, but cannot be used alone. Lacks tables and diagrams to facilitate studying. Facts outlining the next step in management are often not discussed. Needs updating. **Summary:** Inadequate as a sole source for Step 2 CK review.

B−

Advanced Life Support for the USMLE Step 2

FLYNN

$24.95   Review

Lippincott Williams & Wilkins, 1999, 2nd ed., 142 pages, ISBN 0781719763

Brief outline format with high-yield topics described in tables or illustrations. **Pros:** Quick, easy read. Emphasis is on high-yield facts. Amusing cartoons highlight key concepts and excellent mnemonics. Great for last-minute review. **Cons:** Not adequate for in-depth review. Needs updating. **Summary:** Worthwhile review for the days right before the exam.

Classic Presentations and Rapid Review for USMLE Step 2

O'CONNELL

$25.00   Review

J&S, 1999, 1st ed., 215 pages, ISBN 1888308052

Light overview organized by specialty, with emphasis on "classic" presentations of commonly seen conditions. Presented in bullet-point format. **Pros:** Good for last-minute studying. **Cons:** Neither comprehensive nor consistent in the material provided on each topic. Information is not overly detailed. No clinical images, ECGs, or clinical case examples. **Summary:** Quick and superficial review.

Insider's Guide to the USMLE Step 2

STANG

$44.95   Review/450 q

Elsevier, 2000, 1st ed., 426 pages, ISBN 0721682790

Contains case-based questions with explanations and includes suggested review topics. **Pros:** "Pop quizzes" after each section encourage retention. Practice test has detailed explanations to answers. **Cons:** Sparse information; may serve as a study guide rather than a review book. Some topics are not relevant to the boards. Questions do not reflect the vignette format on Step 2. **Summary:** A well-organized but not overly detailed comprehensive review. Some content is irrelevant to Step 2.

Kaplanmedical.com
KAPLAN
$149–$499

Compilation of online programs for Step 2 review, including a large test bank. **Pros:** Questions can be arranged by topic or randomly to simulate the real exam. Tests are timed to simulate boards conditions. Extensive number of questions in vignette format. Content level of questions reflects the boards test. Explanations are thorough, and the text now reports the national average for each question. Allows students to identify strong and weak points. **Cons:** Very expensive. Online lectures can be difficult to watch for extensive periods of time. **Summary:** A good source of questions with thorough explanations, but the price may be prohibitive for many.

USMLEWorld.com
USMLE World
$90–$175

Test bank with more than 2000 questions. Similar to the Kaplan test bank as described above. **Pros:** Well-written questions with explanations. Cheaper than Kaplan. Questions tend to be more difficult than those on the actual exam, but many students find this an advantage during preparation. **Cons:** Some questions are overly picky. **Summary:** An excellent source of questions that is cheaper than Kaplan.

USMLEasy.com
McGraw-Hill
$99–$199

Comprehensive test bank with more than 3300 questions and explanations. Similar in style to the Kaplan question bank described above. **Pros:** Large number of questions. Mimics the CBT format. Cheaper than Kaplan. Access is often free through medical libraries. **Cons:** Questions can be more obscure than those appearing on the actual exam. Questions overlap with those of the PreTest series of review books. **Summary:** A fair source of questions that may be good for supplemental review, especially in preparation for clerkship shelf exams.

REVIEW RESOURCES

ONLINE REVIEW

Step-Up to Medicine

AGABEGI

$37.95   Review

Lippincott Williams & Wilkins, 2005, 1st ed., 516 pages, ISBN 0781747872

Comprehensive review of commonly tested diseases and topics in internal medicine organized in an outline format. Includes a color atlas and an appendix on interpreting x-rays, ECGs, and physical exam findings. **Pros:** Very comprehensive, with informative tables and diagrams to help synthesize information. Includes occasional clinical vignettes that correlate with the topic being discussed. Quick facts to remember are included in the margins of each page. **Cons:** Very lengthy. Geared more toward clerkship preparation than Step 2 review. **Summary:** Good book packed with useful information for the wards, but may be too lengthy and detailed for Step 2.

High-Yield Internal Medicine

NIRULA

$26.95   Review

Lippincott Williams & Wilkins, 2006, 3rd ed., 128 pages, ISBN 0781781698

Core review of internal medicine in outline format. **Pros:** Focus is on high-yield diseases and symptoms. Quick and easy read. **Cons:** Not comprehensive. Some mistakes in formulas. Needs more illustrations. No index. **Summary:** Good, fast review presented in a format that allows for quick and repetitive readings. Use as a supplement, not as a primary study source.

First Aid for the Medicine Clerkship

STEAD

$34.95   Review

McGraw-Hill, 2005, 2nd ed., 416 pages, ISBN 0071448756

High-yield review of symptoms and diseases. **Pros:** Comprehensive review; well organized by symptoms with good illustrations, scenarios, diagrams, algorithms, and mnemonics. **Cons:** May not be suited to the reader who prefers information arranged in text form. May be too basic for certain topics. **Summary:** Excellent, concise review of medicine.

REVIEW RESOURCES

INTERNAL MEDICINE

B+ *PreTest Medicine*   *$24.95*   Test/500 q

BERK

McGraw-Hill, 2006, 11th ed., 356 pages, ISBN 0071455531

Question-and-answer format organized by medical subspecialty. **Pros:**
Organization by subspecialty helps pinpoint weak areas. Good num-
ber of vignette-style questions, with detailed explanations. **Cons:**
Many questions are more detailed than needed for the boards and are
geared more toward the shelf exam. Few illustrations. **Summary:**
Solid source of challenging review questions.

B+ *Underground Clinical Vignettes: Emergency Medicine*   *$17.95*   Review

BHUSHAN

Lippincott Williams & Wilkins, 2005, 3rd ed., 120 pages, ISBN
1405104198

Clinical vignette review of emergency medicine topics. **Pros:** Recently
revised and updated. Well organized by focus points: pathogenesis, epidemiology, management, complications, and associated diseases. Well
illustrated, and includes high-yield "minicases" and links to the UCV
Clinical/Basic Color Atlas. **Cons:** Not comprehensive; use as a supplement. **Summary:** Organized and easy-to-read supplement to studying.

B+ *Underground Clinical Vignettes: Internal Medicine,*   *$17.95 each* Review
Vols. I and II

BHUSHAN

Lippincott Williams & Wilkins, 2005, 3rd ed., ISBN 1405104201,
140510421X

Clinical vignette review of common topics in internal medicine. **Pros:**
Recently revised and updated. Well organized by focus points: pathogenesis, epidemiology, management, complications, and associated
diseases. Vignettes mirror the boards-style presentation of questions.
Cons: Not comprehensive; use as a supplement. **Summary:** Organized and easy-to-read supplement to studying.

B+ *Platinum Vignettes: Internal Medicine*   *$23.95*   Review

BROCHERT

Elsevier, 2002, 1st ed., 102 pages, ISBN 1560535318

Clinical vignette review of common topics in internal medicine. **Pros:**
Well-written cases similar to boards-type vignettes. Well illustrated.
Discussion is organized by pathophysiology, diagnosis and treatment,
and more high-yield facts. **Cons:** Expensive for amount of material.
Not comprehensive; use as a supplement. **Summary:** Organized and
easy-to-read supplement to studying.

Platinum Vignettes: Internal Medicine Subspecialties
BROCHERT

$23.95   Review

Elsevier, 2002, 1st ed., 105 pages, ISBN 1560535377

Clinical vignette review of common topics in the internal medicine subspecialties. **Pros:** Information is taught through the presentation of common clinical cases. Explanations are organized by pathophysiology, diagnosis and treatment, and more high-yield facts. **Cons:** Expensive for amount of material. Not comprehensive; use as a supplement. **Summary:** Organized and easy-to-read supplement to studying.

A&L's Review of Internal Medicine
GOLDLIST

$34.95   Test/1100+ q

McGraw-Hill, 2002, 3rd ed., 276 pages, ISBN 007138524X

General review with questions and answers divided by subspecialty. **Pros:** Well-written vignette questions reflect the boards format. Representative of the content of the boards. Complete explanations. Well illustrated. **Cons:** Questions are shorter, and some nonvignette questions are more straightforward than those on the exam. **Summary:** Good source of questions that accurately reflect the multistep nature of boards questions.

Blueprints Clinical Cases in Medicine
LI

$29.95   Test/200 q

Lippincott Williams & Wilkins, 2007, 2nd ed., 418 pages, ISBN 1405104910

Compendium of vignette-type cases arranged by symptom followed by related questions and answers. **Pros:** Excellent companion to the Blueprints series. Focuses on high-yield cases. Easy to read with nice illustrations and review of management. **Cons:** Not comprehensive; use as a supplement for review. Better suited to clerkship preparation than to Step 2. **Summary:** Organized and easy-to-read supplement. Adds clinical correlates to the Blueprints series. Best if used with the Blueprints text.

PreTest Preventive Medicine and Public Health
RATELLE

$24.95   Test/500 q

McGraw-Hill, 2000, 9th ed., 238 pages, ISBN 0071359621

Question-and-answer review of epidemiology, biostatistics, and preventive medicine. **Pros:** Majority of test questions appropriately simulate boards content and difficulty. Good explanations. **Cons:** Some questions contain too many calculations. The biostatistics chapter is too detailed. Few vignettes. **Summary:** Good question-and-answer review for a low-yield topic.

REVIEW RESOURCES

INTERNAL MEDICINE

B+ ***Medical Secrets***   **$36.95**   Review
ZOLLO
Elsevier, 2004, 4th ed., 480 pages, ISBN 1560533870
Question-and-answer style typical of the Secrets series. **Pros:** Covers a
great deal of clinically relevant information. Concise answers are
given with pearls, tips, and memory aids. **Cons:** Too lengthy and detailed for USMLE review. **Summary:** May be most appropriate for
wards use. Not a focused review.

B ***Medicine Recall***   **$32.95**   Review
BERGIN
**Lippincott Williams & Wilkins, 2003, 2nd ed., 1035 pages, ISBN
0781736765**
Standard Recall-series question-and-answer format, organized by medical specialty. **Pros:** Addresses a broad range of high-yield clinical topics. Good format for self-quizzing. Appropriate level of detail. **Cons:**
No vignettes and no images; requires significant time commitment.
Style simulates questions asked on rounds, not those on Step 2. **Summary:** Style may be more conducive to wards than to boards preparation. Use as a supplement to other resources.

B ***In A Page Emergency Medicine***   **$31.95**   Review
CATERINO
**Lippincott Williams & Wilkins, 2003, 1st ed., 316 pages,
ISBN 1405103574**
Collection of short, one-page summaries of 250 medical emergencies
discussed in terms of etiology, differential diagnosis, presentation, di-
agnostic tests, treatment, and disposition. **Pros:** Concise and high
yield. Covers a wide variety of emergencies seen in the ER. **Cons:**
Text is crowded and somewhat confusing. No images or diagrams.
Summary: Good for use during the emergency medicine clerkship,
but may not be appropriate for Step 2 review.

B ***Blueprints Clinical Cases in Family Medicine***   **$29.95**   Test/200 q
CHANG
**Lippincott Williams & Wilkins, 2006, 2nd ed., 437 pages,
ISBN 1405104953**
Compendium of vignette-type cases arranged by symptom followed by
related questions and answers. **Pros:** Excellent companion to the
Blueprints series. Focuses on high-yield cases. Easy to read with nice
illustrations and review of management. **Cons:** Not comprehensive;
use as a supplement for review. **Summary:** Organized and easy-to-read
supplement. Adds clinical correlates to the Blueprints series. Best if
used with the Blueprints text.

REVIEW RESOURCES

INTERNAL MEDICINE

B ***Internal Medicine Pearls***
HEFFNER
$41.95 Review
Elsevier, 2001, 2nd ed., 249 pages, ISBN 1560534044
Detailed clinical vignettes with laboratory and radiographic findings followed by a discussion of clinically important pearls. **Pros:** High-quality, realistic vignettes. Questions focus on decision making and management. **Cons:** Selected topics; not comprehensive. Discussions may be too detailed for purposes of review. Miscellaneous details. **Summary:** Good, clinically focused supplement for review.

B ***In A Page Medicine***
KAHAN
$31.95 Review
Lippincott Williams & Wilkins, 2003, 1st ed., 275 pages, ISBN 1405103256
One-page reviews of 211 diseases discussed by etiology, epidemiology, signs/symptoms, differential diagnosis, diagnostic tests, treatment, and prognosis. **Pros:** Fast and concise review of high-yield information on common diseases. **Cons:** Text is crowded onto one page without any images or diagrams. **Summary:** Useful for quick study on the wards, but may not be comprehensive enough for Step 2.

B ***Blueprints Q & A Step 2 Medicine***
SHINAR
$17.95 Test/200 q
Lippincott Williams & Wilkins, 2004, 2nd ed., 153 pages, ISBN 1405103892
Two hundred vignette-style questions. **Pros:** Nice companion to the Blueprints series. Focuses on high-yield topics. Explanations are easy to follow. **Cons:** Not comprehensive; use as a supplement for review. Expensive; includes few questions given the cost of the book. **Summary:** Organized and easy-to-read supplement. Adds clinical correlates to the Blueprints series.

B ***First Aid for the Emergency Medical Clerkship***
STEAD
$34.95 Review
McGraw-Hill, 2006, 2nd ed., 484 pages, ISBN 007144873X
High-yield review of symptoms and diseases. **Pros:** Comprehensive review; well organized by symptoms with good illustrations, scenarios, diagrams, algorithms, and mnemonics. **Cons:** May not be suited to the reader who prefers information arranged in text form. **Summary:** Excellent review of emergency medicine and nice presentation of high-yield topics for Step 2 preparation, but not intended for boards review.

Blueprints in Medicine   ***$36.95***   Review/89 q
YOUNG
Lippincott Williams & Wilkins, 2007, 4th ed., 403 pages,
ISBN 1405105003
Text review of internal medicine organized by common diseases and
common symptoms. Question-and-answer section with explanations.
Pros: Well-organized, concise review. Easy reading. Differential diag-
noses for symptoms are helpful. Good charts and diagrams. **Cons:**
Few illustrations. Has some superfluous details; some areas are too
broad and simplistic to be useful for testing purposes. **Summary:**
Good primary boards review for internal medicine, although poorly il-
lustrated.

A⁻

Blueprints in Neurology
DRISLANE

$34.95   Review

Lippincott Williams & Wilkins, 2006, 2nd ed., 225 pages,
ISBN 1405104635

Review of neurology by disease and symptom with a brief exam. **Pros:** Reviews high-yield topics of a complex discipline and is easy to follow. Good use of tables, images, and diagrams. Questions in the exam are similar to those found on both the shelf exam and Step 2. **Cons:** Lengthy. **Summary:** Excellent review of high-yield material for the wards and Step 2.

B⁺

PreTest Neurology
ANSCHEL

$24.95   Test/500 q

McGraw-Hill, 2006, 6th ed., 340 pages, ISBN 0071455507

Question-and-answer review of neurology. **Pros:** Thorough coverage of neurology topics with a good number of clinical vignettes. Good emphasis on common topics, and thorough explanation of answers. Good practice for interpreting common head CTs/MRIs that might be tested. **Cons:** Some questions may be more detailed than needed for the boards. **Summary:** Good source of test questions for rapid review of neurology.

B⁺

Underground Clinical Vignettes: Neurology
BHUSHAN

$17.95   Review

Lippincott Williams & Wilkins, 2005, 3rd ed., 112 pages,
ISBN 1405109228

Clinical vignette review of high-yield topics in neurology. **Pros:** Recently revised and updated. Well organized by focus points: pathogenesis, epidemiology, management, complications, and associated diseases. Well illustrated, and includes "minicases," links to a color atlas supplement, and updated treatments. **Cons:** Not comprehensive; use as a supplement to review. **Summary:** Organized and easy-to-read supplement to studying. Lengthy for dedicated review of neurology.

REVIEW RESOURCES

NEUROLOGY

B ***Neurology Recall***   *$32.95*   Review

MILLER

Lippincott Williams & Wilkins, 2003, 2nd ed., 377 pages, ISBN
0781745888

Brief question-and-answer format. **Pros:** Many important facts are reviewed; useful for self-quizzing. **Cons:** Not a comprehensive review.
Lengthy and lacks illustrations. Concepts are not integrated. **Summary:** Good for review of some high-yield concepts, but not a stand-
alone resource for this topic.

B ***Neurology Secrets***   *$39.95*   Review

ROLAK

Elsevier, 2005, 4th ed., 456 pages, ISBN 1560536217

Secrets-series question-and-answer format. **Pros:** Concise review of
many high-yield topics. Good use of clinical images. Quick question-
and-answer approach. **Cons:** No clinical vignettes; instead offers lists
of questions that might be posed on the wards. Does not have a structured format and leaves out important information. Relatively expensive and lengthy. Not a reference book. **Summary:** Overall, good content for self-quizzing and study, but does not substitute for a formal
review or practice tests. More appropriate for clerkship than for boards
review.

B ***Blueprints Clinical Cases in Neurology***   *$29.95*   Review

SHETH

Lippincott Williams & Wilkins, 2007, 2nd ed., 390 pages,
ISBN 1405104945

Compendium of vignette-type cases organized by symptom followed
by related question and answers. **Pros:** Excellent companion to the
Blueprints subspecialty series. Focuses on high-yield cases. Easy to
read, with nice illustrations and review of management. **Cons:** Not
comprehensive; use as a supplement. Few illustrations. **Summary:** Organized and easy to read. Adds clinical correlates to the Blueprints series.

B ***Neurology Pearls***   *$41.95*   Review

WACLAWIK

Elsevier, 2000, 1st ed., 228 pages, ISBN 1560532610

Detailed clinical vignettes, including laboratory and test results and
radiographic findings, followed by a discussion of diagnosis and emphasis on important pearls. **Pros:** High-quality vignettes on many important neurologic conditions. **Cons:** Requires significant time investment. **Summary:** Challenging clinical scenarios to supplement a
more structured topic review.

A⁻

Underground Clinical Vignettes: OB/GYN   *$17.95*   Review

BHUSHAN

Lippincott Williams & Wilkins, 2005, 3rd ed., 120 pages,
ISBN 1405104236

Clinical vignette review of frequently tested diseases in obstetrics and gynecology. **Pros:** Recently revised and updated. Well organized by focus points: pathogenesis, epidemiology, management, complications, and associated diseases. Well illustrated. Easy read and stresses high-yield facts. **Cons:** Not comprehensive; use as a supplement. **Summary:** Well-organized and easy-to-read practice vignettes.

A⁻

Platinum Vignettes: Obstetrics and Gynecology   *$23.95*   Review

BROCHERT

Elsevier, 2002, 1st ed., 102 pages, ISBN 1560535326

Clinical vignette review of common topics in obstetrics and gynecology. **Pros:** Well-written cases are similar to boards-type vignettes. Discussion is organized by pathophysiology, diagnosis and treatment, and more high-yield facts. **Cons:** Expensive for amount of material. Not comprehensive; use as a supplement. Few illustrations. **Summary:** Organized and easy-to-read supplement to studying.

A⁻

Blueprints Clinical Cases in Obstetrics and Gynecology   *$29.95*   Test/200 q

CAUGHEY

Lippincott Williams & Wilkins, 2007, 2nd ed., 418 pages,
ISBN 1405104902

Compendium of vignette-type cases arranged by symptom followed by related questions and answers. **Pros:** Excellent companion to the Blueprints series. Focuses on high-yield cases. Easy to read, with nice illustrations and review of management. **Cons:** Not comprehensive; use as a supplement. **Summary:** Organized and easy-to-read supplement. Adds clinical correlates to the Blueprints series.

A⁻

Blueprints in Obstetrics and Gynecology   *$35.95*   Review/149 q

CAUGHEY

Lippincott Williams & Wilkins, 2003, 3rd ed., 352 pages,
ISBN 1405103310

Text review with tables and illustrations. Includes a short exam with explanations. **Pros:** Strong emphasis on high-yield topics with concise text, clear diagrams, and many classic illustrations. Easy read. Appropriate for both clinical clerkship and Step 2 preparation. **Cons:** Some topics are overly detailed, while some are not detailed enough. **Summary:** Overall, a good choice for boards and wards preparation.

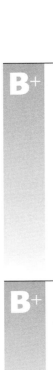

B+   ***NMS Obstetrics and Gynecology***   **$36.95**   Review/500 q

MORGAN

Lippincott Williams & Wilkins, 2004, 5th ed., 512 pages,
ISBN 0781726794

Detailed outline of OB/GYN with few tables and diagrams. **Pros:** Comprehensive review for both wards and boards. Final exam is relatively good, with complete explanations. **Cons:** Dense and lengthy OB/GYN review. Many questions do not reflect the boards format. Lacks illustrations. **Summary:** Complete review with questions and discussion. Too ambitious for exam preparation alone; more helpful if used throughout the clerkship.

B+   ***High-Yield Obstetrics and Gynecology***   **$26.95**   Review

SAKALA

Lippincott Williams & Wilkins, 2006, 2nd ed., 194 pages,
ISBN 078179630X

Review of high-yield topics in outline format. Clinical scenarios at the end of each chapter highlight key points. **Pros:** Easy read with good discussion of high-yield topics. **Cons:** Lacks depth. No practice questions. **Summary:** A quick but superficial review.

B+   ***First Aid for the OB/GYN Clerkship***   **$34.95**   Review

STEAD

McGraw-Hill, 2007, 2nd ed., 291 pages, ISBN 0071448748

High-yield review of symptoms and diseases. **Pros:** Comprehensive review with nice diagrams, images, charts, algorithms, and mnemonics. **Cons:** Lengthy review. **Summary:** Excellent review of OB/GYN, but lengthy for boards review.

B+   ***Case Files: Obstetrics and Gynecology Review***   **$29.95**   Review

TOY

McGraw-Hill, 2007, 2nd ed., 414 pages, ISBN 0071463011

Review of OB/GYN in case format with questions and answers following each vignette. **Pros:** Cases reflect high-yield topics and are arranged in an easy-to-follow format. **Cons:** Some topics are either not covered or given only brief treatment. Few diagrams and images. Lengthy and time-consuming for one topic. Explanations are terse. **Summary:** Good review of the subject in clinical vignette format, but may be too detailed for Step 2 review.

B+

Blueprints Q & A Step 2 Obstetrics & Gynecology $19.95   Test/200 q
TRAN

Lippincott Williams & Wilkins, 2005, 2nd ed., 153 pages,
ISBN 1405103906

One hundred vignette-style questions. **Pros:** Nice companion to the
Blueprints series. Focuses on high-yield topics. Explanations are easy
to follow. **Cons:** Not comprehensive; use as a supplement for review.
Sparse images. Some questions are esoteric and not boards-like. **Summary:** Organized and easy-to-read supplement. Adds clinical correlates to the Blueprints series.

B

Obstetrics and Gynecology Secrets $36.95   Review
BADER

Elsevier, 2004, 3rd ed., 432 pages, ISBN 0323034152

Secrets-series question-and-answer format, organized by topic within
OB/GYN. **Pros:** Good coverage of many high-yield, clinically relevant
topics. **Cons:** Detailed; not useful for rapid review. No vignettes; few
illustrations and images. **Summary:** Good clinical content, but does
not serve as a formal topic review. Better for use during clerkship than
for Step 2 preparation.

B

BRS Obstetrics and Gynecology $32.95   Review/500 q
SAKALA

Lippincott Williams & Wilkins, 2000, 2nd ed., 443 pages, ISBN
0683307436

General review text with questions at the end of the chapters and a
comprehensive exam at the end of the book. **Pros:** Appropriate content for boards and wards study. New edition offers more detail on
pregnancy complications and a new STD chapter. **Cons:** Some sections are overly detailed with few diagrams. Questions offer few clinical vignettes. **Summary:** Appropriate content review, but more helpful for wards than for boards.

B

PreTest Obstetrics and Gynecology $24.95   Test/500 q
SCHNEIDER

McGraw-Hill, 2003, 11th ed., 354 pages, ISBN 0071458107

Question-and-answer review with detailed explanations for OB/GYN.
Pros: Organization by subtopic may be useful for studying weak areas.
Good content emphasis. Generally well illustrated. **Cons:** Some questions are too difficult or detailed. Vignette-based questions are short
and simplistic compared to Step 2 content. **Summary:** Decent source
of questions to supplement topic study, especially for addressing specific areas of weakness.

REVIEW RESOURCES

OB/GYN

Obstetrics and Gynecology Recall $32.95 Review/350 q
BOURGEOIS
Lippincott Williams & Wilkins, 2004, 2nd ed., 582 pages, ISBN 0781748798
Recall-series question-and-answer style. **Pros:** Two-column format makes it useful for self-quizzing. Reviews many high-yield concepts and facts. **Cons:** Questions emphasize individual facts but do not integrate concepts. No vignettes or images. Spotty coverage of some topics. **Summary:** Useful for review of selected concepts, but not a comprehensive source for USMLE preparation. More appropriate for clerkship than for boards.

A⁻

Underground Clinical Vignettes: Pediatrics
BHUSHAN

$17.95   Review

Lippincott Williams & Wilkins, 2005, 3rd ed., 120 pages,
ISBN 1405104244

Clinical vignette review of frequently tested topics in pediatrics. **Pros:** Recently revised and updated. Well organized by focus points: pathogenesis, epidemiology, management, complications, and associated diseases. Well illustrated, and the new edition includes "minicases" to broaden subject material and present more high-yield information. **Cons:** Not comprehensive; use as a supplement to text review. **Summary:** Well organized and easy to read, but meant as a supplement for review.

A⁻

Platinum Vignettes: Pediatrics
BROCHERT

$23.95   Review

Elsevier, 2002, 1st ed., 100 pages, ISBN 1560535334

Clinical vignette review of common topics in pediatrics. **Pros:** Well-written cases are similar to boards-type vignettes. Well illustrated. Discussion is organized by pathophysiology, diagnosis and treatment, and more high-yield facts. **Cons:** Expensive for amount of material. Not comprehensive; use as a supplement. **Summary:** Organized and easy-to-read supplement to studying.

A⁻

PreTest Pediatrics
YETMAN

$24.95   Test/500 q

McGraw-Hill, 2006, 11th ed., 388 pages, ISBN 0071455523

Question-and-answer review with detailed discussion. **Pros:** Organization by organ system is useful for pinpointing weaknesses. Strong, thorough explanations. Fair number of vignette-style questions. Well illustrated. **Cons:** Some questions are too detailed or emphasize low-yield topics. **Summary:** Good source of questions and review for pediatrics. Solid content with good illustrations, although not entirely in Step 2 format.

B⁺

Blueprints Q & A Step 2 Pediatrics
FOTI

$17.95   Test/100 q

Lippincott Williams & Wilkins, 2004, 2nd ed., 240 pages,
ISBN 1405103914

Two hundred vignette-style questions. **Pros:** Nice companion to the Blueprints series. Focuses on high-yield topics. Explanations are easy to follow. **Cons:** Not comprehensive; use as a supplement for review. Sparse images. **Summary:** Organized and easy-to-read supplement. Adds clinical correlates to the Blueprints series.

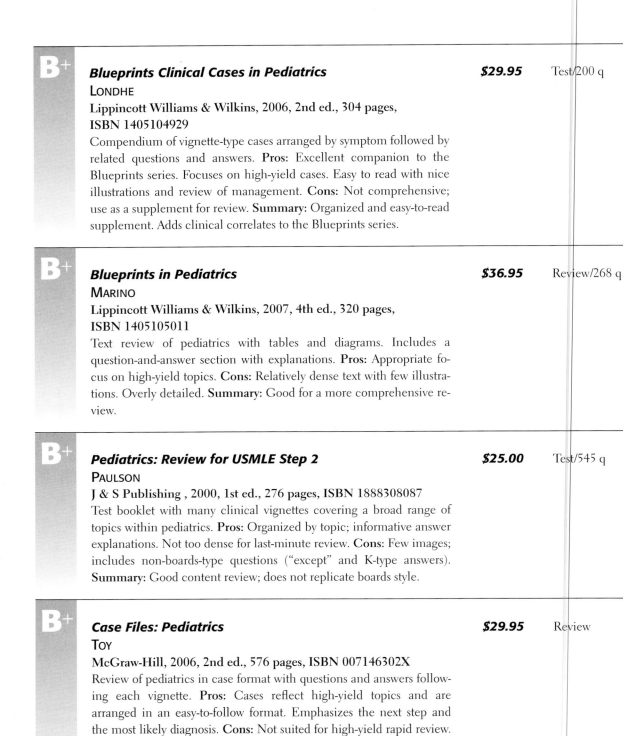

Blueprints Clinical Cases in Pediatrics $29.95 Test/200 q
LONDHE

Lippincott Williams & Wilkins, 2006, 2nd ed., 304 pages,
ISBN 1405104929

Compendium of vignette-type cases arranged by symptom followed by
related questions and answers. **Pros:** Excellent companion to the
Blueprints series. Focuses on high-yield cases. Easy to read with nice
illustrations and review of management. **Cons:** Not comprehensive;
use as a supplement for review. **Summary:** Organized and easy-to-read
supplement. Adds clinical correlates to the Blueprints series.

Blueprints in Pediatrics $36.95 Review/268 q
MARINO

Lippincott Williams & Wilkins, 2007, 4th ed., 320 pages,
ISBN 1405105011

Text review of pediatrics with tables and diagrams. Includes a
question-and-answer section with explanations. **Pros:** Appropriate focus on high-yield topics. **Cons:** Relatively dense text with few illustrations. Overly detailed. **Summary:** Good for a more comprehensive review.

Pediatrics: Review for USMLE Step 2 $25.00 Test/545 q
PAULSON

J & S Publishing , 2000, 1st ed., 276 pages, ISBN 1888308087

Test booklet with many clinical vignettes covering a broad range of
topics within pediatrics. **Pros:** Organized by topic; informative answer
explanations. Not too dense for last-minute review. **Cons:** Few images;
includes non-boards-type questions ("except" and K-type answers).
Summary: Good content review; does not replicate boards style.

Case Files: Pediatrics $29.95 Review
TOY

McGraw-Hill, 2006, 2nd ed., 576 pages, ISBN 007146302X

Review of pediatrics in case format with questions and answers following each vignette. **Pros:** Cases reflect high-yield topics and are
arranged in an easy-to-follow format. Emphasizes the next step and
the most likely diagnosis. **Cons:** Not suited for high-yield rapid review.
Summary: Excellent review with emphasis on vignette-style case presentation and important boards-type answers, but may be too detailed
for a stand-alone boards review book.

A&L's Review of Pediatrics
VIESSMAN

$34.95   Test/1000+ q

McGraw-Hill, 2004, 6th ed., 250 pages, ISBN 0838503039

Question-and-answer review of pediatrics with detailed explanations. **Pros:** Questions focus on boards-relevant content. The last chapter includes excellent vignette-based questions. Thorough, well-written explanations. Nice primer on test-taking strategies. **Cons:** Non-vignette-based questions are shorter and more straightforward than those on Step 2. Some questions may be too detailed for Step 2 preparation. Poorly illustrated. **Summary:** Excellent, concise review with appropriate content and good discussions, but the majority of questions do not reflect Step 2 style.

In A Page Pediatrics
KAHAN

$31.95   Review

Lippincott Williams & Wilkins, 2003, 1st ed., 294 pages, ISBN 1405103264

One-page reviews of 228 diseases/topics discussed by etiology, epidemiology, signs/symptoms, differential diagnosis, diagnostic tests, treatment, and prognosis. **Pros:** Fast and concise review of high-yield information on common diseases. **Cons:** Text is crowded onto one page, without any images or diagrams. Includes low-yield topics. **Summary:** Useful for quick study on the wards, but too time intensive for Step 2 review.

NMS Pediatrics
DWORKIN

$34.95   Review/166+ q

Lippincott Williams & Wilkins, 2001, 4th ed., 768 pages, ISBN 0683306375

General review of pediatrics in outline format. Includes questions at the end of each chapter. **Pros:** Thorough, detailed review of pediatrics. Boldfacing highlights key points. Case studies and a comprehensive exam (also provided on CD-ROM) at the end of the book are helpful. Good discussion. **Cons:** Dense, lengthy text. Lacks good illustrations of any kind. **Summary:** Thorough review, but more appropriate for clerkships than for Step 2 review.

Pediatrics Recall
MCGAHREN

$32.95   Review

Lippincott Williams & Wilkins, 2002, 2nd ed., 461 pages, ISBN 0781726115

Concise question-and-answer format typical of the Recall series. **Pros:** Two-column format makes self-quizzing easy. Emphasizes diagnosis and management. **Cons:** Requires time commitment. Not all topics are covered thoroughly. No vignettes. **Summary:** Useful material, but does not provide a systematic review or substitute for practice tests.

Pediatric Secrets $36.95 Review
POLIN
Elsevier, 2005, 4th ed., 670 pages, ISBN 1560536276
Question-and-answer format typical of the Secrets series, organized by
pediatric subspecialty. **Pros:** Thorough discussion of a wide variety of
clinical topics. **Cons:** Detailed content geared toward the wards; re-
quires a large time investment. No images or illustrations. **Summary:**
Too detailed for USMLE review. Better suited to clerkship.

A⁻

Underground Clinical Vignettes: Psychiatry

$17.95   Review

BHUSHAN

Lippincott Williams & Wilkins, 2005, 3rd ed., 128 pages,
ISBN 1405104252

Clinical vignette review of frequently tested topics in psychiatry. **Pros:** Well organized by focus points: pathogenesis, epidemiology, management, and associated diseases. Well illustrated, and includes "mini-cases" that present high-yield information. **Cons:** Not comprehensive; use as a supplement. **Summary:** Organized and easy-to-read practice vignettes.

A⁻

Platinum Vignettes: Psychiatry

$23.95   Review

BROCHERT

Elsevier, 2002, 1st ed., 102 pages, ISBN 1560535342

Clinical vignette review of common topics in psychiatry. **Pros:** Well-written cases are similar to boards-type vignettes. Well illustrated. Discussion is organized by pathophysiology, diagnosis and treatment, and more high-yield facts. **Cons:** Not comprehensive; use as a supplement. **Summary:** Organized and easy-to-read supplement to studying.

A⁻

Blueprints Clinical Cases in Psychiatry

$25.95   Test/200 q

HOBLYN

Lippincott Williams & Wilkins, 2007, 2nd ed., 304 pages,
ISBN 1405104961

Compendium of vignette-type cases arranged by symptom followed by related questions and answers. **Pros:** Excellent companion to the Blueprints series. Focuses on high-yield cases. Easy to read with nice illustrations and review of management. **Cons:** Not comprehensive; use as a supplement for review. **Summary:** Organized and easy-to-read supplement. Adds clinical correlates to the Blueprints series.

A⁻

Blueprints in Psychiatry

$23.95   Review/74 q

MURPHY

Lippincott Williams & Wilkins, 2007, 4th ed., 144 pages,
ISBN 140510502X

Brief text review of psychiatry with DSM-IV criteria. Includes a brief question-and-answer section at the end of the book. **Pros:** Clear, concise review of psychiatry with helpful tables. Good coverage of high-yield topics, including the pharmacology section. Quick read. **Cons:** Too general in certain areas. **Summary:** Rapid review with appropriate coverage of high-yield topics.

A⁻

PreTest Psychiatry
PAN

$24.95   Test/500 q

McGraw-Hill, 2006, 11th ed., 320 pages, ISBN 007145554X
Question-and-answer review of topics in psychiatry. **Pros:** Questions are well written and organized. Most questions have appropriate content level. Good explanations. **Cons:** Too few vignette-type questions. Some questions are too detailed. **Summary:** Good source of questions and review for psychiatry and Step 2, although the format may not reflect the actual test.

B⁺

High-Yield Psychiatry
FADEM

$24.95   Review

Lippincott Williams & Wilkins, 2003, 2nd ed., 150 pages, ISBN 0781742684
Brief outline-format review of psychiatry. **Pros:** Quick read with clinical vignettes scattered throughout. Concise tables. **Cons:** Not enough detail for in-depth review. **Summary:** Excellent, quick review of psychiatry for use as an additional study source. Similar to *High-Yield Behavioral Sciences* by the same author.

B⁺

A&L's Review of Psychiatry
ORANSKY

$34.95   Test/900+ q

McGraw-Hill, 2002, 7th ed., 304 pages, ISBN 0071402535
General review of psychiatry with questions and answers. **Pros:** Includes 114 vignette-style questions appropriate for boards review. Appropriate content emphasis; thorough explanations. The new edition features updated treatment and management sections. **Cons:** Questions are shorter and more straightforward than those of the boards. **Summary:** Decent boards review for psychiatry, but does not reflect boards format.

B⁺

Case Files: Psychiatry
TOY

$29.95   Review

McGraw-Hill, 2006, 2nd ed., 408 pages, ISBN 0071462821
Review of psychology in case format with questions and answers following each vignette. **Pros:** Cases reflect high-yield topics and are arranged in an easy-to-follow format. Emphasizes the next step, the most likely diagnosis, and the best initial treatment. **Cons:** Not suited to high-yield rapid review, and may be too detailed for Step 2 review. **Summary:** Excellent subject review with emphasis on vignette-style case presentation and important boards-type answers. Great for the wards, and a good supplement for the boards.

B+

Psychiatry
TUCKER

$25.95   Review/500 q

Biotest, 2002, 1st ed., 194 pages, ISBN 1893720101

Thorough review of psychiatry in outline format with questions. **Pros:** Many high-yield tables; questions are included at the end of each chapter with a reference to the text or explanations. **Cons:** Few illustrations, dense and lengthy, and lacking in vignette-style questions. **Summary:** Fairly comprehensive review of psychiatry with an emphasis on high-yield topics, but many questions do not reflect Step 2 style.

B

Psychiatry Made Ridiculously Simple
GOOD

$13.95   Review

MedMaster, 2005, 4th ed., 98 pages, ISBN 0940780682

Part of the "Made Ridiculously Simple" series. **Pros:** Comprehensive, fast read with nice tables and entertaining illustrations to highlight key points. **Cons:** Some areas are not detailed enough; other areas are too verbose. Not boards oriented. **Summary:** Good, fast review, but more helpful for clerkship than for boards.

B

Blueprints Q & A Step 2 Psychiatry
McLOONE

$17.95   Test/200 q

Lippincott Williams & Wilkins, 2004, 2nd ed., 240 pages, ISBN 1405103922

Two hundred vignette-style questions. **Pros:** Nice companion to the Blueprints series. Focuses on high-yield topics. Explanations are easy to follow. **Cons:** Not comprehensive; use as a supplement for review. Sparse images. Some questions are esoteric and not boards-like. **Summary:** Organized and easy-to-read supplement. Adds clinical correlates to the Blueprints series.

B

NMS Psychiatry
SCULLY

$39.95   Review/500 q

Lippincott Williams & Wilkins, 2007, 5th ed., 339 pages, ISBN 0781765145

General review of topics in outline format with questions at the end of each chapter and a comprehensive final exam. **Pros:** Well-written text with concise disease discussions. Includes an expanded pharmacology section. Questions test appropriate content and have complete explanations, and the new edition offers more vignette-style questions. Good companion text for clerkship. **Cons:** Not enough vignette-style questions. Lengthy for purposes of boards review. **Summary:** Detailed review that requires time commitment. Good single choice for clerkship study, but may be too long for Step 2 review.

REVIEW RESOURCES

PSYCHIATRY

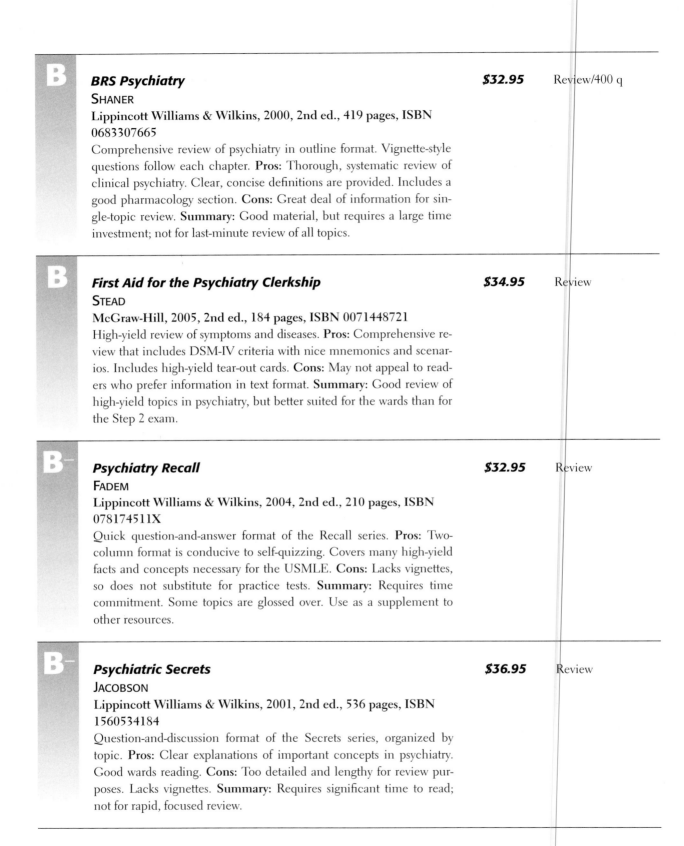

B

BRS Psychiatry
SHANER
Lippincott Williams & Wilkins, 2000, 2nd ed., 419 pages, ISBN 0683307665

$32.95   Review/400 q

Comprehensive review of psychiatry in outline format. Vignette-style questions follow each chapter. **Pros:** Thorough, systematic review of clinical psychiatry. Clear, concise definitions are provided. Includes a good pharmacology section. **Cons:** Great deal of information for single-topic review. **Summary:** Good material, but requires a large time investment; not for last-minute review of all topics.

B

First Aid for the Psychiatry Clerkship
STEAD
McGraw-Hill, 2005, 2nd ed., 184 pages, ISBN 0071448721

$34.95   Review

High-yield review of symptoms and diseases. **Pros:** Comprehensive review that includes DSM-IV criteria with nice mnemonics and scenarios. Includes high-yield tear-out cards. **Cons:** May not appeal to readers who prefer information in text format. **Summary:** Good review of high-yield topics in psychiatry, but better suited for the wards than for the Step 2 exam.

B–

Psychiatry Recall
FADEM
Lippincott Williams & Wilkins, 2004, 2nd ed., 210 pages, ISBN 078174511X

$32.95   Review

Quick question-and-answer format of the Recall series. **Pros:** Two-column format is conducive to self-quizzing. Covers many high-yield facts and concepts necessary for the USMLE. **Cons:** Lacks vignettes, so does not substitute for practice tests. **Summary:** Requires time commitment. Some topics are glossed over. Use as a supplement to other resources.

B–

Psychiatric Secrets
JACOBSON
Lippincott Williams & Wilkins, 2001, 2nd ed., 536 pages, ISBN 1560534184

$36.95   Review

Question-and-discussion format of the Secrets series, organized by topic. **Pros:** Clear explanations of important concepts in psychiatry. Good wards reading. **Cons:** Too detailed and lengthy for review purposes. Lacks vignettes. **Summary:** Requires significant time to read; not for rapid, focused review.

B⁻

Saint-Frances Guide to Psychiatry   **$28.95**   Review
McCarthy
Lippincott Williams & Wilkins, 2000, 3rd ed., 279 pages, ISBN
0683306618
Comprehensive text review of psychiatry. **Pros:** Thorough; outline format is easy to read and follow. Portable. Clinical correlates stress key
points. **Cons:** Lengthy. Some areas have superfluous information. Not
geared toward the boards. **Summary:** Nice review of psychiatry with
helpful correlates that emphasize key points, but may be more helpful
for clerkship than for the boards.

Underground Clinical Vignettes: Surgery
BHUSHAN

$17.95   Review

Lippincott Williams & Wilkins, 2005, 3rd ed., 178 pages,
ISBN 1405104260

Clinical vignette review of frequently tested surgical topics. **Pros:** Recently revised and updated. Well organized by focus points: pathogenesis, epidemiology, management, complications, and associated diseases. Well illustrated and includes "minicases" that present high-yield information. **Cons:** Not comprehensive; use as a supplement to review. **Summary:** Well-organized and easy-to-read practice vignettes.

Platinum Vignettes: Surgery and Trauma
BROCHERT

$23.95   Review

Elsevier, 2002, 1st ed., 102 pages, ISBN 1560535350

Clinical vignette review of common topics in surgery and trauma medicine. **Pros:** Well-written cases similar to boards-type vignettes. Well illustrated. Discussion is organized by pathophysiology, diagnosis and treatment, and more high-yield facts. **Cons:** Expensive for amount of material. Not comprehensive; use as a supplement. **Summary:** Organized and easy-to-read supplement to studying.

Platinum Vignettes: Surgical Subspecialties
BROCHERT

$23.95   Review

Elsevier, 2002, 1st ed., 105 pages, ISBN 1560535385

Clinical vignette review of common topics in the surgical subspecialties. **Pros:** Well-written cases similar to boards-type vignettes. Well illustrated. Discussion is organized by pathophysiology, diagnosis and treatment, and more high-yield facts. **Cons:** Expensive for amount of material. Not comprehensive; use as a supplement. **Summary:** Organized and easy-to-read supplement to studying.

PreTest Surgery
KAO

$24.95   Test/500 q

McGraw-Hill, 2006, 11th ed., 382 pages, ISBN 0071457704

Review of topics in general surgery in question-and-answer format. **Pros:** Predominantly case based. Well organized by subspecialty. **Cons:** Many questions are too detailed or esoteric and do not reflect boards style. Some explanations are overly detailed. **Summary:** Thorough review, but questions may be beyond the level needed for Step 2 preparation.

Case Files: Surgery
TOY

$29.95   Review

McGraw-Hill, 2006, 2nd ed., 504 pages, ISBN 0071463046

Review of surgery in case format with questions and answers following each vignette. **Pros:** Cases reflect high-yield topics and are arranged in an easy-to-follow format. Emphasizes the next step and the most likely diagnosis. **Cons:** Not suited to high-yield rapid review, and may be too detailed for Step 2 preparation. **Summary:** Excellent review with emphasis on vignette-style case presentation and important boards-type answers. Great for the wards, and a good supplement for boards study.

NMS Surgery
JARRELL

$34.95   Review/350 q

Lippincott Williams & Wilkins, 2000, 4th ed., 699 pages, ISBN 0683306154

Outline review of general surgery and surgical subspecialties. **Pros:** Well organized and thorough. Vignette-style questions are included after each chapter with good explanations. **Cons:** Dense, detailed text. Few tables or illustrations. **Summary:** Comprehensive surgery review, but very time-consuming. More appropriate for clerkship than for boards review.

In A Page Surgery
KAHAN

$31.95   Review

Lippincott Williams & Wilkins, 2003, 1st ed., 206 pages, ISBN 1405103655

One-page reviews of 154 diseases/topics discussed by etiology, epidemiology, signs/symptoms, differential diagnosis, diagnostic tests, treatment, and prognosis. **Pros:** Fast and concise review of high-yield information on common diseases. **Cons:** Text is crowded onto one page without any images or diagrams. Includes low-yield topics. **Summary:** Useful for quick study on the wards, but too time intensive for Step 2 review.

Blueprints in Surgery
KARP

$36.95   Review/62 q

Lippincott Williams & Wilkins, 2007, 4th ed., 214 pages, ISBN 1405104996

Short text review of general surgery with tables and diagrams. Brief question-and-answer section is included. **Pros:** Well organized. Easy to read with strong focus on high-yield topics. Clear diagrams. **Cons:** Some sections are overly detailed (e.g., anatomy), while others are occasionally too simplistic. Too few illustrations. **Summary:** Concise review of surgery, but not ideal for Step 2 preparation.

B **Blueprints Clinical Cases in Surgery**   **$29.95**   Test/200 q

LI

Lippincott Williams & Wilkins, 2007, 2nd ed., 415 pages,
ISBN 1405104937

Compendium of vignette-type cases arranged by symptom followed by
related questions and answers. **Pros:** Excellent companion to the
Blueprints series. Focuses on high-yield cases. Easy to read with nice
illustrations and review of management. **Cons:** Not comprehensive;
use as a supplement for review. **Summary:** Organized and easy-to-read
supplement. Adds clinical correlates to the Blueprints series.

B **Blueprints Q & A Step 2 Surgery**   **$17.95**   Test/200 q

NELSON

Lippincott Williams & Wilkins, 2004, 2nd ed., 169 pages,
ISBN 1405103930

Two hundred vignette-style questions. **Pros:** Nice companion to the
Blueprints series. Focuses on high-yield topics. Explanations are easy
to follow. **Cons:** Not comprehensive; use as a supplement for review.
Sparse images. Some questions are esoteric and not boards-like. Expensive, and includes few questions given the cost of the book. **Summary:** Organized and easy-to-read supplement. Adds clinical correlates to the Blueprints series.

B **High-Yield Surgery**   **$26.95**   Review

NIRULA

Lippincott Williams & Wilkins, 2006, 2nd ed., 160 pages,
ISBN 0781776562

Outline review of most common general surgery topics. **Pros:** Concise; useful for quick topic review. Well organized. **Cons:** Information
can be superficial. Some topics are omitted. No practice questions.
Summary: Lean text for rapid review.

B **A&L's Review of Surgery**   **$34.95**   Test/1000+ q

WAPNICK

McGraw-Hill, 2002, 320 pages, ISBN 0071378146

General review of surgery with questions and answers. **Pros:** Good
clinical emphasis. Many vignette-style questions. Explanations are
thorough. **Cons:** Some questions are too short, and style does not reflect that of the Step 2 exam. Questions are highly variable in difficulty and are often far too detailed. Few illustrations. **Summary:**
Good content for the exam; however, much too detailed for clerkship
and Step 2 review.

B⁻ Surgical Recall
BLACKBOURNE

$34.95   Review

Lippincott Williams & Wilkins, 2002, 3rd ed., 745 pages, ISBN 0781729734

Question-and-answer format, as with other Recall-series books. **Pros:** Questions emphasize important, high-yield clinical concepts. Columns allow self-testing. Fast review. Good preparation for "pimping" on rounds. **Cons:** Not boards-type questions. Poorly organized. Spotty coverage of some topics. **Summary:** Useful adjunct to a more organized topic review. Much more appropriate for clerkship than for boards review.

B⁻ BRS General Surgery
CRABTREE

$29.95   Review/375 q

Lippincott Williams & Wilkins, 2000, 1st ed., 564 pages, ISBN 0683306367

Comprehensive review in outline format, organized by topic or organ. **Pros:** Appropriate clinical emphasis for boards and wards. Includes vignette-style review questions at the end of each chapter. **Cons:** Lengthy for single-topic review. Some information is not specific enough to be useful. Few images or illustrations. **Summary:** Overall, a strong review resource. Requires time commitment, so may not be suited to rapid review.

B⁻ BRS Surgical Specialties
CRABTREE

$32.95   Review/150 q

Lippincott Williams & Wilkins, 2000, 1st ed., 852 pages, ISBN 0781730503

Focused review of topics in the surgical subspecialties in outline format. **Pros:** Good emphasis for boards and wards. Good use of illustrations. Vignette-style review questions. **Cons:** Some information may be redundant from review of other topics, and some information may be beyond the scope of the Step 2 exam. **Summary:** For the advanced surgery student.

B⁻ Abernathy's Surgical Secrets
HARKEN

$36.95   Review

Elsevier, 2005, 5th ed., 473 pages, ISBN 0323034160

Question-and-answer Secrets-series format. **Pros:** Discussions are up to date and thorough. **Cons:** Too detailed for the purposes of the USMLE, yet not comprehensive. **Summary:** Not a well-organized review. Better suited to clerkship than to boards preparation.

Pocket Surgery

$34.95   Review

MOSCA

Lippincott Williams & Wilkins, 2002, 1st, 144 pages, ISBN 0781735793

Review of high-yield surgical material in outline format. **Pros:** Fast, easy read. Portable. Highlights high-yield information in "fact boxes." **Cons:** Some material is not detailed enough. No illustrations. **Summary:** Good for rapid review during clerkship. Does not contain enough detailed information to be used as a single study source for the boards.

A

Dermatology for Boards and Wards
AYALA

$20.95   Review

Lippincott Williams & Wilkins, 2001, 1st ed., 96 pages,
0632045728

Brief book with pictures of dermatologic findings **Pros:** Brief, with pictures of high-yield topics. **Cons:** Minimal explanations. **Summary:** Short book with pictures of high-yield dermatologic diagnoses and findings.

A⁻

First Aid for the International Medical Graduate
CHANDER

$29.95   Review

McGraw-Hill, 2002, 2nd ed., 295 pages, ISBN 0071385320

High-yield review for the IMG on how to pass the USMLE boards and adapt to medical culture in the United States. **Pros:** Comprehensive, well-organized review. **Cons:** Some readers may need to obtain additional information from other sources. **Summary:** Excellent review of material for the IMG. Best used as a primer for boards review.

A⁻

The IMG's Guide to Mastering the USMLE & Residency
CHANDER

$39.95   Test/500 q

McGraw-Hill, 2000, 1st ed., 310 pages, ISBN 0071347240

Comprehensive guide for IMGs that navigates the complicated process of training in the United States. Includes information on visas, USMLE and TOEFL exams, the Step 2 CS exam, and applying to residencies, with emphasis on overcoming the many obstacles that IMGs face along the way. Also provides practical advice on establishing a home in the United States, residency survival skills, and finding a job.

Commercial preparation courses can be helpful for some students, but these courses are expensive and require significant time commitment. They are usually effective in organizing study material for students who feel overwhelmed by the volume of material. Note that multiweek courses may be quite intense and may thus leave limited time for independent study. Also note that some commercial courses are designed for first-time test takers while others focus on students who are repeating the examination. In addition, some courses focus on IMGs who want to take all three Steps in a limited amount of time. Student experience and satisfaction with review courses are highly variable. We suggest that you discuss options with recent graduates of the review courses you are considering. Course content and structure can change rapidly. Some student opinions can be found in discussion groups on the World Wide Web. Below is contact information for some Step 2 commercial review courses.

Falcon Physician Reviews
1431 Greenway Drive, #800
Irving, TX 75038
(214) 632-5466
info@falconreviews.com
www.falconreviews.com

Kaplan Medical
700 South Flower Street
Los Angeles, CA 90017
(800) KAP-TEST (800-527-8378)
www.kaptest.com

Northwestern Medical Review
P.O. Box 22174
East Lansing, MI 48909-2174
(866) MedPass (866-633-7277)
registrar@northwesternmedicalreview.com
http://northwesternmedicalreview.com

Postgraduate Medical Review Education (PMRE)
1909 Tyler Street, Suite 305
Hollywood, FL 33020
(800) 323-6430
sales@pmre.com
www.pmre.com

Youel's Prep, Inc.
P.O. Box 31479
Palm Beach Gardens, FL 33420
(800) 645-3985
Fax: (561) 622-4858
info@youelsprep.com
www.youelsprep.com

APPENDIX

Abbreviations and Symbols

Abbreviation	Meaning
A-a	alveolar-arterial (oxygen gradient)
ABG	arterial blood gas
ABI	ankle-brachial index
ABVD	Adriamycin (doxorubicin), bleomycin, vinblastine, dacarbazine
ACA	anterior cerebral artery
ACC	American College of Cardiology
ACE	angiotensin-converting enzyme
ACEI	angiotensin-converting enzyme inhibitor
ACh	acetylcholine
ACLS	advanced cardiac life support
ACTH	adrenocorticotropic hormone
AD	Alzheimer's disease
ADA	American Diabetes Association
ADH	antidiuretic hormone
ADHD	attention-deficit hyperactivity disorder
AF	atrial fibrillation
AFI	amniotic fluid index
AFP	α-fetoprotein
AHA	American Heart Association
AIDS	acquired immunodeficiency virus
ALL	acute lymphocytic leukemia
ALS	amyotrophic lateral sclerosis
ALT	alanine aminotransferase
AMA	American Medical Association
AML	acute myelogenous leukemia
ANA	antinuclear antibody
ANCA	antineutrophil cytoplasmic antibody
AOA	American Osteopathic Association
AP	anteroposterior
aPTT	activated partial thromboplastin time
AR	attributable risk
ARB	angiotensin receptor blocker
ARC	Appalachian Regional Commission
ARDS	acute respiratory distress syndrome
ARF	acute renal failure
5-ASA	5-aminosalicylic acid

Abbreviation	Meaning
ASA	acetylsalicylic acid
ASCUS	atypical squamous cells of undetermined significance
ASD	atrial septal defect
ASO	antistreptolysin O
AST	aspartate aminotransferase
ATN	acute tubular necrosis
AV	atrioventricular
AVM	arteriovenous malformation
AVN	avascular necrosis
AVNRT	atrioventricular nodal reentry tachycardia
AXR	abdominal x-ray
AZT	azidothymidine (zidovudine)
BID	twice a day
BMI	body mass index
BP	blood pressure
BPH	benign prostatic hyperplasia
bpm	beat per minute
BPP	biophysical profile
BPPV	benign paroxysmal positional vertigo
BSA	body surface area
BT	bleeding time
BUN	blood urea nitrogen
CABG	coronary artery bypass graft
CAD	coronary artery disease
CaEDTA	calcium disodium edetate
CALLA	common ALL antigen
CBC	complete blood count
CBT	cognitive-behavioral therapy, computer-based testing
CCS	computer-based case simulations
CD	cluster of differentiation
CEA	carcinoembryonic antigen
CF	cystic fibrosis
cGMP	cyclic guanosine monophosphate
CHF	congestive heart failure
CHOP	cytoxan, Adriamycin (doxorubicin), Oncovin (vincristine), prednisone
CIN	candidate identification number, cervical intraepithelial neoplasia

Abbreviation	Meaning
CK	creatine kinase, Clinical Knowledge
CK-MB	creatine kinase, MB fraction
CLL	chronic lymphocytic leukemia
CML	chronic myelogenous leukemia
CMP	cytidine monophosphate
CMV	cytomegalovirus
CN	cranial nerve
CNS	central nervous system
COGME	Council on Graduate Medical Education
COMT	catechol-O-methyltransferase
COPD	chronic obstructive pulmonary disease
CPAP	continuous positive airway pressure
CPK	creatine phosphokinase
CRP	C-reactive protein
CS	Clinical Skills
CSF	cerebrospinal fluid
CST	contraction stress test
CT	computed tomography
CXR	chest x-ray
D&C	dilation and curettage
DCIS	ductal carcinoma in situ
DDAVP	1-deamino (8-D-arginine) vasopressin
DES	diethylstilbestrol
DEXA	dual-energy x-ray absorptiometry
DHEAS	dehydroepiandrosterone sulfate
DHS	Department of Homeland Security
DI	diabetes insipidus
DIC	disseminated intravascular coagulation
DIP	distal interphalangeal (joint)
DKA	diabetic ketoacidosis
DL_{CO}	diffusing capacity of carbon monoxide
DM	diabetes mellitus
DMARD	disease-modifying antirheumatic drug
DMD	Duchenne muscular dystrophy
DNA	deoxyribonucleic acid
DNase	deoxyribonuclease
DNI	do not intubate
DNR	do not resuscitate
DPOA	durable power of attorney
DRE	digital rectal examination
DS	double strength
DSM	Diagnostic and Statistical Manual (of Mental Disorders)
DTaP	diphtheria, tetanus, acellular pertussis (vaccine)
DTR	deep tendon reflex
DTs	delirium tremens
DVT	deep venous thrombosis
EBV	Epstein-Barr virus
ECFMG	Educational Commission for Foreign Medical Graduates

Abbreviation	Meaning
ECG	electrocardiography
ECT	electroconvulsive therapy
ED	erectile dysfunction
EEG	electroencephalography
EF	ejection fraction
EGD	esophagogastroduodenoscopy
ELISA	enzyme-linked immunosorbent assay
EMG	electromyography
ENT	ears, nose, and throat
EPS	extrapyramidal symptom(s)
ER	emergency room, estrogen receptor
ERAS	Electronic Residency Application Service
ERCP	endoscopic retrograde cholangiopancreatography
ESR	erythrocyte sedimentation rate
ESWL	extracorporeal shock-wave lithotripsy
ETEC	enterotoxic E. coli
EtOH	ethanol
FAP	familial adenomatous polyposis
FAST	focused abdominal sonography for trauma
Fe_{Na}	fractional excretion of sodium
FEV_1	forced expiratory volume in one second
FFP	fresh frozen plasma
FiO_2	fraction of inspired oxygen
FNA	fine-needle aspiration
FOBT	fecal occult blood test
FSH	follicle-stimulating hormone
FSMB	Federation of State Medical Boards
FTA-ABS	fluorescent treponemal antibody absorption (test)
FTT	failure to thrive
5-FU	5-fluorouracil
FUO	fever of unknown origin
FVC	forced vital capacity
G6PD	glucose-6-phosphate dehydrogenase
GA	gestational age
GAS	group A streptococcus
GBM	glomerular basement membrane
GBS	group B streptococcus, Guillain-Barré syndrome
GC	gonorrhea and chlamydia (screen)
G-CSF	granulocyte colony-stimulating factor
GERD	gastroesophageal reflux disease
GFR	glomerular filtration rate
GGT	gamma-glutamyl transferase
GH	growth hormone
GI	gastrointestinal
GNR	gram-negative rod
GnRH	gonadotropin-releasing hormone
GTD	gestational trophoblastic disease
GU	genitourinary

Abbreviation	Meaning
GVHD	graft-versus-host disease
H&P	history and physical
HAV	hepatitis A virus
Hb	hemoglobin
HbA_{1C}	hemoglobin A_{1C}
HBcAb	hepatitis B core antibody
HbO_2	hyperbaric oxygen
HBsAb	hepatitis B surface antibody
HBsAg	hepatitis B surface antigen
HBV	hepatitis B virus
hCG	human chorionic gonadotropin
HCTZ	hydrochlorothiazide
HCV	hepatitis C virus
HDL	high-density lipoprotein
HDV	hepatitis D virus
HHNK	hyperosmolar hyperglycemic nonketotic (coma)
HHS	Health and Human Services
HHV	human herpesvirus
Hib	Haemophilus influenzae type B (vaccine)
HIDA	hepato-iminodiacetic acid (scan)
HIV	human immunodeficiency virus
HLA	human leukocyte antigen
HMG-CoA	hydroxymethylglutaryl coenzyme A
HNPCC	hereditary nonpolyposis colorectal cancer
hpf	high-power field
HPL	human placental lactogen
HPSAs	Health Professional Shortage Areas
HPV	human papillomavirus
HRT	hormone replacement therapy
HSV	herpes simplex virus
HUS	hemolytic-uremic syndrome
HVA	homovanillic acid
IBD	inflammatory bowel disease
IBS	irritable bowel syndrome
ICD	implantable cardiac defibrillator
ICP	intracranial pressure
ICU	intensive care unit
I/E	inspiratory/expiratory (ratio)
IFN	interferon
IFN-α	α-interferon
Ig	immunoglobulin
IGF	insulin-like growth factor
IHSS	idiopathic hypertrophic subaortic stenosis
IM	intramuscular
IMED	International Medical Education Directory
IMG	international medical graduate
INH	isoniazid
INR	International Normalized Ratio
I/O	input/output

Abbreviation	Meaning
IPV	inactivated polio vaccine
IR	incidence rate
ITP	idiopathic thrombocytopenic purpura
IUD	intrauterine device
IUGR	intrauterine growth rate
IV	intravenous
IVC	inferior vena cava
IVF	in vitro fertilization
IVIG	intravenous immunoglobulin
IVP	intravenous pyelography
JNC-7	Joint National Committee on Prevention, Detection, Evaluation, and Treatment of High Blood Pressure
JRA	juvenile rheumatoid arthritis
JVD	jugular venous distention
JVP	jugular venous pressure
KOH	potassium hydroxide
KUB	kidney, ureter, bladder
LBBB	left bundle branch block
LBP	low back pain
LCL	lateral collateral ligament
LDH	lactate dehydrogenase
LDL	low-density lipoprotein
LEEP	loop electrosurgical excision procedure
LES	lower esophageal sphincter
LFT	liver function test
LH	luteinizing hormone
LLQ	left lower quadrant
LMN	lower motor neuron
LMP	last menstrual period
LMWH	low-molecular-weight heparin
LP	lumbar puncture
LR	lactated Ringer's
LVEDP	left ventricular end-diastolic pressure
LVH	left ventricular hypertrophy
MAC	membrane attack complex, *Mycobacterium avium* complex
MAOI	monoamine oxidase inhibitor
MCA	middle cerebral artery
MCHC	mean corpuscular hemoglobin concentration
MCL	medial collateral ligament
MCP	metacarpophalangeal (joint)
MCV	mean corpuscular volume
MDE	major depressive episode
MEN	multiple endocrine neoplasia
$MgSO_4$	magnesium sulfate
MGUS	monoclonal gammopathy of undetermined significance
MHC	major histocompatibility complex
MHPSAs	Mental Health Professional Shortage Areas

Abbreviation	Meaning
MI	myocardial infarction
MIBG	metaiodobenzylguanidine
MMR	measles, mumps, rubella (vaccine)
MoM	multiple of the median
MRA	magnetic resonance angiography
MRI	magnetic resonance imaging
MS	multiple sclerosis
MSAFP	maternal serum α-fetoprotein
MTP	metatarsophalangeal (joint)
MUA/Ps	Medically Underserved Areas and Populations
MuSK	muscle-specific kinase
MVA	motor vehicle accident
$NaHCO_3$	sodium bicarbonate
NBME	National Board of Medical Examiners
NF	neurofibromatosis
NG	nasogastric
NKH	nonketotic hyperglycemia
NPO	nil per os (nothing by mouth)
NPV	negative predictive value
NS	normal saline
NSAID	nonsteroidal anti-inflammatory drug
NSCLC	non–small cell lung cancer
NST	nonstress test
NYHA	New York Heart Association
O&P	ova and parasites
OCD	obsessive-compulsive disorder
OCP	oral contraceptive pill
OR	odds ratio, operating room
ORIF	open reduction and internal fixation
$PaCO_2$	partial pressure of carbon dioxide in arterial blood
PaO_2	partial pressure of oxygen in arterial blood
PAS	periodic acid–Schiff
PCA	posterior cerebral artery
PCKD	polycystic kidney disease
PCL	posterior cruciate ligament
PCO_2	partial pressure of carbon dioxide
PCOS	polycystic ovarian syndrome
PCP	phencyclidine hydrochloride, *Pneumocystis carinii* pneumonia
PCR	polymerase chain reaction
PCWP	pulmonary capillary wedge pressure
PDA	patent ductus arteriosus
PDE	phosphodiesterase
PEA	pulseless electrical activity
PEEP	positive end-expiratory pressure
PFT	pulmonary function test
PG	prostaglandin
PID	pelvic inflammatory disease
PIP	proximal interphalangeal (joint)
PIV	parainfluenza virus

Abbreviation	Meaning
PMI	point of maximal impulse
PML	promyelocytic leukemia
PMN	polymorphonuclear (leukocyte)
PO	per os (by mouth)
PO_2	partial pressure of oxygen
POC	product of conception
P_{PA}	pulmonary arterial pressure
PPD	purified protein derivative (of tuberculin)
PPI	proton pump inhibitor
PPV	pneumococcal polysaccharide vaccine, positive predictive value
PR	progesterone receptor
PROM	premature rupture of membranes
PSA	prostate-specific antigen
PT	prothrombin time
PTCA	percutaneous transluminal coronary angioplasty
PTH	parathyroid hormone
PTHrP	parathyroid hormone–related protein
PTSD	post-traumatic stress disorder
PTT	partial thromboplastin time
PUD	peptic ulcer disease
PUVA	psoralen plus ultraviolet A
PVC	premature ventricular contraction
PVR	peripheral vascular resistance
QD	once a day
QID	four times a day
RA	rheumatoid arthritis
RAIU	radioactive iodine uptake
RBBB	right bundle branch block
RBC	red blood cell
RCT	randomized controlled trial
RDS	respiratory distress syndrome
RDW	red cell distribution width
RF	rheumatoid factor
RLQ	right lower quadrant
RNA	ribonucleic acid
ROM	range of motion, rupture of membranes
RPR	rapid plasma reagin
RR	relative risk, respiratory rate
RSV	respiratory syncytial virus
RTA	renal tubular acidosis
RUQ	right upper quadrant
RVH	right ventricular hypertrophy
SA	sinoatrial
SAAG	serum-ascites albumin gradient
SAB	spontaneous abortion
SAH	subarachnoid hemorrhage
SaO_2	oxygen saturation in arterial blood
SBO	small bowel obstruction
SCLC	small cell lung cancer

Abbreviation	Meaning
SCPE	slipped capital femoral epiphysis
SD	standard deviation
SES	socioeconomic status
SEVIS	Student and Exchange Visitor Information System
SEVP	Student and Exchange Visitor Program
SIADH	syndrome of inappropriate secretion of antidiuretic hormone
SIL	squamous intraepithelial lesion
SIRS	systemic inflammatory response syndrome
SJS	Stevens-Johnson syndrome
SLE	systemic lupus erythematosus
SPEP	serum protein electrophoresis
SQ	subcutaneous
SRPs	sponsoring residency programs
SS	single strength
SSRI	selective serotonin reuptake inhibitor
STD	sexually transmitted disease
SVT	supraventricular tachycardia
T_3	triiodothyronine
T3RU	T_3 resin uptake
T_4	thyroxine
TA	temporal arteritis
TAH/BSO	total abdominal hysterectomy and bilateral salpingo-oophorectomy
TB	tuberculosis
TBG	thyroxine-binding globulin
3TC	dideoxythiacytidine (lamivudine)
TCA	tricyclic antidepressant
TdT	terminal deoxynucleotidyl transferase
TEE	transesophageal echocardiography
TEF	tracheoesophageal fistula
TEN	toxic epidermal necrolysis
TENS	transcutaneous electrical nerve stimulation
TFT	thyroid function test
TIA	transient ischemic attack
TIBC	total iron-binding capacity
TID	three times a day

Abbreviation	Meaning
TIPS	transjugular intrahepatic portosystemic shunt
TLC	total lung capacity
TMNG	toxic multinodular goiter
TMP-SMX	trimethoprim-sulfamethoxazole
TNF	tumor necrosis factor
TNM	tumor, node, metastasis (staging)
TOEFL	Test of English as a Foreign Language
tPA	tissue plasminogen activator
TPN	total parenteral nutrition
TPO	thyroid peroxidase
TSH	thyroid-stimulating hormone
TSS	toxic shock syndrome
TSST	toxic shock syndrome toxin
TTP	thrombotic thrombocytopenic purpura
TURP	transurethral resection of the prostate
TV	tidal volume
UA	urinalysis
UMN	upper motor neuron
U_{Na}	urinary sodium
UPEP	urine protein electrophoresis
URI	upper respiratory infection
USDA	United States Department of Agriculture
USIA	United States Information Agency
USMLE	United States Medical Licensing Examination
UTI	urinary tract infection
UV	ultraviolet
VDRL	Venereal Disease Research Laboratory
VIN	vulvar intraepithelial neoplasia
VLDL	very low density lipoprotein
VMA	vanillylmandelic acid
V/Q	ventilation-perfusion (ratio)
vWD	von Willebrand's disease
vWF	von Willebrand's factor
VZV	varicella-zoster virus
WHO	World Health Organization

NOTES

INDEX

Arthus reaction, 74
Asbestosis, 415
Asperger's syndrome, 399
Aspergillus, 205, 217, 234
Asthma, 415–416
    medications for, 416, 417
Astrocytoma, 200, 288
"Athlete's foot," 90
Atrial fibrillation, 42, 44, 45
    management of, 42
Atrial flutter, 44, 45
Atrial hypertrophy, 42
Atrial septal defect (ASD),
    356–357
Atrial tachycardia, multifocal, 44
Atrioventricular (AV) block, 42, 43
Atrioventricular nodal reentry
    tachycardia (AVNRT), 44
Atrioventricular reciprocating
    tachycardia (AVRT), 45
Attention-deficit hyperactivity dis-
    order (ADHD), 398
Auspitz sign, 77
Austin Flint murmur, 63
Autism spectrum disorders,
    398–399

B

Bacillus anthracis, 236–237
Bacillus cereus, 147
Bacterial vaginosis, 342–343
Bagassosis, 414
Baker's cysts, 257
Barlow's maneuver, 248
Barrett's esophagus, 142, 144, 200
Basal cell carcinoma (BCC),
    99–101
    types of, 100
Becker muscular dystrophy, DMD
    vs. 247
Beck's triad, 62
Behavioral counseling, 131
Behçet's disease, 80
Bell's palsy, 231
Benign paroxysmal positional ver-
    tigo (BPPV), 280
Benign prostatic hyperplasia
    (BPH), 446–447
Berger's disease (IgA nephropathy),
    439
Berylliosis, 415
β-blockers, 60, 63, 76
    for hypothyroidism, 112
Biliary colic, 161–162

Bipolar disorders, 394
Bird fancier's lung, 414
Bishop score, 302
Blackwater fever, 228
Bladder cancer, 448
Blunt and deceleration trauma,
    454–455
    abdomen/pelvis, 454–455
    chest, 454
Body dysmorphic disorder, 408
Bone and mineral disorders,
    114–117
    hyperparathyroidism, 116–117
    osteoporosis, 114–115
    Paget's disease, 115, 116
Bordetella pertussis, 377
Borrelia, 212
Borrelia burgdorferi, 230
Boxer's fracture, 244
Bradyarrhythmias, 42, 43
Brain abscess, 214
Breast disorders, 326–329
    breast cancer, 328–329
    fibroadenoma, 327
    fibrocystic change, 326–327
    mastitis, 326
Broca's aphasia, 290
Bronchiectasis, 416–417
Bronchiolitis, 372–373
Brudzinski's sign, 211, 376
Budd-Chiari syndrome, 168
Bulimia nervosa, 403–404
Bullous pemphigoid, 81–82
Burkitt's lymphoma, 191
Burns, 458–459
Bursitis, 240–241

C

C1 esterase deficiency (hereditary
    angioedema), 370
Ca^{2+} channel blockers, 60
CAGE questionnaire, 401
Calcinosis, 259
Calymmatobacterium granulomatis
    (granuloma inguinale-
    donovanosis), 223, 341
Campylobacter, 147, 148, 256
Campylobacter jejuni, 283
Candida, 217, 234
Candida albicans, 87, 141, 218
Candidal thrush, 216
Carbon monoxide poisoning,
    459–460
Carcinoid syndrome, 150

Cardiac life support basics, 455,
    456
Cardiac tamponade, 62
Cardiobacterium, 235
Cardiomyopathy, 42–43, 47–48
    differential diagnosis of, 46
    dilated, 42–43, 47
    hypertrophic, 47–48
    restrictive, 48
Cardiovascular, high-yield facts in,
    39–67
    acute coronary syndromes,
        53–56
        ST-elevation myocardial in-
            farction (STEMI), 53–56
        unstable angina/non-ST-eleva-
            tion myocardial infarction
            (NSTEMI), 53
    arrhythmias, 42
        bradyarrhythmias and conduc-
            tion abnormalities, 42, 43
        tachyarrhythmias, 42
    cardiomyopathy, 42–43, 47–48
        differential diagnosis of, 46
        dilated, 42–43, 47
        hypertrophic, 47–48
        restrictive, 48
    congestive heart failure (CHF),
        48–52
        acute management of, 50
        AHA/ACC classification and
            treatment of, 49
        causes of, 49
        diastolic dysfunction, 52
        left-sided vs. right-sided, 50
        NYHA functional classifica-
            tion of, 50
        systolic dysfunction, 49–51
    coronary artery disease (CAD),
        52–53
        angina pectoris, 52–53
        major risk factors for, 52
    electrocardiogram, 41–42
        axis, 41
        chamber enlargement, 42
        intervals, 42
        measurements, 41
        rate, 41
        rhythm, 41
        waveforms, 42
    hypercholesterolemia, 56–57
        lipid-lowering agents, 57
        risk stratification and target
            LDL, 57
    hypertension, 58–61

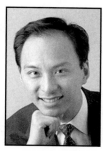
Tao Le, MD

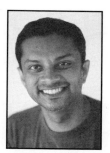
Vikas Bhushan, MD

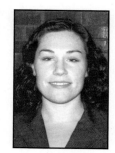
Julia Skapik

Tao Le, MD, MHS

Tao has been a well-recognized figure in medical education for the past 14 years. As senior editor, he has led the expansion of *First Aid* into a global educational series. In addition, he is the founder of the *USMLERx* online test bank series as well as a cofounder of the *Underground Clinical Vignettes* series. As a medical student, he was editor-in-chief of the University of California, San Francisco *Synapse,* a university newspaper with a weekly circulation of 9000. Tao earned his medical degree from the University of California, San Francisco, in 1996 and completed his residency training in internal medicine at Yale University and fellowship training at Johns Hopkins University. At Yale, he was a regular guest lecturer on the USMLE review courses and an adviser to the Yale University School of Medicine curriculum committee. Tao subsequently went on to cofound Medsn and served as its chief medical officer. He is currently conducting research in asthma education as section chief of adult allergy and immunology at the University of Louisville.

Vikas Bhushan, MD

Vikas is an author, editor, entrepreneur, and roaming teleradiologist who divides his days between Los Angeles, Maui, and balmy remote locales with abundant bandwidth. In 1992 he conceived and authored the original *First Aid for the USMLE Step 1,* and in 1998 he originated and coauthored the *Underground Clinical Vignettes* series. His entrepreneurial adventures include a successful software company; a medical publishing enterprise (S2S); an e-learning company (Medsn); and, most recently, an ER teleradiology venture (24/7 Radiology). His eclectic interests include medical informatics, independent film, humanism, Urdu poetry, world music, South Asian diasporic culture, and avoiding a day job. He has also coproduced a music documentary on qawwali; coproduced and edited *Shabash 2.0: The Hip Guide to All Things South Asian in North America* (available at www.artwallah.org/shabash); and is now completing a CD/book project on Sufi poetry translated into four languages. Vikas completed a bachelor's degree in biochemistry from the University of California, Berkeley; an MD with thesis from the University of California, San Francisco; and a radiology residency from the University of California, Los Angeles.

Julia Skapik

Julia is currently completing her MPH at the Johns Hopkins Bloomberg School of Public Health before returning to the Johns Hopkins School of Medicine. Originally from Licking County, Ohio, she attended New College of Florida, graduating with dual BAs in biology and psychology in 2001. Subsequently, she spent a year at the FDA in Bethesda performing viral and vaccine neurovirulence research. Since then, she has worked on many research projects, primarily examining medical errors. She is also the author of the chapter "Psychotic Disorders, Severe Mental Illness, and HIV Infection" in the *Comprehensive Textbook of AIDS Psychiatry* to be published in September 2007. She also serves as the 2007–2008 Health Policy Action Committee chair for the American Medical Student Association. This is her first *First Aid* publication, and she can be contacted at julia@jhmi.edu.

ABOUT THE AUTHORS